Primary Healthcare: Theory and Practice

Primary Healthcare: Theory and Practice

Danna Carson

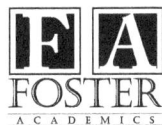

FA
FOSTER
ACADEMICS

www.fosteracademics.com

www.fosteracademics.com

FA
FOSTER
ACADEMICS

Cataloging-in-Publication Data

Primary healthcare : theory and practice / edited by Danna Carson.
    p. cm.
Includes bibliographical references and index.
ISBN 978-1-63242-580-5
1. Primary care (Medicine). 2. Medical care. I. Carson, Danna.
RA427.9 .P75 2019
362.1--dc23

Foster Academics,
118-35 Queens Blvd., Suite 400,
Forest Hills, NY 11375, USA

ISBN 978-1-63242-580-5 (Hardback)

Contents

Permissions

List of Contributors

Index

Preface

Primary healthcare is defined as the essential healthcare, which allows the facilitation of universal healthcare for all individuals and families in a community. It is one of the primary objectives of the World Health Organization's goal of Health for all. The five considerations that are central to the achievement of this goal are reducing social disparities in health, service delivery reforms to meet people's needs, public policy reforms, leadership reforms and increasing stakeholder participation. The approach to primary healthcare also strives to account for disparities in resources and local priority health problems. In developing countries, diseases responsible for high rates of infant and child mortality are targeted. Oral rehydration therapy, immunization, family planning, female education and food supplementation are certain key issues under the broad framework of primary healthcare. The topics included in this book on primary healthcare are of the utmost significance and bound to provide incredible insights to readers. Some of the diverse topics covered in this book address the varied branches that fall under this category. This book will serve as a reference to a broad spectrum of readers.

Various studies have approached the subject by analyzing it with a single perspective, but the present book provides diverse methodologies and techniques to address this field. This book contains theories and applications needed for understanding the subject from different perspectives. The aim is to keep the readers informed about the progresses in the field; therefore, the contributions were carefully examined to compile novel researches by specialists from across the globe.

Indeed, the job of the editor is the most crucial and challenging in compiling all chapters into a single book. In the end, I would extend my sincere thanks to the chapter authors for their profound work. I am also thankful for the support provided by my family and colleagues during the compilation of this book.

Editor

An Educational Intervention in Primary School Students Regarding Sun Protection

Saridi M[1], Toska A[1], Rekleiti M[1], Sarafis P[2], Zoukas L[3], Souliotis K[4]* and Birbas K[5]

[1]Department of Nursing, General Hospital of Korinthos, Greece
[2]Faculty of Nursing, Technological Educational Institute, Lamia, Greece
[3]Department of Gynecology, General Hospital of Korinthos, Greece
[4]Faculty of Social Sciences, University of Peloponnese, Korinthos, Greece
[5]Faculty of Nursing, National and Kapodistrian, University of Athens, Greece

Abstract

Background: Epidemiological data have established a correlation between prolonged sun exposure during childhood and adolescence and occurrence of malign melanoma later in life. The aim of the present study was to investigate knowledge and attitudes of primary school students regarding sun protection measures and sun-related risks before and after an educational intervention.

Methods: It is a descriptive randomized pilot study of two stages with comparison of the results before and after an educational intervention. Sixty students aged 8-12 years from a coastal area participated in this study. Students first completed an anonymous questionnaire and after that took part in an intervention program. After 15 days the same students completed the questionnaire again. Data analysis was performed using the SPSS 17.0 and statistical significance was set to 0.05.

Results: Students' awareness and knowledge level about sun-related risks and sun protection measures before the implementation of the intervention was satisfactory. Regarding sun protection factor, students' knowledge levels also increased and 55% of them answered correctly. The students' attitudes after the intervention showed some improvement, yet without any significant variation. There were no changes regarding the use of sunglasses and wearing appropriate clothing (hat, long-sleeve shirts, etc.). The proportion of children who used a sunscreen with SPF 30+ was significantly higher in students after the intervention (p<0.001). Sunburn incidence was found to be high. 35% of the students reported having at least one sunburn in the past summer. Children after the intervention had significantly higher knowledge scores compared to those before the program but the score in attitudes was not so high.

Conclusions: This pilot study showed that a similar intervention in a larger sample could increase and expand the students' knowledge about sun protection.

Keywords: Sun protection; Sun exposure; Sun block; Melanoma; Sunburn

Introduction

Solar light, entering the Earth's atmosphere, is filtered by the ozone layer which is at the stratosphere and absorbs most of the UVR by transforming it to heat. Ozone depletion in the last decades has resulted in a 1-3% annual increase in skin cancer cases worldwide [1,2]. Solar radiation risks are widely known and well-established in the literature. Solar radiation may have direct effects on the kin (redness, sunburn, etc.) that occur within hours or days after exposure, or long-term effects (squamous-cell carcinoma, basal-cell carcinoma, malign melanoma) that occur after prolonged exposure for many years [3].

Epidemiological data have established a correlation between prolonged sun exposure during childhood and adolescence and occurrence of malign melanoma later in life. Sunburn incidence in these age-groups is also a risk factor for skin cancer [4,5]. Children and adolescents are the main target groups of educational interventions in countries with high skin cancer incidence, such as Australia, New Zealand and USA. WHO and CDC have launched in the last decade similar programs that have been used as an example for other countries that wish to implement similar interventions too [6-9].

Relative studies and interventions have highlighted the students' awareness about sun-related risks and sun protection measures as well. They have also investigated the students' attitudes, beliefs and behaviours regarding sun exposure and sun protection. It has been documented that providing systematic and continuous information can change erroneous attitudes and lead to wiser behaviours [8-10].

The aim of the present study was to investigate knowledge and attitudes of primary school students regarding sun protection measures and sun-related risks before and after an educational intervention. It is a pilot study and its findings will be the basis for a full-scale study in the future. The present study will provide some useful insight about methodological problems and difficulties that may arise during planning, implementation, data collection and assessment of the intervention.

Material and Methods

Research planning

The present study is a pilot study that will be used as a guideline for a large-scale epidemiological study. It is a descriptive randomized study of two stages with comparison of the results before and after an educational intervention. One hundred and twenty students aged 8-12 years were our sample. They attended a school in the prefecture

*Corresponding author: Kyriakos Souliotis, Assistant Professor of Health Policy, Faculty of Social Sciences University of Peloponnese, Korinth, Greece, E-mail: soulioti@hol.gr

of Korinthia which was later excluded from the final large-scale study. Response rate was 98% and the study took place from January 2009 until March 2009.

Inclusion/Exclusion criteria -Ethics

In this study, the sample comprised of elementary school students (n=120) aged 8-12 years. Their school was in an urban area and was later excluded from the final large-scale study. The students attended the Fourth, Fifth and Sixth grades. The Greek Pedagogical Institute granted approval. Informed consent was granted by the students' parents and the students themselves. Two non-Greek students had to be excluded due to poor Greek language skills. Strict anonymity was preserved. The school principal also granted permission. No banners or other advertising material was included in the intervention.

Data collection

The students had to complete a questionnaire that was administered to them before and after the intervention. In January 2009 students were administered the questionnaires for the first time. After that, the educational intervention took place, and then, in March, the same questionnaire was re-administered to them, in order to assess any changes in their awareness and attitudes regarding sun protection. Completion of the questionnaires took one school hour during the 'Flexible Zone' hours. The intervention took place after the collection of the questionnaires, and the researchers came back to the school 40 days later and administered the same questionnaires in order to assess the intervention's effectiveness.

Instruments

Questionnaire: The literature review did not provide us with a questionnaire specifically designed for this particular age-group (8-12 years old students). Consequently, the researchers had to develop a special questionnaire drawing from the Intersun programme, developed by the WHO [8]. The relevant Australian programme (Sun Smart) also played a role in the development of our instrument [7].

The questions, apart from the demographics, aimed at assessing the students' knowledge about sun-related risks and sun protection measures. The questionnaire included 21 items. Demographics included age, gender, nationality, place of residence and distance from the beach. Personal data that are important for someone's attitude towards sun protection, such as complexion, eye colour, freckles and moles on the skin were also included. The students' knowledge about sun-related risks and sun protection measures were also investigated. The biggest part of the questionnaire (items 10-21) was about daily sun-protection, especially in the summer. The questionnaire had also been pilot-tested on 50 same-age students and all necessary amendments had been made. Internal cohesion reliability was assessed by Cronbach's alpha which was 0.79. Alpha reliability of the attitude-related items was rs= 0.78. Face validity was deemed satisfactory by four specialists (one statistician, two university professors and one PhD candidate in Health Education).

Educational intervention: The intervention programme was designed along the lines of the Australian SunSmart [7] programme, which is tailored for this particular age group. It included a presentation about positive and negative effects of sun radiation on humans and extensive information about ozone and its protective role against UVR. After that, students were informed in detail about sun protection measures. The intervention focused on the correct sun protection factor a sunscreen for children should have, and on applying correctly the sunscreen.

Statistical analysis

Means and standard deviations were used for the description of quantitative variables. Absolute (N) and relative (%) frequencies were used for the qualitative variables. In order to compare quantitative variables among two groups, Student's t-test was used, whereas for comparison among three or more groups parametric analysis (ANOVA) was used. Significance levels were bilateral and statistical significance was set to 0.05. The SPSS 17.0 software was used for the analysis.

Results

Demographics

The average age of the sample (n =120) was 9.9 years (±1.1), while 58% (n=75) were females and 42% (n=50) were males. Moreover, 80% (n=24) of the students were Greek, while 20% (n=24) were of non-Greek nationality. 26% (n=32) of the participants belonged to the high-risk group. More specifically, the high-risk group included children who had four out of five high-risk characteristics (fair complexion, light-coloured eyes or hair, freckles and moles) (Table 1).

Awareness and knowledge

Students' awareness and knowledge level about sun-related risks and sun protection measures before the implementation of the intervention was satisfactory. After the intervention, there was an overall increase in knowledge levels. More specifically, before the intervention, 82% of the participants knew that the sun's heat is at its peak between 10.00 a.m. and 16.00 p.m., 92% were aware that sunscreen can help prevent sunburns and 75% knew that excessive sun exposure may cause skin and eye damage. Yet only 25% of them knew that sunscreens for children should have a sun protection factor of 50. After the implementation of the programme, there was a positive shift in the students' knowledge levels. More specifically, 91% of the students knew when the sun's heat is at its peak, 95% had learned that sunscreen can prevent sunburns and 85% knew that excessive sun exposure may lead to skin and eye damage. Regarding sun protection factor, students' knowledge levels also increased and 55% of them answered correctly.

There was also a significant difference regarding knowledge levels among children of different age. More specifically, after Bonferroni Correction was applied, students aged 10 years outscored both students aged less than 9 years (p<0.001), and students aged 9-10 years (p<0.001), as well.

Also there was no statistically significant difference regarding knowledge levels between females and males. The males' percentage of

		N	%
High-risk group	No	88	74
	Yes	32	26
Your complexion is	Fair, prone to sunburns	30	25
	Darker, sunburns are rare	90	75
Your eye-colour is	light	24	20
	dark	96	80
Your hair-colour is	light	28	23
	dark	92	77
Do you have freckles on your face/body?	No	88	80.6
	Yes	32	19.4
Do you have any moles on your face/body?	No	88	74
	Yes	32	26

Table 1: Individual characteristics.

overall right answers increased significantly (2.8 ± 0.9 vs 3.2 ± 0.9), and so did the females' right answers (2.9 ± 0.8 vs 3.4 ± 0.8).

Attitudes

The students' attitudes after the intervention showed some improvement, yet without any significant variation (Table 2). It seems that there was a significant difference regarding applying sun protection measures before and after the intervention (Table 3). More specifically, children after the intervention said they applied sun protection measures more often than before the programme.

There were no changes regarding the use of sunglasses and wearing appropriate clothing (hat, long-sleeve shirts, etc.). The proportion of children who used a sunscreen with Sun Protection Factor (SPF) 30+ was significantly higher in students after the intervention (p<0.001). On the other hand, sunscreen use was higher among students when asked before the intervention (78.2% vs 65.5%). The percentage of children who re-applied sunscreen after getting out of the sea was much higher after the intervention, while when asked if they continue to apply sunscreen even after getting a tan the percentage was significantly lower among children when asked after the intervention (29.7% vs 54.8%).

In what regards the children's activities and protection measures

before and after the intervention, when asked after the programme, they said they took more protection measures compared to before the programme. More specifically, before the intervention children said that they used to take more protection measures compared to their answers after the intervention, mainly when they play at the park (22.5% vs 20.1%), during Physical Exercise (P.E.) class (17% vs 15.6%) and when they go hiking to the mountain (15.2% vs 1.6%). Even when they go the beach/pool, it seems that more children used to take protection measures (67.5% vs 66.2%) before the intervention, although this does not seem to be statistically significant (p=0.092).

Sunburn incidence was found to be high. 35% of the students reported having at least one sunburn in the past summer. This answer was not assessed after the intervention, since it wasn't summer yet and because this was a pilot-study in order for the intervention to be standardized.

Correlations

There was a significant difference in knowledge levels in accordance with a child's place of residence and its distance from the beach. After Bonferroni Correction was applied, it was found that students who lived 15-20km away from the beach had lower scores compared to those who lived 0-5 km, 10-15 km, 20 and over km away from the beach (p<0.001, p=0.005 and p=0.015 respectively). Moreover, students living in urban areas outscored those who lived in semi-urban areas (2.9 ± 0.9 VS 2.7 ± 0.8. P=0.001, Pearson's x^2 test).

The correlation between attitude and gender showed that both males and females had slightly worse attitudes towards protection measures after the intervention. Specifically, males and females do not usually wear a hat and appropriate clothes (p<0.001).On the other hand, use of sunscreen with SPF 30+ showed an important (p<0.001) increase (males: 33.2% vs 47.2%; females: 26.2% vs 62.9%). Re-application of sunscreen was also higher. In this case, males reported they re-applied sunscreen every two hours, after the intervention, (30.7% vs 33.8%, p=0.030), but females did not show any significant change (30.2% vs 31.2%, p=0.337).

Correlation between knowledge and age showed that younger students had gained much more knowledge after the intervention. It was also found that children less than 9 years of age took protection measures when playing at the park (15.1% vs 23.4%) and when they used to go to the mountain (8.4% vs 14%), compared to children 10 years and older. Males took significantly (p<0.001) less protection measures than females when they used to go to the beach (65.3% vs 73.5%) and during P.E. class (13.8% vs 21.7%).

Correlation between attitudes and nationality showed that Greek students had had better sun-related attitude than students of non-Greek nationality. Also, students that did not belong to a high-risk group had had better attitude regarding protection measures.

Finally, it was found that children after the intervention had significantly higher knowledge scores compared to those before the programme, regardless of whether they belonged to a high-risk group or not.

Regarding the high-risk group, there was a difference in using protection measures among students before and after the intervention. More specifically, when asked after the intervention, high-risk children said that they used to wear less often long trousers (19.1% vs 2.7%), sunglasses (38.4% vs 31.4%) and apply sunscreen (77.5% vs 65.9%) compared to their answers before the intervention. On the other hand, after the intervention, high-risk students said that they would

| | Measurements | | | | |
| | Before | | After | | P Student's t-test |
	mean	SD	mean	SD	
Attitude score	21.6	3.45	23.71	3.48	<0.001

Table 2: Overall attitude before and after intervention.

| | | Percentage | | P Pearson's x^2 test |
| | | Before | After | |
		%	%	
Do you wear a hat when under the sun?	Always	33.1	42.3	<0.001
Do you wear long trousers and long-sleeve shirts when under the sun?	Always	18.7	7.9	<0.001
Do you usually stay in the shade when at the beach?	Always	45.2	49.0	0.049
Do you wear sun-glasses?	Always	38.5	33.9	0.009
Do you use sunscreen?	Always	64.0	75.3	<0.001
What is the SPF of your sunscreen?	I never used one/ Lower than 15	8.8	9.0	<0.001
	15	15.3	14.5	
	30	29.7	54.8	
	I do not know	46.2	21.6	
Do you re-apply sunscreen at the beach?	Every 2 hours	30.5	32.5	0.037
When tan, do you use keep using sunscreen?	Always	59	52.6	<0.001
Do you like to get a tan?	No	57.4	34.2	<0.001
	Yes	26.5	39.5	
	I don't care	16.1	26.3	

Table 3: Attitude before and after intervention.

use sunscreen with SPF 30+ much more than before the intervention (27.2% vs 60.6%). Similarly, after the intervention the percentage of high-risk students who would re-apply sunscreen every two hours was much higher than before (28.3% vs 43.2%). Also, after the intervention the percentage of high-risk students who wanted to be tan, was again higher (25.4% vs 51%).

Discussion

The present study investigated the changes in knowledge and attitudes of students after an educational intervention. Also, it examined whether the questionnaire was easily understood by the students, in order to be administered to a larger sample without any significant methodological problems.

The implementation of prevention and educational programmes within primary education is an important part of Health Education in many countries. In Greece, some health promotion programmes have taken place during the last years, although it seems that sun protection is not a top priority for the Ministry of Health yet. Nevertheless, sun protection is a priority for many other countries, and also for the WHO and the CDC, and multiple prevention programmess have been launched and taken place in schools [6-9].

The international literature has established that systematic and well-coordinated programmes that focus on large population groups can have better results than sporadic, isolated interventions. The 8-12 age-group seems to be the best option for educational interventions aiming at knowledge improvement and healthier behaviours through attitude change [11-13].

Our demographic results showed that the number of males and females was almost the same. Almost 20% of the participants were of non-Greek nationality, something that shows that Greece has become essentially multicultural. In the larger study, it is expected that knowledge and attitudes will vary according to nationality, as well. This hypothesis is based on the assumption that other characteristics (e.g. phototype) and different clothing in other cultures may have an effect on the foreigners' attitude towards sun exposure and sun protection measures [14-16].

The students' knowledge level was high even before the intervention, but it got significantly higher after the intervention, something that confirms that this programme could be useful for a larger student sample. Our findings are in agreement with those of other studies that have reported high knowledge scores regarding sun protection measures [15-20]. Also, although before the intervention the students' knowledge about sun protection factors was low (25%), after the intervention it increased to 55%, since the programme was specifically aiming at enhancing knowledge about SPF. Similar studies from Spain, the US, New Zealand and Turkey have found lower knowledge levels regarding SPF [21-24]. Several international studies have shown an improvement regarding choosing the appropriate sunscreen, similarly to the present study. Finally, older age students seem to have higher knowledge levels, as expected, since knowledge accumulates over time [10-15].

The students' attitude showed some improvement after the intervention, although not a very significant one. Nevertheless, this was an encouraging sign for the present study. This finding could be attributed to the fact that new and healthier behavioral patterns cannot be adopted by children just on account of more knowledge, since family, peer and school influence play an important role in adopting wiser behaviors, as other studies have also shown [15,18,25].

Sunburn incidence is a well-known risk factor for sun-related

damages, according to the literature. In the present study, a significant percentage of the participants (35%) reported having at least one sunburn in the past summer. Other studies have also found similar percentages [20,26-30]. In the present study, it wasn't feasible to assess whether the intervention had reduced sunburn incidence, because it took place before the summer. The forthcoming full-scale study will include a full assessment. Similar interventions worldwide have been shown to reduce sunburn incidence among young person's [26,28,31-33].

Distance between place of residence and the beach was also found to be a significant factor affecting knowledge and attitudes. Students who lived relatively away from the beach in semi-urban areas had, in general, low knowledge levels and did not take sun protection measures, compared to students who lived closer to the beach and had more frequent exposure to the sun. On the other hand, children from rural areas have prolonged exposure to the sun because they may help their parents at the farm or play outdoors [34,35].

This pilot study showed that educational interventions yield better results when implemented at a young age, a finding confirmed by other international studies. Interventions should be aimed at previously documented knowledge gaps and deficiencies and try to accomplish specific targets. The main target of the present study was to enhance the students' knowledge about sun protection factors (SPF), appropriate use of sunscreens and sun-related risks. The long-term target was to make students adopt healthier attitudes and behavior towards sun exposure. The present pilot study used a small sample and was followed by a full-scale study with a sample of 5000 students.

Conclusion

This pilot study showed that a similar intervention in a larger sample could increase and expand the students' knowledge about sun protection. The study was also used as a means of assessing the questionnaire and, in this respect, no methodological problems arose during all the stages of the study.

It is noteworthy that such interventions should be systematic and continuous, since a simple one-time presentation cannot expand the students' knowledge. Systematic up-to-date information is required, and developing interventions specifically designed for each age-group is also essential. In order for such interventions to be successful, social, school and family environment should be included and should actively participate. Parents and teachers should also be informed, since students are by and large influenced by family and school environment.

References

1. Zepp RG, Erickson DJ 3rd, Paul ND, Sulzberger B (2011) Effects of solar UV radiation and climate change on biogeochemical cycling: interactions and feedbacks. Photochem Photobiol Sci 10: 261-279.

2. Zerefos CS, Meleti C, Balis DS, Bais AF, Gillotay D (2000) On changes of spectral UV-B in the 90's in Europe. Advances in Space Research 26: 1971-1978.

3. Arola A, Lakkala K, Bais A, Kaurola J, Meleti C, et al. (2003) Factors affecting short- and long-term changes of spectral UV irradiance at two European stations. Journal of Geophysical Research 108.

4. Armstrong BK, Kricker A (2001) The epidemiology of UV induced skin cancer. J Photochem Photobiol B 63: 8-18.

5. Siegel R, Naishadham D, Jemal A (2012) Cancer statistics, 2012. CA Cancer J Clin 62: 10-29.

6. Cancer Society of New Zealand (2006) Sample Sun Protection Policy for Primary Schools. Wellington, New Zealand: Cancer Society of New Zealand.

7. Anti-Cancer Council of Victoria (2002) SunSmart Program 2003-2006. Victoria, Anti-Cancer Foundation of Victoria: 1-48.

8. World Health Organization (2003) Sun Protection and Schools: How to Make a Difference. Geneva: World Health Organization.

9. CDC (2003) Counseling to prevent skin cancer: recommendations and rationale of the US Preventive Services Task Force. MMWR 52: 13-17.

10. Dadlani C, Orlow SJ (2008) Planning for a brighter future: a review of sun protection and barriers to behavioral change in children and adolescents. Dermatol Online J 14: 1.

11. Horsley L, Charlton A, Waterman C (2002) Current action for skin cancer risk reduction in English schools: pupils' behaviour in relation to sunburn. Health Educ Res 17: 715-731.

12. Buller DB, Buller MK, Reynolds KD (2006) A survey of sun protection policy and education in secondary schools. J Am Acad Dermatol 54: 427-432.

13. Eakin P, Maddock J, Techur-Pedro A, Kaliko R, Derauf DC (2004) Sun protection policy in elementary schools in Hawaii. Prev Chronic Dis 1: A05.

14. Saraiya M, Hall HI, Uhler RJ (2002) Sunburn prevalence among adults in the United States, 1999. Am J Prev Med 23: 91-97.

15. de Vries H, Lezwijn J, Hol M, Honing C (2005) Skin cancer prevention: behaviour and motives of Dutch adolescents. Eur J Cancer Prev 14: 39-50.

16. Hill D, Dixon H (1999) Promoting sun protection in children: rationale and challenges. Health Educ Behav 26: 409-417.

17. Dixon H, Borland R, Hill D (1999) Sun protection and sunburn in primary school children: the influence of age, gender, and coloring. Prev Med 28: 119-130.

18. Saridi M, Toska A, Rekleiti M, Wozniak G, Liachopoulou A, et al. (2012) Sun-protection habits of primary students in a coastal area of Greece. J Skin Cancer 2012: 629652.

19. Piperakis SM, Papadimitriou V, Piperakis MM, Zisis P (2003) Understanding Greek primary school children's comprehension of sun exposure. Journal of Science Education and Technology 12: 135-142.

20. LaBat K, De Long M, Gahring SA (2005) A Longitudinal Study of Sun-Protective Attitudes and Behaviors. Family and Consumer Sciences Research Journal 33: 240-254.

21. Gilaberte Y, Alonso JP, Teruel MP, Granizo C, Gállego J (2008) Evaluation of a health promotion intervention for skin cancer prevention in Spain: the SolSano program. Health Promot Int 23: 209-219.

22. Wright C, Reeder AI, Gray A, Cox B (2008) Child sun protection: sun-related attitudes mediate the association between children's knowledge and behaviours. J Paediatr Child Health 44: 692-698.

23. Ergul S, Ozeren E (2011) Sun protection behavior and individual risk factors of Turkish Primary School Students associated with skin cancer: a questionnaire-based study. Asian Pac J Cancer Prev 12: 765-770.

24. Geller AC, Cantor M, Miller DR, Kenausis K, Rosseel K, et al. (2002) The Environmental Protection Agency's National SunWise School Program: sunprotection education in US schools (1999-2000). J Am Acad Dermatol 46: 683-689.

25. Geller AC, Rutsch L, Kenausis K, Selzer P, Zhang Z (2003) Can an hour or two of sun protection education keep the sunburn away? Evaluation of the Environmental Protection Agency's Sunwise School Program. Environ Health 2: 13.

26. Richtig E, Jung E, Asbäck K, Trapp M, Hofmann-Wellenhof R (2009) Knowledge and perception of melanocytic nevi and sunburn in young children. Pediatr Dermatol 26: 519-523.

27. Cokkinides V, Weinstock M, Glanz K, Albano J, Ward E, et al. (2006) Trends in sunburns, sun protection practices, and attitudes toward sun exposure protection and tanning among US adolescents, 1998-2004. Pediatrics 118: 853-864.

28. Davis KJ, Cokkinides VE, Weinstock MA, O'Connell MC, Wingo PA (2002) Summer sunburn and sun exposure among US youths ages 11 to 18: national prevalence and associated factors. Pediatrics 110: 27-35.

29. Lowe JB, Borland R, Stanton WR, Baade P, White V, et al. (2000) Sun-safe behavior among secondary school students in Australia. Health Educ Res 15: 271-281.

30. Girgis A, Sanson-Fisher RW, Tripodi DA, Golding T (1993) Evaluation of interventions to improve solar protection in primary schools. Health Educ Q 20: 275-287.

31. Richards R, McGee R, Knight RG (2001) Sunburn and sun protection among New Zealand adolescents over a summer weekend. Aust N Z J Public Health 25: 352-354.

32. Milne E, Jacoby P, Giles-Corti B, Cross D, Johnston R, et al. (2006) The impact of the kidskin sun protection intervention on summer suntan and reported sun exposure: was it sustained? Prev Med 42: 14-20.

33. Banks BA, Silverman RA, Schwartz RH, Tunnessen WW Jr (1992) Attitudes of teenagers toward sun exposure and sunscreen use. Pediatrics 89: 40-42.

34. Aalborg J, Morelli JG, Mokrohisky ST, Asdigian NL, Byers TE, et al. (2009) Tanning and increased nevus development in very-light-skinned children without red hair. Arch Dermatol 145: 989-996.

35. Saridi M, Bourdaki E, Rekleiti M (2014) Young students' knowledge about sun protection and its relation with sunburn incidence. A systematic review. Health Science Journal 8: 4-21.

Cardiovascular Risk and Physical Activity: Simulated Analysis in General Practice Patients based on a Risk Score System

Maria Scatigna[1]*, Maria De Felice[1], Anna R. Giuliani[1], Fabio Samani[2], Luigi Canciani[2], Leila Fabiani[1]

[1]Department of Medicine, Health and Environmental Sciences, University of L'Aquila - Italy
[2]Health Search – Italy

Abstract

Aim: This cross-sectional study was aimed at evaluating the association between physical activity (PA), overweight and CV risk in a large sample of Italian general practice patients and forecast the impact of increasing PA in a general population.

Methods: Regression analysis on single CV risk factors and stratification of global risk score have been carried out on 45,862 records with normal/overweight and active/inactive conditions as primary explanatory variables. Moreover a hypothetical attributable risk was calculated on the basis of expected cases.

Results: HDL cholesterol resulted the risk factor most correlated with PA. Systolic blood pressure and fasting plasma glucose levels seemed to be more correlated to overweight than to PA. Active women and men would respectively have a 15% and 17% lower probability of experiencing a major cardiovascular event in the subsequent ten years than their inactive counterparts, adjusting for overweight. If inactive subjects became active at the lowest level, 818.8 cases/100,000 men and 201.5 cases/100,000 women aged 35-69 years would be protected during the same period.

Conclusion: As counsellors for active lifestyle, general practitioners could contribute in reducing the absolute number of CV major events in the 'healthy' general population.

Keywords: CVD risk; Physical activity; General practice

Introduction

Cardiovascular diseases (CVDs), including myocardial infarction and stroke, are the major causes of morbidity, disability and mortality in Italy and were responsible for the deaths of 97,953 men and 126,531 women in 2008. The most important risk factors for these diseases are hypertension, hypercholesterolemia, diabetes, smoking, a sedentary lifestyle, and obesity [1].

Various methods of evaluating cardiovascular risk have been developed, beginning with the American Framingham score [2]. In relation to coronary heart diseases, the Framingham score can be calculated on the basis of age, gender, systolic and diastolic pressure, smoking habits, total cholesterolemia, high-density lipoprotein (HDL) cholesterol, the presence/absence of diabetes, and the electrocardiographic (ECG) presence/absence of left ventricular hypertrophy. Another method of classifying the risk of CVD is the European Systematic Coronary Risk Evaluation (SCORE), in which coloured charts indicate the 10-year risk of subjects aged 40-65 years on the basis of their gender, cholesterol levels, systolic pressure, and smoking status [3].

The individual score used in the Italian Project Cuore not only allows a precise risk estimate (unlike the class estimates used in the charts), but also takes into account continuous values for age, systolic blood pressure, total cholesterolemia and HDL cholesterol, and considers the prescription of anti-hypertensive drugs (yes/no) [4]. The score applies to subjects aged 35-69 years, and indicates the percentage of people of the same age and gender, and with the same characteristics, who are likely to experience a first major cardiovascular event (myocardial infarction or stroke) in the subsequent ten years. This score provides general practitioners (GPs) with an important opportunity to discuss possible preventive action with their patients because it is known that appropriate preventive and clinical interventions can considerably reduce the morbidity and mortality associated with CVD.

Within other risk estimation systems: ASSIGN had the main advantages of the addition of an area indicator of social deprivation and

family history of coronary heart disease; QRISK was developed using a substantial amount of data from pooled general practice databases; the Prospective Cardiovascular Munster (PROCAM) function is derived from a relatively small sample; some consider it to be underpowered in women; Reynolds Risk Scores were developed primarily to incorporate C-reactive protein (CRP), wich is now know to be a strong predictor of CVD risk [5].

Physical exercise plays a fundamental role in reducing the risk of coronary disease and all-cause mortality, and has been evaluated in many studies [6-15]. A meta-analysis by Sattelmair et al. showed that, in comparison with no exercise, a minimum of moderately intense physical activity (PA) (150 minutes/week) leads to a 14% reduction in the risk of coronary disease (relative risk [RR] 0.86, 95% confidence interval [CI] 0.77-0.96), and a reduction of 20% (RR 0.80, 95% CI 0.74-0.88) if the exercise is increased to 300 minutes/week) [14]. A review by other authors has shown that high levels of PA play a significantly protective role against coronary disease (RR 0.73, 95% CI 0.66-0.88; p < 0.00001), and other studies have shown that an increase in PA or fitness over time reduces mortality due to coronary diseases as well as all-cause mortality [12,16-22].

The aims of this study were: firstly to evaluate the association between PA levels and overweight (as predictors) and CV risk single factors and global score (as health outcomes); secondly to forecast the impact on the general population of a physical inactivity reduction by

*Corresponding author: Maria Scatigna, Department of Medicine, Health and Environment Sciences, University of L'Aquila, Italy, E-mail: maria.scatigna@cc.univaq.it

calculating the expected cases of a CV major events and the 'theoretical' attributable risk in a GP population.

Method and Materials

Study design and data source

This cross-sectional study involved a sample of general practice patients observed in 2007. The data were provided by Health Search, a research institute of the Italian Society of General Medicine (SIGM) that was founded in 1998 and is based on a network of researchers who use Millewin© software to manage and record clinical data [23-25]. The GPs regularly send clinical data to a centralised database recognised as containing complete information concerning the main aspects of healthcare information. The geographic distribution of the GPs is homogeneous and a previous study on indicator variables of GPs clinical practice and use of computerised records demonstrated that the patients' population can be considered representative of the Italian population as a whole and the database is not biased by the characteristics of the GPs, so it can be used for research purposes [26].

Outcomes and determinant variables

The variables assessing CV risk factors were considered independently and as part of a score estimating the "absolute global risk" of experiencing a first major coronary or cerebrovascular event within ten years. This score has been calculated on the basis of Project Cuore method, suitable for subjects aged 35-69 years, by means of a mathematical function that included gender, age, systolic blood pressure (SBP), total cholesterol, HDL cholesterol, smoking habits, diabetes, and hypertension treatment [4].

Primary explanatory variables were BMI-based weight category and PA. Using the international body mass index (BMI) cut-off values, the patients were classified as being "underweight/normal weight", "overweight" or "obese" [27]. PA was self-reported by the patients and classified by the GPs at the time of recording using coded examples of the intensity of work and leisure time PA, as established by Millewin© software: *inactive*, at work he/she remains predominantly in a sitting position, with no need to get up (employee, medical, textile worker, etc..) and spents his/her leisure time only in sedentary activities (television, reading, cinema); *low active*, at work he/she stands up or walks a lot, but does not move loads (normal housework, salesman, bartender, postman, etc..) and spents his/her leisure time walking, riding a bike, gardening, bowling, dancing, etc. for less than 4 hours per week; *active,* at work he/she walks and moves loads a lot (heavy housework, painter, bricklayer, laborer, mechanic, etc.) and spents his/her leisure time walking, bicycling, gardening, bowling, dancing, etc. for more than 4 hours per week; *higly active*, at work he/she moves heavy weights (unloader, porter, etc.) and/or practices competitive sports that imply systematic and heavy training.

Sample

The cardiovascular risk score has been calculated on 45,862 patients aged 35-49 years. Data on BMI and PA were available, respectively, only for 41,896 and 37,481 subjects.

Data analysis

The data were processed using Stata/IC 12.1 software.

Separate gender-based multiple regression models were used to analyse four continuous variables (total cholesterol, HDL cholesterol, fasting plasma glucose - FPG and systolic blood pressure - SBP) in terms of the categorical variables of BMI-based weight classification,

PA, and age class [28]. This analysis excluded the subjects receiving specific pharmacological treatment (i.e. lipid-lowering treatment for high total and low HDL cholesterol, anti-diabetic treatment for high FPG, or anti-hypertensive treatment for high SBP).

Mean individual scores and their 95% confidence intervals were calculated in the different BMI-based weight classification and PA categories and Student's t-test was used to verify the significance of the differences.

Subsequently, assuming that, in the worst scenario, the patients' overweight doesn't decrease and PA habits doesn't improve in the following ten years, the calculation of absolute number of foreseeable cases was simulated on the basis of the individual scores. Using this approach we estimated the hypothtical relative risk (RR) of exposure to the different levels of PA (low-active *vs* inactive; active/high active *vs* inactive) relating to 37,015 records, adjusting by BMI-based weight category (Mantel-Haenszel stratification and the chi-squared test). Finally, also the hypothetical population attributable risk (AR) was calculated.

Using the information from Palmieri et al. study cohort about the level of SBP, Total and HDL cholesterol as quantitive variables and considering the whole sample size for the calculation, the study power resulted higher than 80% [4].

The database complies with European Union guidelines on the use of medical data for medical research. The protocol of this study was approved by the Scientific and Ethical Advisory Board of Health Search.

Results

Comparison of the four multiple regression models showed that, taking into account the simultaneous effect of age, HDL cholesterol seemed to be correlated to overweight and PA (Table 1). In comparison with the normal weight subjects, the overweight and obese males showed an estimated reduction in HDL cholesterol levels of 4.97 mg/dL ($p < 0.001$) and 8.37 mg/dL ($p < 0.001$), and the overweight and obese females showed reductions of 5.48 mg/dL ($p < 0.001$) and 9.57 mg/dL ($p < 0.001$). In comparison with the inactive subjects, the estimated increase in HDL cholesterol was 0.40 mg/dL (n.s.) in low-active males, and 1.92 mg/dL ($p < 0.01$) in active/high active males; the corresponding values for the females were 0.28 mg/dL (n.s.) and 1.38 mg/dL ($p < 0.001$).

Weight had a significant influence on FPG levels in both genders: an estimated increase in overweight and obese males of respectively 2.93 mg/dL ($p < 0.001$) and 7.05 mg/dL ($p < 0.001$), and in overweight and obese females of respectively 3.59 mg/dL ($p < 0.001$) and 7.78 mg/dL ($p < 0.001$). FPG seemed not to be significantly correlated with PA both in males and in females.

Among the overweight and obese subjects, there were significant increases in SBP of respectively 3.29 mmHg ($p < 0.001$) and 6.91 mmHg ($p < 0.001$) in males, and respectively 3.71 mmHg ($p < 0.001$) and 7.79 mmHg ($p < 0.001$) in females. As for FPG, no-significant association has been found between SBP and PA.

In the total cholesterol model, age seemed to be the most important variable, particularly among the women: in comparison with the reference age group (35-39 years), the estimated increases in the three subsequent age groups were 10.00 mg/dL ($p < 0.001$), 27.00 mg/dL ($p < 0.001$) and 31.10 mg/dL ($p < 0.001$). This trend was not found among the males: the corresponding increases were 9.66 mg/dL ($p < 0.001$), 12.79 mg/dL ($p < 0.001$) and 5.93 mg/dL ($p < 0.001$). In respect to the weight

Dependent variables	Total cholesterol[1] (mg/dL)		HDL cholesterol[1] (mg/dL)		FPG[2] (mg/dL)		SBP[3] (mmHg)	
Independent variables	β coeff	P value	β coeff	P value	β coeff	P value	β coeff	P value
Males								
BMI								
Overweight vs normal weight	3.93	***	-4.97	***	2.93	***	3.29	***
Obese vs normal weight	-0.13	n.s.	-8.37	***	7.05	***	6.91	***
Physical activity								
Low active vs Inactive	1.59	*	0.4	n.s.	-0.18	n.s.	-0.05	n.s.
Active/High active vs Inactive	3.82	***	1.92	**	-0.45	n.s.	0.23	n.s.
Age								
40-49 vs 35-39 years	9.66	***	1.01	***	2.75	***	0.83	n.s.
50-59 vs 35-39 years	12.79	***	1.92	***	6.71	***	2.96	***
59-69 vs 35-39 years	5.93	***	2.75	***	10.12	***	5.79	***
No.	16,621		16,621		15,404		10,762	
R²	1.4%		7.0%		7.1%		5.9%	
F test	***		***		***		***	
Females								
Weight								
Overweight vs normal weight	3.9	***	-5.48	***	3.59	***	3.71	***
Obese vs normal weight	-0.28	n.s.	-9.57	***	7.78	***	7.79	***
Physical activity								
Low active vs Inactive	1.05	n.s.	0.28	n.s.	0.06	n.s.	-0.24	n.s.
Active/High active vs Inactive	1.77	*	1.38	***	-0.26	n.s.	0.69	n.s.
Age								
40-49 vs 35-39 years	10.00	***	0.06	n.s.	2.35	***	3.86	***
50-59 vs 35-39 years	27.00	***	0.81	*	5.45	***	8.94	***
59-69 vs 35-39 years	31.10	***	0.75	n.s.	8.4	***	13.1	***
No.	18,029		18,029		17,636		12,218	
R²	8.5%		7.4%		9.9%		14.5%	
F test	***		***		***		***	

Table 1: Multiple regression analyses on four biological dependent variables by age, BMI and physical activity in GPs' patients
* = p < 0.05, ** = p< 0.01, *** = p < 0.001
Analyses carried on patients: 1Not receiving lipid-lowering treatment; 2Not receiving anti-diabetic treatment; 3Not receiving anti-hypertensive treatment
HDL = High-Density Lipoprotein, **FPG** = Fasting Plasma Glucose, **SBP** = Systolic Blood Pressure

status, cholesterol seemed more associated with overweight (males 3.93 mg/dL, p < 0.001; females 3.90 mg/dL, p < 0.001) than with obesity (males -013 mg/dL, n.s.; females -0.28 mg/dL, n.s.). There was also an apparently non-protective trend in the case of PA: in comparison with the inactive patients, the males active/high active had a total cholesterol level that was 3.82 mg/dL higher (p < 0.001), and the female's low-active had a level that was 1.77 mg/dL higher (p < 0.05).

The mean expected number of major cardiovascular events per 100 patients in the subsequent ten years was 9.20 (95% CI: 9.09-9.31) among men, and 3.25 (95% CI: 3.21-3.30) among women. Comparing PA categories, emerged a significant difference between inactive and active/high active patients, higher in men (about two expected events, 9.84 vs 7.86, p < 0.001) than in women (about one expected event 3.46 vs 2.67 and 1.63, p < 0.001) (Table 2).

The differences between the BMI-based weight categories were more marked in the patients of both genders: more than four expected cases between the obese and normal weight in males (11.20 vs 6.99, p < 0.001) and two cases and a half in women (4.64 vs 2.15, p < 0.001) (Table 2).

Table 3 and Figure 1 show the results of the simulated analysis based on expected number of major events in the next 10-years by PA levels. Only the active/high active sub-group had a significantly lower 'theoretical' risk than the inactive sub-group, with an RR of 0.76 (95% CI 0.60-0.98) among the females and 0.80 (95% CI 0.71-0.90) among the males. That is to say, in the absence of an active style improvement in the

Expected percentage of cases over 10 years	Males	Females
No.	17,948	19,533
No physical activity	9.84 (9.62-10.06)	3.46 (3.38-3.54)
Light physical activity	9.61 (9.42-9.81)	3.19 (3.11-3.27)
Moderate/intense physical activity	7.86 (7.65-8.08)	2.67 (2.56-2.78)
No.	20,012	21,884
Underweight/normal weight	6.99 (6.80-7.18)	2.15 (2.10-2.21)
Overweight	9.38 (9.21-9.54)	3.65 (3.57-3.74)
Obese	11.20 (11.10-11.61)	4.64 (4.53-4.76)

Table 2: Cardiovascular risk score by physical activity and BMI: mean values and 95% confidence intervals.

sample, it is estimated that active/high active women and men would respectively have a 23% and 20% lower probability of experiencing a major cardiovascular event. If the additional effect of overweight is taken into account, this protective effect decreased as the overweight-adjusted RR was 0.85 (95% CI 0.66-1.01) among the women and 0.83 (95% 0.73-0.94) among the men (i.e. active/high active women and men would respectively have a 15% and 17% lower probability of experiencing a major cardiovascular event). Furthermore, the Mantel-Haenszel analysis showed that stratifying variable was not statistically significant, and so the protective effect of an active/high active lifestyle was maintained in the overweight and obese subjects.

In terms of impact, the population RA was 6.2% (p < 0.05) among the women and 8.9% (p < 0.001) among the men. Given the estimated

	Females				Males			
	Crude relative risk			Population attributable risk	Crude relative risk			Population attributable risk
	RR	95% CI			RR	95% CI		
Inactive	1				1			
Low active	0.927	0.786	1.094	3.7 %	0.977	0.879	1.085	1.3 %
Active / High active	0.765	0.597	0.981	6.2 %	0.800	0.707	0.906	8.9 %
	Stratified RR				Stratified RR			
	RR	IC 95			RR	IC 95		
Inactive	1				1			
Low active	0.980	0.931	1.157		0.998	0.899	1.109	
Active / High active	0.847	0.660	1.088		0.829	0.732	0.939	

Table 3: Hypothetical relative risk and population attributable risk of cardiovascular major events by physical activity level. Crude RR and RR stratified by BMI-based weight classification (Mantel-Haenszel method).

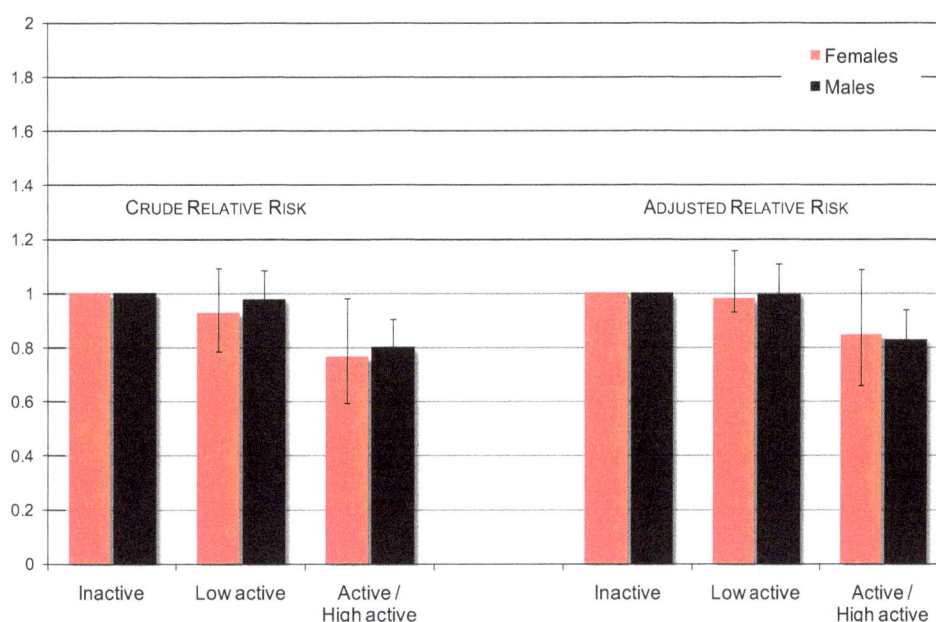

Figure 1: Hypothetical relative risk of cardiovascular major events by physical activity level, Crude RR and RR stratified by BMI-based weight classification (Mantel-Haenszel method).

10-year incidence of 9.20 cases per 100 men and 3.25 cases per women, it can be calculated that, if the inactive subjects became active/high active, 818.8 cases/100,000 men and 201.5 cases/100,000 women aged 35-69 years would be saved in the same period.

Discussion

In comparison with the data of the surveillance national study 'Progressi delle Aziende Sanitarie per la Salute in Italia' (PASSI) which used computer-assisted telephone interviewing (CATI) in a national sample of about 15,000 subjects, our sample had a higher prevalence of diseases in the corresponding age classes: 10% higher in the case of overweight/obesity, 6% higher in the case of hypertension, and about twice as high in the case of diabetes [29,30]. Furthermore, the percentage of current smokers was lower and the percentage of ex-smokers higher, probably because they had stopped smoking after the occurrence of clinical events, the diagnosis of disease or medical counselling [29]. Hinrichs et al. have confirmed that GPs behave differently in terms of recommending PA, and tend to concentrate more on educating patients with chronic diseases [31].

However, despite the limitations described above, our findings

are useful because our sample was larger than that of the PASSI study. Furthermore, unlike our study, the PASSI study used self-reported data based on patient's recall rather than laboratory data or medical diagnoses also for the clinical variables, and for this reason, there may be a selection bias insofar as more healthy participants are probably more willing to respond to a questionnaire.

The patients in our sample did not engage in much PA, particularly the women: less than a quarter of the study sample (22.2%) was active/high active (15.8% of the women, and 29.3% of the men).

It is necessary to point out a methodological limitation relating to the assessment of PA, which was based on the GPs' skill in categorisation on the basis of the patients' self-reports, and not evaluated about its reliability and validity.

Self-reported PA measures have many sources of measurement error due to the cognitive tasks associated with recall, incomplete ascertainment across the spectrum of intensity and physical activity contexts, and possibly the tendency to provide socially desirable responses For that, researchers have long sought alternative measurement approaches by means of technological devices that directly measure human movement (e.g. pedometers, accelerometers).

Nevertheless, these devices have their own set of limitations and sources of measurement error, and there are specific times and circumstances in which self-report measure of PA remains the most appropriate approach, particularly in the context of surveillance and public health [32]. For example, in our study, the formulation of the PA category for the assessment corresponds exactly to the health education message (simple and understandable) that GPs should use to communicate reccomandation about PA healthy levels to the general population and that he/she should assess.

A further limitation in the present study is that ins't possible to know for sure when the data on CVD risk factors, PA and weight status have been collected, since the practitionnairs update the database in a continous way. For example, exposure data (PA) could have been collected after CVD risk factors and not before, or simultaneously. So, we can't exclude that the patient could change his/her behaviour after the GP's counselling due to the risk awareness. But that is a advantage condition that should be considered as confirming condition of our results: that means that the preventable cases could be more that those calculated since a portion could have been hidden by an inducted increasing of PA level.

The regression analyses (Table 1) showed that HDL cholesterol was more clearly associated with PA (particularly in men) and overweight status (particularly in women) than the other intermediate risk factors: the models for total cholesterol, FPG and SBP seemed to be less clear and sometimes contradictory. The meta-analysis of Kelley et al. also found that PA had a greater effect on HDL cholesterol, although it revealed a significant effect on all blood lipids. In the same way the results of the study of Parraga-Martinez et al. will provide extremely useful information about the effectiveness of the proposed strategy (counselling and lifestyles as PA) of improving compliance in the prevention and management of cardiovascular disease based on increased control of lipid profile plasma levels [33,34]. Conversely, Liira et al. demonstrated that PA had no effect on HDL cholesterol or other cardiovascular outcomes [35]. Overweight seems to have a transversal effect on all of the parameters, probably because it is less subject to errors and dishomogeneity as it is directly measured in the GPs' surgeries in order to calculate the patients' BMI.

The trend of total cholesterol is inconsistent between genders, and the greatest difference was observed when comparing the youngest age group (35-39 years) with those above the age of 50 years in females: the tripling in levels is probably related to the hormonal changes that occur after menopause. It cannot be excluded that the models of total cholesterol may have involved inverse causality due to the partially clinical/diagnostic character of the GP data (i.e. patients may have been more active because they received GP counselling to reduce a high level of total cholesterol).

Aadahl et al. also found that, unlike other parameters (e.g. diastolic pressure, overweight, waist circumference), SBP was not significantly affected by a change in the level of PA [36]. However, the absence of any apparent protective effect of PA on SBP may also be due to limitations in the method of data collection method: e.g. the lack of information about 'spontaneous' or everyday activities (work, domestic chores) previously pointed out by Churilla and Ford [37]. Furthermore, the published studies describing reduced hypertension levels in more physically active subjects were longitudinal and/or experimental, and compared the effects using dose-response analyses and more precisely defined thresholds for the intensity and frequency of exercise [38,39]. In the same way, we couldn't adjust the PA influence by nutritional intakes as in major studies on diabetes risk [40]. Those might be the reasons for the absence of significance in the regression terms about SBP and FPG.

Moreover in present study, no information about family history of diabetes was available. Again, this limit could explain the poor relationship between impairment in glycemic control and PA, since Ciccone and coll highlighted that family history of diabetes accounts for an increase in cardiovascular risk of individuals even if such subjects have no signs of pre-diabetes or diabetes. It should be interesting to study the role of PA in reducing the hidden risk attributable to that genetically determined condition and potential mediating mechanisms involving other CV risk factors [41].

The hypothetical risk reduction attributable to moderate/intense PA in our simulated analysis (15% in men and 17% in women) is comparable with that found by Sofi et al., although these authors considered a specific disease category (coronary diseases) and activity (leisure time activity): 27% for intense activity vs none, and 12% for moderate activity vs none [12]. Although the hypothetical RR and AR calculated on the basis of PA are not so high, it needs to be borne in mind that PA/inactivity is a risk factor that concerns everyone in the population and, as in the case of nutritional epidemiology (everyone eats, and the consumption of certain foods and nutritional intake is transversal), even small variations in such risk indices correspond to a high number of cases in absolute terms (and a considerable cost for national health services).

Moreover, the absolute number of preventable cases in the general 'healthy' population would be higher.

An approach very similar to our simulated risk calculation has been recently used by Mallaina and coll in a study predicting the impact of smoking cessation in term of cardiovascular risk reduction in a wide European sample, carried-out, exactly as ours, with a cross-sectional data collection and in the primary care setting [42].

Our study, it should be clear, only gives clues to aetiological factors, without any intention to confirm the causal associations, since it has a cross-sectional design, not longitudinal. By using the CV risk score (with an algorithm based on a previous Italian cohort study) we simply forecasted how many expected cases of CV major events probably could be avoided in the GPs population, while a huge amount of scientific literature focuses on second-level healthcare facilities (specialist).

It is a demonstration of the usefulness of data collection on behavioural risk factors in the general medical practice and highligths the strategic role of GPs as observators, counsellors and, so, as public health promoters.

Acknowledgements

We would like to thank Dr. Davide Grassi, Research Fellow at the Department of Internal Medicine of the University of L'Aquila, for his help in collecting the bibliographical material;

Dr. Serena Pecchioli, Statistician of Health Search, a research institute of the Italian Society of General Medicine (SIMG), who extracted the data; Dr Gianfranco Poccia, Diabetologist of L'Aquila, for his expertise concerning outlier biological values.

Competing Interests

The Author's declare that they have no competing interests.

Author's contribution statement (individual contribution to the manuscript)

Maria Scatigna took part in study designing, performed the statistical analysis and drafted the manuscript; Maria De Felice contributed to analysis and interpretation of data, drafted the manuscript and revisited it critically for plausibility of clinical content; Anna R. Giuliani took part in the sequence alignment and revisited manuscript critically for epidemiological content; Fabio Samani contributed to acquire data from Health Search Institute and gave final approval of the manuscript; Luigi Canciani contributed to acquire data from Health Search Institute and critically revisited manuscript for epidemiological content; Leila Fabiani conceived the study, participated in designing and coordinated the manuscript.

References

1. Relazione sullo Stato Sanitario del Paese (2010) Ministero della salute Direzione Generale del Sistema Informativo e Statistico Sanitario.

2. Wilson PW, D'Agostino RB, Levy D, Belanger AM, Silbershatz H, et al. (1998) Prediction of coronary heart disease using risk factor categories. Circulation 97: 1837- 1847.

3. Conroy RM , Pyörälä K, Fitzgerald AP, Sans S, Menotti A, et al. (2003) Estimation of ten-year risk of fatal cardiovascular disease in Europe: the SCORE project. Eur Heart J 24: 987- 1003.

4. Palmieri L, Panico S, Vanuzzo D, Ferrario M, Pilotto L, et al. (2004) Evaluation of the global cardiovascular absolute risk: The Progetto CUORE individual score. Ann Ist Super Sanita 40: 393-399.

5. Cooney MT, Cooney HC, Dudina A, Graham IM (2010) Assessment of cardiovascular risk. Curr Hypertens Rep 2: 384-393.

6. Bull FC, Armstrong TP, Dixon T, Ham S, Neiman A, et al. (2004) Physical inactivity. In: Lopez AD, Rodgers A, Murray CJL, Ezzati M, editors. Comparative Quantification of Health Risks. Global and Regional Burden of Disease Attributable to Selected Major Risk Factors. Geneva: World Health Organization: 729-882.

7. Berlin JA, Colditz GA (1990) A meta-analysis of physical activity in the prevention of coronary heart disease. Am J Epidemiol 32: 62-628.

8. Eaton CB (1992) Relation of physical activity and cardiovascular fitness to coronary heart disease. Part I: A meta-analysis of the independent relation of physical activity and coronary heart disease. J Am Board Fam Pract. 5: 31-42.

9. Pate RR, Pratt M, Blair SN, Haskell WL, Macera CA, et al (1995) Physical activity and public health. A recommendation from the Centers for Disease Control and Prevention and the American College of Sports Medicine. JAMA 273: 402-407.

10. Williams PT (2001) Physical fitness and activity as separate heart disease risk factors: a meta-analysis. Med Sci Sports Exerc 33: 754-756 .

11. Oguma Y, Shinoda-Tagawa T (2004) Physical activity decreases cardiovascular disease risk in women: review and meta-analysis. Am J Prev Med 26: 407-418.

12. Sofi F, Capalbo A, Cesari F, Abbate R, Gensini GF (2008) Physical activity during leisure time and primary prevention of coronary heart disease: An updated meta-analysis of cohort studies. Eur J Cardiovasc Prev Rehabil 5: 247-257.

13. Physical activity guidelines advisory committee report (2008) Washington, DC: Physical activity guidelines advisory committee 2008.

14. Sattelmair J, Pertman J, Ding EL, Kohl HW 3rd, Haskell W, et al. (2011) Dose response between physical activity and risk of coronary heart disease: A meta-analysis. Circulation 24: 789-795.

15. Petersen CB, Grønbæk M, Helge JW, Thygesen LC, Schnohr P, et al. (2012) Changes in physical activity in leisure time and the risk of myocardial infarction, ischemic heart disease, and all-cause mortality. Eur J Epidemiol 27: 91-99.

16. Blair SN, Kohl HW 3rd, Barlow CE, Paffenbarger RS Jr, Gibbons LW, et al. (1995) Changes in physical fitness and all-cause mortality. A prospective study of healthy and unhealthy men. JAMA 273: 1093-1098.

17. Wannamethee SG, Shaper AG, Walker M (1998) Changes in physical activity, mortality, and incidence of coronary heart disease in older men. Lancet 35: 1603- 1608.

18. Gregg EW, Cauley JA, Stone K, Thompson TJ, Bauer DC, et al. (2003) Relationship of changes in physical activity and mortality among older women. JAMA 289: 2379-2386.

19. Erikssen G, Liestøl K, Bjørnholt J, Thaulow E, Sandvik L, et al. (1998) Changes in physical fitness and changes in mortality. Lancet 352: 759-762.

20. Andersen LB, Schnohr P, Schroll M, Hein HO (2000) All-cause mortality associated with physical activity during leisure time, work, sports, and cycling to work. Arch Intern Med 60: 162-1628.

21. Schnohr P , Scharling H, Jensen JS (2003) Changes in leisure-time physical activity and risk of death: an observational study of 7,000 men and women. Am J Epidemiol 58: 639-644.

22. Byberg L, Melhus H, Gedeborg R, Sundström J, Ahlbom A, et al. (2009) Total mortality after changes in leisure time physical activity in 50 year old men: 35 year follow-up of population based cohort. Br J Sports Med 43: 482.

23. Fabiani L, Scatigna M, Panopoulou K, Sabatini A, Sessa E, et al (2004) Health Search – Istituto di ricerca della Società italiana di Medicina Generale; la realizzazione di un database per la ricerca in medicina generale Epidemiol Prev 28: 156-162.

24. Millennium S.R.L. Firenze, Italia. http://www.millewin.it consulted on 2 May 2012.

25. Samani F, Del Zotti F, Garavina I, Negri F, Cioffi M. Dalla formazione alla ricerca. SIMG 1999:7-11.

26. Niccolai C, Nardi R, Samani F, Ventriglia G (2001) Health Search: chi sono i ricercatori? SIMG 1: 5-6.

27. [No authors listed] (2000) Obesity: preventing and managing the global epidemic. Report of a WHO consultation. World Health Organ Tech Rep Ser 894: 253.

28. University of California, Los Angeles – UCLA Regression with Stata.

29. Istituto Superiore di Sanità (2010) Epicentro. Rapporto Nazionale PASSI.

30. Trinito MO, Bertozzi N, Bietta C, Binkin N, De Giacomi G, et al (2006) Analisi di alcuni fattori di rischio cardiovascolari nella popolazione delle ASL partecipanti allo studio PASSI. Not Ist Super Sanità 19.

31. Hinrichs T, Moschny A, Klaassen-Mielke R, Trampisch U, Thiem U, et al (2011) General practitioner advice on physical activity: analyses in a cohort of older primary health care patients (getABI). BMC Fam Pract 12: 26.

32. Troiano RP , Pettee Gabriel KK, Welk GJ, Owen N, Sternfeld B (2012) Reported physical activity and sedentary behavior: why do you ask? J Phys Act Health 9 Suppl: S68-S75.

33. Kelley GA, Kelley KS, Tran ZV (2005) Exercise, lipids, and lipoproteins in older adults: a meta-analysis. Prev Cardiol 8: 206-224.

34. Parraga-Martinez I, Rabanales-Soto J, Tellez-Lapeira JM, Escobar-Rabadan F, Villena-Ferrer A, et al (2015) Effectiveness of a combined strategy to improve therapeutic complianceand degree of control among patients with hypercholesterolemia: A randomised clinical trial. BMC Cardiovascular Disorders 15: 8.

35. Liira H, Engberg E, Leppavuori J, From S, Kautiainen H, Liiira J, et al (2014) Exercise intervention and health checks for middle-age men with elevated cardiovascular risk: a randomized controlled trial. Scandinavian J of Primary Health Care. 32: 156-162.

36. Aadahl M, von Huth Smith L, Pisinger C, Toft UN, Glümer C, et al. (2009) Five-year change in physical activity is associated with changes in cardiovascular disease risk factors: the Inter99 study. Prev Med 48: 326-333 .

37. Churilla JR, Ford ES (2010) Comparing physical activity patterns of hypertensive and nonhypertensive US adults. Am J Hypertens 23: 987-993.

38. Lee IM, Sesso HD, Paffenbarger RS Jr (2000) Physical activity and coronary heart disease risk in men: does the duration of exercise episodes predict risk? Circulation 02: 981-986.

39. Cornelissen VA, Fagard RH, Coeckelberghs E, Vanhees L (2011) Impact of resistance training on blood pressure and other cardiovascular risk factors: a meta-analysis of randomized, controlled trials. Hypertension 58: 950-958.

40. Lindström J, Ilanne-Parikka P, Peltonen M, Aunola S, Eriksson JG, et al (2006) Finnish Diabetes Prevention Study Group. Sustained reduction in the incidence of type 2 diabetes by lifestyle intervention: follow-up of the Finnish Diabetes Prevention Study. Lancet. Nov 368: 673-679.

41. Ciccone MM, Scicchitano P, Cameli M, Cecere A, Cortese F, et al. (2014) Endothelial Function in Pre-diabetes, Diabetes and Diabetic Cardiomyopathy: A Review. J Diabetes Metab 5: 364.

42. Mallaina P, Lionis C, Rol H, Imperiali R, Burgess A, et al. (2013) Smoking cessation and the risk of cardiovascular disease outcomes predicted from established risk scores: results of the Cardiovascular Risk Assessment among Smokers in Primary Care in Europe (CV-ASPIRE) study. BMC Public Health 3: 362.

3

An Observational Comparative Study of Cardiac Index Estimated by FloTrac and Intermittent Thermo Dilution in Off-Pump Coronary Artery Bypass Grafting

Manender Kumar Singla[1]*, Kanwalpreet Sodhi[2], Anupam Shrivastava[3], Kishore C Mukherjee[4], Sonia Saini[1] and Manpreet Singh Salooja[4]

[1]Department of Cardiac Anesthesia, SPS Apollo Hospital, Ludhiana, India
[2]Department of Critical Care, SPS Apollo Hospital, Ludhiana, India
[3]Department of Anesthesia and Critical Care, SPS Apollo Hospital, Ludhiana, India
[4]Department of Cardiothoracic and Vascular Surgery, SPS Apollo Hospital, Ludhiana, India

Abstract

Objective: The purpose of this study was to determine the correlation between cardiac index (CI) measurements made using intermittent thermodilution (ITD) technique by pulmonary artery catheter (PAC) and arterial pulse-contour analysis by FloTrac.

Design: Prospective observational study.

Setting: Cardiac surgery unit in a 350 bedded tertiary care hospital in India. Participants: 31 adult patients undergoing elective off-pump coronary artery bypass grafting (OPCABG) Interventions: CI measurements performed by the two different methods at six time points during the surgery (before skin incision, during grafting of left anterior descending artery, obtuse marginal artery and right coronary/ posterior descending artery, after protamine administration and after shifting the patient to recovery room).

Measurements and results: The techniques a weak correlation at all six time points during the OPCABG. The mean bias of 0.85 L/min/m2 and precision of 0.55 was found in the study population. The percentage error calculated using Critchley s criteria was found to be 46%.

Conclusion: CI measurements obtained using FloTrac showed a limited correlation with those acquired by ITD technique at different stages of OPCABG. Further studies are required in other patient populations and clinical situations.

Keywords: FloTrac; Bypass grafting; Coronary artery

Abbreviations: CO: Cardiac Output; ITD: Intermittent Thermo Dilution Technique; PAC: Pulmonary Artery Catheter; IABP: Intra-Aortic Balloon Pump; LOA: Limits of Agreement; CI: Cardiac Index; OPCABG: Off-Pump Coronary Artery Bypass Grafting

Introduction

The use of Off Pump Coronary Artery Bypass Grafting (OPCABG) is gaining widespread acceptance as the preferred choice for myocardial revascularization [1,2]. However, during OPCABG, hemodynamic instability is common and thus, maintaining an adequate cardiac output (CO) plays a pivotal role in the peri-operative management of these patients [3-5]. Traditionally, CO monitoring has been accomplished by the Intermittent Thermodilution Technique (ITD) using Pulmonary Artery Catheter (PAC) [6]. Considering its potential advantage of providing additional information about cardiac filling pressures, pulmonary artery pressures and mixed venous oxygen saturation, PAC still remains the favored technique by many clinicians [7]. However, the routine use of PAC has been questioned in the literature for the lack of statistical evidence of its benefit and associated problems such as longer time required for its placement, cost, intermittent nature leading to potential for delay and rare complications like pulmonary artery rupture [8].

Various lesser invasive techniques have been developed such as transthoracic bioimpedence, pulse dye densitometry, Doppler and pulse wave contour analysis [7,9]. FloTrac by Edwards Life sciences is one of such devices based on the pulse contour analysis that estimates the cardiac output by beat to beat stroke volume analysis, based on Windkessel model described by Otto Frank in 1899 [10].

Major advantages with the device are the ability to measure cardiac output using any existent arterial line and elimination of the need for system calibration. The drawbacks include inability to provide other hemodynamic parameters as measured by PAC and limitation of its use in situations of arterial wave artifacts, aortic incompetence, severe peripheral vasoconstriction, irregular pulse and patients on Intra-Aortic Balloon Pump (IABP) [11].

Numerous studies in literature have produced inconsistent results with cardiac output measured using the conventional ITD and newer FloTrac methods in different clinical settings. The present study was aimed at analysis of clinical agreement between the ITD technique and FloTrac device for the estimation of cardiac index (CI).

Material and Methods

The study was approved by the hospital ethics committee and written informed consent was taken from all the patients enrolled in the study. The study included patients planned for elective OPCABG.

*Corresponding author: Dr. Manender Kumar Singla, Department of Cardiac Anesthesia, SPS Apollo Hospital, Ludhiana, India,
E-mail: drmksingla@yahoo.com

Patients with concomitant valvular heart disease, arrhythmias or intra-aortic balloon pump during pre-operative and intra-operative period were excluded from the study. The patient group for the study comprised of 32 consecutive patients planned for elective OPCABG in our institution without the concomitant problems. In all the study patients, CO was monitored using both the techniques in question i.e. by ITD method and FloTrac technique. Pre-operative evaluation of the patients was performed a day before surgery. Patients were reassured and premedicated with oral lorazepam 2 mg and ranitidine 150 mg at the bed time and on the morning of surgery. For the patients on beta blockers, half the regular dose was given on the morning of surgery. All other cardiac medications including anti-hypertensive and nitrates were continued till the morning of surgery. In the operating room, routine monitoring was started with 5 lead ECG and pulse oximetry. Under local anaesthesia with 1% lignocaine, a 14/16G cannula was inserted in right antecubital vein and right radial artery was cannulated with 20G cannula which was connected to FloTrac sensor for cardiac output estimation. The anesthesia was induced with midazolam 0.03mg/kg, fentanyl 4 mcg/kg and propofol 1% in the dose of 1.5-2 mg/kg. Endotracheal intubation was facilitated with rocuronium 0.6 mg/kg. After induction 7.5 Fr PAC was inserted into the right internal jugular vein and right femoral artery was cannulated with 16G cannula. Other intra-operative monitoring included nasopharyngeal temperature and end tidal $CO2$. Anesthesia was maintained with 0.5-2% isoflurane with oxygen-air mixture in ratio of 1:1, fentanyl and rocuronium. Normothermia was maintained throughout the procedure with the help of warm intravenous fluids, forced air warmers and circulating warm water mattress under the patient. Heparin was administered in the dose of 1500 IU/Kg and repeated as required to maintain the activating clotting time more than 250 seconds during myocardial revascularization. Medtronic octopus was used to stabilize the heart during beating heart surgery. During the grafting, the inotropes, intravenous fluids or vasodilators were used to maintain the hemodynamics as per the discretion of the attending anesthesiologist. On completion of revascularization, protamine was used to neutralize the effect of heparin. The patients were shifted to cardiac recovery room on completion of surgery and extubated as per the institutional weaning protocol.

For the purpose of the study, cardiac output values were estimated by thermo dilution Method by PAC and by FloTrac. Cardiac index values were derived and termed as CI by Thermo dilution Technique (CITD) and CI by FloTrac Technique (CIFT). The measurements were recorded at six time points (T1-T6) i.e. before skin incision (T1), during grafting of left anterior descending artery (T2), obtuse marginal artery (T3) and right coronary Artery/posterior descending artery (T4), after protamine administration (T5) and just after shifting the patient to cardiac recovery room (T6). During grafting, CI values were obtained after the arteriotomy and placement of the shunt. For CITD by PAC, an average of 3 values was taken not deviating more than 20% that were obtained within 3 minutes. For each injection, 10 ml of 0.9% normal saline at room temperature was used and each injection was completed in less than 3 seconds. CIFT was directly recorded from the Vigileo monitor.

Statistics

The results obtained were analyzed by MedCalc 11.0 and SPSS 16.0 software for windows. Bland and Altmann analysis, which is used for assessing the agreement between 2 measurements of the same clinical variable by two different techniques, was used [12]. According to it, bias is defined as the average difference between the two measures and limits of agreement (LOA) is 2SD (standard deviation) of the bias. A paired t-test was applied to test the mean difference between the two groups. A p-value of <0.05 depicted statistically significant difference between the CI values recorded by two different techniques.

Critchley's criteria were also applied [13]. According to it, the limit of acceptance for calculated Percentage error is 30% and the value more than 30% indicates poor agreement between the two techniques.

Results

A total of 32 patients were included in the study. One patient was electively converted to On-pump CABG because of poor quality of target vessels and thus was excluded from the Study. Thus the study group included 31 adult patients who underwent OPCABG at our Institution. Left anterior descending artery was grafted in all the patients. Anastomoses to obtuse marginal and right coronary artery/posterior descending artery were performed in 28 and 24 patients respectively.

The demographic profile and patient characteristics are as shown in (Table 1). There were 23 males and 8 females. The mean left ventricular ejection fraction was 48.87 ± 7.7% (Figure 1).

Represents the mean values of CI plotted against their respective

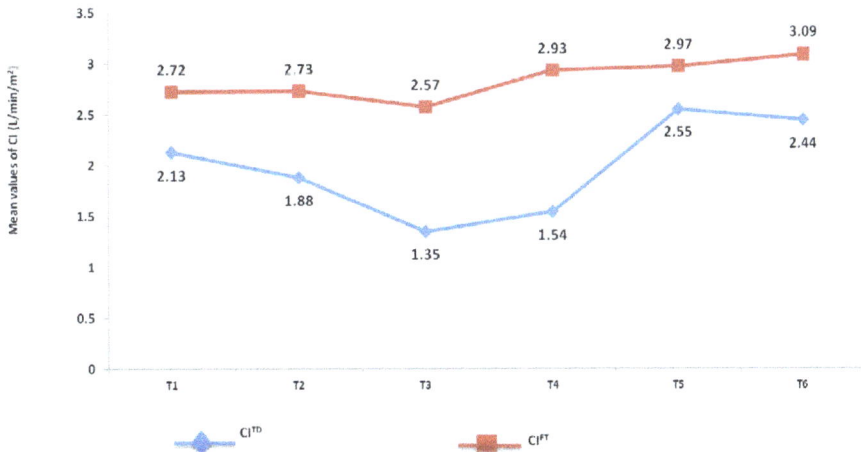

Figure 1: Graph showing mean values of CI at different time points.

time points. The mean values of CI at all six time points during our study and correlation between these 2 sets of values are as mentioned in (Table 2). It is evident that the 2 techniques exhibit a weak correlation at all the six stages of the surgery. A paired t-test to test the mean difference between the 2 study techniques shows p-values of much lesser than 0.05, suggesting a statistically significant difference between the CI values calculated by the 2 methods at all six time points. Bland-Altman analysis of CITD and CIFT showed the mean bias and limits

of agreement (2 SD) expressed in L/min/m2 at their respective time points to be 0.59 ± 0.95, 0.85 ± 1.14, 1.22 ± 1.20, 1.39 ± 0.99, 0.42 ± 1.23, and 0.65 ± 1.17 (Table 3). Figures 2-7 show the Bland-Altman plots, where the differences between CI values measured by the 2 methods are plotted against their mean values. The mean bias of 0.85 L/min/m2 and precision of 0.55 was found in the study population. The overall CI in the present study was 2.41 ± 0.48 L/min/m2. The percentage error using the calculation recommended by Critchley is 46% which is well above the accepted limit of 30%.

Discussion

The present study on 31 patients showed a weak correlation and a statistically significant difference between the two methods of CO monitoring at six different stages of OPCABG. OPCABG is increasingly being performed as an alternative to the standard CPB assisted procedure and aims at reduction in peri-operative morbidity [14]. This new approach requires accurate hemodynamic monitoring because surgical

	Mean ± SD
Age (yrs.)	65.65 ± 10.14
Weight (kg)	66.58 ± 11.42
Height (cm)	166.26 ± 8.75
Body surface area (m2)	1.74 ± 0.17
Left ventricular ejection fraction (%)	48.87 ± 7.71
Sex (Male: Female)	23:08

Table 1: Demographic data and patient characteristics.

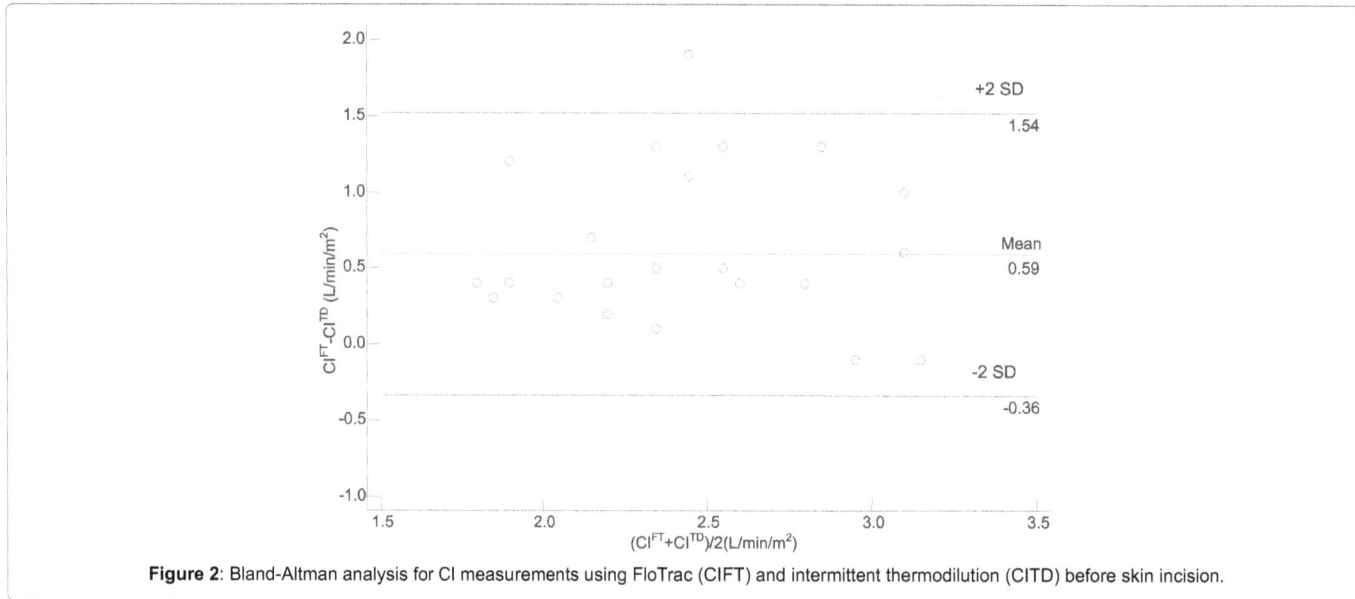

Figure 2: Bland-Altman analysis for CI measurements using FloTrac (CIFT) and intermittent thermodilution (CITD) before skin incision.

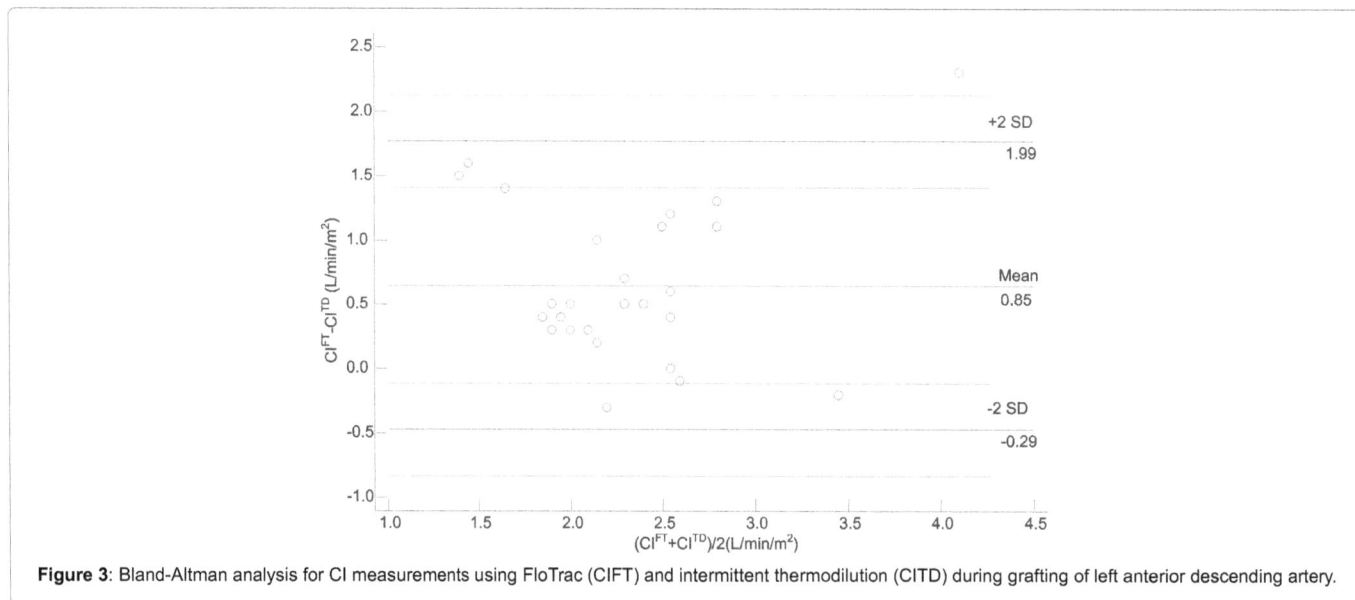

Figure 3: Bland-Altman analysis for CI measurements using FloTrac (CIFT) and intermittent thermodilution (CITD) during grafting of left anterior descending artery.

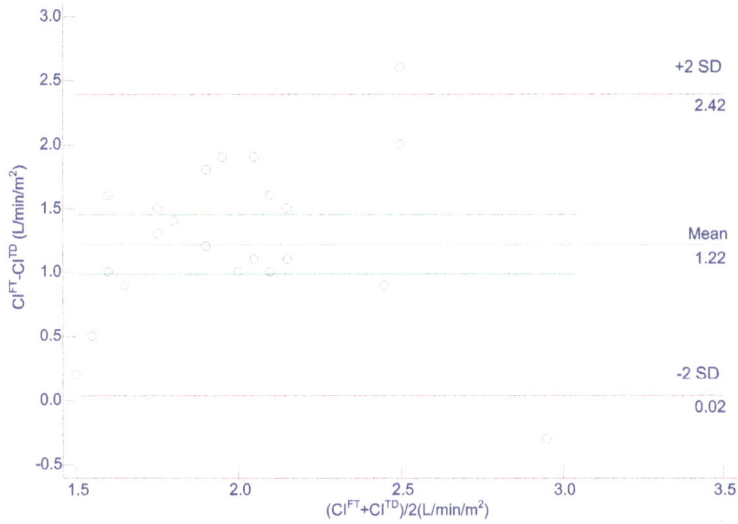

Figure 4: Bland-Altman analysis for CI measurements using FloTrac (CIFT) and intermittent thermodilution (CITD) during grafting of obtuse marginal artery.

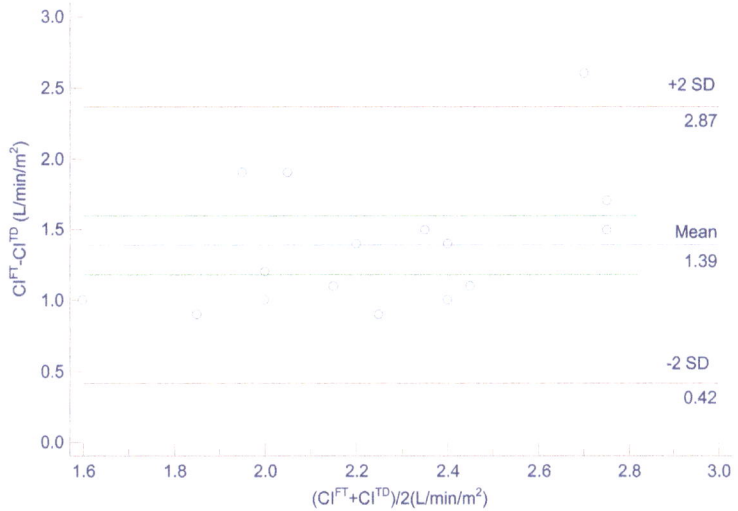

Figure 5: Bland-Altman analysis for CI measurements using FloTrac (CIFT) and intermittent thermodilution (CITD) during grafting of right coronary/posterior descending artery.

Variable → Time points I ↓	CI^{TD} (L/min/m2)	CI^{FT} (L/min/m2)	Correlation Coefficient
T1 (n = 31)	2.12 ± 0.46	2.72 ± 0.45	0.46
T2 (n = 31)	1.89 ± 0.63	2.73 ± 0.58	0.56
T3 (n = 28)	1.35 ± 0.42	2.57 ± 0.49	0.14
T4 (n = 24)	1.54 ± 0.31	2.92 ± 0.52	0.38
T5 (n = 31)	2.55 ± 0.56	2.97 ± 0.41	0.22
T6 (n = 31)	2.44 ± 0.62	3.09 ± 0.41	0.42

(Abbreviations: CI^{TD}- Cardiac index measured by intermittent thermodilution technique, CI^{FT}- cardiac index measured by FloTrac, T1- before incision, T2- left anterior descending artery grafting, T3- obtuse marginal grafting, T4- right coronary/ posterior descending artery grafting, T5- after protamine administration, T6- after shifting the patient to recovery room)

Table 2: Correlation between CI^{TD} and CI^{FT} at different time points

manipulations, unprotected myocardial ischemia and use of stabilizers on the beating heart can provoke abrupt hemodynamic changes. As a principal determinant of oxygen delivery and perfusion pressure,

CO represents an important hemodynamic variable. Its measurement offers potentially useful information to the cardiac anesthesiologists in the peri-operative period in the patients undergoing cardiac surgical procedures [9,15].

Since being introduced in 1970, intermittent thermo dilution technique by PAC has been considered the gold standard for the measurement of CO [10]. Apart from calculating CO, PAC provides data about the cardiac filling pressures such as central venous pressure, pulmonary artery pressure, pulmonary artery occlusion pressure, systemic vascular resistance, pulmonary vascular resistance and mixed venous oxygen saturation. This additional information can be a valuable tool particularly in the management of hemodynamically unstable patients [7]. The use of PAC has been increasingly criticised because of its invasiveness and unclear evidence of its benefit.7 CO estimation by ITD method fails to detect rapid and transient hemodynamic changes that may occur especially during OPCABG [16]. Other limitations of ITD technique include the potential for development of arrhythmias,

Variable→ Time Points I ↓	No. of Data Pairs	CI (L/min/m²) (Mean ±SD)	Bias (Limits of Agreement) (2SD) (L/min/m²)	95% Confidence Interval of the Difference (L/min/m²) Upper	Lower	p-value
T1	31	2.42 ± 0.455	0.59 (0.95)	0.76	0.42	0.000
T2	31	2.31 ± 0.60	0.85 (1.14)	1.06	0.64	0.000
T3	28	1.96 ± 0.45	1.22 (1.20)	1.45	0.98	0.000
T4	24	2.23 ± 0.42	1.39 (0.99)	1.60	1.18	0.000
T5	31	2.76 ± 0.48	0.42 (1.23)	0.64	0.19	0.001
T6	31	2.76 ± 0.52	0.65 (1.17)	0.86	0.43	0.000

(Abbreviations: T1- before incision, T2- left anterior descending artery grafting, T3- obtuse marginal grafting, T4- right coronary/ posterior descending artery grafting, T5- after protamine administration, T6- after shifting the patient to recovery room)

Table 3: Statistical analysis of comparison of CI^{TD} and CI^{FT}.

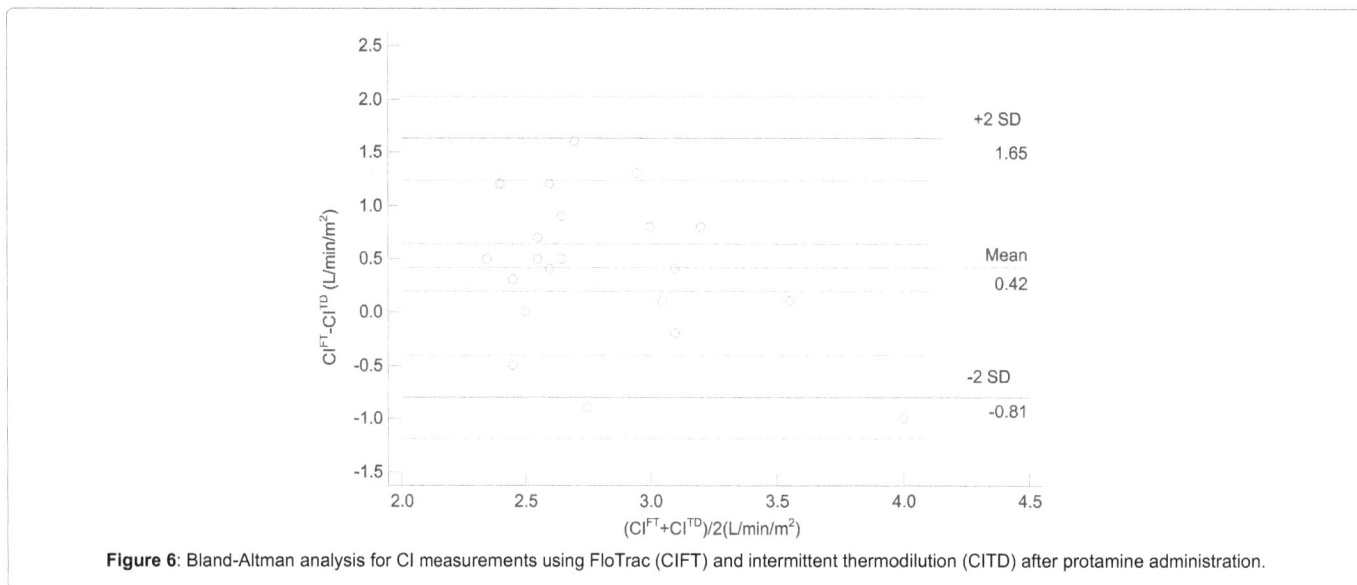

Figure 6: Bland-Altman analysis for CI measurements using FloTrac (CIFT) and intermittent thermodilution (CITD) after protamine administration.

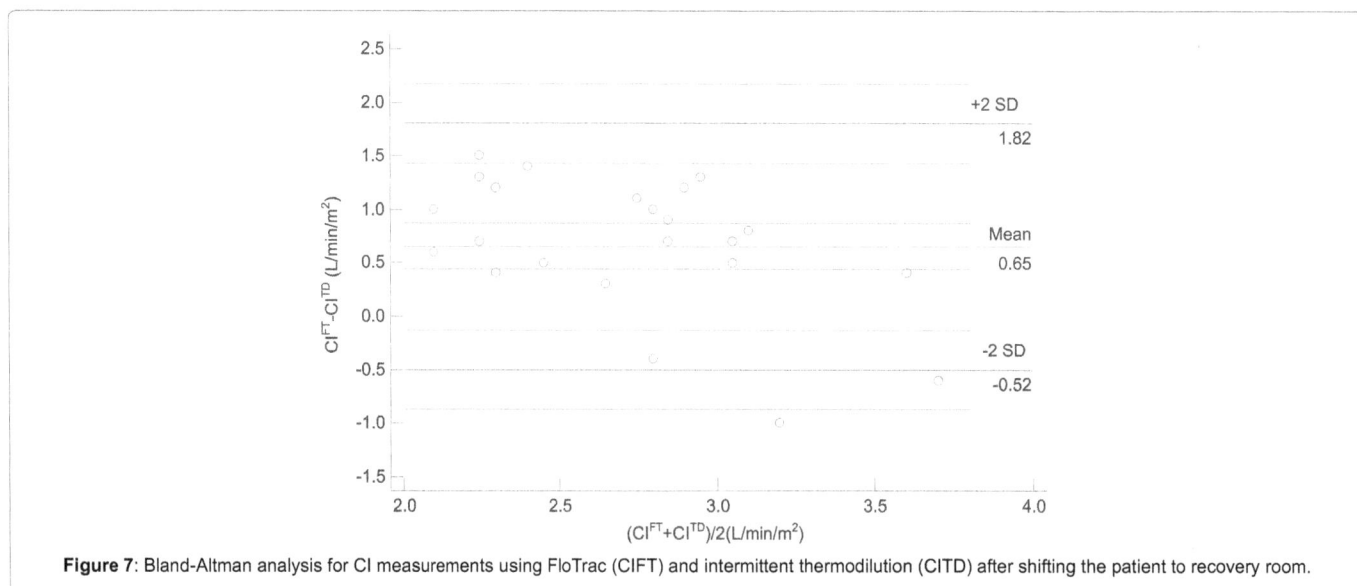

Figure 7: Bland-Altman analysis for CI measurements using FloTrac (CIFT) and intermittent thermodilution (CITD) after shifting the patient to recovery room.

valvular lesions and rupture of pulmonary artery [17]. Sandham et al. demonstrated that the use of PAC was associated with an increased risk of pulmonary embolism in patients undergoing major cardiac surgery [18]. The accuracy of CO by ITD method can be influenced by factors such as timing of injection within the respiratory cycle, temperature of injectate, speed of injection and placement of catheter [19,20]. These limitations along with the desire for lesser invasive technologies have driven the development of various arterial pulse contour based devices.

The arterial pressure waveform analysis has come a long way from the description of Windkessel model by Otto Frank in 1899 to the model by Erlangen and Hoober (1904) and Wesseling et al. [13]. Most of the pulse contour analysis techniques are explicitly or implicitly based on this Windkessel model [11]. In 2005, Edwards Life sciences introduced a novel device naming FloTrac for arterial pressure waveform CO estimation [10]. It consists of a special transducer that can be attached to an existing arterial cannula on one end and to a processing/display unit (Vigileo) on the other end. CO is calculated from an arterial pressure based algorithm that utilizes the relationship between pulse pressure and stroke volume. The arterial pressure waveform is assessed at 100 hertz and standard deviation of pulse pressure is determined over 20 seconds window. The algorithm takes two additional factors into account, i.e., vessel compliance (influenced by age, gender, height and weight) and peripheral resistance effects (determined from arterial waveform characteristics) [21]. The FloTrac has some unique features that are appealing to the clinician. First, the system can theoretically be used with any arterial line and there is no need to put a specifically designed proprietary catheter. The second major feature is the fact that FloTrac system does not require external calibration. The FloTrac analysis algorithm does its own calibration based on patient demographics and waveform characteristics [9]. Possible limitations of this device may be the inability to measure CO in situations of arterial wave artifacts, aortic incompetence, and severe peripheral vasoconstriction, compromise of arterial catheter and irregular pulse as in dysrhythmias and concomitant use of IABP [11].

Many studies have been published in the literature questioning the efficacy of FloTrac in a variety of cardiac operations and critical care units. Critchley and Critchley proposed that the acceptance of any method of determination of CO should be judged against the accuracy of the reference method which is till date considered being the ITD method obtained by PAC [22]. Since the measurement of this physiological variable generally lacks precision, error of +10-20% are common even for the reference method. Applying the same error limit to the new method results in a combined percentage error of +28.3% (calculated using Pythagorean approach). Thus it was recommended that limits of agreement between the new and the reference technique of up to +30% should be accepted. In our study, we analyzed 176 pairs of CI measured by FloTrac and ITD at six stages of OPCABG in 31 patients. A statistically significant (p<0.05) weak correlation was found between the two methods at all the six time points. On applying the Critchleyns criteria, a percentage error of 46% was revealed in the study that is well above the accepted limit.

One of the earliest studies done by Sander et al in 30 patients undergoing CABG analyzed 108 pairs of CO measured by FloTrac and ITD [23]. It measured a high bias (0.6 L/min, (LOA) of - 2.2 to 3.4 L/min). Percentage error in this study using Critchleyns criteria is 30% that is such higher than the accepted limit of 30%. Another study by Manecke and Auger reported a positive correlation between the 2 techniques with a mean bias of 0.55 (LOA-1.96) L/min in 50 postoperative cardiac surgical patients [24]. Opdam et al. in their pilot study involved 251 measurements in 6 patients and showed limited correlation [21]. Our study also showed similar results with limited correlation at all six stages of surgery, with a mean bias of 0.85 L/min/m2 and a precision of 0.55. However the major limitation in the study by Opdam was that 66% of all the calculations were done in only one patient. Mehta et al compared the CO values estimated by FloTrac and ITD in 12 patients undergoing OPCABG at various time points and concluded that good agreement existed between the 2 techniques [11]. However, the percentage error found in this study was 29% that is again closer to the accepted limit of 30%. The major limitation of the study was a small number of patients. Zimmermann et al. analyzed 192 data

pairs of CO estimated by FloTrac and ITD at seven predefined time points during elective CABG [25]. They concluded that FloTrac seems sufficiently accurate when considering 30% limit of agreement and not applying the 20% criteria. Mayer et al. measured CI in 40 patients undergoing elective cardiac surgery and analyzed 244 data pairs and found the high percentage error of 46% [7]. de Waal and colleagues also compared ITD and FloTrac and found a percentage error of 33% [26]. Lorsomradee et al. compared FloTrac with continuous thermo dilution method (CCO) and found that pulse contour analysis was able to reflect CO measured with CCO technique in patients undergoing uncomplicated CABG [27]. However, the pulse contour was less reliable in some situations like during sternotomy and phenylephrine administration. Similar alterations were also observed when the arterial pressure waveform is changed as in patients with aortic insufficiency and in patients on IABP. Many other studies involving other different subsets of patients have produced inconsistent results when the CO was measured with thermodilution and pulse contour analysis techniques [4-6,14-16,22,28-32]. Thus, although FloTrac method has many potential advantages including non-invasiveness, simplicity, no need for external calibration and minimal operator intervention, it still has many limitations in a variety of situations. Also the higher bias found particularly during settings of acute hemodynamic changes further questions the use of this technology in the dynamic settings of OPCABG.

Thus we conclude that CO estimation by FloTrac does not appear to adequately agree with ITD technique in patients undergoing OPCABG. However, it can be particularly recommended in situations where invasive CO monitoring is not an option and tracking of changes in CO are more important than absolute values of CO such as in management of hemodynamically unstable patients in emergency department. As the study population in our study was relatively small, more studies are required in the future to authenticate the usefulness of pulse contour analysis method.

Limitations of the Study

We must acknowledge some of the limitations in our study. A limitation of our study is that we do not know the true CI. We only assume that CO calculated by ITD method represents a reliable estimation of the true CI. Another limitation of this study is that the use of radial artery for estimation of CI by FloTrac and vasopressor administration for maintaining the hemodynamics in the intra-operative period might have influenced the accuracy of CO estimation due to vasoconstriction in variety of situations during OPCABG. Our study also suffers from the potential weakness that all the measurements made by these methods may not have been in real time with respect to each other as ITD involves 3 different injections and CO is then averaged over these 3 values.

Acknowledgement

We sincerely thank Ms. Namita Bansal, M.Sc. (Statistics), statistician, and Department of Quality Assurance, Satguru Partap Singh Apollo Hospitals, Ludhiana for her great and valuable support in the data analysis.

References

1. Ashok V, Nishkantha A, Leong KH, Luo HD, El-Oakley RM, et al. (2005) Off-pump coronary artery bypass grafting is a safe and effective treatment modality for Asian patients requiring coronary revascularization. Singapore Med J 46: 15-20.

2. Chassot PG, van der Linden P, Zaugg M, Mueller XM, Spahn DR (2004) Off-pump coronary artery bypass surgery: Physiology and anesthetic management. Br J Anaesth 92: 400-413.

3. Nierich AP, Diephuis J, Jansen EWL, Borst C, Knape JTA (2000) Heart

displacement during off-pump CABG: How well is it tolerated? Ann Thorac Surg 70: 466-472.

4. Paarmann H, Groesdonk HV, Sedemund-Adib B, Hanke T, Heinze H, et al. (2011) Lack of agreement between pulmonary arterial thermo dilution cardiac output and the pressure recording analytical method in postoperative cardiac surgery patients. Br J Anaesth 106: 475-481.

5. Halvorsen PS, Sokolov A, Cvancarova M, Hol PK, Lundblad R, et al. (2007) Continuous cardiac output during off-pump coronary artery bypass surgery: Pulse contour analyses vs. pulmonary artery thermo dilution. Br J Anaesth 99: 484-492.

6. Paarmann H, Fassl J, Kiefer H, Ender J, Groesdonk HV (2010) Lack of agreement between esophageal Doppler cardiac output measurements and continuous pulse contour analysis during off-pump cardiac surgery. Appl Cardiopulm Pathophysiol 14: 16-20.

7. Mayer J, Boldt J, Schöllhorn T, Röhm KD, Mengistu AM, et al. (2007) Semi-invasive monitoring of cardiac output by a new device using arterial pressure waveform analysis: A comparison with intermittent pulmonary artery thermo dilution in patients undergoing cardiac surgery. Br J Anaesth 98: 176-182.

8. Manecke GR (2010) The FloTrac device should be used to follow cardiac output in cardiac surgical patients. J Cardiothorac Vasc Anesth 24: 706-708.

9. Pugsley J, Lerner AB (2010) Cardiac output monitoring: Is there a gold standard and how do the newer technologies compare? Semin Cardiothorac Vasc Anesth 14: 274-282.

10. Singh S, Taylor MA (2010) The FloTrac device should not be used to follow cardiac output in cardiac surgical patients. J Cardiothorac Vasc Anesth 24: 709-711.

11. Mehta Y, Chand RK, Sawhney R, Bhise M, Singh A, et al. (2008) Cardiac output Monitoring: comparison of a new arterial pressure waveform analysis to the bolus thermo dilution technique in patients undergoing off-pump coronary artery bypass surgery. J Cardiothorac Vasc Anesth 22: 394-399.

12. Bland JM, Altman DG (1999) Measuring agreement in method comparison studies. Stat Methods Med Res 8: 135-160.

13. Critchley LA, Critchley JA (1999) A meta-analysis of studies using bias and precision statistics to compare cardiac output measurement techniques. J Clin Monit Comput 15: 85-91.

14. Wouters PF, Quaghebeur B, Sergeant P, Hemelrijck JV, Vandermeersch E (2005) Cardiac output monitoring using a brachial arterial catheter during off-pump coronary artery bypass grafting. J Cardiothorac Vasc Anesth 19: 160-164.

15. Chakravarthy M, Patil TA, Jayaprakash K, Kalligudd P, Prabhakumar D, et al. (2007) Comparison of simultaneous estimation of cardiac output by four techniques in patients undergoing off-pump coronary artery bypass surgery--A prospective observational study. Ann Card Anaesth 10: 121-126.

16. Halvorsen PS, Espinoza A, Lundblad R, Cvancarova M, Hol PK, et al. (2006) Agreement between PiCCO pulse-contour analysis, pulmonal artery thermo dilution and transthoracic thermo dilution during off-pump coronary artery by-pass surgery. Acta Anaesthesiol Scand 50: 1050-1057.

17. Schuerholz T, Meyer MC, Friedrich L, Przemeck M, Sümpelmann R, et al. (2006) Reliability of continuous cardiac output determination by pulse-contour analysis in porcine septic shock. Acta Anaesthesiol Scand 50: 407-413.

18. Sandham JD, Hull RD, Brant RF, Knox L, Pineo GF, et al. (2003) A randomized, controlled trial of the use of pulmonary-artery catheters in high-risk surgical patients. N Eng J Med 348: 5-14.

19. Pinsky MR (2001) A rose by any other name: cardiac output. Crit Care Med 29: 2021-2022.

20. Morris AH, Chapman RH, Gardner RM (1984) Frequency of technical problems encountered in the measurement of pulmonary artery wedge pressure. Crit Care Med 12: 164-170

21. .Opdam HI, Wan L, Bellomo R (2007) A pilot assessment of the FloTrac cardiac output monitoring system. Intensive Care Med 33: 344-349.

22. Compton FD, Zukunft B, Hoffmann C, Zidek W, Schaefer JH (2008) Performance of a minimally invasive uncalibrated cardiac output monitoring system (Flotrac/Vigileo) in haemodynamically unstable patients. Br J Anaesth 100: 451-456.

23. Sander M, Spies CD, Grubitzsch H, Foer A, Muller M, et al. (2006) Comparison of uncalibrated arterial waveform analysis in cardiac surgery patients with thermo dilution cardiac output measurements. Crit Care 10: R164.

24. Manecke GR Jr, Auger WR (2007) Cardiac output determination from the arterial pressure wave: clinical testing of a novel algorithm that does not require calibration. J Cardiothorac Vasc Anesth 21: 3-7.

25. Zimmermann A, Kufner C, Hofbauer S, Steinwendner J, Hitzl W, et al. (2008) The accuracy of the Vigileo/FloTrac continuous cardiac output monitor. J Cardiothorac Vasc Anesth 22: 388-393

26. .Waal EE, Kalkman CJ, Rex S, Buhre WF (2007) Validation of a new arterial pulse contour based cardiac output device. Crit Care Med 35: 1904-1909.

27. Lorsomradee S, Lorsomradee S, Cromheecke S, De Hert SG (2007) Uncalibrated arterial pulse contour analysis versus continuous thermo dilution technique: Effects of alterations in arterial waveform. J Cardiothorac Vasc Anesth; 21: 636-643.

28. Mayer J, Boldt J, Poland R, Peterson A, Manecke GR (2006) Continuous arterial pressure waveform-based cardiac output using the FloTrac/Vigileo: A review and metaanalysis. J Cardiothorac Vasc Anesth 23: 401-406.

29. Buhre W, Weyland A, Kazmaier S, Hanekop GG, Baryalei MM, et al. (1999) Comparison of cardiac output assessed by pulse-contour analysis and thermo dilution in patients undergoing minimally invasive direct coronary artery bypass grafting. J Cardiothorac Vasc Anesth 13: 437-440.

30. Button D, Weibel L, Reuthebuch O, Genoni M, Zollinger A, et al. (2007) Clinical evaluation of the FloTrac/VigileoTM system and two established continuous cardiac output monitoring devices in patients undergoing cardiac surgery. Br J Anaesth 99: 329-336.

31. Ostergaard M, Nielsen J, Rasmussen JP, Berthelsen PG (2006) Cardiac output—pulse contour analysis vs. pulmonary artery thermo dilution. Acta Anaesthesiol Scand 50: 1044-1049.

32. Breukers RM, Sepehrkhouy S, Spiegelenberg SR, Groeneveld AB (2007) Cardiac output measured by a new arterial pressure waveform analysis method without calibration compared with thermo dilution after cardiac surgery. J Cardiothorac Vasc Anesth 21: 632-635.

4

Assessment of Risky Sexual Behaviour and Associated Factors among Jimma University of Kitto Furdisa Campus Students, Jimma Town, Oromia Region, South West of Ethiopia, 2015

Samuel Abdu A*, Habtamu Tesfaye M, Bekana FeKecha H

Department of Nursing, Jimma University, Ethiopia

Abstract

Background: Risky sexual behaviors including early sexual debut, unprotected sexual intercourse, multiple sexual partner and changing sexual partners, occur in broader context.

Objective: To assess risky sexual behaviors and associated factors among Jimma university of Kitto Furdisa students, Jimma zone, Jimma town, Kitto Furdisa in 2015.

Method: Cross-sectional study was conducted on 407 undergraduate Engineering students of Jimma university of Kitto Furdisa students and with sampling technique of Stratified random sampling technique. Data was collected through self-administered questionnaire and analyzed using SPSS. For significant statistical association between dependent and independent variable chi-square test was employed and data was presented using table as needed.

Results: A total of 407 questionnaires were distributed and 356 returned which makes the response rate 87.5%. 250 (70.2%) were male, majority 263 (73.9%) were in the age range of 20-24 years, 304 (85.4%) of them were aware of risk sexual behavior, 65 (32.9%) had their first sexual intercourse at the age 15-19 years followed by 46 (23.4%) at the age 20-24 year and 83 (42.1%) were do not remember their first sexual intercourse. Age, previous place residence and academic year are significantly associated with risky sexual behavior at $p < 0.05$.

Conclusion: This study revealed that there is risky sexual behavior among JIT students. Thus, continuous health information's to create awareness on condom utilization and anticipation of future risks should be provided by Anti-HIV/ AIDS club of Jimma University of Kitto Furdisa Campus Students, Peer-club of students and student clinic.

Keywords: Risky behaviour; Jimma University; Kitto Furdisa campus

Introduction

Youths are especially at risk firstly because they are adventurous and very sexually active, being at an age where sexual hits and conquests are perceived as important for self-esteem. Secondly they have multiple sexual partners, and are more likely to practice innovative sexual and risky techniques. Thirdly students are financially insecure. Therefore finical incentives form older men exert strong influence towards their acceptance of risky sexual behaviours especially as regards to non-condom as other study have also indicated [1].

Risky sexual behaviours including early sexual debut, unprotected sexual intercourse, multiple sexual partner and changing sexual partners, occur in broader context. The intensity of involvement in sexual risk behaviour ranges from no sexual relationship to unprotect in sexual intercourse with multiple partner and prostitution. Sexually active teenagers who exhibits few positive or pre-socially behaviours such as involvement in organized action at School or in the community are at high risk for outcomes such as early sexual activity and pregnancy during their teenage years [2]. The trends in sexual activity younger ages are increasing alarmingly in the world. In many countries the majority of young age people are sexually active before age of 20 and premarital sex is common among 15-19 years old [3].

In 2008, young people aged 15-24 years accounted for 42% of new HIV infection in people aged 15 and older and nearly 805 of this live in sub-Saharan Africa [4]. As part the young age bracket, undergraduate University students are in an important group exposed to range risky behaviours. The increased privacy afforded by living outside of their parents. Home provides greater opportunity for sexual expression risk behaviours among undergraduate may be further worsened by the fact that they mostly live in campuses without boundaries or security peer-pressure, economic problems and lack of youth friendly recreational facilities [5].

In the 2006 year almost two third of infection with HIV were in Sub-Saharan countries; Ethiopia is one of the countries where HIV/ AIDS is fuelling and striking its population of all ages including adolescents. World Health Organization estimated that, the people with newly acquired infections of HIV between the age of 15 and 24 years mainly through unsafe sexual practice [6].

Despite public health effort to educate individuals about risk behaviours and provide solution to reduce or avoid sexually transmitted diseases (STDs) young people continue to contract HIV and/or STDs at an alarming rate. Rate of HIV continue to rise among young adult ages 15 to 24 that accounted for approximately 14% of all HIV new cases in the USA during 2005 [7].

A study done on knowledge and attitude of college students of Kerala towards HIV/AIDS,STDS and sexualities in India 45% knew as AIDS is not curable at present 34.5% were aware of symptoms of STDS and AIDS. Even boys were afraid of donating blood at blood Bank and receiving injection from governmental hospital. Because they associative with lack of aseptic precautions with increased risk of acquiring infections including HIV however, 55% of then believer as

*Corresponding author: Samuel Abdu A, Department of Nursing, Jimma University, Ethiopia, E-mail: samuelabdu2004@gmail.com

AIDS is curable disease. It was believed by the study subjects that Boys engaged in premarital sex than girls [8].

According to study conducted in risk of HIV and sexual risk behaviours in USA, Turkey and South Africa, Those sexually active 27.6% of the USA female students compared with 2.1% south African and none of the Turkish students had their first sexual intercourse before age of 15 31.1% of USA, 9.7% of Turkish and 10.6% of south Africa male students had their sexual debut before the age of 15 [3].

The study conducted on pattern of risky sexual behaviour and associated factors among undergraduate students of porter court university river state Nigeria revealed More than half them 52% had either by friend or girlfriend and 52% have had sex with someone 33.6% of them had their sex for the first time at age range of 5-19 years 3.2% 5-9years, 5.1% 10-14 years 25.3% 15-19 years and 14.1% 20-24 years and 52.3% above 24 years 23.5% had sex with someone in the month preceding the study and 13.4% had one sexual partner girl Boyfriend topped the list of person respondents had sex with and only 31.8% of them used a form of protection [9].

A study done in Zambia shows 48% of the first sex done for the desire to experiment 18% due to peer pressure, 3.6 need of money, 5.4% preparation for marriage and 2.2% forced the largest group of school girls 65% had their first sexual intercoms between the age of 15 and 17 years [9,10].

As across-sectional study done on pattern of sexual risk behaviour among undergraduate university students in Ethiopia revealed 28% students had sexual intercourse at once more proportion of male students ever had sexual intercourse compared to females 4.8% 22.8% of those students had their sexual debit after they joined university. About 6% of students with sexual partners half of the males with sexual experience had intercourse with commercial sex workers about 60% of students had used condom rarely [11].

As study done in Jimma University in 2009, 26.9% ever had sexual intercourse 75.6% started sexual intercourse during their secondary school from those 51% had sex with the last 12 months and 28.3% had multiple sexual partners, consistent condom use with non-regular partner was 69.1%. Lack of parental control, substance use, peer pressure campus and outside environment were identified as predisposing factors; males were about three times more likely to ever had sexual intercourse as compared to females. Majority 68% had first sexual intercourse with boyfriend or girlfriend 48.1% had their first sexual intercourse with individuals of same age females were more likely to have first sex with individuals who were about five year or older than them [12].

Another study done on risky sexual behaviour and predisposing factors among students of Jimma University in 2012 the following result were obtained 26.9% had ever sexual intercourse the mean age at first intercourse was 17+2.7years. Most, 75.6% started sexual intercourse during secondary school. Among those who ever had sexual intercourse, 51% had sex in their last 12 months of the study period and 28.3% had multiple sexual partners. Consistent condom use with non-regular partners in the last 12 months of the study time was 69.1% Lack of prenatal control, peer pressure, campus and outside environment were identified as predisposing factors [12].

However; to what extent the risky sexual behaviour exist among Jimma university students, particularly among Kitto Furdisa Campus regular students is not known, thus this study is aimed to assess the risky sexual behaviour of undergraduate students.

Materials and Methods

Study area

This study was conducted at Jimma university of Kitto Furdisa, found in Oromia regional state, Jimma zone, Jimma town in Kitto Furdisa Kebele which is located 352 km south west of Addis Ababa. Kitto Furdisa was one of Jimma university branch, which is established 4 years back and today teaches different department such as civil, water and pre engineering. The total population of university was 9960 students (which projected from the technology Institute (Faculty) register office of 2nd semester data of students of 2014/2015.

Study period

This study was conducted from May 25-June 30, 2015.

Study design

Institutional based cross sectional study design.

Population

Source population: All Jimma university of Kitto Furdisa students.

Study population: All Selected regular Jimma university of Kitto Furdisa students.

Sample size determination and sampling technique

Sample size: Single population estimation parameter is used to calculate sample size.

$$n = \frac{(z\alpha/2)^2 \times pq}{d^2}$$

$$n = \frac{(1.96)^2 \times 0.5 \times 0.5}{(0.05)^2}$$

=384

Where, n: minimum sample size

p: Estimate of the prevalence rate for the population

d: The margin of sampling error tolerated (5%)

zα/2: The standard normal variable at 1-2% confidence level is mostly 5%.

But the source population (N) is <10,000; the sample size will be modified using the correction formula.

$$nf = \frac{n}{N^{1+n}}$$

$$= \frac{384}{\frac{1+384}{9960}}$$

$$= \frac{384}{\frac{9960+384}{9960}}$$

$$= \frac{384}{\frac{10344}{9960}}$$

$$= \frac{384 \times 9960}{10344}$$

=370

Where, nf: Final sample size

Ni: Initial sample size

N: Total population

Add 10% for non-respondents=10% of sample size+sample size

$$=37+370$$

$$=407$$

Sampling technique

Stratified random sampling technique: Students were stratified by their year (batch) and final study subjects will be selected from each year by statistical sample size proportion allocation as follows:

$$ni = \frac{NI \times n}{N}$$

Where, N: Total population

Ni: Population size in each stratum

ni: Sample to be drawn from each stratum

n: Total sample size to be drawn from total population

$$\text{Firstyear}: \ ni = \frac{Ni \times n}{N} = \frac{1871 \times 407}{9960} = 76$$

$$\text{Second Year}: \ ni = \frac{Ni \times n}{N} = \frac{1440 \times 407}{9960} = 59$$

$$\text{Third Year}: \ ni = \frac{Ni \times n}{N} = \frac{1791 \times 407}{9960} = 73$$

$$\text{Fourth Year}: \ ni = \frac{Ni \times n}{N} = \frac{2759 \times 407}{9960} = 113$$

$$\text{Fifth Year}: \ ni = \frac{Ni \times n}{N} = \frac{2099 \times 407}{9960} = 86$$

Total sample size: 76+59+73+113+86=407

Inclusion and exclusion criteria

Inclusion: All students learn regular academic years at Jimma university of Kitto Furdisa, present during data collection and volunteer to participate was included in study.

Exclusion criteria: All students those were absent during data collection, not volunteer during data collection excluded from the study.

Study variable

Independent variables: • Age

- Sex
- Previous place of residence
- Income
- Use of substance
- Condom use

Dependent variable: Risky sexual behavior.

Data collection techniques

Data was collected using semi structured self-administered questionnaire designed in English language.

Data collection instruments

Data was collected through semi structured opened and closed-ended questionnaires. The questionnaire was pre tested before duplicating to get valuable information. It was structured as closed ended questionnaire and was developed and adapted after review of relevant literatures and arranged according to particular objective it can address.

Data analysis

Data analysis was made by principal investigator using scientific calculator. Frequency and percentage of each variable will be presented using table. Chi square -test will be done to understand the association (Table 1).

Ethical consideration

Ethical approval was obtained from the college of health science office. Permission also obtained from Jimma university of Kitto Furdisa administration. Once permission is obtained from responsible body, verbal informed obtained from participant of this research study, clear information about purpose of study, their confidentiality, the name of participant didn't includes in questionnaires, and the right participant have to withdraw themselves at any time during the interview.

S. No.	Factors		Non-risky behavior	Risky Behavior	Total	X^2/P value
1	Age	15-19	41 (75.9)	13 (24.1)	54	X^2=2 P=0.012
		20-24	227 (86.3)	36 (13.7)	263	
		25-29	38 (97.4)	1 (2.6)	39	
2	Sex	Male	215 (86.0)	35 (14.0)	250	X^2=1 P=0.970
		Female	91 (85.8)	15 (14.2)	106	
3	Previous place of residence	Urban	193 (88.9)	24 (11.1)	217	X^2=1 P=0.043
		Rural	113 (81.3)	26 (18.7)	139	
4	Monthly income	<250 (ETB)	154 (88.5)	20 (11.5)	174	X^2=2
		250-500 (ETB)	82 (87.2)	12 (12.8)	94	
		>500 (ETB)	70 (79.5)	18 (20.5)	88	P=0.131
5	Academic year	1 year	53 (74.6)	18 (25.4)	71	X^2=4
		2 years	48 (87.3)	7 (12.7)	55	
		3 years	53 (77.9)	15 (22.1)	68	
		4 years	84 (94.4)	5 (5.6)	89	P=0.001
		5 years	68 (93.2)	5 (6.8)	73	

Table 1: Distribution of factors associated with risky sexual behavior among Jimma University Kitto Furdisa campus, Jimma, Ethiopia May 2015.

Results

A total of 407 questionnaires were distributed and 356 were returned filled correctly which gives the response rate of 87.46%. From 356 study respondents 250 (70.2%) were males and 106 (29.8) were females. majority 263 (73.9%) in age range of 20-24 years followed by age from 15-19 years-54 (15.2%). Concerning ethnicity, majority were Oromo 142 (39.9%) followed by Ahmara- 111 (31.2%). Regarding the religion majority of them were Orthodox 195 (54.8%) followed by Muslim and protestant 70 (19.7%). Concerning their resident area, majority of them were from urban217 (61.0%) and rural 139 (39.0%). With regard to monthly income, majority 174 (48.9%) had <250 Ethiopian birr monthly followed by 250-500 birr 94 (26.4%).

Awareness of risky sexual behavior

Out of 356 study participants about 306 (86.0%) were aware about risky sexual behaviour, 341 (95.8%) were aware of its impacts on social and human health, majority 205 (75.37%) had got information from class room lesson while 120 (44.12%) students have got from their parents.

The students in this study considered risky sexual behaviour in different ways. Of the 356 study respondents 294 (82.6%) considered sex with multiple partner. 313 (87.9%) considered sex without condom use. 308 (86.5%) considered sex after substance use as risky sexual behavior 0.253 (71.1%) considered risky sexual behaviour as having sex with commercial sex workers. 255 (71.6%) of them said sex through anal and oral is considered as risky behaviour.

Concerning the outcome of risky sexual behaviour, majority 340 (95.5%) indicated STI including HIV/AIDS as a great impact; Even though, separation from family or relatives were reported as social impacts.

Discussion

33.0% had their first sexual intercourse at age range of 15-19 years among these 37.0% males and 63.0% females. This was greater than the study conducted at Jimma University main campus which was 26.9%. A study done in Zambia showed the largest group of school girls 65% had their first sexual intercoms between the age of 15 and 17 years [10]. This difference might be due to the cultural different in that time and know.

Concerning the reason of starting sexual intercourse 46.7% due to peer pressure, 28.42% due to desire to had sexual experiment, 10.66% were forced to do, 9.64% were preparation for marriage and 4.56% due to need of money [12]. This finding was differ from the study conducted in Zambia showed 48% of the first sex done for the desire to experiment and 18% due to peer pressure [5]. This difference might be due to students were spent most of their time with their peers which might influence their behaviour.

Among 59.2% respondents who had used condom, 74.7% had always used during sexual contact and 25.3% had used occasionally. Similar study conducted in Ethiopia walaita Sodo University revealed that 54.0% used condom always whereas 25.0% used occasionally [13].

Conclusion

This study also assessed pattern of substance use which was 356 (29.35%) among these 76.3% males and 23.7% females. 53.33% respondents had used alcohol, 24.76% had consumed or chewed chat and 10.48% have used Hashish. It differ from other study conducted in Ethiopia Bahir Dar City private College which revealed 25% of respondents used alcohol and 18.0% have used chat. The difference might be due to life or living situation of the study respondents.

Age, previous place of residence and academic year had significant statistical association with risky sexual behaviour. Similar study conducted in Jimma University main campus showed lack of parental control, substance use, peer pressure in campus and outside environment were identified as predisposing factors for risky sexual behaviour.

Acknowledgement

I would like to extend my deep appreciation to Jimma University Kitto Furdisa campus student and staffs.

I am grateful to Jimma University College of health sciences department of nursing, who has given me this chance and fund this paper work.

References

1. World Health Organization (1999) Adolescent program. Geneva.

2. Renee ES, Jennifer AO, Robert WB (2002) Adolescent sexual behavior and sexual health. Pediatr Rev 23.

3. UNICEF, USAIDS and WHO (2002) Young people and HIV/AIDS opportunity in crisis.

4. Tura G, Alemseged F, Dejene (2012) Risky sexual behavior and predisposing factors among students of Jimma University, Ethiopia. Ethiop J Health Sci 22: 170-180.

5. Dingeta TOL, Assefa N (2012) Pattern of risky sexual behavior. Pan Afr Med J 12: 33.

6. Lal SS, Vasan RS, Sankara Sarma P, Thankappan KR (2000) Knowledge and attitude of college students in Kerala towards HIV/AIDS, sexually transmitted diseases and sexuality. Natl Med J India 13: 231-236.

7. Abdulrahman IJ, Peter KOB, Olukemi AE (2012) Pattern of risky sexual behavior and associated factors among undergraduate students of the University of Port Harcourt, Rivers State, Nigeria. Pan Afr Med J 12: 97.

8. Jejeebhoy SJ (1998) Adolescent sexual and reproductive behavior: A review of the evidence from India. Soc Sci Med 46:1275-1290.

9. Dingeta T, Oljira L, Assefa N (2012) Patterns of sexual risk behavior among undergraduate university students in Ethiopia: A cross-sectional study. Pan Afr Med J 12: 33.

10. MC Daid D (2003) Risky Awareness and behavior patterns. Western Health Board, pp: 13-18.

11. Eshete H, Sahlu T (1996) The progression of HIV/AIDS in Ethiopia. J Health Develop 10: 17-90.

12. Tura G, Alemseged F, Dejene S (2012) Risky sexual behavior and predisposing factors among students of Jimma University, Ethiopia. Ethiop J Health Sci 22: 170-180.

13. Yohannes B, Gelibo T, Tarekegn M (2013) Prevalence and associated factors of sexually transmitted infections among students of Wolaita Sodo University, Southern Ethiopia. Intern J Sci Tech Res 2: 86-94.

5

Common Aeroallergens by Skin Prick Test among the Population in Two Different Regions

Siti Nadzrah Y[1], Zulkiflee AB[2]* and Prepageran N[2]

[1]Faculty of Medicine, University of Malaya, Malaysia
[2]Department of Otorhinolaryngology, Faculty of Medicine, University of Malaya, Malaysia

Abstract

Objectives: The purpose of this study primarily was to determine and characterise the common allergens found using skin prick test both in Malaysia and the Netherlands.

Study Design: This is retrospective cross-sectional descriptive study which the data was collected from two different hospitals.

Methodology: The study population included patients with history of atopy and / or diagnosed with any forms of allergy, mainly nasal allergy that were referred for skin prick test.

Results: In 284 respondents, the Asians showed significantly (p<0.001) higher percentage of positive response towards most of the subgroups of aeroallergen especially house dust mite (82.4%) as compared to the Europeans (41.2%). More than half (84.3%) of the Asian population had positive test responses to one or more aeroallergens and the highest prevalence was for house dust mite, 69% - 78% (*Dermatophagoides pteronyssinus, Dermatophagoides farinae* and *Blomia sp.*) followed by cat fur (40.6%) and *Alternaria sp.* (38.2%). Even the European has higher prevalence of positive response towards house dust mite subgroup (24.7%) in comparison with fungi and epidermals with 3.9% and 8.8% respectively (p<0.001). However, the prevalence for both Bermuda grass and grain pollen (20.9%) in Europe were more or less the same with house dust mite, 21% - 25% (*Dermatophagoides pteronyssinus* and *Dermatophagoides farinae*). The least frequent aeroallergen for both Asia and Europe was dog hair (30.6% and 1.7% respectively).

Conclusions: House dust mites are the most common aeroallergens in the two different regions.

Introduction

Allergy is an immune-mediated hypersensitivity reaction involving specific recognition of a particular allergen and the production of specific immunoglobulins, usually of isotype E (IgE) [1]. This hypersensitivity reaction is often described as type 1 allergic reaction. An allergic reaction of this kind can be manifested in the lungs (allergic asthma), in the eyes and nose (conjunctivitis and allergic rhinitis), or in the skin (atopic eczema). Among those, allergic rhinitis is considered the most common manifestation, furthermore aeroallergens are important contributing factors causing the symptoms in allergic rhinitis [2,3].

Various aeroallergens from animals or plants play an important role in the early development of asthma and allergy[4]. Exposure to aeroallergens increases the risk of sensitisation and the development of allergic respiratory complaints [5]. Many studies have shown that the distribution and pattern of aeroallergen is significantly different in different countries and even in different parts of a country [6,7]. Herbal geography, climate and temperature are responsible for the variations [8]. Among these, climate affects many aspects of allergy and allergen exposure, including the type and frequency of allergens in any particular geographic location, exposure to food and insect allergens, cross-reactivity among allergens, and the prevalence of allergy-related diseases [9-27].

The incidence of allergy is increasing throughout the world with increasing trend of skin prick test positivity [2]. In the latter decades of the twentieth century, there was a rise in the prevalence of allergy, particularly in children, not only in the Netherlands but also in other western countries [28-30]. According to the National Institute of Allergy and Infectious Diseases, as many as 50 million people in the United States suffer from various types of allergies [31]. Of these, 20.3 million have asthma, a chronic lung disease often triggered by allergies.

These allergic conditions affect all ages in all countries, with signs and symptoms and types of allergens changing according to the ages of the sufferer [2]. In Malaysia, one out of three people is allergic to something and it is expected to affect 50% of Malaysians by the year 2020 [32]. Around 50% of world's teenagers were already suffering from airway allergies such as allergic rhinitis [33]. In addition, a study from the Netherlands done in year 2002 also reported the prevalence of 'nasal allergy' in adults has risen since 1992 [34].

Allergy is one of the common disorders that have major influence on quality of life which also contributes to academic and occupational absenteeism with significant impact on health care expenditure [35-39]. Therefore, it is useful to identify the common allergens that provoke allergic reaction so that prevention from exposure to these allergens can be made to reduce the potential health catastrophe from occurring.

The purpose of this study primarily was to determine and characterise the common allergens found using skin prick test both in Malaysia and the Netherlands. The secondary objective was to compare the allergens between two countries, which were an emerging developing country in Asia like Malaysia and developed country in Europe like the Netherlands; with different economical, lifestyle and climate.

*Corresponding author: Zulkiflee AB, Department of Otorhinolaryngology, Faculty of Medicine, University of Malaya, Malaysia, E-mail: abzulkiflee@yahoo.com

Methodology

This was a hospital-based retrospective cross-sectional descriptive study that was carried out in University of Malaya Medical Centre (UMMC), Malaysia and University Medical Centre Utrecht (UMCU), in the Netherlands. Both of this centres are the tertiary centre in both countries. The study population included patients with history of atopy and / or diagnosed with any forms of allergy, mainly nasal allergy who were referred for skin prick test. Patients who was on anti-allergic drugs had went through an appropriate wash out period according to the types of drugs taken. Subsequently, the skin prick test was performed by the attending physician excluded those with previous history of severe allergy (anaphylactic shock) or persistant skin disease such as dermographism, atopic dermatitis and eczema.

Skin Prick Test

It was carried out on the flexor aspect of forearm avoiding the wrist and antecubital fossa. The forearm was coded with a marker pen for the allergens to be tested spacing the tests out at about 3 cm. A drop of the extract was deposited on the indicated position. The skin was then pricked vertically through each drop using a standardised prick test needle (Stallepoint). The extract solution was wiped away with a tissue paper. Result was read after 15 to 20 minutes.

Allergen tested

All patients underwent skin prick test (SPT) with at least 10 common regional allergenic extracts. Eleven and twelve common regional allergen extracts were performed in UMMC and UMCU respectively. These allergens were chosen according to the prevalence of each aeroallergens in each region (Table 1). Histamine and normal saline solution were used as positive and negative controls, respectively. The aeroallergens tested were classified into indoor or outdoor aeroallergens and subdivided four groups as reflected below in Table:

Definition of a positive skin test response

For analysis of the skin prick test data, an allergen-specific skin test response was considered to be positive if there was associated erythema of 3 centimetre diameter even with or without the presence of wheal. If there were wheals present, the wheals of the allergen extracts were compared with the wheals of the controls of which the positive control was histamine and the negative control was saline. Sensitisation should be considered as positive as soon as the allergen extract's diameter was: superior to negative control (saline) wheal diameter by at least 3mm; and at least equal to half of the positive control (histamine) wheal diameter

The size of the wheal does not indicate the severity of symptoms. The patient was considered to have positive skin prick test towards different subgroup of aeroallergen when there is a positive response to at least one of the aeroallergen in that category. Three patients were excluded from the study because of the positive response to negative control.

Data collection and statistical analysis

Allergy data from April 2007 to September 2009 were obtained from the Department of Otorhinolaryngology in UMMC and UMCU. Collected data included demographics (age, gender, and race) and skin prick test results were entered and analysed using the SPSS version 16.0 software. More than 50% data feather extract was unavailable. Therefore, those were excluded from analysis. Unavailable data for other allergens were treated as a missing data for each case. The chi-square test was used to assess the association between categorical variables and test the univariate association between demographic characteristics and positive skin prick test. The significant level was pre-set at 0.05.

Results

(Table 2) showed the distributions of respondents aged 5 to 84 years by demographic backgrounds and skin prick test (SPT) responses. Of

Asia		Europe	
Aeroallergen tested	Unavailable data, n(%)	Aeroallergen tested	Unavailable data, n(%)
House Dust Mite		**House Dust Mite**	
Blomia sp.*	15 (14.7)	Dermatophagoides farinae*	0 (0.0)
Dermatophagoides farinae*	0 (0.0)	Dermatophagoides pteronyssinus*	0 (0.0)
Dermatophagoides pteronyssinus*	0 (0.0)		
Fungi		**Fungi**	
Alternaria sp.†	0 (0.0)	Fungi mix 1*	1 (0.5)
Aspergillus mix*	0 (0.0)	Fungi mix 2†	1 (0.5)
Cladosporium sp.*	0 (0.0)		
Penicillium mix*	0 (0.0)		
Yeast mix†	0 (0.0)		
Pollens		**Pollens**	
Bermuda grass†	0 (0.0)	Grain pollen†	0 (0.0)
		Bermuda grass†	0 (0.0)
		Weed pollen†	0 (0.0)
		Seasonal tree pollen†	0 (0.0)
		Non-seasonal tree pollen†	1 (0.5)
Epidermals		**Epidermals**	
Cat fur*	1 (1.0)	Cat fur*	2 (1.1)
Dog hair*	30 (29.4)	Dog hair*	1 (0.5)
		Feather†	116 (63.7)

*indoor aeroallergens
†outdoor aeroallergens

Table 1: Subdivision and classification of aeroallergens tested and the proportions of missing data for each aeroallergen in both regions.

| Characteristic | Skin Prick Test (SPT) | | | | | | p-value |
| | Total | | Positive | | Negative | | |
	n	%	n	%	n	%	
All respondents	284	100.0	161	56.7	123	43.3	
Gender							
Female	141	49.6	78	48.4	63	51.2	0.643
Male	143	50.4	83	51.6	60	48.8	
Age group							
0 to 4	0	0.0	0	0.0	0	0.0	< 0.001
5 to 14	27	9.5	24	14.9	3	2.4	
15 to 24	68	23.9	50	31.1	18	14.6	
25 to 34	55	19.4	30	18.6	25	20.3	
35 to 44	43	15.1	18	11.2	25	20.3	
45 to 54	37	13.0	18	11.2	19	15.4	
55 to 64	35	12.3	15	9.3	20	16.3	
65 to 74	15	5.3	5	3.1	10	8.1	
75 to 84	4	1.4	1	0.6	3	2.4	
Region of residence							
Asia	102	35.9	86	53.4	16	13.0	< 0.001
Europe	182	64.1	75	46.6	107	87.0	

Table 2: Distribution of respondents by background characteristics and skin prick test (SPT) responses in both regions.

the total sample (284 respondents), majority of them were European (64.1%) and only 35.9% were Asian. However, there were fair distributions of respondents in terms of gender with 50.4% of them were male and 49.6% were female. Majority of the respondents were between 15 to 44 years of age with the mean of 36.17 ± 1.044 [S.E] (median 33.07).

About 57% of the total sample have positive skin prick test with the Asian showing higher proportion of positive response (53.4%) as compared to the European (46.6%). Even among Asians (Figure 1), there were higher percentage of respondents with positive response, 84.3% (p<0.001). In contrast, a negative skin prick test (SPT) response was greater among the respondents in Europe with 87.0%. (Table 2) also showed that there were significant difference (p<0.001) in skin prick test response among the different age group with higher positive response among the teenagers and young adults aged 15 to 24 years (31.1% had positive skin prick test). There was no significant difference in skin prick test (SPT) response between both genders.

As shown in (Figure 1), the Asians showed significantly (p<0.001) higher percentage of positive response towards most of the subgroups of aeroallergen especially house dust mite (82.4%) as compared to the Europeans (41.2%). Similar pattern can be observed in the skin prick

test (SPT) response to individual aeroallergens as depicted in (Table 3). More than half (84.3%) of the Asian population had positive test responses to one or more aeroallergens and the highest prevalence was for house dust mite, 69% - 78% (*Dermatophagoides pteronyssinus*, *Dermatophagoides farinae* and *Blomia sp.*) followed by cat fur (40.6%) and *Alternaria sp.* (38.2%).

| Aeroallergen tested | Positive skin prick test (SPT) responses | |
	Asia, n (%)	**Europe**, n (%)
Indoor aeroallergen		
House Dust Mite		
Blomia sp.	60 (69.0)	-
Dermatophagoides farinae	79 (77.5)	38 (20.9)
Dermatophagoides pteronyssinus	80 (78.4)	45 (24.7)
Epidermals		
Cat fur	41 (40.6)	14 (7.8)
Dog hair	22 (30.6)	3 (1.7)
Fungi / Moulds		
Fungus mix 1	-	5 (2.8)
Aspergillus sp.	38 (37.3)	-
Penicillium mix	37 (36.3)	-
Chladosporium sp.	35 (34.3)	-
At least one indoor aeroallergen	86 (84.3)	50 (27.5)
Outdoor aeroallergen		
Pollens		
Bermuda grass	35 (34.3)	38 (20.9)
Grain pollen	-	38 (20.9)
Weed pollen	-	7 (3.8)
Seasonal tree pollen	-	22 (12.1)
Non-seasonal tree pollen	-	24 (13.3)
Fungi / Moulds		
Alternaria sp.	39 (38.2)	-
Yeast mix	35 (34.3)	-
Fungus mix 2	-	4 (2.2)
At least one outdoor aeroallergen	42 (41.2)	55 (30.2)
At least one indoor or outdoor allergen	86 (84.3)	74 (40.7)

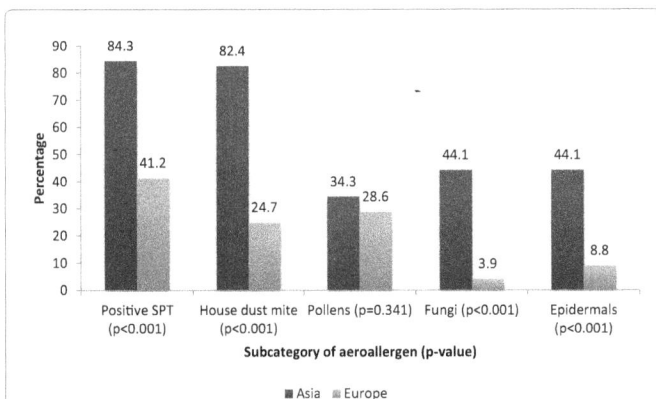

Figure 1: Distribution of positive skin prick test (SPT) response towards different subgroups of aeroallergens tested among the population in both regions.

Table 3: Percentages of positive skin prick test (SPT) responses among the population in both regions aged 5 to 84 years.

Even the European has higher prevalence of positive response towards house dust mite subgroup (24.7%) in comparison with fungi and epidermals with 3.9% and 8.8% respectively (p<0.001). However, the prevalence for both Bermuda grass and grain pollen (20.9%) in Europe were more or less the same with house dust mite, 21% - 25% (*Dermatophagoides pteronyssinus* and *Dermatophagoides farinae*). The least frequent aeroallergen for both Asia and Europe was dog hair (30.6% and 1.7% respectively).

A positive to at least one outdoor aeroallergen was slightly more common than a positive test response to at least one indoor aeroallergen in Europe (30.2% vs 27.5%). In comparison with Asia, the reverse pattern was observed whereby a positive test response to at least one indoor aeroallergen was greater than to outdoor aeroallergen (84.3% vs 41.2%). There was insignificant finding in positive skin prick test (SPT) response towards pollens among the population in both regions. (Figure 1)

Discussion

Exposure to allergens is an important triggering factor for the development of allergic sensitization and skin prick test is useful in detecting sensitization to allergen [40-42]. In Asia, it was believed that the prevalence of allergic disease, including food allergy was low [43]. In contrast, this study has shown that majority of Asian with personal history of atopy revealed positive allergic sensitisation to at least one category or subgroup of aeroallergen through skin prick test (SPT) which was consistence with a study from Thailand [44,45].

Negative skin prick response was higher in the Europe although prevalence of nasal allergies appeared to be higher in Western Europe as compared with Eastern Europe and South and Central Asia [46]. However, the result of SPT can varied from 24.9 – 81.6% depending on the diversity of populations tested with regard to the lifestyle, either urban or rural and mobility [47-49].

Aeroallergen is the most common sensitising allergens with variation from area to area with different geo-climate condition [50]. House dust mites (mainly *Dermatophagoides pteronyssinus*) constitute the major sensitising aeroallergen in both Asia and Europe [51,52]. The result was expected for Asia because of the humid climate and moderate temperature in most of the countries [45,51,53]. In a region with four seasons, house dust mites thrive in summer and die during winter. Nevertheless, they will continue thriving even in the coldest of months in a warm and humid house [53].

Although in some countries indoor aeroallergens are the important trigger of nasal allergic symptoms but generally pollens were proven in other study to be the aeroallergens with the highest sensitisation rates among Europeans [54-56]. In this study, pollens were the second most prevalent aeroallergen causing sensitisation in Europe. While the most important pollens causing allergy differ in each geographical area, grass pollen had the highest rate of sensitisation in both regions which was about 35% in Asia and 21% in Europe. The same figure was found in a German study for grass pollen (23.9%) [57,58].

Highest rates of sensitisation to fungi or moulds were found in tropical countries like Singapore and Malaysia, emphasising the role of a climate factor [49-59]. Highest degree of sensitisation to Alternaria sp. was found in Asia supporting the findings of other studies [49,60,61]. This study also supported the facts of high prevalence of Aspergillus sp. and Penicillium sp. in Asia and the low rate of sensitisation to moulds reported across Europe [61,62].

Allergens from cat and dog dander are found in almost every home,

even in the house without resident pets [63]. The sensitisation rate to cat fur was much higher than to dog hair [64,65]. Cats are more likely to cause allergic reactions than dogs because they always lick themselves and spend more time in the house close to humans [52].

Significant association between different age group and positive skin prick test response was also found in this study with higher proportions at age 15 to 44 years with the peaks in the second decade of life among the Asian and the third decade of life among the European supporting the findings in NHANES II and III[61]. Significant correlation between region of residence of the respondents and positive skin prick test response was also observed in this study.

Unfortunately, insignificant correlation between sex and positive skin test responses in this study was proved otherwise in NHANES II and III with higher prevalence of positive skin test responses among male subjects at each decade of life [61]. It is because male subjects have higher levels of serum IgE than female subjects at any give age in the general population, but whether sex influences sensitisation primarily through a genetic or an environmental pathway is controversial [66,67].

Conclusion

There was significant difference in skin prick test (SPT) responses towards different group of aeroallergens in regions with diverse geo-climate. Yet, house dust mites were still the commonest aeroallergen causing allergic sensitisation.

Acknowledgments

We would like to express utmost gratitude to Dr A.M Lo Galbo and colleagues in UMC Utrecht, Netherland. The authors have no conflict of interest to declare and an ethical approval was not essential as it was just data analysis.

References

1. Johansson SG, Bieber T, Dahl R, Friedmann PS, Lanier BQ, et al (2004) Revised nomenclature for allergy for global use: Report of the Nomenclature Review Committee of the World Allergy Organization, October 2003. J Allergy Clin Immunol 113: 832-836.

2. Soegiarto G, Mai Shihah A (2007) Allergic sensitisation among Surabaya school children and undergraduate students. World Allergy Organisation 646: 207.

3. Sibbald B, Rink E (1991) Epidemiology of seasonal and perennial rhinitis: clinical presentation and medical history. Thorax 46: 895-901.

4. Guilbert TW, Morgan WJ, Zeiger RS, Bacharier LB, Boehmer SJ, et al. (2004) Atopic characteristics of children with recurrent wheezing at high risk for the development of childhood asthma. J Allergy Clin Immunol 114: 1282-1287.

5. Johansson SG, Hourihane JO, Bousquet J, Bruijnzeel-Koomen C, Dreborg S, et al. (2001) A revised nomenclature for allergy. An EAACI position statement from the EAACI nomenclature task force. Allergy 56: 813-824.

6. Bousquet PJ, Chinn S, Janson C, Kogevinas M, Burney P, et al. (2007) Geographical variation in the prevalence of positive skin tests to environmental aeroallergens in the European Community Respiratory Health Survey I. Allergy 62: 301-309.

7. Arnedo-Pena A, García-Marcos L, García Hernández G, Aguinagua Ontoso I, González Díaz C, et al. (2005) [Time trends and geographical variations in the prevalence of symptoms of allergic rhinitis in 6-7-year-old children from eight areas of Spain according to the ISAAC]. An Pediatr (Barc) 62: 229-236.

8. Sener O, Kim YK, Ceylan S, Ozanguc N, Yoo TJ,et al. (2003) Comparison of skin tests to aeroallergens in Ankara and Seoul. J Investig Allergol Clin Immunol 13: 202-208.

9. Truong C, Palmé AE, Felber F (2007) Recent invasion of the mountain birch Betula pubescens ssp. tortuosa above the treeline due to climate change: genetic and ecological study in northern Sweden. J Evol Biol 20: 369-380.

10. Confalonieri U, Menne B, Akhtar R, Ebi M, Hauengue RS, et al (2007) Impacts, Adaptation and Vulnerability. Contribution of Working Group II to the Fourth Assessment Report of the Intergovernmental Panel on Climate Change. Cambridge, UK: Cambridge University Press: 391-431.

11. Wayne P, Foster S, Connolly J, Bazzaz F, Epstein P (2002) Production of allergenic pollen by ragweed (Ambrosia artemisiifolia L.) is increased in CO2-enriched atmospheres. Ann Allergy Asthma Immunol 88: 279-282.

12. Garci´a-Mozo H, Gala´n C, Jato V, Belmonte J, Diaz de la Guardia C,et al (2006). Quercus pollen season dynamics in the Iberian Peninsula: response to meteorological parameters and possible consequences of climate change. Ann Agric Environ Med 13: 209-224.

13. Beggs PJ, Bambrick HJ (2005) Is the global rise of asthma an early impact of anthropogenic climate change? Environ Health Perspect 113: 915-919.

14. Williams R (2005) Climate change blamed for rise in hay fever. Nature 434: 1059.

15. Galán C, García-Mozo H, Vázquez L, Ruiz L, de la Guardia CD, et al. (2005) Heat requirement for the onset of the Olea europaea L. pollen season in several sites in Andalusia and the effect of the expected future climate change. Int J Biometeorol 49: 184-188.

16. Weryszko-Chmielewska E, Puc M, Piotrowska K (2006) Effect of meteorological factors on Betula, Fraxinus and Quercus pollen concentrations in the atmosphere of Lublin and Szczecin, Poland. Ann Agric Environ Med 13: 243-249.

17. Puc M, Wolski T (2002) Betula and Populus pollen counts and meteorological conditions in Szczecin, Poland. Ann Agric Environ Med 9: 65-69.

18. Laaidi K (2001) Predicting days of high allergenic risk during Betula pollination using weather types. Int J Biometeorol 45: 124-132.

19. Gilmour MI, Jaakkola MS, London SJ, Nel AE, Rogers CA (2006) How exposure to environmental tobacco smoke, outdoor air pollutants, and increased pollen burdens influences the incidence of asthma. Environ Health Perspect 114: 627-633.

20. Moorcroft PR, Pacala SW, Lewis MA (2006) Potential role of natural enemies during tree range expansions following climate change. J Theor Biol 241: 601-616.

21. Ziska LH, Gebhard DE, Frenz DA, Faulkner S, Singer BD, et al. (2003) Cities as harbingers of climate change: common ragweed, urbanization, and public health. J Allergy Clin Immunol 111: 290-295.

22. Emberlin J, Detandt M, Gehrig R, Jaeger S, Nolard N,et al (2002). Responses in the start of Betula (birch) pollen seasons to recent changes in spring temperatures across Europe. Int J Biometeorol 46:159-170.

23. Peteet D (2000) Sensitivity and rapidity of vegetational response to abrupt climate change. Proc Natl Acad Sci U S A 97: 1359-1361.

24. Stach A, Garci´a-Mozo H, Prieto-Baena JC, Czarnecka-Operacz M, Jenerowicz D, et al (2007). Prevalence of Artemisia species pollinosis in western Poland: impact of climate change on aerobiological trends, 1995-2004. J Investig Allergol Clin Immunol. 17: 39-47.

25. Breton MC, Garneau M, Fortier I, Guay F, Louis J (2006) Relationship between climate, pollen concentrations of Ambrosia and medical consultations for allergic rhinitis in Montreal 1994-2002. Sci Total Environ 370: 39-50.

26. Schneiter D, Bernard B, Defila C, Gehrig R (2002) [Effect of climatic changes on the phenology of plants and the presence of pollen in the air in Switzerland]. Allerg Immunol (Paris) 34: 113-116.

27. Steinman HA, Donson H, Kawalski M, Toerien A, Potter PC (2003) Bronchial hyper-responsiveness and atopy in urban, peri-urban and rural South African children. Pediatr Allergy Immunol 14: 383-393.

28. van der Wal MF, Uitenbroek DG, Verhoeff AP (2000) [Increased proportion of elementary school children with asthmatic symptoms in the Netherlands, 1984/85-1994/95; a literature review]. Ned Tijdschr Geneeskd 144: 1780-1785.

29. Downs SH, Marks GB, Sporik R, Belosouva EG, Car NG, et al. (2001) Continued increase in the prevalence of asthma and atopy. Arch Dis Child 84: 20-23.

30. Kuehni CE, Davis A, Brooke AM, Silverman M (2001) Are all wheezing disorders in very young (preschool) children increasing in prevalence? Lancet 357: 1821-1825.

31. Burney P (2002) The changing prevalence of asthma? Thorax 57 Suppl 2: II36-36II39.

32. Nelson HS (2000) The importance of allergens in the development of asthma and the persistence of symptoms. J Allergy Clin Immunol 105: S628-632.

33. Warner JO, Kaliner MA, Crisci CD, Del Giacco S, Frew AJ, et al. (2006) Allergy practice worldwide: a report by the World Allergy Organization Specialty and Training Council. Int Arch Allergy Immunol 139: 166-174.

34. American College of Allergy (2006) Asthma and Immunology. Allergy.

35. van Schayck CP, Smit HA (2005) The prevalence of asthma in children: a reversing trend. Eur Respir J 26: 647-650.

36. Smit HA, van Schayck CP (2006) [Recent changes in the prevalence of asthma in children]. Ned Tijdschr Geneeskd 150: 233-236.

37. Downs SH, Marks GB, Sporik R, Belosouva EG, Car NG, et al. (2001) Continued increase in the prevalence of asthma and atopy. Arch Dis Child 84: 20-23.

38. Kuehni CE, Davis A, Brooke AM, Silverman M (2001) Are all wheezing disorders in very young (preschool) children increasing in prevalence? Lancet 357: 1821-1825.

39. Blanc PD, Trupin L, Eisner M, Earnest G, Katz PP, et al. (2001) The work impact of asthma and rhinitis: findings from a population-based survey. J Clin Epidemiol 54: 610-618.

40. Sampson HA (2001) Utility of food-specific IgE concentrations in predicting symptomatic food allergy. J Allergy Clin Immunol 107: 891-896.

41. Skolnick HS, Conover-Walker MK, Koerner CB, Sampson HA, Burks W, et al. (2001) The natural history of peanut allergy. J Allergy Clin Immunol 107: 367-374.

42. Hill DJ, Hosking CS, Reyes-Benito LV (2001) Reducing the need for food allergen challenges in young children: a comparison of in vitro with in vivo tests. Clin Exp Allergy 31: 1031-1035.

43. Turkeltaub PC, Gergen PJ (1989) The risk of adverse reactions from percutaneous prick-puncture allergen skin testing, venipuncture, and body measurements: data from the second National Health and Nutrition Examination Survey 1976-80 (NHANES II). J Allergy Clin Immunol 84: 886-890.

44. [No authors listed] (1998) Worldwide variation in prevalence of symptoms of asthma, allergic rhinoconjunctivitis, and atopic eczema: ISAAC. The International Study of Asthma and Allergies in Childhood (ISAAC) Steering Committee. Lancet 351: 1225-1232.

45. Pumhirun P, Towiwat P, Mahakit P (1997) Aeroallergen sensitivity of Thai patients with allergic rhinitis. Asian Pac J Allergy Immunol 15: 183-185.

46. Arrigo C (2005) Epidemiology and economics of allergy treatment. Clinical and Experimental Allergy Reviews 5: 36-39.

47. Ontiveros CR, López SM, Cerino JR (1995) Aeroallergens detected by skin prick test in children with respiratory allergy (asthma and rhinitis); from the south of Mexico City. Alergia e Inmunol Pediatr 4: 112-116.

48. Dottorini ML, Bruni B, Peccini F, Bottini P, Pini L, et al. (2007) Skin prick-test reactivity to aeroallergens and allergic symptoms in an urban population of central Italy: a longitudinal study. Clin Exp Allergy 37: 188-196.

49. Calabria CW, Dice JP, Hagan LL (2007) Prevalence of positive skin test responses to 53 allergens in patients with rhinitis symptoms. Allergy Asthma Proc 28: 442-448.

50. Pawankar (2008) State of World Allergy Report 2008: Allergy and Chronic Respiratory Diseases. World Allergy Organ J 1: S4-S17.

51. Yeoh SM, Kuo IC, Wang DY, Liam CK, Sam CK, De Bruyne JA, et al. Sensitization profiles of Malaysian and Singaporean subjects to allergens from Dermatophagoides pteronyssinus and Blomia tropicalis. Int Arch Allergy Immunol 132: 215-220.

52. Airborne allergens. National Institute of Allergy and Infectious Diseases, NIH 2003; Publication No. 03-7045.

53. Arbes SJ Jr, Cohn RD, Yin M, Muilenberg ML, Burge HA, et al. (2003) House dust mite allergen in US beds: results from the First National Survey of Lead and Allergens in Housing. J Allergy Clin Immunol 111: 408-414.

54. Rabito FA, Iqbal S, Holt E, Grimsley LF, Islam TM, et al. (2007) Prevalence of indoor allergen exposures among New Orleans children with asthma. J Urban Health 84: 782-792.

55. Custovic A, Taggart SC, Woodcock A (1994) House dust mite and cat allergen in different indoor environments. Clin Exp Allergy 24: 1164-1168.

56. Solomon WR, Platts-Mills TAE (1998) Aerobiology and inhalant allergens. In: Middleton E, Reed ChE, Ellis EF, Adkinson NF, editors. Allergy Principles and Practice. USA: Mosby : 367-403.

57. Kuehr J, Karmaus W, Frischer T, Hendel-Kramer A, Weiss K, et al. (1992) Longitudinal variability of skin prick test results. Clin Exp Allergy 22: 839-844.

58. Kidon MI, See Y, Goh A, Chay OM, Balakrishnan A (2004) Aeroallergen sensitization in pediatric allergic rhinitis in Singapore: is air-conditioning a factor in the tropics? Pediatr Allergy Immunol 15: 340-343.

59. Wan Ishlah L, Gendeh BS (2005) Skin prick test reactivity to common airborne pollens and molds in allergic rhinitis patients. Med J Malaysia 60: 194-200.

60. Taksey J, Craig TJ (2001) Allergy test results of a rural and small-city population compared with those of an urban population. J Am Osteopath Assoc 101: S4

61. Arbes SJ Jr, Gergen PJ, Elliott L, Zeldin DC (2005) Prevalences of positive skin test responses to 10 common allergens in the US population: results from the third National Health and Nutrition Examination Survey. J Allergy Clin Immunol 116: 377-383.

62. Bavbek S, Erkekol FO, Ceter T (2006) Sensitization to Alternaria and Cladosporium in patients with respiratory allergy and outdoor counts of mold spores in Ankara atmosphere, Turkey. J Asthma 43: 421-426.

63. Bierman C.W (1998) Environmental Control of Asthma. Medscape General Medicine 2:13.

64. Hon KLE, Leung TF, Ching G (2008)Patterns of food and aeroallergen sensitisation in childhood eczema. Acta Paediatrica 2008 97: 1734-1737.

65. Hon KLE, Leung TF, Lam MCA (2007) Which aeroallergens are associated with eczema severity? Clinical and Experimental Dermatology 32: 401-404.

66. Barbee RA, Halonen M, Lebowitz M, Burrows B (1981) Distribution of IgE in a community population sample: correlations with age, sex, and allergen skin test reactivity. J Allergy Clin Immunol 68: 106-11.

67. Robert Chobot (1935) The significance of tobacco reactions in allergic children. Journal of allergy: 383-386.

6

Conditions of Palliative Home Care: The Case of Family Physicians in Switzerland

Vanessa Alvarado[1], Brigitte Liebig[2]*

[1]*University of Applied Sciences, Applied Psychology, Riggenbachstrasse 16, Olten, 4600, Switzerland*
[2]*University of Applied Sciences, Applied Psychology, Riggenbachstrasse 16, Olten, 4600, Switzerland*

Abstract

Family physicians (FPs) play a key role in the treatment and care for terminally ill men and women. However, little is known about the conditions and challenges of FPs services in this domain. Aim of this article is to identify, how FPs can be supported in palliative home care in Switzerland by the availability of guidelines and advance directives, community-based palliative care structures, education and training, as well as remuneration of palliative home care services.

Case studies in three Swiss cantons, namely Lucerne (LU), Vaud (VD), and Ticino (TI) are the basis of the following investigation. They not only represent French, Italian and German language regions but differ considerably with respect to the history of palliative care. Within and between cantons documents, questionnaires and expert interviews are analyzed thematically with the help of content-analysis.

The results illustrate considerable shortcomings with respect to the backing of FPs palliative home care services. The availability and use of guidelines as well as advance directives is rather small in general practice, and FPs care and treatment at the end of life is only marginally supported by ambulant care structures, especially in rural areas. Also the coordination of services and collaboration between specialists and generalists is poorly developed. Furthermore FPs possibilities to acquire competencies in palliative care are strongly limited, and palliative home care provided by FPs is poorly financed.

The results draw a rather bleak picture with respect to the support of FPs palliative home care services in Switzerland today. Though considerable steps towards implementing palliative care have been made in recent years in general, conditions for FPs medical services have to get improved strongly. Major efforts have to be made to foster the recognition and implementation throughout Switzerland.

Introduction[1]

Family physicians (FPs) play a key role in community-based palliative care (CBPC) in many European countries [1,2]. In palliative home care and in nursing homes FPs care not only for oncological patients, but for patients with terminal organ failures, with degenerative neurologic diseases, or for multi-morbid and/or geriatric patients [3]. Best symptom-management, advance care planning, the collaboration with families, ambulant services and medical specialists, as well as the organization of transitions between different care settings (home, hospital, retirement and nursing homes or specialized care services), pose highest demands on FPs' services [4,5]. Demands increase since palliative care services at home constitute a specific work environment: Due to their solitary practice FPs only have restricted opportunities to refer to social guidance by peers, and rely strongly on their very own competencies. The proof and the availability of information and of other medical resources in the environment are therefore highly important factors for the quality of care [6]. However, while specialized palliative care already has gathered attention, the recognition and implementation of palliative home care is still underdeveloped [1].

Community-based palliative care in Europe and in Switzerland

The development of CBPC is crucial to measure up to the expectations and wishes of patients [7], of who most wish to spend their end of life at home. Due to these wishes, but also to the demographic aging of societies, and to the need for cost-effective medical services the intention to increase and strengthen CBPC is an issue that is on the agenda in many countries. In Europe a 'Taskforce on Primary and Community Palliative Care' exists since 2011[8]. Early efforts to increase and strengthen CBPC are especially known from Great Britain and Ireland. The Golden Standard Framework, established in England in 2000, was one of the first guidelines available on European level aiming on the improvement of end-of-life care [9]. As a recent report shows [10] the reinforcement of CBPC is also on the agenda of other European Countries: Besides England and Ireland also Germany, Scotland, Serbia and Albania have invested into national palliative care strategies with a strong focus on primary or community-based care. Practice-oriented programs to foster CBPC have been established in other European countries as well. But aside from these efforts there are still many countries where palliative care as a part of primary care has to be acknowledged and promoted [10,11].

Community-based palliative care in Switzerland

As in other European countries the promotion of CBPC is an important public health issue in Switzerland [10]. While generally a broad range of activities to establish palliative care can be noted since the 1980ies, the need for new strategies to assure cost-effectiveness

[1]This publication is based on the study "Decision-making in general practice settings at the end of life ", which has been carried out in the Swiss national research program 67 "end of life" and financed by the Swiss National Research Foundation (project-ID.: 406740-139270). We thank Karine Darbellay, Chiara Piccini, Klaus Bally, Heike Gudat, Peter Voll and Antonella Carassa for their support and the anonymous peer reviewers for their constructive feedback.

***Corresponding author:** Brigitte Liebig, University of Applied Sciences, Applied Psychology, Riggenbachstr. 16, Olten, 4600, Switzerland, E-mail:brigitte.liebig@fhnw.ch

constantly increases. According to the Swiss Federal Office of Public Health about 75-80% of patients, who require palliative care services in Switzerland can be looked after by means of primary care today [12,13].

However, the establishment of CBPC all over the country is far from being achieved. Quite basically, the Swiss language regions differ remarkably with respect to the information about and the backing of palliative care [14]. The German, French and Italian speaking regions show considerably different attitudes towards life preservation, the alleviation of pain and other symptoms, very similar to those found in Germany, France and Italy [15] and also with respect to palliative care structures a comparison between Switzerland and other European countries reveals Switzerland to be a "Europe in miniature"[14].

Further, the federalist organization of the Swiss health system makes it difficult to define uniform standards. Strong differences across cantons exist also with respect to the legal status of palliative care. While 6 of 26 Swiss cantons do not provide any legal basis for palliative care others mention palliative care as an aspect of public health (e.g. Vaud), or as a patient's right (e.g. Lucerne) [16]. Obviously the legal framing of palliative care affects its development and implementation in the cantons: a legal basis expresses a public interest of the legislative body and empowers cantonal health authorities to take action for installing a comprehensive palliative care system. Of course, measures can also be taken without a legal basis, but a cantonal legislation expresses the officially recognized value of palliative care[2,3].

Starting from the profound lack of information and knowledge about FPs as important actors in CBPC, this article aims to highlight some of the specific conditions and challenges for the provision of palliative home care by FPs in Switzerland.

Methods

The empirical study has been conducted by the University of Applied Sciences Northwestern Switzerland, School of Applied Psychology, in collaboration with the University of Basel, the University of Lugano and the University of Applied Sciences and Arts Western Switzerland. In order to identify the backing of FPs services in palliative home care in more depth, the analysis focuses on 3 selected cantons, namely Lucerne (LU), Vaud (VD), and Ticino (TI), which do not only represent French, Italian and German speaking regions in Switzerland but differ considerably with respect to the history of implementing palliative care. Within these cantons most important supply structures for FPs palliative home care services, as they have been used in the course of first general evaluations of palliative care on national level [13], were surveyed. These were defined as a) the availability of guidelines and recommendations for FPs, b) provisional structures in CBPC (such as mobile palliative care teams, ambulatories as well as the number of specialized FPs and nurses), c) the availability of training and further education for FPs, and finally d) the financial backing of FPs services.

In the course of the 3 cantonal case studies a data set has been generated on the basis of (a) documents about health care policies and provisional structures in CBPC[4], and (b) 10 expert interviews with 7 FPs, 2 nurses and a project leader of a cantonal palliative care project,

[2] Personal communication of Prof. Bernhard Waldmann, Université de Fribourg, Switzerland

[3] Personal communication of Pia Coppex, Swiss conference of cantonal health directorates

[4] As numerous documents have been used for the analysis, it is not possible to list all of them. For each canton all the available documents on palliative care have been looked at, as e.g. "Inventaire donées sur les soins palliatifs" for the canton Vaud, "Detail Konzept Palliative Care" for the canton Lucerne, and "Rapporto Annuale" for the canton Ticino.

1)	How do you evaluate the conditions for FPs providing palliative care in your canton? Please answer with respect to the following aspects:
	a. degree of information among population on the provision of palliative care
	b. degree of information among FPs regarding medico-ethical guidelines and advanced directives, as well as regarding aspects of palliative medicine
	c. area of coverage and the quality of community based palliative care structures (especially at home)
	d. area coverage and quality of specialized palliative care structures / offers (in clinics, nursing homes, and hospices)
	e. financing of palliative care provided by FPs
	f. possibilities of education and training for FPs and community nurses in the domain of palliative medicine
	g. collaboration between FPs and specialized physicians as well as with institutions of specialized palliative care
	h. attitude towards palliative care among the (regional) population (e.g. favourable or negative)
	i. Is there a region/a community in your canton, where no/nearly no palliative care is provided (This questions has only been put to cantonal representatives)
2)	Which are the specific challenges/problems for FPs in Switzerland resp. in your canton in community based palliative care?
3)	Which measures can be taken in order to strengthen FPs in the domain of palliative care in Switzerland resp. your canton?

Table 1: Items of the questionnaire.

all of them providing expert knowledge in the field of palliative care. Further (c), data were generated by a semi-standardized questionnaire with open questions for 15 representatives of national and cantonal health care services and policy actors (for items see table 1). all participants got the same questionnaire, but as questions were open, different qualitative data could be gathered.

The questionnaire started from core issues concerning supply structures and asked for a general evaluation of the status quo, while the interview guideline for experienced FPs and nurses concentrated on supply structures, as well as requirements and challenges in palliative home care. Interview guidelines and questionnaires where agreed on by a supervisory board and translated in three languages (French, Italian, German). Collection of data was conducted from February till June 2013. Within and between cantons documents, questionnaires and expert interviews got analyzed thematically with the help of content-analysis [17]. This is an interpretative technique which allows the identification of key issues within text material on the basis of a systematic and controlled reduction and abstraction. Smallest text units got paraphrased, generalized and integrated into core statements in orientation at the above mentioned questions of our study.

Results and Discussion

Low distribution of guidelines and advance directives

Ethical guidelines, professional rules of conduct and standards are known as practical aids for health care professionals making difficult treatment decisions. They aim on assuring an appropriate allocation of medical and nursing care and foster ethical competence among health professionals [18]. Especially advance directives can influence decision-making at the end of life, when eschewing certain medical interventions for FPs [19]. The revised Swiss Civil Code confers a legal status to these instruments from 2013 on [20][5].

As our analysis shows, the availability and visibility of

[5] According to Swiss law physicians have to follow advance directives of patients and the order of possible representatives since January 2013.

guidelines is still rather small for FPs, who report to be rather rarely informed, especially in the French and Italian part of Switzerland. Correspondingly, also the application of guidelines is described as rather rare. Especially the older generation of FPs relies primarily on professional experience, while they assess the practical use of guidelines rather critically. Challenges exist also with respect to the implementation of advance directives in CBPC: information about this tool seems not only low among Swiss citizens [14], but also among FPs as CBPC providers. Neither FPs in the Ticino (TI) nor in Vaud (VD) report a high visibility of advance directives: Quite contrary, the frequency of using advance directives is described as low, even in hospitals. The small degree of implementation seems to explain, why respondents in French and Italian speaking Switzerland report, that advance directives are rarely used. Or, as an expert from canton Vaud (VD) explains: "Advance directives are a problem. Generally FPs are uneasy about them". However, in the German speaking part of Switzerland advance directives seem to be more popular: "What the patient has written in his/her living will is an important guideline for us", claims a FP from Lucerne (LU). The results of the present study reaffirm statements from other publications in Switzerland, where regional differences regarding the dissemination of and dealing with advance directives are described as strong [14,21].

Provisional structures

Marginal supply of FPs by ambulant care structures

To be able to guarantee an extensive palliative service system and to meet the needs of all patients, FPs rely on support by ambulatory and further supporting provisional structures, such as mobile palliative care teams (MPCTs) or specialized nurses [22]. Yet, these supply structures differ strongly across Switzerland: Cantonal health offices evaluate the ambulatory provisional structures in palliative care still as insufficient and provided by to many different actors. Better conditions exist with respect to palliative ambulatories, which are often provided by hospitals. Ambulatory services are provided in several cantons (e.g. Ticino), whereas other regions do not provide palliative ambulatories at all (e.g. Basel or Valais) [15].

The different situation of palliative care in the three Swiss cantons studied here is inter alia attributable to the specific history of its implementation. Switzerland constitutes an intersection of different national European influences, which find their expression in different regional developments. As for Ticino the development of palliative care started already in the late 1980ies: First offers developed in PC concerned palliative home care service, a tradition that seems to contribute to a rather good standing of CBPC in this canton. In canton Vaud (VD) PC started with the foundation of stationary services in 1988; today this canton provides very good specialized PC, and since 2003 also an extensive offer of MPCTs has been realized [12]. In the German speaking canton Lucerne (LU) the implementation of PC started during the last decade: up till today it offers only a poor degree of specialized care in clinics, nursing homes, or hospices, and a rather week offer with respect to CBPC services [23].

Besides cantonal differences considerable divides exist along urban and rural areas with respect to the provision of PC structures. This applies especially to the canton Lucerne (LU), which is generally worse supplied than the two other cantons. However, experts claim noticeable changes within the last few years: even if in some regions only weakly developed CBPC structures are offered, the positive impact of the Swiss national promotion program for PC starting 2010 [13] can be registered almost everywhere.

Lack of coordination between palliative care services

Well managed and integrated health care services are essential, if efficiency and cost-control, as well as high quality of care for patients shall be achieved [24]. While in the canton Lucerne (LU) support and resources for CBPC as well as specialized care is very rare, the canton Ticino (TI) apparently can rely on good coordination between different actors of primary and specialized palliative care. In the canton Vaud (VD) palliative care supply structures are provided comparatively well, while they are not very well coordinated with the field of CBPC. The case of Vaud shows that even well-established provisional structures in palliative care do not necessarily guarantee well-coordinated health care services. As experts from Vaud (VD) report, the knowledge about MPCTs in general practice is still small, and the division of labor between FPs and mobile teams is quite often unclear: "FPs do not necessarily collaborate with mobile palliative care teams or other peer physicians." Also the coordination of services and collaboration between specialists and generalists is poorly developed due to time constraints and professional attitudes; especially the relation between oncologists and FPs seems rather competitive-dialogue between these professionals in the course of treatment and care is still rare.

The lack of coordination between specialized care providers and CBPC is a problem that is widely reported by interviewees. As a FP claims: "You have to put the pieces together; it is not the case that one team is responsible for everything, as for instance in England. Here, palliative care is not that holistic". Also health care representatives estimate a higher degree of inter-professional collaboration between PC providers as highly important.

Limited education and training opportunities

Since 2010 considerable action has been taken in order to integrate palliative care into the medical curriculum [11]: these initiatives include inter alia the distribution of a guideline for further education programs on national level. However, our document analysis shows that the quality of formation in PC remains very heterogeneous between cantons: While in Ticino (TI) and Vaud (VD) it is possible to attend courses at a university level, in Lucerne (LU) education and training opportunities are mainly provided by hospitals, nursing homes, or NGOs such as CARITAS. And even if efforts are made to homogenize the catalogue of competencies on a national level, the quality of competences generated by education programs is rarely checked, e.g. by certification. Due to a lack of formal education, palliative care is widely practiced still rather individually or 'hands on'.

Especially for FPs possibilities to acquire competencies seem very limited. Mainly three constraints are mentioned by our respondents in this context: Firstly and most important, FPs do have very spare time for further education and training in palliative care due to a large number of medical obligations. Secondly, courses in PC are competing with numerous other offers in further education and training, while at the same time credit points gathered in (further) education in PC are comparatively few. Thirdly, the lack of knowledge about palliative care skills does contribute to a lack of recognition of formally acquired competencies. As experts report, some physicians still define palliative care as a rather 'naturally given' human competence, and therefore not an issue of formal learning. In everyday practice experience and 'tacit knowledge' [25] is considered to be mainly transferred by experienced colleagues and in peer intervision - and constructed in opposition to formal educational contents.

Lack of appropriate remuneration

Finally, while specialized palliative care generates hospital charges, palliative home care provided by FPs is poorly financed; parts of their medical PC services are even not represented in the Swiss tariff for medical activities (TARMED). This cut across to the fact that palliative home care activities are very complex and especially time consuming: As it is stated provocatively by a representative of a Swiss professional medical association: "A washing machine repairmen gets better rewarded for home visits than we do".

Some interviewees interpret the insufficient financial support for palliative care by generalists as resulting from the dominance of an attitude, which associates medical practice primarily with 'cure' [26]. Also in primary care the medical approach seems still based on this paradigm of cure, instead promoting patients well-being primarily by care. An FP states: "It is correct to say 'we try to cure' and to work curatively, but it should also be okay to say 'death is part of life' and there have to be created financial spaces for this last phase of life to be able to provide good palliative care".

As our data show, FPs services are not remunerated at all if they are related to activities apart from immediate contact to the patient. These activities include the coordination between care providers, such as between home care nurses, volunteers, social services and psychologists, advice and support for relatives, inter-professional dialogue between FPs and specialized doctors in hospitals or private surgery, as well as many other activities. So for example in canton Vaud (VD) services of MPCTs are financed by a cantonal budget, but administrative expenditures to coordinate palliative home care by FPs and other services lack remuneration.

Conclusions

Our data draw a rather bleak picture with respect to the support of FPs palliative home care services in Switzerland today. Though considerable steps towards implementing palliative care have been made in recent years in general [13] conditions for FPs medical services have to get strongly improved.

To begin with, the shortcomings are related to the lack of a unitary development of CBPC in Switzerland, the cantonal different mixture of law and 'soft law' in this field, but also to the absence of guidelines directed to FPs in palliative home care, or the lack of visibility of advance directives for this group of professionals. More than that, our findings highlight the cantonal different backing of FPs services by provisional palliative care structures, especially with respect to MPCTs or professional support and collaboration. In all three cantons surveyed here, palliative care structures do not reflect a continuum of specialization, as it is recommended by the European Association for Palliative Care [27]. Especially in Swiss rural areas FPs are acting rather alone and cannot rely on support by a developed palliative care network. Further, our data show considerable challenges related to the use of training and/or further education in palliative care, which varies regionally and across cantons, while at the same time there exists no specific training for generalists. The lack of knowledge and skills on community level constitutes an important barrier to the quality and recognition of palliative care in general. But also the remuneration of FPs services still is far from appropriate and reflects the lack of recognition.

In 2004 the World Health Organization (WHO) claimed, that high quality care at the end of life must be understood as a basic human right [28]. Our study shows that strong efforts have to be made by health policy on national, cantonal and municipal level, to promote the public understanding and acceptance of palliative care also in Switzerland [9]. Especially the development of CBPC services seems elementary in order to fulfill expectations and wishes of patients, of whom the majority prefers to die at home [7]. FPs are main target groups for political action if accessibility of palliative care for every patient shall be guaranteed. The availability of and information on guidelines and advance directives in general practice, the support of FPs services by ambulant as well as specialized services, and the development of their competencies and skills therefore have to become highest priority in public health policies. And: FPs services in palliative care have to be based on adequate remuneration, in order to allow recognition and implementation throughout Switzerland.

References

1. Schneider N, Mitchell G K, Murray S A (2010) Palliative care in urgent need of recognition and development in general practice: the example of Germany. BMC Family Practice 11:66.

2. Meeussen K, Van den Block L, Echteld M, Bossuyt, N, Bilsen, J et al. (2011) Advance care planning in Belgium and the Netherlands: a nationwide retrospective study via sentinel networks of general practitioners. J Pain Symptom Manage 42 : 565-577.

3. Murray SA, Kendall M, Boyd K, Sheikh A (2005) Illness trajectories and palliative care. BMJ 330: 1007–1011.

4. Alsop A (2010) Collaborative working in end-of-life care: developing a guide for health and social care professionals. Int J Palliat Nurs 16:120-5.

5. Jensen H I, Ammentorp J, Erlandsen M, Ording H (2011) Withholding or withdrawing therapy in intensive care units: an analysis of collaboration among healthcare professionals. Intensive Care Med 37 :1696-705.

6. Geneau R, Lehoux P, Pineault R, Lamarche P (2008) Understanding the work of general practitioners: a social science perspective on the context of medical decision making in primary care. BMC Family Practice 9:12.

7. Murray SA, Boyd K, Sheikh A, Thomas K, Higginson I J (2004) Developing Primary Palliative Care. BMJ 329:1056-1057.

8. The Irish Hospice Foundation (2011) Primary Palliative Care in Ireland. Identifying improvements in primary care to support the care of those in their year of life.

9. Hansford, P, Meehan, H (2007) Gold Standards Framework: Improving Community Care. End of Life Care 1: 56-61.

10. European Association of Palliative Care [EAPC] (2014) Promoting palliative care in the community: producing a toolkit to improve and develop primary palliative care in different countries internationally. Report of the Taskforce in Primary Palliative Care. 29:101–111.

11. Centeno C, Lynch T, Donea O, Rocafort J, Clark D (2013) EAPC Atlas of Palliative Care 2013 – Full Edition. Milano: EAPC (European Association of Palliative Care).

12. Binder J, von Wartburg L (2009) Nationale Strategie Palliative Care 2010-2012. Bundesamt für Gesundheit [BAG/FOPH] und Schweizerische Konferenz der kantonalen Gesundheitsdirektorinnen und –direktoren, Bern.

13. Von Wartburg L, Näf F (2012) Nationale Strategie Palliative Care 2013-2015. Bundesamt für Gesundheit (BAG) und Schweizerische Konferenz der kantonalen Gesundheitsdirektorinnen und –direktoren (GDK): Bern.

14. Vodoz V (2010) Palliative Care 2009 Eine Studie im Auftrag des Bundesamtes für Gesundheit BAG. GfK Custom Research.

15. Fischer S, Bosshard G, Faisst K, Gutzwiler F (2005) Swiss doctors' attitudes towards end-of-life decisions and their determinants, in Swiss Med Wkly. 135:370-376.

16. Wyss N, Coppex P (2013) Stand und Umsetzung von Palliative Care in den Kantonen 2013. Ergebnisbericht vom 11. Juni 2013.

17. Mayring P (2000) Qualitative Inhaltsanalyse. Grundlagen und Techniken, 7. Aufl. Weinheim.

18. Reiter-Theil S, Mertz M, Meyer-Zehnder B, Pargger H (2011) Klinische Ethik als Partnerschaft – oder wie eine ethische Leitlinie für den patientengerechten

Einsatz von Ressourcen entwickelt und implementiert werden kann. Ethik Med 23: 93-105.

19. Abarshi E, Echteld M, Donker G, Van den Block L, Onwuteaka-Philipsen B et al. (2011) Discussing end-of-life issues in the last months of life: a nationwide study among general practitioners. J Palliat Med 14:323-330.

20. Hausheer H, Aebi-Müller R, Geiser T (2010) Das neue Erwachsenenschutzrecht. Bern.

21. Swiss National Advisory Commission on Biomedical Ethics (2011) Patientenverfügung. Ethische Erwägungen zum neuen Erwachsenenschutzrecht unter besonderer Berücksichtigung der Demenz. Stellungnahme Nr. 17: Bern.

22. Radbruch L, Payne S (2011b) Standards und Richtlinien für Hospiz- und Palliativversorgung in Europa: Teil 2. Weissbuch zu Empfehlungen der Europäischen Gesellschaft für Palliative Care (EAPC). Zeitschrift für Palliativmedizin 12: 260-270.

23. Alvarado V, Liebig B (2013) Unterstützung und Ressourcen der hausärztlichen Palliativversorgung - ein Vergleich dreier Schweizer Kantone, pallative.ch, Zeitschrift der Schweiz. Ges. für palliative Medizin, Pflege und Begleitung. 3: 32-37.

24. Martin-Moreno J, Harris M, Gorgojo L, Clark D, Normand C et al. (2008) Palliative Care in the European Union. Study Report by the Policy Department Economic and Scientific Policy.

25. Polanyi M (1966) The Tacit Dimension, New York: Doubleday & Company Inc.

26. Apesosa-Varano E C, Barker J C, Hinton L (2011) Curing and Caring: The Work of Primary Care Physicians With Dementia Patients. Qualitative Health Research 21 :1469-1483.

27. Radbruch L, Payne S (2011a) Standards und Richtlinien für Hospiz- und Palliativversorgung in Europa: Teil 1. Weissbuch zu Empfehlungen der Europäischen Gesellschaft für Palliative Care (EAPC). Zeitschrift für Palliativmedizin 12: 216-227.

28. World Health Organization (2004) Palliative Care: The Solid Facts.

7

Congruence between Staff and Lead Physician's Ability to Adapt to Change in a Pediatric Medical Home Project

Caprice Knapp[1]*, Vanessa Madden[1], Hanny Lane[1], Ruth Gubernick[2], Steven Kairys[3], Cristina Pelaez-Velez[4], Lee Sanders[5] and Lindsay Thompson[6]

[1]Department of Health Outcomes and Policy, Gainesville, FL, USA
[2]Gubernick-RSG Consulting, Cherry Hill NJ, USA
[3]School of Public Health, University of Medicine and Dentistry of New Jersey, Newark, NJ, USA
[4]University of South Florida, Department of Pediatrics, Tampa, FL, USA
[5]Center for Health Policy, Stanford University, Stanford, CA, USA
[6]Department of Pediatrics and Health Outcomes and Policy, Gainesville, FL, USA

Abstract

Objective: In the era of continuous quality improvement, practices must be ready to implement new ideas and processes. Alignment between staff and practice leadership is crucial to implementation. This study assesses the level of congruence that physician leaders and staff report about their ability to adapt to change.

Methods: Survey data were collected from staff working in 20 Florida pediatric practices and a physician leader from each practice. Both surveys assessed adaptive reserve which measures the ability of the practice to adapt to change by asking questions about their willingness to make changes, problem solving skills, communication, and general team dynamics. Overall, 170 staff members completed the staff survey with a response rate of 42.6% and twenty lead physicians completed the physician leader survey for a response rate of 100%. Descriptive, bivariate, and multivariate analyses were conducted.

Results: Among all staff, 30% were in high levels of agreement with their lead physician while 23.5% were in low levels of agreement with their lead physician. Practices with older staff were found to be the most aligned. Practices with one to three physicians were associated with decreased odds of congruence (Odds ratio=0.16). Staff ages 41 to 50 were associated with increased odds of congruence versus their younger counterparts (OR=5.77).

Conclusions: Adaptive reserve inventory and alignment should be seen as an investment and a priority by practices, medical home facilitators, and policymakers. A team approach is essential for patient-centered medical home implementation. Staff should be considered stakeholders in the medical home transformation and their feedback should be sought throughout the process and acted on in a timely manner.

Keywords: Medical home; Pediatrics; CHIPRA; Staff; Survey; Adaptive reserve

Introduction

Medical home is a philosophy and model of health care that has been in existence since the 1960s when the American Academy of Pediatrics first began to describe a centralized place for a child's medical records [1,2]. It has evolved and is now described as a highly sought-out model of care that is accessible, coordinated, comprehensive, family-centered, compassionate, culturally competent, and continuous [3,5]. Recently, the medical home model has been touted as a way to transform primary care in the United States, with the aims of reducing costs and improving quality. Medical home projects are underway in almost every state, in several federal agencies, and endorsed by the Affordable Care Act [6,7]. As more projects are undertaken, more evidence emerges; however, most of the literature is focused on adults with limited evidence in pediatrics. Further, Homer's 2008 systematic review of medical literature noted that none of the 33 studies reviewed evaluated medical home in a comprehensive manner [8].

Transforming to a medical home is challenging as it involves changes that occur at the patient, provider, and health system level. A practice's environment can be described in many ways including shared values, mission, standards, and adaptive reserve [9,10]. Adaptive reserve is described as a "practice's capacity for organizational learning and development" [11]. Practices with high levels of adaptive reserve are characterized by having healthy relationships, strong leadership, and shared vision [11]. Interviews conducted with staff at 36 family practices

that participated in a national medical home transformation project noted that adaptive reserve was present in successful transformations and referred to it as a "practice's most precious resource... and [it] must be supported and strengthened" [11].

To our knowledge, no studies of adaptive reserve in pediatric primary care practices exist. The current study addresses this gap in the literature. Our study uses data from 20 pediatric practices participating in the Florida Pediatric Medical Home Demonstration Project to 1) describe adaptive reserve, 2) evaluate adaptive reserve congruence between staff and lead physician, and 3) estimate the association between adaptive reserve congruence and medical homeness. We hypothesize that greater adaptive reserve congruence between the staff and lead physician will be associated with greater medical homeness.

*Corresponding author: Caprice Knapp, Department of Health Outcomes and Policy, Gainesville, FL, USA, 1329 SW 16th St, Gainesville Florida 32610, USA, E-mail: caprice1@ufl.edu

Sample and Methods

Sample

Florida's Pediatric Medical Home Demonstration project is a funded component of the state's Children's Health Insurance Program Reauthorization (CHIPRA) grant. The five-year Pediatric Medical Home Demonstration project began in July 2011 with the recruitment of 20 practices from around the state. Practices received no enhanced payment to participate, but were given incentives such as discounted prices to several online learning modules offered by the American Academy of Pediatrics (AAP) and earned credit toward Part 4 Maintenance of Certification. There are two parts to the Pediatric Medical Home Demonstration project: 1) a facilitated quality improvement intervention led by the AAP's Quality Improvement Innovation Network(QuIIN) [12] and 2) a four-year independent, multi-stakeholder evaluation of the aforementioned intervention. The four-year evaluation includes annual surveys with the practice staff, its three-person core project team, the lead physician, and parents whose children receive care at the practices; on-site interviews; and analysis of practice-level results of several CHIPRA measures [13].

Staff and lead physician surveys conducted at baseline were used for this study. In year one of the evaluation, between October and November 2011, staff at each of the 20 practices were given a packet. All staff, regardless of position, were included. The packet included the survey, instructions for submission, and a return envelope. A personal identifier, chosen by the respondent, was to be entered on the cover of the survey to track the responses longitudinally. No incentives were given. It was requested that staff mail back the survey within 14 days. Reminders were sent via email at two, four, and six weeks. Flyers were posted in common areas of the practices to encourage staff participation. Overall, 170 surveys were completed (response rate of 42.6%).

Lead physician surveys were collected between August and September 2011. Surveys were emailed to the 20 lead physicians. Surveys could be completed electronically or printed and returned by mail or fax. Again, no incentives were given. Overall, 20 lead physicians completed the survey (response rate 100%).

Two supplemental datasets were used in this study 1) data from the practice's original project application (which was submitted by the lead physician) and 2) data from the core project team's annual survey. Items on the application asked about the practice's characteristics such as estimated caseload and ownership. Items on the core clinical team survey asked about the medical home characteristics of the practice. This study was approved by the Institutional Review Board at the University of Florida (#80-2011).

Survey measures

Congruence between staff and lead physician adaptive reserve is the primary outcome in this study. Adaptive reserve was measured with the 23-item scale from the Trans for MED Practice Environment Checklist [14]. Topics covered include willingness to change, problem solving, communication, and team dynamics. Items were scored using a five-point Likert scale. Total adaptive reserve was transformed to a 100 point scale where 100 indicates the highest level of adaptive reserve. Congruence between staff and lead physician adaptive reserve was calculated by subtracting the mean staff reported adaptive reserve score from the lead physician reported adaptive reserve score and taking the absolute value. Non-zero differences indicate incongruence while a zero difference indicate the staff and lead physician reported

the same adaptive reserve score. Congruence scores were also separated into high and low levels using the 50th percentile of the distribution of scores as the cutoff. Congruence was categorized as high-high, low-high, high-low, and low-low (staff-lead physician, respectively).

Degree of medical homeness was assessed by the Medical Home Index (MHI) [15]. The MHI includes six domains: Organizational Capacity, Chronic Condition Management, Care Coordination, Community Outreach, Data Management, and Quality Improvement. Domains were scored from 1 to 8, with higher scores indicating that the practice had more characteristics of a patient-centered medical home. Total medical home score encompassed the scores on all six domains and ranged from 0 to 100, where 100 signified that a practice reported achieving every element of the medical home model.

Finally, several staff and practice level characteristics were included in the analyses. Staff characteristics gleaned from the staff surveys included age, gender, years worked in the practice, race, and position (clinical or non-clinical). Clinical position was defined as physicians, social workers, nurses, and physician assistants while non-clinical was defined as staff in areas such as finance, billing, office management, administrative assistants, and medical recordkeeping. Practice characteristics, collected from the original application,included self-reported percentage of pediatric patients enrolled in Medicaid or Florida's Children's Health Insurance Program (CHIP), percentage of pediatric patients enrolled in Medicaid or Florida's CHIP with special healthcare needs, practice size, practice location, practice region, and number of full time equivalent employees.

Analyses

Summary statistics were produced to describe the staff characteristics, practice characteristics, and item-level congruence scores.

Congruence between the total adaptive reserve score of the staff and lead physician was tested using Cohen's kappa to measure the rate of inter-observer agreement. Agreement ranged from 0 (poor), 0.01-0.20 (slight), 0.21-0.40 (fair), 0.41-0.60 (moderate), 0.61-0.80 (substantial), 0.81-0.99 (almost perfect), to 1 (perfect) [16]. Bivariate tests (z-scores) were conducted to determine if the level of agreement (high and low) statistically varied between the lead physician and the staff.

Logistic regression was performed to determine associations between high-high congruence and the aforementioned staff and practice characteristics. A binary dependent variable was constructed and equals one when the agreement was high-high, and zero otherwise. A second multivariate regression was performed to determine the association between medical homeness and congruence. The aforementioned staff and practice characteristics were also included in this model. An ordinary least squares regression was estimated with total MHI score as the dependent variable.

To account for any unobserved effect common to staff working at the same practice, the standard errors estimated in all the models were controlled for by clustering at the practice level. This approach is consistently used in other patient-centered medical home evaluations [14,17]. All analyses were conducted using Stata [18].

Results

Sample characteristics

Staff in the sample was primarily female (86.5%), White non-Hispanic (57.3%), and had been working in the practice for less than five years (63.2%) (Table 1). The staff was equally distributed in age, and the number of non-clinical staff (80) was more than the number of clinical staff (69).

Practice characteristics

Table 2 shows that most of the practices in the sample were large practices and that most were in urban areas. Mean percentage of pediatric patients in the practices that were enrolled in Medicaid or Florida's CHIP was 58.7%, and the mean percentage of those patients who had special healthcare needs was 31.3%. The mean number of full time equivalent employees in the practices was 15. Mean MHI scores by domain are presented in Figure 1. Mean total MHI score is 39.83 out of 100 (standard deviation (SD) 15.04), and across the practices, ranged from 14.29 to 80.

Congruence

Mean staff-reported adaptive reserve was 63.41 (SD=0.18; Median=66.30), while mean lead-physician reported adaptive reserve was higher at 68.34 (SD=0.08; Median=69.57). Table 3 presents the mean congruence scores for the 23 items in the adaptive reserve scale. Items are ranked from least to most congruence. "Most people in this practice are willing to change how they do things in response to feedback from other," had the least congruence (0.14). "People in this practice operate as a real team," "After trying something new, we take time to think about how it worked," and "People are aware of how their actions affect others in this practice," were the three items with the most congruence (0.01).

Congruence kappa values

	Frequency	Percent
Age	**152**	
Age 20-30	38	25.0%
Age 31-40	36	23.7%
Age 41-50	40	26.3%
Age 50+	38	25.0%
Gender	**156**	
Male	21	13.5%
Female	135	86.5%
Race	**150**	
White	86	57.3%
Black	21	14.0%
Hispanic	32	21.3%
Asian	7	4.7%
Other Race	4	2.7%
Position at Practice	**149**	
Nurse- RN, LPN	24	16.1%
Social Worker	1	0.7%
Clinician-PA, ARNP, MD, DO	44	29.5%
Administrative-Secretary, Finance, Records, Office Manager	43	28.9%
Other Position	37	24.8%
Clinical Staff Positions	69	46.3%
Non-Clinical Staff Positions	80	53.7%
Number of Years worked at Practice	**152**	
Worked 0-5 years	96	63.2%
Worked 6-10 years	24	15.8%
Worked 11-15 years	14	9.2%
Worked 16-20 years	11	7.2%
Worked 20+ years	7	4.6%

Table 1: Staff characteristics.

Variable	Frequency	Percent
Practice Size		
Solo	5	25%
Small Practice	6	30%
Large Practice	9	45%
Practice Location		
Urban	13	65%
Suburban	7	35%
Practice Region		
North	5	25%
Central	8	40%
South	7	35%
	Mean	**Standard Deviation**
Percent of pediatric patients enrolled in Medicaid/CHIP	58.70	22.27
Percent Pediatric patients enrolled in Medicaid/CHIP that have special health care needs	31.34	20.20
Number of Full Time Employees	15	13

Table 2: Practice Characteristics.

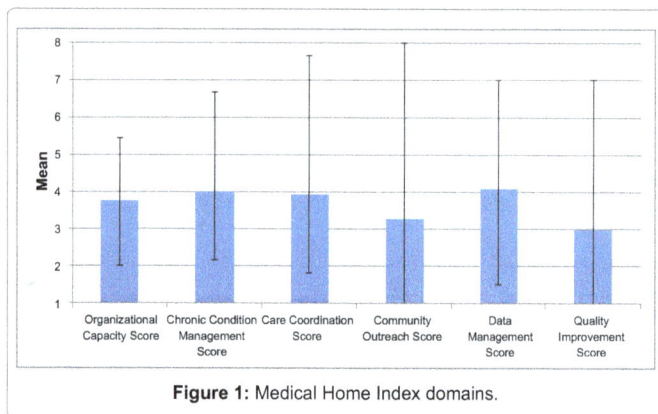

Figure 1: Medical Home Index domains.

Figure 2 presents the kappa value as well as the distributions across the dichotomized levels of agreement (high and low). Thirty percent of the staff members were in high levels of agreement with their lead physician and 23.5% were in low levels of agreement with their lead physician. Agreement was mixed for 46.4% of the staff (17.6% High-Low and 28.8% Low-High). The kappa value was 0.08 (Z=1.05; Probability>Z=0.15).

Multivariate results

Table 4 presents the results of the logistic regression where the binary agreement variable (1=high-high, and 0=otherwise) is the dependent variable. Results suggest that staff aged 41 to 50, as opposed to the referent group (aged 20 to 30), are associated with almost six times the odds of being in the high-high agreement category (Odds ratio=5.78). Small and large sized practices, as opposed to solo practices, are significantly less likely to be associated with high-high agreement (Odds ratios=0.161 and 0.039, respectively).

Table 5 shows the results of the ordinary least squared regression where the dependent variable is the total MHI score. Three variables were found to be significantly associated with the MHI score. Non-clinical positions are associated with a 3.128 decrease in the MHI total score. A one unit increase in the number of full time employees is associated with a 0.358 increase in the MHI total score. A one percentage point increase in the percent of patients enrolled in Medicaid or CHIP that has a special health care need is associated with a 0.550 increase in the MHI total score.

Rank	Item Description	Mean Score
1	Most people in this practice are willing to change how they do things in response to feedback from others.	0.14
2	People in this practice have the information that they need to do their jobs well	0.13
3	Leadership in this practice creates an environment where things can be accomplished.	0.12
4	Difficult problems are solved through face-to-face discussions in this practice.	0.11
5	People in our practice actively seek new ways to improve how we do things.	0.10
6	Leadership strongly supports practice change efforts.	0.08
7	The practice leadership makes sure that we have the time and space necessary to discuss changes to improve care.	0.08
8	People at all levels of this office openly talk about what is and isn't working.	0.08
9	Practice leadership promotes an environment that is an enjoyable place to work.	0.07
10	Mistakes have led to positive changes here.	0.06
11	This practice encourages everyone (front office staff, clinical staff, nurses, and clinicians) to share ideas.	0.06
12	Most of the people who work in our practice seem to enjoy their work.	0.05
13	We regularly take time to reflect on how we do things.	0.04
14	This practice learns from its mistakes.	0.03
15	This practice is a place of joy and hope.	0.03
16	I have many opportunities to grow in my work.	0.03
17	It is hard to get things to change in our practice.	0.03
18	When we experience a problem in the practice we make a serious effort to figure out what's really going on.	0.02
19	I can rely on the other people in this practice to do their jobs well.	0.02
20	We regularly take time to consider ways to improve how we do things.	0.02
21	People in this practice operate as a real team.	0.01
22	After trying something new, we take time to think about how it worked.	0.01
23	People are aware of how their actions affect others in this practice.	0.01

Note: Mean Score is calculated by first subtracting staff adaptive reserve score from practice adaptive reserve score for each item. Then for each item that difference is averaged and put in absolute values. Finally the items are ranked from least congruence to most congruence, where a larger mean score means the difference between practice and staff adaptive reserve scores is greatest, i.e. least congruent

Table 3: Rank of the 23 Items of the Adaptive Reserve.

Discussion

Results from our descriptive and multivariate analyses extend the pediatric medical home literature in several ways. Taking an inventory of adaptive reserve is an important first step in developing strategies to improve needed alignment. Results from our adaptive reserve item level congruence analyses point to several areas where the practices could focus their efforts on improving alignment between staff and lead physician. For example, incongruence was noted for the statement "Difficult problems are solved through face-to-face discussions." Setting aside a time to routinely meet face-to-face with the staff likely allows for reflection, problem solving, planning, and information sharing. This may seem difficult given the competing demands on time, but could reap benefits in the short and long term [19,20]. Strategies for the individual items will vary in duration and intensity. However, these human interactions should be considered investments, just as is purchasing an electronic medical record system.

Congruence across all practices in our study was slight (kappa=0.08). This points to needed adjustments at the practice level and to groups of practices seeking to transform themselves to a medical home. Medical home facilitators should be trained to measure and address adaptive reserve by including this topic in their curriculum. For example, AHRQ created a guide on developing and running a practice facilitator program in 2011 [21]. Although the term adaptive reserve is not mentioned specifically, the guide notes that facilitators should be trained in "concepts and strategies for empowering staff and building organizational capacity." Likewise, the NCQA recently introduce its NCQA PCMH Content Expert Certification [22]. It is unclear if that certification program emphasizes the human infrastructure that is needed to become a medical home, but this may be another platform to ensure that the issue is addressed.

Our multivariate findings suggest more alignment between staff and lead physician with older staff and less alignment in practices with more than one physician.

The latter finding is somewhat expected since aligning staff and physician adaptive reserve should be easier when there is only one physician in the practice. When there is more than one physician in a practice these physicians might have different management styles, personalities, and practice patterns all of which could affect adaptive reserve. In a multi-physician practice, subtle challenges might also emerge, through ownership or title for example, where only one physician is the lead physician. Practices with multiple physicians may also have to implement strategies to align themselves before working on staff alignment. Older staff might be better aligned with their lead physician because they understand the importance of, and need for, change. Older staff may also be more perceptive to their leaders' style and understand the benefits that can come from alignment.

Although not statistically significant, results from our multivariate model suggest that greater differences between staff and lead physician adaptive reserve scores were associated with a decrease in the total MHI score. Our hypothesis was not confirmed, however, it is possible that longitudinal data might yield different results. Future research should investigate how adaptive reserve congruence changes as practices journey through the medical home transformation process.

Limitations exist in our study that merit mentioning. Our response rate for the staff survey was 42.6%, which is comparable to other surveys of health care workers [23]. Unfortunately, we do not have any information about the non-responders. The lead physician's adaptive reserve score may not be representative of the organization's adaptive reserve. In a large group practice the lead physician may be able to influence the local practice environment but there may be

	Odds Ratio
	High-High Agreement
Years Worked in Practice	
6-10 years	1.174
	(0.645)
11-15 years	2.742
	(1.692)
16-20 years	3.043
	(2.532)
20+ years	1.644
	(1.318)
Age	
30 to 40 years old	1.596
	(0.862)
41 to 50 years old	5.777***
	(4.015)
50+ years old	0.961
	(0.654)
Race	
Black	0.470
	(0.408)
Hispanic	3.126
	(1.939)
Asian	4.432
	(6.015)
Other race categories	0.196
	(0.254)
Clinic Position	
Non-clinician	2.784
	(1.508)
Sex	
Male	1.192
	(0.657)
Practice Size	
Small (3 or less)	0.161**
	(0.139)
Large practice (more than 3)	0.039***
	(0.0423)
Practice Region	
Suburban	0.220
	(0.207)
North	2.655
	(2.480)
South	1.225
	(1.213
Number of Full time Employees	1.050
	(0.054)
% of patients enrolled in Medicaid/CHIP	1.018
	(0.023)
% of patients enrolled in Medicaid/CHIP that have special healthcare needs	0.994
	(0.023)
Number of Observations	169

Note: **=significant at the 5% level, ***=significant at the 1% level. Practice and Staff Adaptive Reserve Score is the dependent variable and is a categorical variable that takes a value of 1 when there is high agreement (Practice and Staff both have high adaptive reserve scores) and 0 when there is low agreement (Practice has high adaptive reserve score and Staff has low adaptive reserve score, vice versa, and Practice and Staff both have low adaptive reserve). Reference groups are: 20 to 30 years old, White, non-Hispanic, clinical staff, 0 to 5 years of experience, solo practice, urban, and central Florida

Table 4: Logistic regression.

	Total MHI Score
Adaptive Reserve Congruence Score	-0.288
	(0.888)
Years Worked in Practice	
6-10 years	-1.094
	(1.394)
11-15 years	-1.631
	(1.313)
16-20 years	(-4.074)
	(2.709)
20+ years	-7.077
	(4.419)
Age	
30 to 40 years old	-0.525
	(0.928)
41 to 50 years old	1.335
	(1.408)
50+ years old	3.097
	(2.033)
Race	
Black	-0.022
	(1.366)
Hispanic	-1.979
	(1.715)
Asian	0.338
	(1.613)
Other race categories	4.866
	(4.446)
Clinic Position	
Non-clinician	-3.128**
	(1.498)
Sex	
Male	-1.525
	(0.795)
Practice Size	
Small (3 or less)	-9.906
	(7.697)
Large practice (more than 3)	-8.233
	(8.022)
Practice Region	
Suburban	0.432
	(3.723)
North	0.634
	(2.430)
South	-6.171
	(5.293)
Number of Full time Employees	0.358***
	(0.135)
% of patients enrolled in Medicaid/CHIP	0.031
	(0.129)
% of patients enrolled in Medicaid/CHIP that have special healthcare needs	0.550***
	(0.061)
R-Squared	0.877
Root MSE	5.630
Number of Observations	169

Note: **=significant at the 5% level, ***=significant at the 1% level. Total MHI Score is the dependent variable and it is out of 80. Practice and Staff Adaptive Reserve Score is a categorical variable that takes a value of 1 when there is high agreement (Practice and Staff both have high adaptive reserve scores) and 0 when there is low agreement (Practice has high adaptive reserve score and Staff has low adaptive reserve score, vice versa, and practice and staff both have low adaptive reserve). Reference groups are: 20 to 30 years old, White, non-Hispanic, clinical staff, 0 to 5 years of experience, solo practice, urban, and central Florida

Table 5: Ordinary Least Squares Regression.

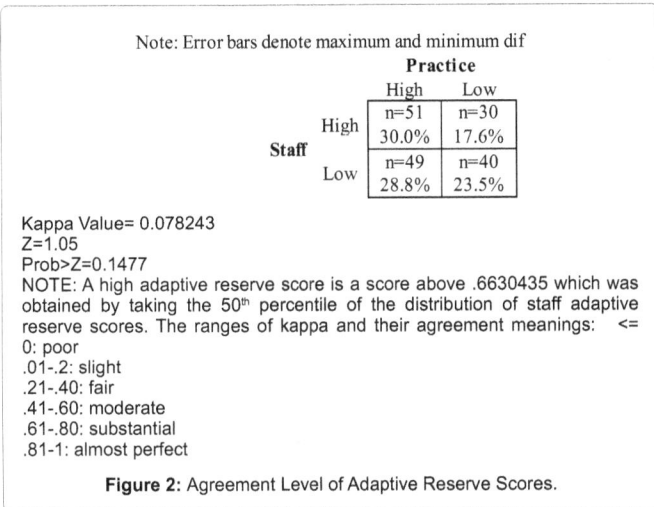

Note: Error bars denote maximum and minimum dif

		Practice	
		High	Low
Staff	High	n=51 30.0%	n=30 17.6%
	Low	n=49 28.8%	n=40 23.5%

Kappa Value= 0.078243
Z=1.05
Prob>Z=0.1477
NOTE: A high adaptive reserve score is a score above .6630435 which was obtained by taking the 50th percentile of the distribution of staff adaptive reserve scores. The ranges of kappa and their agreement meanings: <= 0: poor
.01-.2: slight
.21-.40: fair
.41-.60: moderate
.61-.80: substantial
.81-1: almost perfect

Figure 2: Agreement Level of Adaptive Reserve Scores.

organizational barriers that affect the staff's perspectives of the global environment. For example, the local practice might be a joyful place to work but the overall organization might be struggling financially and this could cause the staff to be stressed. In this case interventions to align the staff and lead physician at the local level might not improve adaptive reserve of the staff. Finally, the MHI was filled out by the core project team and the staff had no input in this measure. Perhaps the staff have different perspectives on whether or not the practice is a medical home.

Despite these limitations our results emphasize the importance of assessing professional experiences in medical home evaluations. Policy makers and health care planners should ensure that professional experiences are assessed and that staff are considered important stakeholders in these projects. Adaptive reserve inventories may inform more appropriately tailored integration of the PCMH model, or at least, they may help forewarn system administrators of potential barriers in its implementation. Practices that do not employ facilitators or participate in a formal facilitation program can still benefit from improving alignment of staff. Disregarding this important concept might affect the long term sustainability of the medical home.

Funding acknowledgment

This document was developed under grant CFDA 93.767 from the U.S. Department of Health and Human Services, Centers for Medicare & Medicaid Services. However, these contents do not necessarily represent the policy of the U.S. Department of Health and Human Services, and you should not assume endorsement by the Federal Government.

References

1. Sia C, Tonniges TF, Osterhus E, Taba S (2004) History of the medical home concept. Pediatrics 113: 1473-1478.

2. Kilo CM, Wasson JH (2010) Practice redesign and the patient-centered medical home: history, promises, and challenges. Health Aff (Millwood) 29: 773-778.

3. (1992) American Academy of Pediatrics Ad Hoc Task Force on Definition of the Medical Home: The medical home. Pediatrics 90: 774.

4. The medical home (2002) Pediatrics. Jul;110: 184-186.

5. American Academy of Family Physicians (2008) Joint principles of the Patient-Centered Medical Home. Del Med J 80: 21-22.

6. http://www.medicalhomeinfo.org/. Accessed March 8, 2013.

7. Patient Protection and Affordable Care Act (2010), 124 Stat. 119.

8. Homer CJ, Klatka K, Romm D, Kuhlthau K, Bloom S, et al. (2008) A review of the evidence for the medical home for children with special health care needs. Pediatrics 122: e922-937.

9. Stroebel CK, McDaniel RR Jr, Crabtree BF, Miller WL, Nutting PA, et al. (2005) How complexity science can inform a reflective process for improvement in primary care practices. Jt Comm J Qual Patient Saf 31: 438-446.

10. Lanham HJ, McDaniel RR, Crabtree BF, Miller WL, Stange KC, et al. (2009) How Improving Practice Relationships Among Clinicians and Nonclinicians Can Improve Quality in Primary Care. Jt Comm J Qual Patient Saf 35: 457-466.

11. Nutting PA, Crabtree BF, Miller WL, Stewart EE, Stange KC, et al. (2010) Journey to the patient-centered medical home: a qualitative analysis of the experiences of practices in the National Demonstration Project. Ann Fam Med 8 Suppl 1: S45-56.

12. American Academy of Pediatrics. Quality Improvement Innovation Networks (QuIIN). 2013

13. Centers for Medicare and Medicaid Services, Center for Medicaid CHIP and Survey & Certification, Children and Adults Health Programs Group. CHIPRA Initial Core Set Technical Specifications Manual 2011. 2011.

14. Jaen CR, Crabtree BF, Palmer RF (2010) Methods for evaluating practice change toward a patient-centered medical home. Ann Fam Med 8 Suppl 1: S9-20; S92.

15. Cooley WC, McAllister JW, Sherrieb K, Clark RE (2003) The Medical Home Index: development and validation of a new practice-level measure of implementation of the Medical Home model. Ambul Pediatr 3: 173-180.

16. Viera AJ, Garrett JM (2005) Understanding interobserver agreement: the kappa statistic. Fam Med 37: 360-363.

17. Lewis SE, Nocon RS, Tang H, Park SY, Vable AM, et al. (2012) Patient-centered medical home characteristics and staff morale in safety net clinics. Arch Intern Med 172: 23-31.

18. Stata Statistical Software: Release 12 [computer program]. College Station, TX: StataCorp LP; 2011.

19. Zickafoose JS, Clark SJ, Sakshaug JW, Chen LM, Hollingsworth JM (2013) Readiness of primary care practices for medical home certification. Pediatrics 131: 473-482.

20. Hollingsworth JM, Saint S, Sakshaug JW, Hayward RA, Zhang L, et al. (2012) Physician practices and readiness for medical home reforms: policy, pitfalls, and possibilities. Health Serv Res 47: 486-508.

21. http://pcmh.ahrq.gov/sites/default/files/attachments/Developing_and_Running_a_Primary_Care_Practice_Facilitation_Program.pdf

22. National Committee for Quality Assurance (2012). PCMH Content Expert Certification (CEC) Handbook. Washington, DC: NCQA

23. Thompson LA, Knapp C, Madden V, Shenkman E (2009) Pediatricians' perceptions of and preferred timing for pediatric palliative care. Pediatrics 123: e777-782.

8

Data Analytics and Operational Data Integration to Reach Out to Rural Masses for Early Detection of Non-Communicable Diseases

Vanishri Arun¹*, Shyam V² and Padma SK¹

¹Department of Information Science and Engineering, Sri Jayachamarajendra College of Engineering, Mysore– 570 006, India
²Forus Health Private Ltd., Bengaluru – 560070, India

Abstract

This paper demonstrates the analysis of healthcare data and integration of operational data to abate the prevalence incidence of non-communicable diseases (NCD). Pilot experiments have been carried out in Suttur village, by screening the masses for early detection of NCDs. An app has been developed to record patient profile onto a tablet. The record is synchronized to update the database on the cloud where the repository is maintained. This provides an efficient way of analysis and statistics to the huge amount of health data. ETL (Extract, Transform and Load) is a process used to extract data from data repository and transform the data based on user requirements and store in a target database as a single repository which helps to achieve goals proactively and on time. The main aim of this paper is to generate reports from the collection of health data by using tools like QlikView for Business Objects as a front end tool for generation of reports and charts, Oracle 11g as backend tool for creation of data repository and Talend Open Studio 5.4 as an ETL tool. We conclude that ETL systems enable a smooth migration from one system to another. By creating an ETL script for each system, data can be stored in a consistent format in the repository. The source system can then be changed, without any impact on the repository or the reporting/analysis systems. Therefore there are phenomenal improvements in turnaround time for data access and reporting. The entire health data can be standardized as there will be one view of information. Health data synced by various sources from different places can be merged to create a more comprehensive information source. This leads to reduction in costs to create and distribute information and reports and also helps in reduction of prevalence incidence of NCDs.

Keywords: Healthcare; Non-Communicable diseases; ETL; Talend open studio; Qlikview

Introduction

The mortality rate due to Non-communicable diseases (NCDs) is increasing and 75% of Indians in rural villages are the victims of NCDs such as Diabetes, Hypertension and Obesity which represent global burden of diseases and cause deaths each year mainly in rural areas [1]. This is in turn affecting the economic conditions of the people. The health-related datasets provide access to patient information to study, analyze and report the health conditions and outcomes for making decisions, policies and to develop processes [2,3].

Data warehouse has been defined by Bill Inmon as a subject-oriented which can be used to analyze a particular subject area, integrated which integrates data from multiple sources, time-variant which enables to retrieve historical data and non-volatile collection of data in support of management's decision making process [4]. Ralph Kimball defines data warehouse as a system that extracts, cleans, conforms, and delivers source data into a dimensional data store and then supports and implements querying and analysis for the purpose of decision makes [5]. In this paper, data warehouse has been modeled to analyze to improve outcomes, safety and patient satisfaction. And accordingly the database is structured. The data warehouse consists of tools to extract data from the multiple operational databases and other external sources, to clean, transform and integrate these data and to load into the data warehouse [6].The health data collected are stored and managed in the warehouse. Data marts present multidimensional views of data to a variety of front end tools like query tools, report writers, analysis tools, and data mining tools [7]. Data warehouse provides an effective way of analysis and statistics to the huge amount of data and helps in decision making. The concept of ETL is followed which means Extract, Transform and Load where data from different sources are extracted, stored in a single repository and analyzed for supporting decision making. Data warehouse enables extraction of information from more than one area and have a single view of information used for

decision making. In healthcare sector, in order to store all the patient data, a tool is used which is a comprehensive Adverse Event (AE) tracking and reporting system which will be used as a source for any ETL tool for generating the report in order to investigate the results and provide regulatory authorities to take necessary actions. Available data sets from the authorities as a source for data analysis and report generation may also be used. Early diagnosis of NCDs is beneficial in enabling less invasive diagnostic evaluation and treatment. It also accelerates the timeline for intervention, reduces the scale and costs of medication and other interventions and May also increases mortality rate or at least delay the onset of symptoms which helps to maximize patient quality of life. Therefore there is a burning need for an effective screening system for early detection, analysis and reporting of NCD in rural areas. Many programs have been launched by the government and Non-governmental organizations to screen the rural masses to identify the individuals at risk and take necessary actions. But the bottleneck for all these programs has been the acute shortage of specialists and experts to screen analyze and report [8].The analysis of the data collected is manually done by Community medicine personnel and reports are generated.

The effectiveness of NCDs screening and utilization of experts time rely on the platform which is offering screening, management of referrals and deskilling. The objective of this work is to develop and

*Corresponding author: Vanishri Arun, Department of Information Science and Engineering, Sri Jayachamarajendra College of Engineering, Mysore–570006, India, E-mail: vanishriarun@gmail.com

measure the efficiency of screening the rural masses for NCDs and the analysis of the information flow, patient referrals and follow-ups providing an intelligent, affordable and accessible system that involves deskilling and optimization.

This study is done in association with the Department of Community Medicine, JSS Hospital, Mysuru, India, which is a 1800-bedded hospital offering comprehensive medical services. JSS Hospital has taken up several projects involving community health survey, health education & treatment for various ailments in Sri Kshethra Suttur village which is situated in Nanjangud Taluk, Mysuru District, Karnataka ,India. It has a population of nearly 5,000. This is an on-going project in which charts and reports are generated to serve various departments of the hospital to take necessary actions or conduct various programs related to the patients' health in the 13 villages of Sri Kshethra Suttur, Mysuru, India. As per guidelines issued by JSS Medical College, screening involves simple clinical examination comprising of relevant questions and easily conducted physical measurements such as demographic details, history of diabetes, history of tobacco and alcohol consumption and measurement of blood pressure, blood sugar, height, abdominal circumference etc. These data stored in the warehouse are then used to periodically generate reports and charts based on queries.

Existing system

Mart is designed for analytical and reporting purposes and also as a data provider for the downstream applications in Reporting and Analytics such as Dashboards/Graphs. Due to the nature of data in the source application there is a possibility of sparsely populated record set in the source application. And as per the regulatory guidelines certain information need to be captured as reported without any corrections to the data [9].

Owing to the above, it is understood that the source data can be incomplete in many instances. This key consideration is being taken into account while populating and accessing the data using ETL process. Existing data (legacy and data that is available on the initial run) will be loaded on the first run. Thereafter, only incremental data will be captured and processed during every subsequent run. Any updates within the case version will be captured and maintained as Slowly Changing Dimensions (SCD) [9].

Fetching the data from various sources requires sequential query fetching and output will be generated as excel sheet which has several drawbacks in which user should know the concept of Database queries and identification of required data in millions of records which is tedious. Since excel sheets are used, it has many limitations which mean it stores only 256 columns. Adding such kind of sheets in millions reduces the performance to fetch the data. Hence to improve this, database concept is used where sequential query fetching for the end users is a tedious job.

Therefore limitations of the existing system are sequential query fetching, redundancy in data and requirement of query language by experts to fetch the data from data base. To overcome these limitations, a system is modeled to develop and measure the efficiency of screening and the analysis of the records using Oracle Schema creation, DDL statements creation, Talend software to create and run jobs and Qlikview for analysis and reporting.

Methodology

This is an ongoing project undertaken in association with the Department of Community medicine, JSS Medical College, Mysuru

and Primary Healthcare Centre, Sri Kshethra Suttur, Nanjangud Taluk, Mysuru, to reach out to the rural masses. Pilot experiments have been carried out in Suttur Mysuru, by screening the masses for early detection and analysis and reporting of non-communicable diseases. An app has been developed to record patient demographics, vitals and other details onto tablets. These tabs are given to Community health workers who covered 13 villages of Suttur, go door-to-door and recorded patient demographics by screening for vitals like BP, Sugar, abdominal circumference, etc., [10]. A total of 150 cases were screened and values were recorded on the tab.

These records are synchronized to update the data warehouse on the cloud where the repository is maintained. The cloud is maintained at Forus Health Pvt. Ltd., Bengaluru. The data warehouse is in a denormalized form with duplications or incomplete entries in the source layer. Then the warehouse is normalized in the staging area where duplicate, redundant and incomplete records are removed or filtered. This normalized and cleansed database (target database) is connected to reporting layer which displays only required data based on the selection criteria of the user which are used for analysis and reporting. Data warehouse are refreshed periodically by extracting, transforming, cleaning and consolidating data from several operational data sources. The data in the warehouse is then used to periodically generate reports, or to rebuild multidimensional views of the data for on-line querying and analysis.

Proposed system

The overall system architecture of the proposed system is as Shown in Figure 1

The system is grouped into the following areas or layers of the warehouse.

Source layer: Source layer contains data from different databases across Suttur villages which are in de-normalized form i.e., databasing with redundant data [11]. Due to some reason a patient record could be entered more than once by the community health worker. This layer is not accessible to end user for report generation.

Staging area: The information in this layer is typically a copy of the source system (or operational system) data along with some cleaning (filtering out error records), control and audit events. Staging area is strictly a Data Warehouse layer and no access will be given to the business users. Therefore reports cannot be run against this area. This area ensures that the window of access to the source system is minimal. At the same time, it is ensured that all the data required for running the daily cycle is available in the Data Warehouse. The frequency of the load is configurable. These processes may apply consistency, standardization of structure, data cleansing, business rule transformation etc. The Centralized Data Warehouse (CDW) layer is generally in the Third Normal Form (3NF) i.e., reduction of duplicate or redundant data [11], in which all the duplicate and redundant records are removed, which can also contain de-normalized tables.

Data mart: It's a subset of Data Warehouse normally referred to as target database. The Data Mart is based on Dimensional modeling which uses the concepts of facts (measures), and dimensions (context) [11]. This is the ideal place for analytical reports and dash boards to be generated. This contains aggregated tables at various levels. This is fully normalized and cleansed required data schema and the reporting layer is directly connected to this database. All the operations performed in the dashboard of the reports will be directly handled by the Data Mart.

Report layer: Finally report layer is the front end of the Data Mart

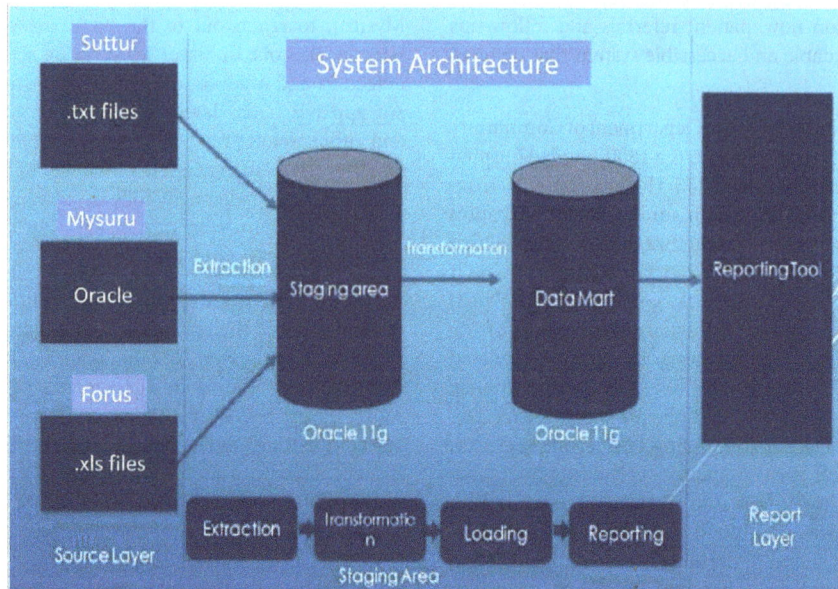

Figure 1: System architecture of Data Warehouse application.

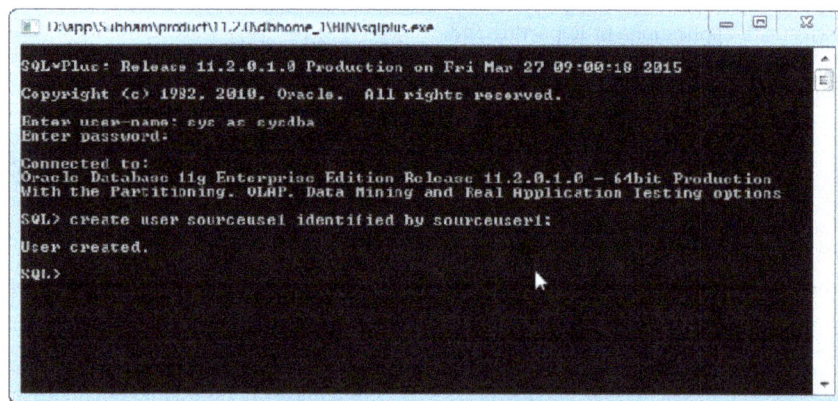

Figure 2: User creation.

for user friendliness which displays only required data based on the selection criteria of the user [12].

Implementation

The following 4 modules are implemented in this application:

1. Oracle Schema creation.

2. Creation of DDL statements.

3. Create and Run jobs using Talend software.

4. Reporting layer

Oracle schema creation

This section explains the creation of Oracle users in order to load the data at various levels (i.e. source, staging and target).

Open the Oracle installed and login to Oracle as system user and create Oracle user by using the syntax below. Use the CREATE USER statement to create and configure a database user, which is an account through which you can log in to the database, and to establish the

means by which Oracle Database permits access by the user as Shown in Figure 2.

Syntax: Create user USERNAME identified by Password;

Once user is created, grant DBA privileges to the user so that user will have the respective privileges to create table and structures.

Syntax: Grant DBA to USERNAME; Shown in Figure 2-4. Data are collected from various community health workers going door-to-door in all the 13 villages of Suttur.The files in different tabs of source will be migrated to staging area with one to one mapping without any change but in single format (Oracle 11g) this staging area is exact replica of source in single format as shown in Fig 4. All the data in staging area are in denormalized form and cleaning/filtering is required to remove duplicate/incomplete records. Some of the fields are Age_group, Hyper_tension, Family_income, etc., which are migrated to staging area without any change.

Staging to target: The data flow between staging and target is depicted in Fig 5 where business logic is applied and all the tables' primary keys of staging area will be moved to the fact table where they

Figure 3: Grant DBA to User.

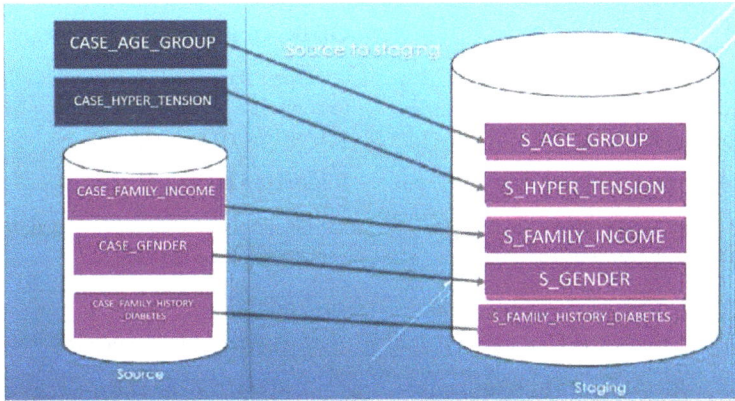

Figure 4: Source to staging data flow.

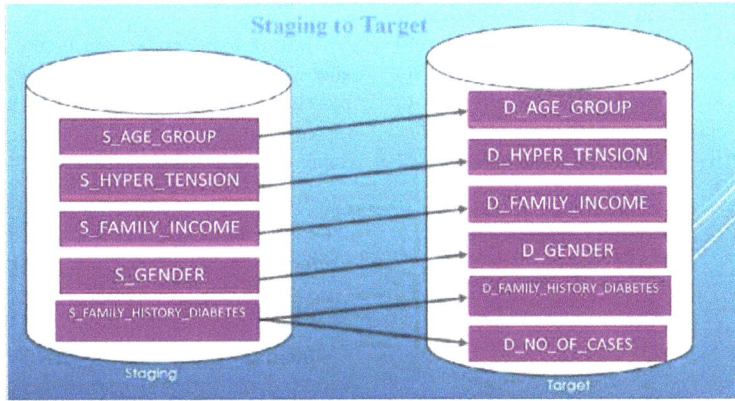

Figure 5: Staging to target dataflow.

act as foreign keys. All cleaned data in normalized form after joining all the required tables will be obtained as star schema structure in target database. For e.g., source S_Age_group which is in denormalized form is transformed into normalized D_Age_group (Figure 5).

Target to reporting: The data flow between target and report layer is depicted in Fig 6 where databases are fetched on the selection criteria

with the help of Business Objects (BO) tools and it will internally fetch the required columns and display the data as an output on the dashboard as per the requirements. For e.g., the normalized fields D_Age_group, D_Hyper_tension, D_Family_income, etc., are ready to be presented to the Report layer. Based on the user query, fields are fetched and related charts and reports are generated (Figure 6).

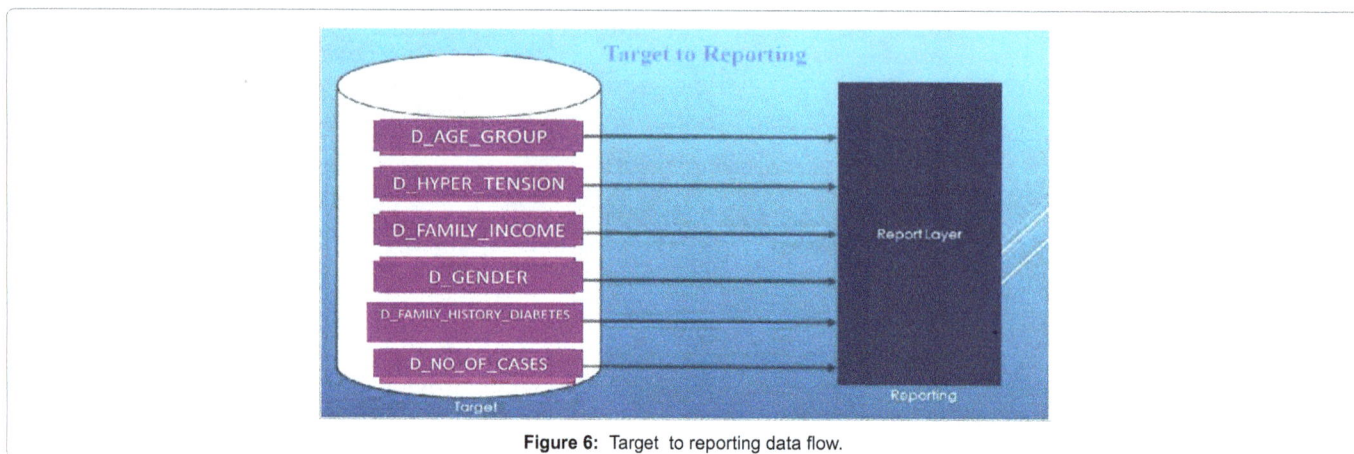

Figure 6: Target to reporting data flow.

Creation of DDL statements: Creation of tables/structures for the Oracle users based on the data modeling design document is done in this step.

Create/import jobs using talent software

Stage jobs creation: Once the source data preparation is done, read data from source and load to the stage. The sources may be database files/text files/excel files. One-to-one mapping from source to staging and no cleaning of data are required. In the query section the data from the source is read by selecting all the columns [13].

Various components are used to read the data from different sources namely:

a. t Oracle input: To reads the data from the data base.

b. t File list: To read the data from textfiles.

c. t File Input Excel: To read the data from excel files.

Once it is all set click the run button in order to read the data from source to staging. After successful run the stage jobs verify the data loaded properly in the stage schema. Similarly load the data from different sources. Once one to one mapping of data loading from source to staging apply the business logics in order to clean the data by selecting only the relevant records in the query section and load into the target database. After reading data from stage schema store data into the target database using Oracle SCD components which allow to change the dimension of the table before loading into the target. After successful run of the target data, verify whether relevant data are loaded

by logging into the target schema database. Ensure that all the data are loaded properly and perform unit testing for the data loaded. Then this should act as a source to the report layer to fetch data. The data loaded successfully can be verified by cross checking the target database details which ensures that Data cleansing and Data denormalizations are done.

ODBC connections from target to report layer

Open Database Connectivity (ODBC) is a protocol that can be used to connect a Microsoft Access database to an external data source such as Oracle/server.

Reporting layer

Once the data source is added, load the data into the front end by performing the following;

1. Open the Qlikview.

2. Design the Qlikview.

3. Reload the configuration.

While reloading the process, it will fetch the data from the target database and display in the front end. The data display can be modified with various selection criteria.

Ensure that Oracle Data Base Connection (ODBC) connection is successful and select the data source of target ODBC and click on load by selecting the various chart types and selection criteria. The data are displayed in report format on the front end as shown in Figures 7-9, Table 1.

Table 1 is the report generated in tabular form for the selected criteria. Totally 150 cases were imported to source layer in denormalized form. After normalization, the total cases were filtered to 145.

Result and Discussion

Main aim of our project is to generate reports by collecting data from various data sources by transforming data from sources and loading in a Data Warehouse repository. Different data, based on various selection criteria can be selected. After data are loaded, verify for the correctness of data by querying in the backend. Thereby the count from target to

Old	M	N	Y	Y	N	Extreme lower	1
Old	M	Y	N	Unknown	Y	Extremelower	1
Old	M	Y	N	Y	Y	Extremelower	1
Old	M	Y	Y	Unknown	Y	Extremelower	1
Old	M	Y	Y	Y	Y	Extremelower	1
Young	F	N	N	N	Y	Extremelower	1
Young	M	N	N	N	Y	Extremelower	1
Young	M	Y	Y	Y	Y	ExtremeLower	1

Table 1: Report in the form of Excel sheet generated for the criteria above.

AGE_GROUP	GENDER	DRINKING HISTORY	SMOKER	HYPER_ TENSION	FAMILYHISTORY DIABETES	FAMILY INCOME	CasesCount
Middle	F	N	N	Y	Y	Extreme Lower	1

Table 2: Case Count =1 with the selected criteria.

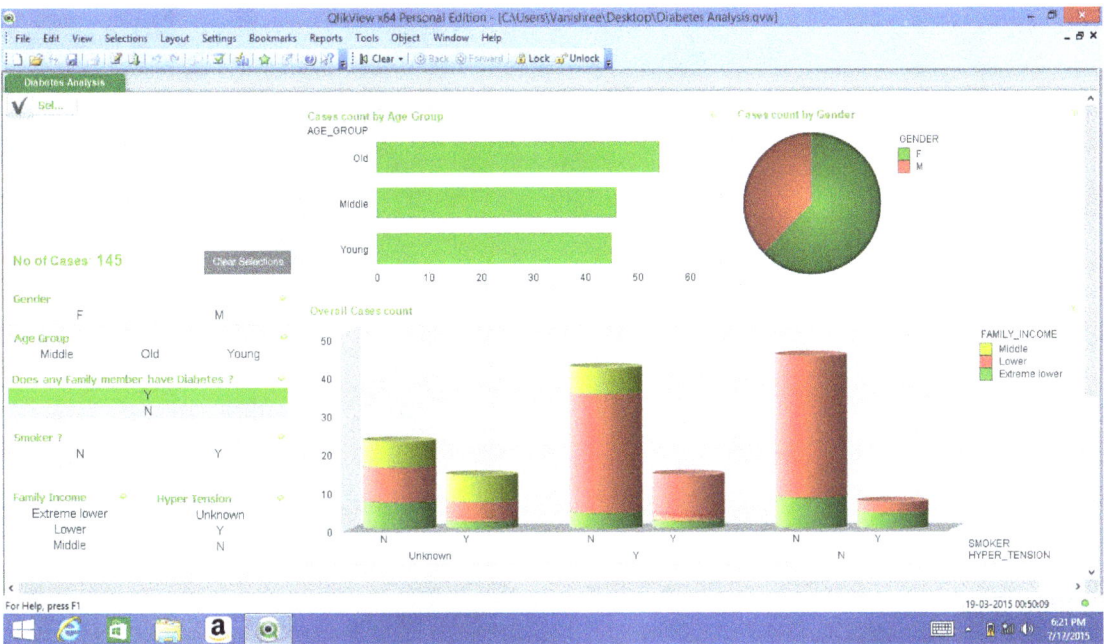

Figure 7: Chart generated without any Criterion with No. of cases = 145.

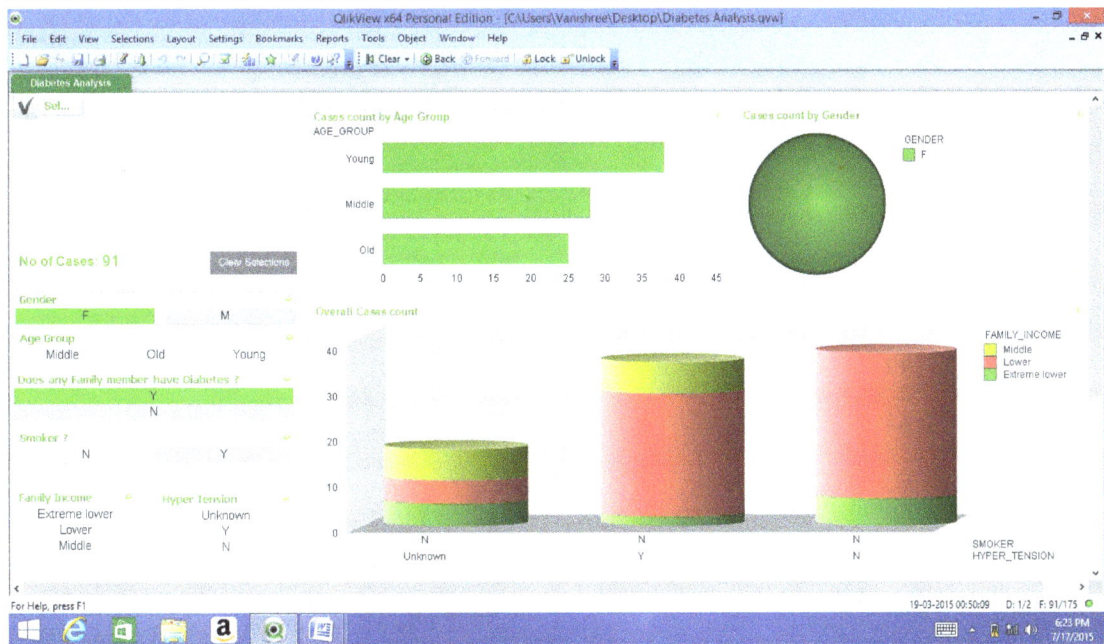

Figure 8: Cases by GENDER="Female".

reporting can be matched. Reports are generated in the form of charts and tables. It is also easy to analyze the report and check the severity of the cases (Table 2).

Table 2 depicts the number of case count with the criteria, Age_ group between 30 and 50 years, Gender being female, with no alcohol and smoking history, BP > 120/80, with a family member being diabetic and economically poor background. This helps the patient to know her health status, the health worker alerts the patient of the complications, clinical intervention and treatment required. It also helps the Department of Community Medicine to have a statistical and disease analysis of these rural areas to take necessary actions.

Conclusion and Future Enhancement

A key use for ETL systems is to enable a smooth migration from one system to another. By creating an ETL script for each system, data can be stored in a consistent format in the data warehouse. The source system can then be changed, without any impact on the data warehouse or the reporting/analysis systems. It has the following advantages:

1.   Phenomenal improvements in turnaround time for data access and reporting.

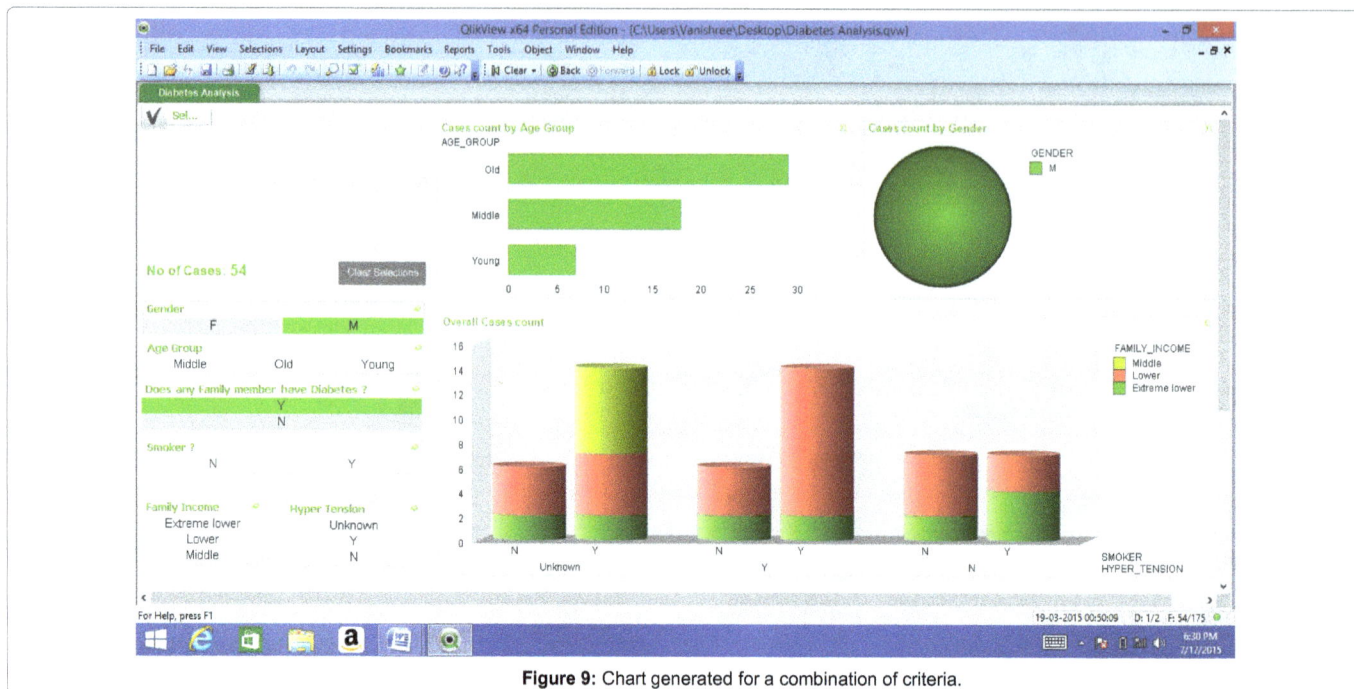

Figure 9: Chart generated for a combination of criteria.

2. Standardizing data across the organization so that there will be one view of information.

3. Merging data from various source systems to create a more comprehensive information source.

4. Reduction in costs to create and distribute information and reports.

5. Helps in informing the public health system of the prevalence of various routine disease conditions.

6. Prepares the health system to respond to unforeseen epidemics so that effective therapy is given at the right time and place.

Since open source software's are used in developing this system, it is sufficient to build the databases through the app which can be installed on tabs. People with minimum computer literacy can use the app and fill in the information where most of the fields have drop-down menus to select options.

As future enhancement, it is intended to port the app on to smart phones which are handy and using the fields available in the data warehouse, predict related diseases to abate the prevalence incidence of various diseases.

References

1. Olivia Namusisi, Juliet N Sekandi, Simon Kasasa, Peter Wasswa, Nicholas T Kamara, et al. (2011) Risk factors for non-communicable diseases in rural Uganda: a pilot surveillance project among diabetes patients at a referral hospital clinic. Pan Afr Med J 10:47.

2. Stead WW, Searle JR, Fessler HE, Smith JW, Shortliffe EH (2011) Biomedical informatics: changing what physicians need to know and how they learn. Acad Med 86: 429–434.

3. Murdoch TB, Detsky AS (2013) The inevitable application of big data to health care. JAMA 309: 1351–1352.

4. W. H. Inmon (2002) "Building The Data Warehouse".Wiley Computer Publishing.

5. Ralph Kimball, Joe Casertam (2004) The Data Warehouse ETL Toolkit.

6. Laura Hadley (2002) Developing a Data Warehouse Architecture.

7. Surajit, Chaudhuri, Umeshwar Dayal (1997) An Overview of Data Warehousing and OLAP Technology.

8. M. G. Deo (2013) "Doctor population ratio for India - The reality". Indian J Med Res 137: 632–635.

9. Marek Wancerz, Paweł Wancerz , " History management of data – slowly changing dimensions".

10. Abdullah A. Aljumah, Mohammed Gulam Ahamad, Mohammad Khubeb Siddiqui (2013) "Application of data mining: Diabetes health care in young and old patients", Journal of King Saud University – Computer and Information Sciences 25: 127–136.

11. https://www.en.wikipedia.org

12. Dario Antonellia, Elena Baralisb, Giulia Brunoa, Tania Cerquitellib, Silvia Chiusanob, et al. (2013) "Analysis of diabetic patients through their examination history". Expert Systems with Applications 40: 4672–4678.

13. Talend Infosense Solution Brief Master Data Management for Health Care Reference Data: White Paper.

9

Depression and Health Risk Behaviors: Towards Optimizing Primary Care Service Strategies for Addressing Risk

Joan Rosenbaum Asarnow[1*,] Luis Roberto Zeledon[2], Elizabeth D'Amico[3], Anne LaBorde[2], Martin Anderson[1], Claudia Avina[4], Talin Arslanian[5], Minh-Chau Do[6], Jessica Harwood[1] and Steven Shoptaw[1]

[1]UCLA School of Medicine, Los Angeles, California 90095, USA
[2]Kaiser Permanente Los Angeles Medical Center, Los Angeles, USA
[3]RAND, California, USA
[4]Harbor-UCLA Medical Center, Torrance, CA 90502, USA
[5]UC Davis School of Medicine, Sacramento, CA 95817, USA
[6]San Diego State/UCSD, San Diego, CA 92182, USA

Abstract

Purpose: Depression and health risk behaviors in adolescents are leading causes of preventable morbidity and mortality. Primary care visits provide prime opportunities to screen and provide preventive services addressing risk behaviors/conditions. This study evaluated the co-occurrence of depression and health risk behaviors (focusing on smoking, drug and alcohol misuse, risky sexual behavior, and obesity-risk) with the goal of informing preventive service strategies.

Methods: Consecutive primary care patients (n=217), ages 13 to 18 years, selected to over-sample for depression, completed a Health Risk Behavior Survey and the Diagnostic Interview Schedule for Children and Adolescents (DISC) depression module.

Results: Youths with DISC-defined past-year depression were significantly more likely to report risk across multiple risk-areas, Wald $X^2(1)$=14.39, p<.001, and to have significantly higher rates of past-month smoking, $X^2(1)$=5.86, p=.02, substance misuse, $X^2(1)$=15.12, p<.001, risky sex, $X^2 (1)$ =5.04, p=.03, but not obesity-risk, $X^2 (1)$ =0.19, p=.66. Cross-sectional predictors of risk behaviors across risk areas were similar. Statistically significant predictors across all risk domains included: youths' expectancies about future risk behavior; attitudes regarding the risk behavior; and risk behaviors in peers/others in their environments.

Conclusions: Depression in adolescents is associated with a cluster of health risk behaviors that likely contribute to the high morbidity and mortality associated with both depression and health risk behaviors. Consistent with the United States National Prevention Strategy (2011) and the focus on integrated behavioral and medical health care, results suggest the value of screening and preventive services using combination strategies that target depression and multiple areas of associated health risk.

Clinical trial: Clinical Trial Registration Information: Reducing Health Risk Behavior and Improving Health in Adolescent Depression. Unique Identifier: NCT00461539. URL: http://www.clinicaltrials.gov.

Keywords: Depression; Health; Sex; Obesity; Smoking; Drug; Marijuana; Alcohol; Primary care

Introduction

Depression is a common problem, associated with significant morbidity and mortality [1]. Primary care is a frequent entry point into the health care system for depressed patients; and most adolescents have access to primary care [1-3]. The United States Preventive Services Task Force recommends primary care screening for depression in adolescents when evaluation and treatment are available(www.uspreventiveservicestaskforce. org/uspstf/uspschdepr.htm) [1]. This recommendation is supported by evidence that providing evidence-based depression care for adolescents through primary care is associated with improved patient outcomes, and consistent with the current emphasis on integrated behavioral and medical health care and Patient Centered Medical Homes [4,5].

Despite the promise of integrated medical and behavioral health care for enhancing access to care, there are a number of barriers to integrating depression and behavioral health care within primary care settings. These include: brief visits, the large number of conditions/behaviors requiring evaluation, provider perceptions of inadequate knowledge; and ambiguity/concerns regarding specialty care linkage. When depression care is offered through primary care, treatment rates are relatively low [4] perhaps related to the general focus on health vs. mental health.

Health risk behaviors (HRBs) such as smoking, substance misuse/abuse, risky sex, and obesity also contribute to adolescent morbidity/mortality and later health problems. Nationwide, tobacco, alcohol and drug abuse are leading preventable causes of death in the United States, [1] nearly half of new STD infections occur among youths ages 15-24 (cdc.gov/healthyyouth/sexualbehaviors), and roughly 28% of youths are overweight/obese. (cdc.gov/healthyyouth/yrbs/pdf/us_obesity_trend_yrbs.pdf). "Problem behavior theory" posits that "problem behavior proneness" is associated with the interaction of personality (attitudes, expectations), perceived environment, and behavior (rates of other problem-behaviors) systems, resulting in the co-occurrence of different HRBs, and is supported by some data indicating associations among HRBs and depression [1,6-11].

*Corresponding author: Joan Rosenbaum Asarnow, Department of Psychiatry, UCLA, Box 956968, 300 Medical Plaza, Suite 3310, CA 90095-6968, USA, E-mail: jasarnow@mednet.ucla.edu

This study evaluates the extent to which depression and four major domains of HRBs tend to co-occur, focusing on four common areas of health risk in adolescents which often extend into adulthood contributing to illness and early mortality: smoking, substance use, risky sexual behavior, and obesity risk. This study builds on prior work [7-11] and expands this work by looking at multiple domains of health risk within a primary care sample. Most prior work has used survey samples and/or examined a more limited range of health-risk areas. We also used brief screening measures that can be adapted for primary care screening programs.

Consistent with "problem behavior theory" and the concept of an underlying "problem-behavior proneness," [6] we predicted that primary care patients with depressive disorders, when compared to less depressed patients, would be significantly more likely to: 1) show a pattern of risk across multiple health-risk domains, and 2) have higher rates of HRBs within each risk-domain. To further inform preventive service strategies, we also conducted exploratory analyses focusing on each area of health-risk and examining whether similar attitudes and social/environmental influences contributed to risk across health risk-domains. If depression and HRBs co-occur and are associated with similar risk-processes, preventive services employing combination strategies that simultaneously target multiple HRBs and risk-processes are likely to be more effective than preventive service strategies that focus on a single risk-area.

Methods

This is the first paper on the 24-7 HEALTH study, a study examining depression and health risk behaviors among primary care patients from two diverse health care organizations purposely selected to include one managed care organization and a medical center accepting a variety of insurance plans. The study was approved by the institutional review boards from both participating organizations. Informed consent was obtained from all parents for youths <18 years, with informed assent from youth; and all youths over 18 years of age. This study reports on results from the baseline assessment. Future publications will focus on the intervention phase of the project.

Consecutive patients, ages 13-18 years inclusive, were invited to participate in the study. To oversample for depression, patients were asked to complete a 4-item depression screener while waiting for their appointments. Screener items included: 1) two Composite International Diagnostic Interview (CIDI) past-year depression items assessing dysphoric mood and anhedonia (as modified for adolescents in prior research); [4] and 2) two parallel items asking about dysphoria and anhedonia "often during the past month". Positive screens on any item resulted in study eligibility, with exclusions for functioning/characteristics that would interfere with study procedures: lives over 1 hour away from site; youth not English-speaking; parents not English or Spanish-speaking.

Screening involved anonymous voluntary questionnaires with no identifiable information, and was done with a waiver of parent informed consent, and most youths (88.7%) agreed to complete the anonymous screener (1324/1493), To enroll in the study, youths had to agree to allow contact with parents for informed consent and be willing to return to the clinic for assessments and the study intervention. Of 491 eligible participants, 279 completed informed consent/assent procedures with youths and parents, and 217 completed the study assessments in an additional clinic-visit. Enrollment occurred between December 2007 and November 2010.

Measures and Procedures

The NIMH Diagnostic Interview Schedule for Children (DISC-IV) depression module, a structured diagnostic interview with established inter-rater and test-retest reliability, was administered by trained interviewers using a computer assisted format [12]. Interviewers were trained, certified, and supervised by a senior staff member trained by the DISC development team. Quality assurance ratings completed on 20% of interviews (randomly selected) indicated strong quality (Mean=1.2, SD=0.54, 3-point scale 1=good to 3=poor).

Due to the sensitive nature of HRB questions, the HRB Survey was completed individually by youths at a private computer station, with assistance available if requested. The HRB Survey used items from the Youth Risk Behavior Survey [13], National Longitudinal Study of Adolescent Health [14], Monitoring the Future [15] and other national surveys [16,17]. Questions asked about: past-month smoking and substance use (alcohol, marijuana, other drugs) and attempts to cut down/quit [15,16]; sex without a condom, number of partners during the prior 6-months,Sexually Transmitted Infections/Diseases (STI/STD), and pregnancy [13,16]. Substance use-related impairment was assessed using the Substance Use Scale of the Problem Oriented Screening Instrument for Teenagers (POSIT) [18]. The Body Mass Index (BMI), based on objective measurement of height and weight by the study assessor, adjusted for sex and age (http://apps.nccd.cdc.gov/dnpabmi/), indexed obesity-risk. We also asked about: 1) expectancies that youth would have the "HRB" in 6-months?" [16,19] 2) attitudes regarding the health risk behavior [16,17,20]; 3) resistance self-efficacy [14,16,19]; 4) perceptions that peers (students in your grade) would have the"risk-behavior"?[19,20]; 5) peer and parent distress if youth engaged in the risk-behavior [16]; and 6) whether youth's best friend, parents, or others they "hung around with" had the risk-behavior [19,21]. Parallel scales assessed variables related to diet, exercise, risky sex, and sex.

A composite HRBI was derived based on the sum of four binary (0/1) HRB indicators: 1) past-month smoking/tobacco use, 2) substance misuse, defined as past-month alcohol use with impairment (POSIT ≥ 1) or illegal drug use (marijuana or other drugs), 3) unprotected sex (without condom) in the past 6-months; 4) obesity risk, defined as BMI-for-age-gender ≥ 85th percentile (http://www.win.niddk.nih.gov/statistics/index.htm). These four risk-indicators also served as risk-indicators for their respective risk-domains.

Statistical Analyses

We present standard descriptive statistics, examined the effects of past-year depressive disorder on the HRBs using logistic regression analyses predicting to dichotomous variables and negative binomial regression analyses predicting to dimensional variables (HRBI, POSIT). Because preliminary analyses indicated that depression was more common in girls (X^2 (1)=11.29, p<.001) and age and Hispanic ethnicity were significantly associated with the HRB measures, analyses adjusted for gender, age, and Hispanic ethnicity. Because we aimed to evaluate overall depression effects and data indicate that subsyndromal depression is associated with increased risk of depressive disorder-onset and impairment levels comparable to those for depressive disorder [22], we collapsed across these categories and compared youths with no depressive disorder to those with disorder broadly-defined to include DISC-definite and intermediate diagnoses. Youths with definite and intermediate diagnoses did not differ significantly on any of the HRB measures and results were similar, with no change in conclusions, when these subgroups were examined separately and when depression was entered as a 3-level variable. Next, we examined the effects of the attitude and social-environmental variables on the binary HRBs using logistic regression. These analyses clarify bivariate associations among the binary HRBs and the predictor variables adjusting for control variables (gender, age, Hispanic ethnicity). Finally, to identify the most parsimonious set of predictors, we used logistic regression with a backwards stepping procedure including all terms significant in the initial analyses and depressive disorder in the model, with variables removed based on their p-values in a descending order and retaining only variables with p-values ≤ 0.10. Statistical analyses were conducted using SPSS, Version 20, except SAS PROC GENMOD was used for negative binomial regression analyses.

Results

The sample included 119 females (55% of sample, mean age=16.01, SD=1.45), and 98 males (45% of sample, mean age=15.90, SD 1.55). Participants were ethnically diverse: 70% endorsed Hispanic/Latino ethnicity, 8% African-American, 3% Asian, 2% Alaskan Native/American Indian, 12% mixed race, and 12% Caucasian. Roughly half of the sample (98/217, 45%) met DISC-criteria for past-year definite (n=51) or intermediate depressive disorder (n=47).

Distribution of risk within the sample

As shown in (Table 1), the HRB domain with the most at-risk youths was obesity. BMI measurements fell in the obese/risk-for-obesity range for 50.2% of youths, 31.3% classified as obese. Substance misuse was

the next most common risk-domain, followed by risky sex, and past-month smoking. Smoking was associated with significantly higher rates of: substance misuse, $X^2(1)$ =45.93, p<.001; and risky sex, $X^2(1)$ =21.00, p<.001; and substance misuse was associated with significantly higher rates of risky sex, $X^2(1)$ =26.74, p<.001. Associations between obesity-risk and the other HRBs were not statistically significant: smoking, $X^2(1)$=0.34, p=.56; substance misuse, $X^2(1)$ =0.40, p=.53; risky sex, $X^2(1)$=2.90, p=.09. Multiple risk indicators were present in 33.6% of the sample: 2 risk areas (20.7%); 3 risk areas (10.1%), four risk areas (2.8%); risk in ≥ 1 area (73.3%).

Depression and HRBs

As predicted, depressive disorder status was a significant predictor of the HRBI, sum of risk levels across the four targeted risk areas (Table 2). Youths with depressive disorder were significantly more likely to report risk across multiple domains, with 45% of depressed youths showing risk in two or more domains vs. 25% of non-depressed youths (Table 2). All youths with risk across all four risk-domains suffered from past-year depression (Figure 1).

Depressive disorder status was significantly associated with most domain-specific risk indicators, specifically: past-month smoking; substance misuse; problematic drug use (drug use with impairment); problematic alcohol use, defined as alcohol use with impairment; substance use-related impairment on the POSIT; risky sexual behavior (without condom) during the preceding 6-months; more sexual

	Total Sample (N=217)		Smoking (N=35)		Substance Misuse (N=68)		Risky Sex (N=61)		Obesity Risk (N=109)	
	f	%	f	%	f	%	f	%	f	%
Smoking	35	16.1%			28	41.2%***	21	34.4%***	16	14.7%
Substance Misuse	76	31.9%	28	80%***			35	57.4%***	32	29.4%
Risky Sex	61	28.1%%	21	60%***	35	51.5%***			25	22.9%
Obesity Risk	109	50.2%	16	45.7%	35	46.1%	25	41%		

*Percentages calculated as percent of youths with HRB in column with co-occurring HRB in row.

Table 1: Risk Across Domains of Health Risk Behavior*.

Variables	NOT DEPRESSED (N=119)		DEPRESSED (N=98)		OR or IRR*	95% CI	X²	p
	f or M	% or SD	f or M	% or SD				
HRBI	1.03	0.90	1.47	1.15	1.5	1.2, 1.9	14.81	.01
HRBI ≥ 2	29	24.4%	44	44.9%	3.6	1.9, 7.0	14.39	.01
Smoking, Past Month	13	10.9%	22	22.4%	2.7	1.2, 6.0	5.86	.02
Sub Misuse, Past Month								
Any Problematic Use	26	21.8%	42	42.9%	3.7	1.9, 7.1	15.12	.01
Problematic Alcohol	19	16.0%	25	25.5%	2.3	1.1, 4.7	4.88	.03
Illegal Drug Use	12	10.1%	29	29.6%	5.0	2.3, 11.1	15.91	.01
Impairment, POSIT	1.11 0	0.22 0-11	1.93 0	2.89 0-12	2.0	1.1, 3.6	5.84	.02
Risky Sex								
No Condom, 6-Mos	27	22.7%	34	34.7%	2.2	1.1, 4.3	5.04	.03
STI/STDs	7	6.4%	12	14.3%	2.5	0.9, 6.9	3.26	.07
#Partners, 3-Mos.	0.37 0	0.64 0-4	0.56 0	0.85 0-5	1.7	1.1, 2.6	6.86	.01
Obesity-Risk, BMI	59	49.6%	50	51.0%	1.1	0.6, 2.0	0.19	.66

*Odds Ratios (OR) reported for logistic regression analyses, incident rate ratios (IRRs) reported for negative binomial regressions which were done for non-categorical variables (HRBI, POSIT, # Partners).

Table 2: Health Risk Behaviors Among Youths with and Without Past-Year Depression.

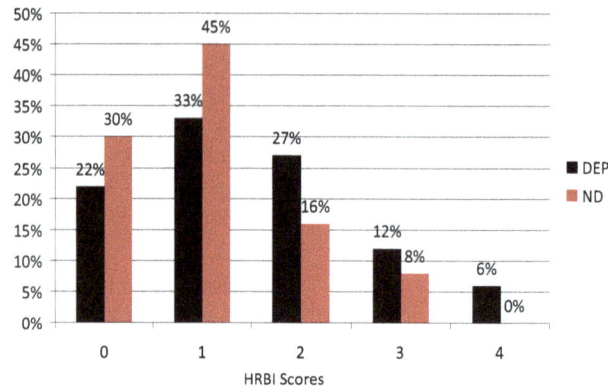

Figure 1: Health Risk Behavior Index (HRBI) Scores for Depressed and Non-Depressed Youths.

Predictor Variables	Smoking				Alcohol				Marijuana				Sexual Behavior				Obesity			
	OR	95% CI	X²	p	OR	95% CI	X²	p	OR	95% CI	X²	p	OR	95% CI	X²	p	OR	95% CI	X²	p
Expect Risk Behavior Next 6 Months Smoking	0.19	0.11, 0.31	41.52	0.01	0.28	0.19, 0.43	35.39	0.01	0.15	0.09, 0.25	51.42	0.01	0.23	0.15, 0.36	39.26	0.01[1]	0.27	0.19, 0.38	53.80	0.01
Resistance Self-Efficacy	0.63	0.55, 0.74	36.39	0.01	0.70	0.62, 0.78	35.37	0.01	0.66	0.58, 0.74	51.48	0.01					1.07	1.01, 1.13	5.04	0.03
Attitudes	1.36	1.20, 1.54	23.30	0.01	1.27	1.16, 1.38	27.00	0.01	1.38	1.25, 1.53	38.98	0.01	0.52	0.36, 0.77	10.95	0.01	1.08	1.03, 1.12	10.41	0.01
% Peers Risk Behavior	1.10	0.95, 1.27	1.67	0.20	1.36	1.17, 1.59	15.90	0.01	1.50	1.29, 1.76	26.00	0.01	1.26	1.09, 1.45	9.94	0.01[1]	1.08	0.95, 1.22	1.41	0.24
Best Friend Risk Behavior	2.17	0.97, 4.84	3.59	0.06	5.18	2.30, 11.64	15.84	0.01	6.83	3.26, 14.28	25.99	0.01					3.86	2.02, 7.37	16.71	0.01
Family Risk Behavior	1.64	0.77, 3.51	1.61	0.20	1.18	0.43, 3.22	0.10	0.75	2.11	0.73, 6.09	1.89	2.11					2.46	1.40, 4.32	9.89	0.01
Time with Others Risk Behavior	0.45	0.29, 0.68	13.85	0.01	0.39	0.26, 0.60	19.02	0.01	0.20	0.12, 0.33	39.85	0.01					0.61	0.43, 0.85	8.53	0.01
Expected Peer Distress	0.66	0.39, 1.11	2.48	0.12	0.52	0.35, 0.77	10.47	0.01	0.50	0.34, 0.72	13.79	0.01					0.99	0.68, 1.15	0.00	0.98
Expected Parent Distress	0.46	0.27, 0.78	8.21	0.01	0.58	0.39, 0.85	7.60	0.01	0.41	0.25, 0.68	12.09	0.01					1.28	0.95, 1.72	2.66	0.10

[1]Question asks about risky sex, defined as sex without a condom

Table 3: Cross-Sectional Predictors of Health Risk Behaviors.

partners within the past 3-months; and marginally associated with increased rates of STI/STDs (Table 2). Rates of obesity were similar across depressed and non-depressed groups.

Descriptive and exploratory analyses of risk in each health-risk domain:

Smoking: Over half the sample (64.1%) reported never having smoked; 35 youths reported past-month smoking, 25 of whom (71.4%) reported ≥ 1 quit attempt. Table 3 presents results of the logistic regression analyses examining associations among the binary HRBs (e.g. post-month smoking) and each attitude and social-environmental variable. These analyses revealed that smoking was significantly associated with: expecting to smoke during the next 6-months; lower resistance self-efficacy/perceived ability to resist smoking; more positive attitudes towards smoking; the amount of time the youth spent with individuals who smoke and perceptions that parents would be upset if youth smoked. When all significant variables and depressive disorder status were entered in the backwards stepping procedure, results indicating a statistically significant effect only for expecting to smoke during the next 6-months, OR 0.36, 95% CI 0.20, 0.68, X²=10.23, p<.001, supporting the strength of the expectancy variable

as a cross-sectional predictor. However, marginal effects for other variables suggest that non-overlapping variance from other variables also contributed to prediction: resistance self-efficacy, OR 0.85, 95% CI 0.70, 1.02, X²=3.07, p<.08; attitudes towards smoking, OR 1.15, 95% CI 0.98, 1.35, X²=2.91, p<.09; hanging around with other smokers, OR 0.61, 95% CI 0.35, 1.06, X²=3.08, p<.08, and older age, OR 1.41, 95% CI 0.98, 2.02, X²=3.44, p<.06.

Alcohol use: Lifetime drinking was reported by 141 youths (65%), 44 (20.3%) reported current drinking with impairment, 22 of whom (20.3%) reported past-month efforts to quit drinking. Statistically significant predictors of problematic drinking included: expecting to drink during the next 6-months; low resistance self-efficacy, more positive attitudes towards drinking; perceptions that peers drank alcohol; having a best friend who drank; hanging around with people who drank; expected that peers would be upset if they found out they drank alcohol; and expected that their parents would be upset if they found out they drank alcohol (Table 3). The final model when depression and all statistically significant variables from the bivariate analyses were included in the model yielded significant effects for expecting to drink, OR 0.51, 95% CI 0.31, 0.83, X²=7.24, p<.007;resistance self-efficacy, OR 0.83, 95% CI 0.72, 0.96, X²=6.38, p<.012; and marginal effects for drinking attitudes, OR 1.10, 95% CI 0.99,1.22, X^2=3.37, p<.07; perceptions that peers drank, OR 0.1.18, 95% CI 0.99, 1.42, X^2=3.37, p<.067; male gender, OR 2.17, 95% CI 0.92, 5.14, X^2=3.12, p<.08; and non-Hispanic ethnicity, OR 2.36, 95% CI 0.91, 6.14, X^2=3.09, p<.08.

Drug use: Ninety-three youths (42.9%) reported lifetime marijuana use; 48 reported past-month use, 29 of whom (60.4%) reported ≥ 1 quit attempt. Other drug use was less common (amphetamines/uppers n=11, 5.1%; ecstasy n=10, 4.6%; hallucinogens n=3, 1.4%) and generally occurred with marijuana use (n=5 past-month marijuana use only, n=32 marijuana and other drugs, $X^2(1)$=39.46, p<.001). Marijuana use was significantly associated with: expecting to use marijuana during next 6 months; low resistance self-efficacy; more positive attitudes towards marijuana; perceptions that peers used marijuana; having a best friend who used marijuana, hanging around with people who used marijuana; and expecting low levels of peer and parent upset if used (Table 3). The final model yielded significant effects for attitudes towards marijuana, OR 1.29, 95% CI 1.13, 1.47, X^2=13.58, p<.001; resistance self-efficacy, OR 0.84, 95% CI 0.72, 0.98, X^2=5.07, p<.03; hanging out with other marijuana-users, OR 0.35, 95% CI 0.17, 0.70, X^2=8.56, p<.003; expected peer distress if used, OR 2.29, 95% CI 1.14, 4.60, X^2=5.43, p<.02; and a marginal effect for expecting to use, OR 0.57, 95% CI 0.31, 1.05, X^2=3.25, p<.07.

Sexual behavior: Eighty-nine youths (40.8%) reported having engaged in sexual intercourse. Fifteen youths (8 girls, 7 boys) endorsed prior pregnancies/getting someone pregnant, with 3 youths reporting >1 pregnancy and one an abortion, and 19 youths (8.8%) reporting STI/STDs. Risky sex (without condoms) was significantly associated with: expecting to have risky sex during next 6 months; more liberal attitudes towards sex; perceptions that peers were engaging in risky sex; perceptions that peers were engaging in sex, OR 1.25, 95% CI 1.10, 1.41, X^2=12.33, p<.01; perceptions that peers had more liberal attitudes towards sex, OR 0.54, 95% CI 0.36, 0.81, X^2=9.16, p<.01; and marginally associated with family attitudes supporting safe sex, OR 2.09, 95% CI 0.93, 4.71, X^2=3.18, p=.08 (Table 3). The final model included significant effects for: expecting to have risky sex, OR 0.23, 95% CI 0.14, 0.36, X^2=38.09, p<.001; perceptions that peers were engaging in sex, OR 1.28, 95% CI 1.08, 1.51, X^2=8.02, p<.005; and older age, OR 1.55, 95% CI 1.15, 2.07, X^2=8.46, p<.004; and a marginal effect for female gender, p<.07.

Obesity-risk: On self-report, 77% of youths (n=167) endorsed having felt overweight in their lifetimes, 122 youths (56.2% of sample) reported current efforts to lose weight. During the past-month, 124 youths (57.1%) reported exercising to lose weight; 91 (41.9%) reported dieting to lose weight. Youths with obesity-risk (objectively-measured BMI) were significantly more likely to report: trying to lose weight ($X^2(3)$=83.68, p<.001), dieting to lose weight ($X^2(1)$ =17.70, p<.001), and exercising to lose weight ($X^2(1)$=18.59, p<.001).

Significant predictors of obesity-risk included: expecting to be overweight; diet self-efficacy; diet attitudes; having an overweight best friend; having overweight parents and siblings; and "hanging out" with overweight people (Table 3). Obesity-risk was not significantly associated with beliefs supporting exercise, self-efficacy for exercise, or perceptions that peers are overweight. The final model included significant effects for expecting to lose weight, OR 0.30, 95% CI 0.21, 0.43, X^2=42.63, p<.001; having an overweight best friend, OR 3.25, 95% CI 1.51, 7.02,X^2=9.05, p<.003; diet attitudes, OR 1.09, 95% CI 1.01, 1.18, X^2=4.81, p<.03; and a marginal trend for obesity risk to be associated with younger age, OR 0.81, 95% CI 0.64, 1.02, X^2=3.16, p<.08.

Conclusions

Consistent with the United States National Prevention Strategy [1], our results support the importance of screening for HRBs. Rates of HRBs were high, with 74% of patients showing risk in ≥ 1 risk-domains. However, as predicted, rates of HRBs were significantly higher among depressed youths and depressed youths were more likely to show multiple areas of health-risk. These data extend prior findings and suggest that elevated levels and patterns of HRBs contribute to the high economic and social costs of depression [7-11]. Depression treatment and course is often complicated by HRBs and extent data indicate that improved depression is associated with reduced HRBs, particularly substance misuse [23-25], underscoring both the need for preventive services targeting risk-reduction in depressed youths and the potential benefits of depression treatment for reducing HRBs.

As predicted and consistent with problem behavior theory [6], some of the most pernicious HRBs clustered together (smoking, substance misuse, risky-sex). For instance, among current smokers in our sample, 80% reported substance misuse, 60% reported engaging in risky sex, and 34% endorsed more than one HRB. These data are consistent with the view that smoking may often be a "gateway" to more extensive drug use and other HRBs and emphasize the potential benefits of intervention strategies that address multiple risk behaviors and the connections between them [6].

Also consistent with problem behavior, social learning, and cognitive-behavioral theory, youths' expectancies that they would engage in the risk-behavior during the next 6-months were significant cross-sectional predictors of the risk- behaviors. This held for all examined risk areas: smoking, substance misuse (alcohol and marijuana), risky sex, and obesity-risk. Attitudes supporting the risk behavior were also significant predictors of the risk behaviors, although attitudes towards diet but not exercise were significant predictors of obesity-risk, and obesity-risk was associated with greater awareness of the benefits of "healthy diet." Lower resistance self- efficacy (perceived difficulty resisting the risk behavior) was significantly associated with smoking, alcohol, marijuana use, and obesity-risk.

Supporting the importance of social/environmental influences, some indicator that peers or others in the environment were engaging in the risk behavior was significantly associated with risk in each of the risk-domains. Youths who smoked were significantly more likely to hang out with other smokers; youths with problematic alcohol and marijuana use were significantly more likely to hang out with others who used these substances and to believe that peers would not be upset if they drank or smoked marijuana; and youths who were overweight were more likely to hang out with others who were overweight, have family members who were overweight, and have a best friend who was overweight. Youths who engaged in risky sex believed that a higher proportion of their peers were having sex and having sex without condoms. Again, compatible with problem behavior theory [6], these data suggest that similar kinds of expectancies, attitudes, and environmental factors contribute to risk across the four risk-domains.

Despite the importance of the peer group during adolescence, when examining substance use and smoking, youths who felt their parents would be upset by smoking or substance misuse were significantly less likely to engage in the risk-behavior. These data support the role that parental values and reactions may play in reducing substance use risk, are consistent with data showing the power of family-based preventive strategies [24], and underscore the important influences of both peers and parents on substance use risk.

Our finding that only a subgroup of youths engaging in risk-behaviors had attempted to quit/reduce the risk-behaviors underscores the challenges for risk-reduction. Quit attempts were reported by 50%, 60.4%, and 71.4% of youths with past-month problematic drinking, marijuana use, and smoking respectively. This finding is consistent with literature showing that youth will make self-change efforts and emphasizes the role that motivational strategies can play in reducing HRBs. California, the state where the study was conducted, has strict laws controlling smoking, economic incentives, a stop-smoking advertising campaign, and a past-month smoking rate which is roughly half of the national average, 6.9% vs. 15.9% (ages 12-17) (www.cdc. gov/tobacco/data_statistics/state_data/state_highlights/2010/states/ california/index.htm). These data and the high rate of quit attempts observed among smokers in this study suggests that these efforts may be increasing motivation to quit.

In contrast, weight reduction appears to be viewed as necessary by a broad group of youths, with weight loss attempts reported by 85.3% of youths with obesity-risk and 44.4% of youths with lower weights. These data suggest that weight loss attempts may play a role in maintaining healthy weight and are often unsuccessful, given the high-rate of weight loss efforts among youths with obesity-risk.

Study limitations include the focus on cross-sectional predictors; future research is needed to examine whether these cross-sectional predictors will predict longitudinal patterns. While strengths of the manuscript include the fact that we sampled patients from two diverse health care organizations, and oversampling for depression allowed us to obtain a large enough sample of youths with depression to address the study aims, results may not generalize to other samples from other health care facilities and using other sampling strategies. Although comparable to similar studies with waivers for parental consent for screening but not broader study participation, response rates were moderate [4]. The sample was recruited to over-select for depression and focused on depression and four areas of health-risk; other research is needed to examine other health-risk and mental health problems. Youths were recruited from consecutive primary care patients and presented at the clinics with a variety of health conditions, as well as for regular check-ups. Future research is needed to evaluate the impact of other health conditions that lead youths to visit health facilities.

Implications and Contributions

Risk behaviors are a leading cause of preventable morbidity and mortality and depression is both a leading cause of disability worldwide and associated with suicide, the third leading cause of death in adolescents and young adults [1]. Study results indicate that depression and HRBs (particularly the cluster of smoking, substance misuse, and risky sex) frequently co-occur and risk across diverse risk-domains was associated with similar constructs. These findings support the value of screening and clinical service strategies that target multiple related risk-conditions, the potential benefits of treatment approaches with flexibility to address both depression and HRBs using clinical decision-making algorithms and/or a modular approach [4], and the value of pediatric collaborative care models for integrating behavioral health within primary care. Such combination strategies that maximize the value of primary care encounters for promoting health and reducing risk are consistent with current guidelines and recommendations and are consistent with our national goal of increasing the quality and years of healthy life [1-3,25-27].

Acknowledgement

Funded by **NIMH grant MH078596**. We wish to thank the youth, families, staff, and colleagues who made this project possible, including Mary Jane Rotheram-Borus, and our DSMB, Donald Guthrie, Gabrielle Carlson, Mark Rapaport.

References

1. U.S. Department of Health and Human Services, Office of the Surgeon General. National Prevention Strategy. In: U.S. Department of Health and Human Services, ed. Rockville, MD: Office of the Surgeon General; 2011.

2. Cheung AH, Zuckerbrot RA, Jensen PS, Ghalib K, Laraque D, et al. (2007) Guidelines for Adolescent Depression in Primary Care (GLAD-PC): II. Treatment and ongoing management. Pediatrics 120: e1313-1326.

3. Wren FJ, Foy JM, Ibeziako PI (2012) Primary care management of child & adolescent depressive disorders. Child AdolescPsychiatrClin N Am 21: 401-419.

4. Asarnow JR, Jaycox LH, Duan N, LaBorde AP, Rea MM, et al. (2005) Effectiveness of a quality improvement intervention for adolescent depression in primary care clinics: a randomized controlled trial. JAMA 293: 311-319.

5. Richardson L, McCauley E, Katon W (2009) Collaborative care for adolescent depression: a pilot study. Gen Hosp Psychiatry 31: 36-45.

6. Jessor R, Chase JA, Donovan JE (1980) Psychosocial correlates of marijuana use and problem drinking in a national sample of adolescents. Am J Public Health 70: 604-613.

7. Katon W, Richardson L, Russo J, McCarty CA, Rockhill C, et al. (2010) Depressive symptoms in adolescence: the association with multiple health risk behaviors. Gen Hosp Psychiatry 32: 233-239.

8. Paxton RJ, Valois RF, Watkins KW, Huebner ES, Drane JW (2007) Associations between depressed mood and clusters of health risk behaviors. Am J Health Behav 31: 272-283.

9. Hallfors DD, Waller MW, Ford CA, Halpern CT, Brodish PH, et al. (2004) Adolescent depression and suicide risk: association with sex and drug behavior. Am J Prev Med 27: 224-231.

10. Shrier LA, Harris SK, Kurland M, Knight JR (2003) Substance use problems and associated psychiatric symptoms among adolescents in primary care. Pediatrics 111: e699-705.

11. Shrier LA, Harris SK, Sternberg M, Beardslee WR (2001) Associations of depression, self-esteem, and substance use with sexual risk among adolescents. Prev Med 33: 179-189.

12. Shaffer D, Fisher P, Lucas CP, Dulcan MK, Schwab-Stone ME (2000) NIMH Diagnostic Interview Schedule for Children Version IV (NIMH DISC-IV): description, differences from previous versions, and reliability of some common diagnoses. J Am Acad Child Adolesc Psychiatry 39: 28-38.

13. Brener ND, Kann L, Kinchen SA, Grunbaum JA, Whalen L, et al. (2004) Methodology of the youth risk behavior surveillance system. MMWR Recomm Rep 53: 1-13.

14. Harris KM, Florey F, Tabor J, Bearman PS, Jones J, et al. (2003) The National Longitudinal Study of Adolescent Health: Research and design [WWW document].

15. Johnston LD, O'Malley PM, Bachman JG, Schulenberg JE (2007) Monitoring the future national survey results on drug use, 1975-2006. Volume I: Secondary school students (NIH Publication No. 07-6205). Bethesda, MD: National Institute on Drug Use.

16. Ghosh-Dastidar B, Longshore DL, Ellickson PL, McCaffrey DF (2004) Modifying pro-drug risk factors in adolescents: results from project ALERT. Health EducBehav 31: 318-334.

17. Bogart LM, Elliott MN, Uyeda K, Hawes-Dawson J, Klein DJ, et al. (2011) Preliminary healthy eating outcomes of SNaX, a pilot community-based intervention for adolescents. J Adolesc Health 48: 196-202.

18. Rahdert E (1991) The Adolescent Assessment/Referral System Manual. In: U.S. Department of Health and Human Services, ed. Rockville, MD: National Institute on Drug Abuse: DHHS pub No. (ADM) 91-1735.

19. Stern SA, Meredith LS, Gholson J, Gore P, D'Amico EJ (2007) Project CHAT: a brief motivational substance abuse intervention for teens in primary care. J Subst Abuse Treat 32: 153-165.

20. Van Haitsma M, Paik A, Laumann EO, Ellingson S, Mahay J, et al. (2004) The sexual organization of the city: University of Chicago Press.

21. Colby SM, Monti PM, O'Leary Tevyaw T, Barnett NP, Spirito A, et al. (2005) Brief motivational intervention for adolescent smokers in medical settings. Addict Behav 30: 865-874.

22. Gotlib IH, Lewinsohn PM, Seeley JR (1995) Symptoms versus a diagnosis of depression: differences in psychosocial functioning. J Consult Clin Psychol 63: 90-100.

23. McKowen JW, Tompson MC, Brown TA, Asarnow JR (2013) Longitudinal associations between depression and problematic substance use in the Youth Partners in Care study. J Clin Child AdolescPsychol 42: 669-680.

24. Bauman KE, Ennett ST, Foshee VA, Pemberton M, King TS, et al. (2002) Influence of a family program on adolescent smoking and drinking prevalence. Prev Sci 3: 35-42.

25. Irwin CE Jr, Adams SH, Park MJ, Newacheck PW (2009) Preventive care for adolescents: few get visits and fewer get services. Pediatrics 123: e565-572.

26. Curry J, Silva S, Rohde P, Ginsburg G, Kennard B, et al. (2012) Onset of alcohol or substance use disorders following treatment for adolescent depression. J Consult Clin Psychol 80: 299-312.

27. Goldstein BI, Shamseddeen W, Spirito A, Emslie G, Clarke G, et al. (2009) Substance use and the treatment of resistant depression in adolescents. J Am Acad Child Adolesc Psychiatry 48: 1182-1192.

10

Estimating Quality of Life in Greek Patients with Hidradenitis Suppurativa

Vassiliki Tzanetakou¹*, Theodora Kanni¹, Kyriakoula Merakou², Anastasia Barbouni² and Evangelos Giamarellos-Bourboulis J¹

¹₂4ᵗʰDepartment of Internal Medicine, University of Athens, Medical School, Greece
Department of Public Health, National School of Public Health, Athens, Greece

Abstract

Background: Hidradenitis suppurativa (HS) is a chronic, relapsing skin disorder causing physical impairment and severe negative effects on patients' quality of life (QoL). The current study aims to estimate the impairment of QoL in HS and the role of disease advancement as a worsening factor.

Patients and Methods: Fifty patients and fifty healthy controls were sex and age matched and completed two questionnaires, the 'Dermatology Life Quality Index' (DLQI) and the 'SF-36v2™ Health Survey' (SF36). Comparisons were carried out between patients of different Hurley stage and between patients and controls' subgroups. The results of both questionnaires were correlated.

Results: According to Hurley system,15 patients manifested first-stage HS,13 second-stage HS, while 22 patients exhibited third-stage disease severity. HS patients experienced greater impact on their QoL compared to healthy controls (total mean DLQI score 13.10 ± 1.19 vs.1.44 ± 0.32, $p<0.001$ and total mean SF36 score 53.13 ± 3.34 vs.79.43 ± 1.38, $p<0.001$). Elevated score was attributed mainly to bodily pain and embarrassment due to skin disease. Patients with advanced stage of disease (Hurley III) obtained significantly higher score compared to patients with milder stage (Hurley I and II) in both questionnaires (mean DLQI score 18.55 ± 1.51 vs. 8.82 ± 1.3, $p<0.001$ and mean SF36 score 40.43 ± 4.44 vs.70.26 ± 3.1,$p<0.001$, respectively). Total DLQI and SF36 scores were excellently correlated ($p<0.01$, Spearman's correlation coefficient -0.771).

Conclusion: Patients with HS suffer a devastating impact on QoL. The phenomenon is greater within advanced disease stages.

Keywords: Hidradenitis suppurativa; Quality of life; Hurley stage; DLQI; SF36

Introduction

Hidradenitis suppurativa (HS) is a chronically recurrent skin disease. HS is characterized by the inflammation of the terminal hair follicle and affects predominantly apocrine gland-bearing regions [1]. HS incidence is estimated at 0.97%, according to the results of a large study conducted in France, while a Danish study estimated HS 1-year prevalence at 1% [2,3]. HS appears to be more common among females with a female/male ratio 3-5:1. The onset of the disease typically occurs after puberty [1].

HS clinical features include deep-seated nodules, polyporous comedones, draining sinuses, abscesses and scarring, while clinical presentation ranges from few, recalcitrant, suppurating lesions to severe, disabling disease. It is mainly localized at axillae, groins, gluteal regions and mammary folds, but also at genitalia, intragluteal region, perineum and scalp. Characteristic lesions, typical localization, chronicity and relapses establish the diagnosis of HS [4].

A well-established and universally accepted therapy does not exist. Current therapeutic options more usually administered to HS patients include antibiotics, retinoids, immunosuppressive treatment and surgery,while the number of studies conducted about the efficacy of biological agents against HS keeps rising [5].

The devastating nature of HS generated the need to provide a measurable way of the impact on the quality of life (QoL).The number of studies performed thus far about the assessment of QoL in HS patients is limited [6-10]. Von der Werth and Jemec measured the impairment of QoL in 114 patients with HS by using the Dermatology Life Quality Index (DLQI) [6]. Wolkenstein et al. evaluated the impact of HS on QoL by administering VQ-Dermato, Skindex-France and Short Form 36 (SF36) questionnaires at 61 patients [7]. In the study conducted by Matusiak et al. the effect of HS on psychological aspects of 52 patients was estimated by multiple questionnaires, including DLQI, Beck Depression Inventory-

Short Form (BDI-SF), Evers et al.'6-Item Scale', EQ-5D, Functional Assessment of Chronic Illness Therapy – Fatigue scale (FACIT-F) and Quality of Life Enjoyment and Satisfaction Questionnaire Short Form (Q-LES-Q-SF) [8]. Esmann and Jemec performed interviews at a total of 12 patients suffering from HS [9]. Onderdijk et al. assessed QoL and depression score in a cohort of 211 patients with HS by DLQI and Major Depression Inventory (MDI) questionnaires [10]. Experience of these studies revealed that HS causes a significant effect on QoL, greater than other dermatologic diseases [6-10].

A commonly asked question is whether these scores, and particularly DLQI, may be a helpful tool for the follow-up of the patients not only in clinical practice but also for patients' assessment in clinical trials. To this end, the current study is the first study, which aims to evaluate the impairment of QoL in HS patients in Greece not only using DLQI but also SF36. The need to introduce SF36 is based on its value on the assessment of physical and mental health.

Patients and Methods

The study was conducted from July 2010 to February 2011 at the outpatient clinic of Immunology of Infections at Attikon University General Hospital in partnership with the Public Health Department of National School of Public Health in Greece.

---

*Corresponding author: Vassiliki Tzanetakou, 4thDepartment of Internal Medicine, University of Athens, Medical School, Greece,
E-mail: tzanetakoub@hotmail.co

The study was approved by the local ethics committee and written informed consent was provided by all studied individuals.

Patients were evaluated in the outpatient clinic and the diagnosis of HS was based on established clinical criteria [11]. For each patient, a brief report form about demographic characteristics, HS history and existence of co-morbidities was completed. Patients with any serious co-existing morbidity, which could affect their QoL and therefore the reliability of the results, were excluded. Finally fifty patients were included in the study and were separated into three groups according to Hurley staging system for HS [12].

Fifty healthy controls from other outpatient clinics of Attikon University General Hospital, who did not meet the criteria for HS, were sex and age matched with HS patients.

Permission for the usage of the Greek official language version of 'Dermatology Life Quality Index' (DLQI) was obtained by Professor Andrew Y. Finlay and for the 'SF-36v2™ Health Survey' (SF36) by Quality Metric Incorporated. Both patients and healthy controls were asked to fill out the questionnaires.

DLQI was the first dermatology-specific instrument to evaluate the impact of skin condition on QoL. It was created in 1994 by Finlay and Khan and it takes one to two minutes to complete. DLQI is a 10-item questionnaire summarized in six sections (symptoms and feelings, daily activities, leisure, work and school, personal relationships, treatment). Total score ranges between 0 and 30, while score for each question between 0 and 3. Higher score indicates greater impairment of QoL (0-1: no effect on QoL; 2-5: small effect; 6-10: moderate effect; 11-20: very large effect; and 21-30:extremely large effect).It is the most widely used tool in dermatology assessing QoL in the majority of relevant studies in patients with dermatologic diseases [13,14].

SF36 was developed by American scientists in health insurance survey. It is a generic instrument and it does not target a specific age group, disease or treatment. SF36 behaves well in a variety of clinical conditions and it is very useful in surveys of general and specific populations. It consists of 36 questions classified into 8 scales (physical function, role-physical, bodily pain, general health, role-emotional, social function, vitality, mental health). Each scale aggregates two to ten items and each item is used in scoring only one scale. The scales of SF36 are classified into two summary measures, physical component including physical function, role-physical, bodily pain and general health, and mental component including role-emotional, social function, vitality and mental health. Total score as well as single scale and item score ranges between 0 and 100. Lower score is considered indicative of greater effect on QoL. SF36 is completed in seven to ten minutes.It is the most studied tool in evaluating QoL and it is considered as the reference instrument by most researchers [14,15].

Results were presented by mean ± standard deviation (SD). Statistical analysis was performed using the Mann-Whitney U test and Spearman's rank correlation coefficient. P<0.05 was considered as statistically significant.

Results

A total of 50 patients (24 male and 26 female) aged 20-64 years (mean age 38.1 ± 12.4 years) were included in the study. The self-reported disease duration was assessed as from 1 to 35 years (mean disease duration 12.0 ± 8.1 years) and the mean age onset was 26.2 ± 11.0 years old ranging from 14 to 57 years old. According to Hurley system,15 patients (30%) manifested first-stage HS,13 patients (26%) second-stage HS and 22 (44%) exhibited third-stage disease severity.

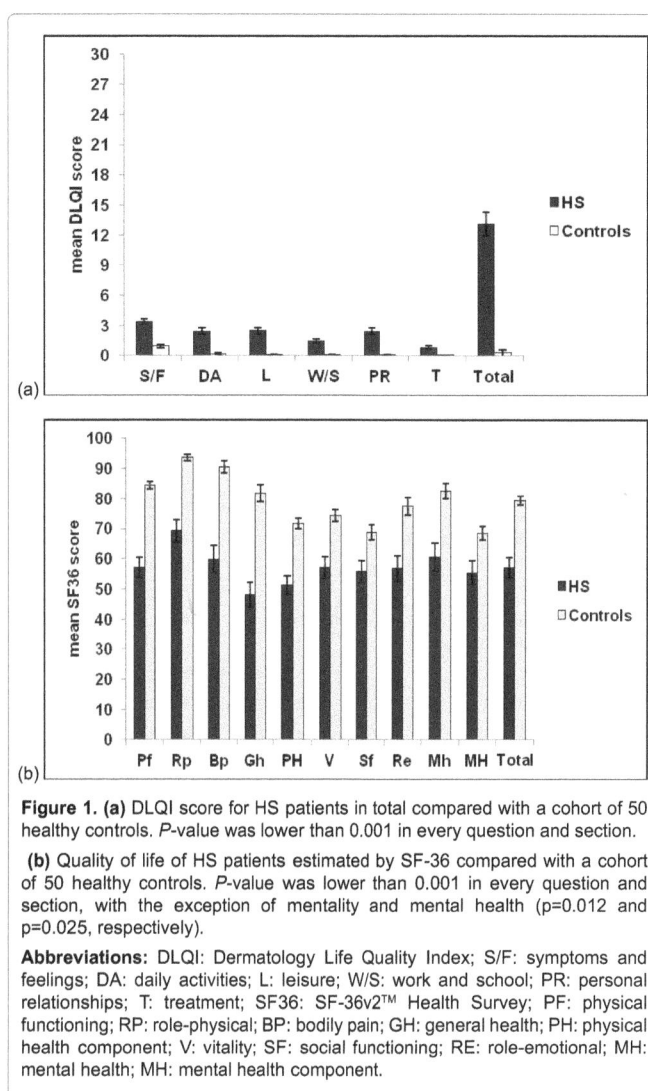

Figure 1. (a) DLQI score for HS patients in total compared with a cohort of 50 healthy controls. *P*-value was lower than 0.001 in every question and section.

(b) Quality of life of HS patients estimated by SF-36 compared with a cohort of 50 healthy controls. *P*-value was lower than 0.001 in every question and section, with the exception of mentality and mental health (p=0.012 and p=0.025, respectively).

Abbreviations: DLQI: Dermatology Life Quality Index; S/F: symptoms and feelings; DA: daily activities; L: leisure; W/S: work and school; PR: personal relationships; T: treatment; SF36: SF-36v2™ Health Survey; PF: physical functioning; RP: role-physical; BP: bodily pain; GH: general health; PH: physical health component; V: vitality; SF: social functioning; RE: role-emotional; MH: mental health; MH: mental health component.

DLQI and SF36 scores for HS patients and for healthy controls are shown in Figure.1. Patients demonstrated a total DLQI score of 13.10 ± 1.19 and a total SF36 score of 57.13 ± 3.34 indicating a very large impairment of QoL.P-value was lower than 0.001 in every question and section of both DLQI and SF36 with the exception of mentality and mental health of SF36 (p=0.012 and p=0.025, respectively) indicating that HS patients experienced greater impact on their QoL in comparison with healthy controls.

Total mean DLQI scores for each particular Hurley stage subgroup are shown in Table 1. HS had a moderate impact on QoL in Hurley I stage patients (total mean score 6.47 ± 1.88), while Hurley II and III patients experienced a very large impairment (total mean score 11.54 ± 1.52 and 18.55 ± 1.5, respectively).The highest score was observed at second question about embarrassment and self-consciousness due to skin condition for all three subgroups.

Hurley stage III patients had significantly greater impact on QoL indicated by markedly elevated score in total mean DLQI and in each section compared with Hurley stage I alone and with Hurley stage I and II together with the exception of clothes selection (p>0.053). Hurley stage I patients differed significantly from Hurley stage II patients in total DLQI score and in three sections including symptoms and

DLQI QUESTIONS AND SECTIONS	HURLEY I (n=15)	HURLEY II (n=13)	HURLEY III (n=22)	HURLEY I vs. II	HURLEY I vs. III	HURLEY II vs. III	HURLEY I, II vs. III
1. Symptoms and feelings	2.00 ± 0.47	3.38 ± 0.37	4.32 ± 0.30	p=0.024	p<0.001	p=0.081	p=0.001
1a. Soreness, pain	0.87 ± 0.26	1.54 ± 0.22	2.14 ± 0.17	p=0.051	p=0.001	p=0.044	p=0.001
1b. Embarrassment	1.13 ± 0.27	1.85 ± 0.19	2.18 ± 0.17	p=0.048	p=0.004	p=0.201	p=0.010
2. Daily activities	1.20 ± 0.44	2.31 ± 0.38	3.41 ± 0.41	p=0.033	p=0.001	p=0.097	p=0.003
2a. Shopping, housework	0.60 ± 0.29	0.69 ± 0.21	1.73 ± 0.25	p=0.343	p=0.007	p=0.010	p=0.001
2b. Clothes selection	0.60 ± 0.19	1.62 ± 0.24	1.68 ± 0.24	p=0.004	p=0.004	p=0.818	p=0.053
3. Leisure	1.00 ± 0.47	2.00 ± 0.34	3.77 ± 0.43	p=0.015	p<0.001	p=0.009	p<0.001
3a. Social and leisure activities	0.60 ± 0.25	1.00 ± 0.23	2.00 ± 0.25	p=0.141	p=0.001	p=0.009	p<0.001
3b. Sports	0.40 ± 0.24	1.00 ± 0.20	1.77 ± 0.24	p=0.014	p=0.001	p=0.032	p=0.001
4. Work and school	0.73 ± 0.28	1.31 ± 0.38	2.05 ± 0.23	p=0.289	p=0.001	p=0.091	p=0.003
5. Personal relationships	1.07 ± 0.47	1.92 ± 0.61	3.73 ± 0.41	p=0.191	p<0.001	p=0.019	p<0.001
5a. Partner, friends, relatives	0.53 ± 0.24	1.15 ± 0.32	1.73 ± 0.26	p=0.112	p=0.004	p=0.168	p=0.009
5b. Sexual difficulties	0.53 ± 0.24	0.77 ± 0.32	2.00 ± 0.23	p=0.666	p<0.001	p=0.006	p<0.001
6. Treatment	0.47 ± 0.19	0.62 ± 0.24	1.27 ± 0.26	p=0.596	p=0.040	p=0.132	p=0.029
Total score	6.47 ± 1.88	11.54 ± 1.52	18.55 ± 1.51	p=0.050	p<0.001	p=0.003	p<0.001

Abbreviations: DLQI: Dermatology Life Quality Index

Table 1: DLQI score (mean ± SD) for each particular Hurley stage group (Hurley I, Hurley II, Hurley III).

SF-36 SCALES AND DIMENSIONS	HURLEY I (n=15)	HURLEY II (n=13)	HURLEY III (n=22)	HURLEY I vs. II	HURLEY I vs. III	HURLEY II vs. III	HURLEY I, II vs. III
1. Physical health	75.10 ± 3.72	65.95 ± 4.71	39.66 ± 4.09	p=0.197	p<0.001	p=0.001	p<0.001
1a. Physical functioning	86.00 ± 3.02	83.85 ± 4.20	49.32 ± 5.25	p=0.814	p<0.001	p=0.002	p<0.001
1b. Role-physical	77.92 ± 6.39	75.48 ± 8.11	38.35 ± 5.60	p=0.852	p<0.001	p<0.001	p<0.001
1c. Bodily pain	69.83 ± 6.53	50.00 ± 7.19	32.16 ± 5.45	p=0.089	p<0.001	p=0.049	p=0.001
1d. General health	66.67 ± 4.09	54.49 ± 4.89	38.83 ± 4.24	p=0.101	p<0.001	p=0.026	p<0.001
2. Mental health	71.10 ± 5.20	68.00 ± 4.90	41.19 ± 5.13	p=0.662	p=0.001	p=0.003	p<0.001
2a. Vitality	66.67 ± 5.68	65.38 ± 4.78	42.90 ± 5.81	p=0.763	p=0.014	p=0.014	p=0.003
2b. Social functioning	74.17 ± 6.84	68.27 ± 5.77	38.07 ± 5.23	p=0.357	p<0.001	p=0.002	p<0.001
2c. Role-emotional	75.56 ± 6.38	77.56 ± 7.45	40.15 ± 6.62	p=0.830	p=0.001	p=0.002	p<0.001
2d. Mental health	68.00 ± 5.97	60.77 ± 6.48	43.64 ± 6.12	p=0.320	p=0.014	p=0.072	p=0.010
Total score	73.10 ± 4.33	66.98 ± 4.42	40.43 ± 4.44	p=0.259	p<0.001	p=0.001	p<0.001

Abbreviations: SF36: SF-36v2™ Health Survey

Table 2: SF-36 score (mean ± SD) for HS patients of different Hurley stage (Hurley I, Hurley II, Hurley III).

feelings, daily activities and leisure. Statistically significant differences were also found between Hurley stage II and III patients in total score, leisure and personal relationships.

The results of SF36 scores in each particular Hurley stage subgroup are presented in Table 2. Total mean SF36 score was assessed as 73.10 ± 4.33 for Hurley I patients, 66.98 ± 4.42 for patients exhibiting Hurley II disease severity and 40.43 ± 4.44 for patients manifesting a third-stage HS. Patients of first-stage HS demonstrated the lowest score at general health scale, while patients of second and third-stage HS at bodily pain scale.

The subgroup of Hurley III patients experienced greater impact on QoL at a statistically significant grade compared with the subgroup of Hurley I alone and to the subgroup of Hurley I and II patients together in SF36 as a total and in each scale. Hurley III patients differed significantly from Hurley stage II patients in total SF36 score and in each scale score with the exception of mental health. No statistically significant differences were seen between Hurley stage I and II patients.

Significant negative statistical correlations were depicted between total DLQI and SF36 scores (Spearman's correlation coefficient -0.771, p<0.001) [Figure 2]. DLQI correlated with physical and mental component of SF36 at a statistically significant grade (Spearman's correlation coefficient -0.740, p<0.001 and -0.752, p<0.001,

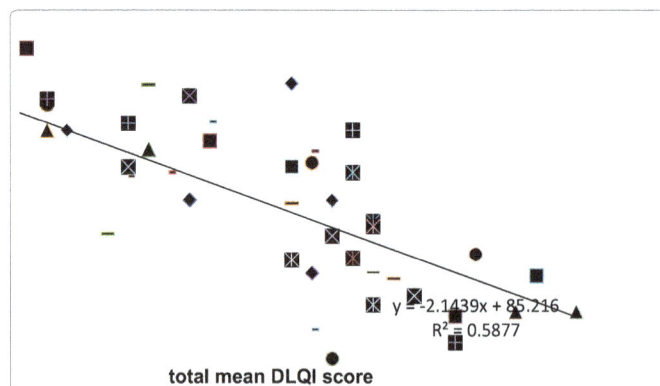

Figure2: Correlation between total mean DLQI and SF36 score. DLQI and SF36 were excellently correlated (Spearman's correlation coefficient -0.771, p<0.001).

Abbreviation: DLQI: Dermatology Life Quality Index, SF36: SF-36v2TM Health Survey.

respectively).

Statistical analysis showed no significant relationship between a variety of factors, including gender, age, disease duration, age at onset, and the score at both questionnaires (p>0.05).

Discussion

The current study is the first study conducted in Greece about the estimation of QoL in patients with HS. The combination of DLQI and SF36 is used for the first time for evaluating QoL in HS patients. The findings reveal a very large impact on QoL of patients suffering from HS.

Total mean DLQI score is in agreement with previously published data from studies conducted in other countries, where it ranged from 8.4 ± 7.5 to 12.7 ± 7.7 [6,8,10,16,17]. Matusiak et al. recorded a total mean DLQI score of 5.77 ± 4.59 for Hurley I patients, 13.10 ± 6.41 for Hurley II and 20.40 ± 6.67 for Hurley III [8]. These results are comparable to our findings.

The second question of DLQI about embarrassment and self-consciousness due to skin condition obtained the highest mean score. In contrast to the results of the current study, von der Werth and Jemec demonstrated that the highest score was observed for the first question about pain, soreness, stinging or itching (mean 1.55 points) [6].

In comparison with the findings of Matusiak et al, both studies recorded that only disease intensity and not gender, age at onset or disease duration played significant role in deterioration of QoL [8]. Contrary to the results of the referred studies, von der Werth and Jemec pointed to a statistically significant relationship between early disease onset and DLQI score [6].

DLQI is the most broadly used questionnaire in dermatology offering the opportunity to compare the effect of several skin diseases on QoL [14]. When comparing DLQI scores obtained for the HS population of the present study with those obtained for other skin disorders, it is apparent that the scores for HS are far greater than those reported for melasma [18,19], acne [13,20,21], psoriasis [22-29], atopic dermatitis [22-24,30,31], vitiligo [13,32-36], alopecia [37], cutaneous lupus erythematosus [38], ichthyosis [39], urticaria [40,41], rosacea [24], contact dermatitis [42].

The importance of using the SF36 questionnaire comes from the potency for detecting the psychosocial impact of the disease whatever fails only with DLQI. This is consistent with the results of using SF36 in other dermatoses [21,43-48].

Wolkenstein et al.have been the only researchers, who used SF36 for assessing QoL in HS patients. With the exception of physical function dimension (mean score 71.3 ± 27.4), the current study demonstrated higher score at the rest of the scales. The lowest score was observed at the scale of vitality in comparison with the present study, where bodily pain was the most negatively influenced scale (mean score 40.4 ± 20.4 vs.48.10 ± 4.2, respectively). Both studies recorded lower scores in SF36 as the disease became more intense. Wolkenstein et al. demonstrated also that early disease onset and long disease duration deteriorated QoL. In the current study, no such relationship was found [7].

Determination of correlation between DLQI and SF36 in HS has not been reported previously. Strong correlations were found between DLQI and other questionnaires including Beck Depression Inventory-Short Form, EQ-5D, EQ-5D-VAS, Functional Assessment of Chronic Illness Therapy – Fatigue scale and Quality of Life Enjoyment and Satisfaction Questionnaire Short Form, with the exception of Evers et al. "6-Item Scale" [8].

As far as correlations between DLQI and SF36 are concerned, the majority of studies about QoL in other skin diseases found that the strongest correlations were between total DLQI and SF36 mental health dimensions. This result could be attributed to the fact that skin diseases mainly affect psychosocial aspects of life [20,43]. However, in the current study, the correlation between total DLQI and SF36 mental health dimensions was as strong as the correlation between total DLQI and SF36 physical dimension. HS patients experience a great impairment of psychosocial aspects of life, but also severe pain and derangement of physical functioning due constant inflammation and location of the lesions [8,9].

DLQI is not only a simple measure for estimating life quality in skin diseases, but it also correlates positively with HS intensity and severity [6,8,14]. With regard to the reasons above, practitioners should be encouraged to use this instrument in everyday clinical practice and in therapeutic trials. The number of therapeutic trials using DLQI as an instrument for estimating patients' course is rising [49-52].

DLQI is focused mainly on patients' functioning. Emotion and mental health is not sufficiently evaluated [14]. This fact must be taken into consideration because of the psychosocial impact of HS. HS patients may suffer from depression, while high stigmatization level and low self-esteem promote isolation [8,9].

On the other hand, SF36 is considered as the instrument of choice for evaluating health-related life quality and it has been used in a wide spectrum of skin diseases. It estimates both physical and mental health and it correlates well with DLQI. The fact that the minimal clinically important difference in dermatology is not exactly known is included in SF36 limitations [14].

Both questionnaires highlighted disparities between Hurley stage I and III patients. DLQI scores reflected better the differences between Hurley stage I and II. Second-stage HS may cause greater impact on function rather than on mental condition compared to first-stage. SF36 was more effective in assessing differences between Hurley II and III patients. Patients suffering from third-stage HS may experience more severe impairment of mental health rather than of skin condition and function. It seems that a combination of DLQI and SF36 usage is more effective in the holistic approach of an HS patient. Bronsard et al. recommended a combination of DLQI and SF36 for evaluating QoL in plaque type psoriasis [53], whereas both et al. SF36 and Skindex-29 for the assessment of QoL in skin diseases [14].

Conclusions

HS is a dermatologic condition causing great impact on QoL. The severity stage of HS according to Hurley classification was found to be the only factor affecting the level of impairment at a statistically significant grade. The usage of both dermatology-specific and generic questionnaires measuring QoL is vital in everyday clinical practice and trials. It is recommended that questionnaires should be filled out at first contact with an HS patient and that their completion may be repeated after treatment. Patients experiencing a high level of impairment should be encouraged to seek psychological advice; formation of supporting groups may also be helpful [9]. The devastating impact on QoL points towards an intensive effort for research for an effective therapeutic method.

References

1. Giamarellos-Bourboulis EJ, Scheinfend N, Pelekanou A (2009) Hidradenitis suppurativa as a chronic inflammatory disorder. Are biological therapies the future therapeutic solution? Expert Rev Dermatol 4: 47-54.

2. Revuz JE, Canoui-Poitrine F, Wolkenstein P, Viallette C, Gabison G, et al. (2008) Prevalence and factors associated with hidradenitis suppurativa: results from two case-control studies. J Am Acad Dermatol 59: 596-601.

3. Jemec GB, Heidenheim M, Nielsen NH (1996) The prevalence of hidradenitis suppurativa and its potential precursor lesions. J Am Acad Dermatol 35: 191-194.

4. Revuz J (2009) Hidradenitis suppurativa. J Eur Acad Dermatol Venereol 23: 985-998.

5. Alikhan A, Lynch PJ, Eisen DB (2009) Hidradenitis suppurativa: a comprehensive review. J Am Acad Dermatol 60: 539-561.

6. von der Werth JM, Jemec GB (2001) Morbidity in patients with hidradenitis suppurativa. Br J Dermatol 144: 809-813.

7. Wolkenstein P, Loundou A, Barrau K, Auquier P, Revuz J; Quality of Life Group of the French Society of Dermatology (2007) Quality of life impairment in hidradenitis suppurativa: a study of 61 cases. J Am Acad Dermatol 56: 621-623.

8. Matusiak L, Bieniek A, Szepietowski JC (2010) Psychophysical aspects of hidradenitis suppurativa. Acta Derm Venereol 90: 264-268.

9. Esmann S, Jemec GB (2011) Psychosocial impact of hidradenitis suppurativa: a qualitative study. Acta Derm Venereol 91: 328-332.

10. Onderdijk AJ, van der Zee HH, Esmann S, Lophaven S, Dufour DN, et al. (2013) Depression in patients with hidradenitis suppurativa. J Eur Acad Dermatol Venereol 27: 473-478.

11. Jemec GBE, Revuz J, Leyden JJ (2006) Hidradenitis suppurativa. Springer, Heidelberg.

12. Roenigk RK, Roenigk HH Jr (1996) Dermatologic surgery. Principles and practice (2ndedn.) Marcel Dekker, New York.

13. Finlay AY, Khan GK (1994) Dermatology Life Quality Index (DLQI)--a simple practical measure for routine clinical use. Clin Exp Dermatol 19: 210-216.

14. Both H, Essink-Bot ML, Busschbach J, Nijsten T (2007) Critical review of generic and dermatology-specific health-related quality of life instruments. J Invest Dermatol 127: 2726-2739.

15. Ware JE Jr, Kosinski M, Gandek B, Aaronson NK, Apolone G, et al. (1998) The factor structure of the SF-36 Health Survey in 10 countries: results from the IQOLA Project. International Quality of Life Assessment. J Clin Epidemiol 51: 1159-1165.

16. Sartorius K, Emtestam L, Jemec GB, Lapins J (2009) Objective scoring of hidradenitis suppurativa reflecting the role of tobacco smoking and obesity. Br J Dermatol 161: 831-839.

17. Sartorius K, Killasli H, Heilborn J, Jemec GB, Lapins J, et al. (2010) Interobserver variability of clinical scores in hidradenitis suppurativa is low. Br J Dermatol 162: 1261-1268.

18. Leeyaphan C, Wanitphakdeedecha R, Manuskiatti W, Kulthanan K (2011) Measuring melasma patients' quality of life using willingness to pay and time trade-off methods in Thai population. BMC Dermatol 11: 16.

19. Pichardo R, Vallejos Q, Feldman SR, Schulz MR, Verma A, et al. (2009) The prevalence of melasma and its association with quality of life in adult male Latino migrant workers. Int J Dermatol 48: 22-26.

20. Takahashi N, Suzukamo Y, Nakamura M, Miyachi Y, Green J, et al. (2006) Japanese version of the Dermatology Life Quality Index: validity and reliability in patients with acne. Health Qual Life Outcomes 4: 46.

21. Klassen AF, Newton JN, Mallon E (2000) Measuring quality of life in people referred for specialist care of acne: comparing generic and disease-specific measures. J Am Acad Dermatol 43: 229-233.

22. Schmitt J, Meurer M, Klon M, Frick KD (2008) Assessment of health state utilities of controlled and uncontrolled psoriasis and atopic eczema: a population-based study. Br J Dermatol 158: 351-359.

23. Lundberg L, Johannesson M, Silverdahl M, Hermansson C, Lindberg M (1999) Quality of life, health-state utilities and willingness to pay in patients with psoriasis and atopic eczema. Br J Dermatol 141: 1067-1075.

24. Langenbruch AK, Beket E, Augustin M (2011) Quality of health care of rosacea in Germany from the patient's perspective: results of the national health care study Rosareal 2009. Dermatology 223: 124-130.

25. Schöffski O, Augustin M, Prinz J, Rauner K, Schubert E, et al. (2007) Costs and quality of life in patients with moderate to severe plaque-type psoriasis in Germany: a multi-center study. J Dtsch Dermatol Ges 5: 209-218.

26. Schäfer I, Hacker J, Rustenbach SJ, Radtke M, Franzke N, et al. (2010) Concordance of the Psoriasis Area and Severity Index (PASI) and patient-reported outcomes in psoriasis treatment. Eur J Dermatol 20: 62-67.

27. Colombo G, Altomare G, Peris K, Martini P, Quarta G, et al. (2008) Moderate and severe plaque psoriasis: cost-of-illness study in Italy. Ther Clin Risk Manag 4: 559-568.

28. Mazzotti E, Barbaranelli C, Picardi A, Abeni D, Pasquini P (2005) Psychometric properties of the Dermatology Life Quality Index (DLQI) in 900 Italian patients with psoriasis. Acta Derm Venereol 85: 409-413.

29. Nijsten T, Meads DM, de Korte J, Sampogna F, Gelfand JM, et al. (2007) Cross-cultural inequivalence of dermatology-specific health-related quality of life instruments in psoriasis patients. J Invest Dermatol 27: 2315-2322.

30. Misery L, Finlay AY, Martin N, Boussetta S, Nguyen C, et al. (2007) Atopic dermatitis: impact on the quality of life of patients and their partners. Dermatology 215: 123-129.

31. Holm EA, Esmann S, Jemec GB (2006) The handicap caused by atopic dermatitis--sick leave and job avoidance. J Eur Acad Dermatol Venereol 20: 255-259.

32. Ongenae K, Van Geel N, De Schepper S, Naeyaert JM (2005) Effect of vitiligo on self-reported health-related quality of life. Br J Dermatol 152: 1165-1172.

33. Kostopoulou P, Jouary T, Quintard B, Ezzedine K, Marques S, et al. (2009) Objective vs. subjective factors in the psychological impact of vitiligo: the experience from a French referral centre. Br J Dermatol 161: 128-133.

34. Kent G, al-Abadie M (1996) Factors affecting responses on Dermatology Life Quality Index items among vitiligo sufferers. Clin Exp Dermatol 21: 330-333.

35. Parsad D, Pandhi R, Dogra S, Kanwar AJ, Kumar B (2003) Dermatology Life Quality Index score in vitiligo and its impact on the treatment outcome. Br J Dermatol 148: 373-374.

36. Radtke MA, Schäfer I, Gajur A, Langenbruch A, Augustin M (2009) Willingness-to-pay and quality of life in patients with vitiligo. Br J Dermatol 161: 134-139.

37. Williamson D, Gonzalez M, Finlay AY (2001) The effect of hair loss on quality of life. J Eur Acad Dermatol Venereol 15: 137-139.

38. Ferraz LB, Almeida FA, Vasconcellos MR, Faccina AS, Ciconelli RM, et al. (2006) The impact of lupus erythematosus cutaneous on the Quality of life: the Brazilian-Portuguese version of DLQI. Qual Life Res 15: 565-570.

39. Gånemo A, Sjöden PO, Johansson E, Vahlquist A, Lindberg M (2004) Health-related quality of life among patients with ichthyosis. Eur J Dermatol 14: 61-66.

40. Liu JB, Yao MZ, Si AL, Xiong LK, Zhou H (2012) Life quality of Chinese patients with chronic urticaria as assessed by the dermatology life quality index. J Eur Acad Dermatol Venereol 26: 1252-1257.

41. Töndury B, Muehleisen B, Ballmer-Weber BK, Hofbauer G, Schmid-Grendelmeier P, et al. (2011) The Pictorial Representation of Illness and Self Measure (PRISM) instrument reveals a high burden of suffering in patients with chronic urticaria. J Investig Allergol Clin Immunol 21: 93-100.

42. Lau MY, Burgess JA, Nixon R, Dharmage SC, Matheson MC (2011) A review of the impact of occupational contact dermatitis on quality of life. J Allergy 2011: 964509.

43. Holm EA, Wulf HC, Stegmann H, Jemec GB (2006) Life quality assessment among patients with atopic eczema. Br J Dermatol 154: 719-725.

44. Maksimović N, Janković S, Marinković J, Sekulović LK, Zivković Z, et al. (2012) Health-related quality of life in patients with atopic dermatitis. J Dermatol 39: 42-47.

45. Kiebert G, Sorensen SV, Revicki D, Fagan SC, Doyle JJ, et al. (2002) Atopic dermatitis is associated with a decrement in health-related quality of life. Int J Dermatol 41: 151-158.

46. Lau MY, Matheson MC, Burgess JA, Dharmage SC, Nixon R (2011) Disease severity and quality of life in a follow-up study of patients with occupational contact dermatitis. Contact Dermatitis 65: 138-145.

47. Oztürkcan S, Ermertcan AT, Eser E, Sahin MT (2006) Cross validation of the Turkish version of dermatology life quality index. Int J Dermatol 45: 1300-1307.

48. He Z, Lu C, Basra MK, Ou A, Yan Y, et al. (2013) Psychometric properties of the Chinese version of Dermatology Life Quality Index (DLQI) in 851 Chinese patients with psoriasis. J Eur Acad Dermatol Venereol 27: 109-115.

49. Cusack C, Buckley C (2006) Etanercept: effective in the management of hidradenitis suppurativa. Br J Dermatol 154: 726-729.

50. Adams DR, Yankura JA, Fogelberg AC, Anderson BE (2010) Treatment of hidradenitis suppurativa with etanercept injection. Arch Dermatol 146: 501-504.

51. Schweiger ES, Riddle CC, Aires DJ (2011) Treatment of hidradenitis suppurativa by photodynamic therapy with aminolevulinic acid: preliminary results. J Drugs Dermatol 10: 381-386.

52. Gulliver WP, Jemec GB, Baker KA (2012) Experience with ustekinumab for the treatment of moderate to severe hidradenitis suppurativa. J Eur Acad Dermatol Venereol 26: 911-914.

53. Bronsard V, Paul C, Prey S, Puzenat E, Gourraud PA, et al. (2010) What are the best outcome measures for assessing quality of life in plaque type psoriasis? A systematic review of the literature. J Eur Acad Dermatol Venereol 24 Suppl 2: 17-22.

11

Evaluation of Preventative Screening for Chronic Disease in a Rural Primary Health Service

Ervin K[1]*, Koschel A[1] and Campi S[2]

[1]*Department of Rural Health, University of Melbourne, Australia*
[2]*Violet Town Bush Nursing Centre, Cowslip St., Violet Town, Australia*

Abstract

Prevention is a key element of primary health care and screening provides the ability to reduce complications and health care burden by early identification of potential disease. There is however little information on the effectiveness or uptake of advice from positive chronic disease screening in rural areas of Australia. This study provides evidence for screening for chronic conditions and uptake of advice to consult their medical practitioner when risk factors were identified.

Community screening in rural Victoria was undertaken with 56 people screened over a six month period from November 2014 to April 2015. Only participants who scored above 12 on the Australian Diabetes type 2 diabetes risk assessment tool (AUSDRISK) who were not regularly engaged with a medical practitioner regarding their diabetes risk or with high blood pressure were asked to participate in the research project. A total of 24 people were screened positive and were advised to attend their medical practitioner. Twenty three participants consented to a follow up interview post participation in screening to determine uptake of advice and outcomes of medical practitioner engagement with a final 20 participants interviewed.

Results demonstrated that the majority of people with a risk of high blood pressure identified during the screening made an appointment with their medical practitioner. Medical practitioners initiated treatment or further testing with these people, ensuring that early intervention would lead to a reduction in complications reducing further burden on the health care system. This early intervention has the potential to avert complications and although the sample was small, it suggests that screening is beneficial and uptake of advice is acted on by those at risk of chronic disease.

Keywords: Screening; Chronic disease; Early intervention

Introduction

Evidence suggests that the engagement of people early is a key to delaying the burdens associated with development of chronic conditions. Interventions in primary health are valuable in assisting the decrease in need for hospitalisations due to chronic conditions and poor management of the same [1,2]. Diabetes is a significant health problem in Australia, but the true burden of the disease is thought to be much greater because many people with diabetes are unaware that they have the condition, or are at significant risk of developing it [3]. It is estimated that as a result of ageing alone, the number of people with type 2 diabetes will double by 2050, while the cost of treating it will quadruple [3]. Diabetes currently accounts for 2.3% of all health care expenditure in Australia [3].

The risk of developing diabetes is measurable. The Australian type 2 diabetes risk assessment tool (AUSDRISK) was developed by the Baker IDI Heart and Diabetes Institute as part of a Commonwealth initiative to assess the risk of type 2 diabetes [4]. The form is a short set of questions measuring lifestyle risk factors and demographic characteristics, only questions that are validated best predictors of the development of diabetes are included in the score. The major factors include age, Aboriginal or Torres Strait Islander status, waist circumference and physical activity.

Similarly, hypertension has long been recognised as an important risk factor for cardiovascular disease and mortality [5]. Hypertension is generally diagnosed, or considered to warrant further follow up, if blood pressure is 140/90 mmHg or higher. The Global Burden of Disease Study (GBD) advocates for prevention, detection, treatment and control of this condition, as a high priority on worldwide health agendas [6]. Hypertension is ranked as the leading single risk factor for GBD, and one barrier identified is the lack of a health care system to identify those at risk for hypertension and cardiovascular disease,

and follow up to monitor and deliver treatment [7]. The most simple diagnostic technique for hypertension is blood pressure measurement using a sphygmanometer and stethoscope or electronic sensor, taking less than 3 minutes [7].

Health screening programs are a strategy used in populations to identify unrecognised disease, performed on people in apparently good health. Health screening interventions are designed to identify disease early to enable early intervention and management and if possible, prevention. Early intervention also involves determining individual's health literacy, which is broadly defined as the skills to access, understand, appraise and apply health information in order to make judgements and decisions about health care [8]. Although health literacy is now ubiquitous in health care settings, it originated from the field of public health in relation to health promotion and primary prevention [9]. Determining health literacy during the health screening process also sets the scene for the commencement of self-management for clients. A key element of self-management is goal setting, which is defined as an agreement between the clinician and client to achieve the required change for optimal health, taking into consideration an individual's preferences, values and needs to achieve the goal[10]. The World Health Organisation sets the criteria for health screening

*Corresponding author: Kaye Ervin, Department of Rural Health, University of Melbourne, Australia, E-mail: ervink@humehealth.org.au

and includes that the conditions screened for should be an important health problem, that it should be treatable, that facilities for diagnosing and treating should be available, and that there should be a test or examination available which is acceptable to the population [11].

There is little, if any, information on the effectiveness of preventative community screening programs, especially in rural settings in Australia, although evaluations of the effectiveness of screening programs in workplace settings have been published [12]. Successful screening programs show evidence that early diagnosis and treatment increases the chance of successfully treating, preventing or managing the disease [13].

A new model of primary health care in rural Victoria, Australia, undertook community health screening for diabetes and hypertension, as do many community health programs. As a new model of care, management were interested to evaluate the effectiveness of community health screening for these conditions – did the population who were identified at risk of diabetes (using the AUSDRISK tool) and those with a blood pressure reading above 140/90 mmHg, seek further evaluation from their medical practitioner? If they did, what was the outcome? If they did not, what barriers prevented further health seeking? The study utilised qualitative and quantitative methods to determine the outcome of the community health screening.

Methodology

The geographical area of the study has a population of 9,486 people spread over an area of 3,302 square kilometres, with three major townships. The townships, vary in population size from 3,100 to 1,080 people [14]. Agriculture is the primary industry in the shire, with a known ageing population and high rates of chronic disease [15]. Apart from the new model of primary health care, there are no publicly funded health agencies in the geographical area.

Participants were recruited in various community settings, including community events and strategic positioning of primary healthcare staff in the three small townships (such as outside local supermarkets). Participants were invited to undertake health screening using the AUSDRISK tool and blood pressure measurement.

Community Health Staff administered the AUSDRISK and measured blood pressure of participants who agreed to health screening. Participants were screened in a seated position. Answers to the AUSDRISK are scored, with a score of 5 or less indicating low risk, 6-11 an intermediate risk and 12 or more high risk.

Participants who were not currently receiving regular care from

their medical practitioner and who scored above 12 on the AUSDRISK or who had a blood pressure reading above 140/90 mmHg, were advised to seek further evaluation from their medical practitioner and invited to participate in the research study. A plain language statement describing the study and contact information for the researcher was provided to all participants who consented. The plain language statement indicated that the participants would be contacted in one month's time to arrange a mutually suitable time to conduct a telephone interview, and to give further consent to participate or withdraw from the study.

Results

A total of 56 people were screened over a six month period. Of the 56 people screened 24 participants were not eligible, 19 of these were already regularly engaged with their medical practitioner. Of the remaining 32 participants identified, 24 were referred to their medical practitioner for follow up (75%). Of the 32 eligible participants;

- 13 recorded an elevated blood pressure (40.6%),
- 1 recorded an irregular pulse (3.1%), and
- 18 recorded an AUSDRISK score above 12 (56.3%).

Of the 24 participants referred to their medical practitioner, 23 (95.8%) agreed to follow up interview by the University of Melbourne researcher. The principal researcher, a nurse and research academic, contacted the consenting participants by telephone. Of the 23 participants who agreed to interview, three could not be contacted leaving a sample of 20 participants. A total of 67 phone calls were made to complete interviews (median 3.3 per person).

Participants who consented were telephoned by the researcher approximately one month after the community screening. After agreeing to an interview time, they were asked three questions – did they visit their medical practitioner as recommended? If they did, what was the outcome of that visit? If they did not, why not? Participants were invited to comment further, but no medical advice was offered by the researcher as there was no existing client/clinician relationship.

Demographic characteristics of the 20 consenting participants are shown in (Table 1). Of the 20 participants, seven had elevated blood pressure, one an irregular heart rate, nine had an AUSDRISK score greater than 12 and the remaining three had both high blood pressure and an elevated AUSDRISK score (Shown in Table 1).

Two participants (10% of the total sample) reported that they did not visit their medical practitioner as recommended. The remaining 18 participants did visit their medical practitioner. The two participants

		n (%)				
Gender	Male	9 (45)				
	Female	11 (55)				
Age (years)	Range	Median (IQR)				
	18-86	60.1 (43-81)				
			Did not visit medical practitioner as recommended	Visited medical practitioner	Further investigation	Further treatment
		n (%)	n (%)	n (%)	n (%)	n (%)
Blood pressure 140/90 or greater		7 (35)	0	7 (100)	7 (100)	5 (71)
AUSDRISK score 12 or greater		9 (45)	2 (22)	7 (77)	3 (43)	0
Irregular heart rate		1 (5)	0	1 (100)	1 (100)	1 (100)
Combined elevated blood pressure and AUSDRISK score		3 (15)	0	3 (100)	3 (100)	3 (100)

Table 1: Demographic characteristics of 20 consenting participants and screening outcomes.

who did not visit their medical practitioner both had elevated AUSDRISK scores as reasons for referral. Both participants provided reasons for not attending their medical practitioner as follows:

"sick of seeing doctors and being treated for so many things. I rattle"

And

"I've had so much wrong with me and it's hard to get around when I don't drive. I have a new doctor and I'm not sure what he's like."

The participant with the irregular heart rate reported that blood pressure medication was increased and specific cardiovascular disease testing was undertaken as a result of her visit to the medical practitioner. As shown in (Table 1), of the participants with elevated blood pressure, two had increases in blood pressure medication, one had medication changed to another type, two were referred to a specialist (one of whom additionally commenced medication) and two had blood tests which resulted in normal results so no further action was taken by their medical practitioners. One of these participants commented that they were happy to have had the screening undertaken.

Of the three participants that had both elevated blood pressure and AUSDRISK scores, two were commenced on new blood pressure medications and one had an increase to cholesterol medication (shown in Table 1).

Of the participants with elevated AUSDRISK scores, three had fasting blood glucose tests with no abnormalities detected and no-one reported any changes to treatment by their medical practitioner (shown in Table 1). Three participants commented that although no further action was taken by their medical practitioner for their elevated AUSDRISK score, they themselves had implemented lifestyle changes as a result.

Discussion

There are very few, if any, similar studies reporting on the outcomes of screening of this kind in the community, particularly in Australian rural communities for comparison of the uptake rates. The uptake proportion of 90% is extremely pleasing in terms of preventative care demonstrating participants desire to achieve healthy lifestyles. An indication of the acceptability of the recommendation of those at risk making an appointment with the medical practitioner was clear, with the majority of those recommendations being taken up.

The two participants who did not visit their medical practitioner both had elevated AUSDRISK scores. One confirmed that travel and access to medical care was a potential barrier, which is widely recognised in the literature as problematic in rural settings [16]. This participant also reported that the relationship with their medical practitioner was new and not fully established.

An interesting result of these interviews was the finding that those with high blood pressure or irregular heart rate had increases in or commenced on medication whilst those with elevated AUSDRISK scores were offered blood testing which resulted in no formal treatment.

Although small, this sample provided some insight into the value of community screening for high blood pressure. Although the value for those with an increased AUSDRISK score was not as clear, due to the long term prediction risk, participants comments suggest that the screening itself was impetus for modifying risk factors in their lifestyle.

Limitation

A limitation of the study is that only de-identified information from the interviews could be provided back to the clinical team, to protect participant's anonymity. This means that the two participants with an AUSDRISK score above 12 who did not visit their medical practitioner as advised, could not be followed up – though this was not the aim of the study. The study simply sought to identify compliance with advice from community health screening, and the outcomes for those who did comply. It was ethically outside the scope of the study to provide further advice to participants at the time of interview as there was no clinician/client relationship.

Conclusion and Recommendations

Most participants, who agreed to undertake health screening in a community setting, sought further evaluation if they were advised to, due to their high risk of diabetes or hypertension. The screening enabled early intervention for those with hypertension but the value for those with a high risk of diabetes is uncertain. It should be remembered that the AUSDRISK tool predicts five year risk of diabetes and that those with a score above 12 warrant continued advice and observation [4].

The results suggest that community screening for hypertension is a valuable use of health resources to implement early intervention which may prevent complications related to this untreated condition.

References

1. Australian Institute for Primary Care. Early intervention in chronic disease in community health services initiative. Statewide Evaluation, Technical and Data Report, 2008.

2. AIHW, Australia's health 2014. 2014: Canberra: AIHW.

3. AIHW, Diabetes: Australian facts 2008. 2008 Canberra: AIHW.

4. Commonwealth Department of Health. Background to the Australian type 2 diabetes risk assessment tool (AUSDRISK) 2015.

5. Bromfield S, Muntner (2013) High bold pressure: The leading global burden of disease (GBD) risk factor and the need for worldwide prevention programs. Current Hypertension Reports 15: 134-136.

6. Kearney P, Whelton M, Reynolds K, Muntner P, Whelton PK, et al. (2005) Global burden of hypertension: Analysis of worldwide data. Lancet 365: 217-23.

7. Perkovic V, Huxley R, Wu Y, Prabhakaran D, MacMahon S, et al. (2007) The burden of blood pressure-related disease: A neglected priority for global health. Hypertension 50: 991-7.

8. Sørensen K, Van den Broucke S, Fullam J, Doyle G, Pelikan J, et al. (2012) Health literacy and public health: A systematic review and integration of definitions and models. BMC Public Health 80: 1-13.

9. Johnson A (2014) Health literacy, does it make a difference? Australian Journal of Advanced Nursing 31: 39-45.

10. Lenzen SA, Daniëls R, van Bokhoven MA, van der Weijden T, Beurskens A, et al. (2015) Setting goals in chronic care: Shared decision making as self management support by the family physician. European Journal of General Practice 21: 138-44.

11. Wilson J, Jungner G (1968) Principles and practice of screening for disease. in WHO chronicle. Geneva: World Health Organisation 16: 318.

12. Bellew B, St George A, King L (2012) Workplace screening programs for chronic disease prevention: An Evidence Check.

13. State Government of Victoria, Population Screening. Viewed 22nd July 2015. Population Screening.

14. Australian Bureau of Statistics. Census QuickStats (2011). "Strathbogie (S) - LGA26430".

15. Strathbogie Health and Community Services Consortium, Strathbogie Health and Community Services Consortium Primary Health Care Funding Proposal.

16. AIHW, Rural, regional and remote health: Indicators of health system performance. 2008: Canberra: AIHW.

12

Exploring Challenges to Primary Occupational Health Care Service for Informal Sector Workers

K Nilvarangkul[1]*, T Phajan[2], U Inmuong[3], JF Smith[3] and P Rithmark[3]

[1]Faculty of Nursing, Khon Kaen University, Thailand
[2]Sirinthon College of Public Health, Khon Kaen, Thailand
[3]Faculty of Public Health, Khon Kaen University, Thailand

Abstract

Informal sector workers are a significant part of the Thai workforce but occupational health service provision for them is under-developed. This multi-method study investigated occupational health policies and service provision in 10 primary health units in four north eastern Thailand provinces. Questionnaires, in-depth interviews and focus group discussions were used to collect data. Descriptive statistics and content analysis were used to analyse quantitative and qualitative data respectively. Results showed limited policy and budget support for such services. Even though service providers' occupational health knowledge overall was good, only two of the units provided such services. They were notable for very good functional relationships with their local administration organizations, community and worker leadership and village health volunteers, plus strong staff commitment to support workers health in their own communities. We suggest that enhancing primary care services for worker health and safety requires development of stronger policy directives, budget provision and management support.

Keywords: Primary occupational health service; Informal sector worker; Primary care unit

Introduction

Thailand is now an upper middle-income country with two thirds of its 65 million populations in the 19-59 year old working age range [1]. In 2015 there were 38.3 million working age people with 21.4 million (55.9%) in informal sector work such as, farmers, home-based silk or cotton workers and contracted sewing factory outworkers; most, 35.5 percent, are in North Eastern Thailand [2]. Although these worker groups are very important to Thailand's economy, producing up to 70 percent of all Thai products, they unfortunately, work outside Thai Labor Law protection, health and safety regulatory frame-works, and without mandated primary care unit (PCU) occupational health services for work-related health and safety needs [3,4].

Informal sector workers work in unsafe environments. For example, 1.4 million workers are exposed to chemical toxicity, 430,000 work with dangerous machinery and equipment and 130,000 work in environments harmful for their vision and hearing. In addition they also have accidental injuries, like sharp cut injuries (63.4%), falls (17%), 6.5 percent have suffered body trauma or had work collisions and 93.5% of women weavers had posture related back, neck arm and hand pain [2,5].

Thai Ministry of Public Health (MOPH) care services and policies focus on industry (formal) sector workers, rather than informal sector workers. However, some provincial health offices have supported training to enhance occupational health care services at PCU level, using the Thai Government Occupational Health Services model [6-8]. In 2007, as part of the Thai health decentralisation process, 22 of 9762 government community health centers were transferred to pilot municipalities and local (sub-district) administrative organizations (LAO) [9,10]. As health and safety PCU services were not well-developed, the Thai National Health Security Office (NASAO) and the Thai Health Foundation (Thai Health) later provided community health funds to support a further pilot series of brief training (2-3 day workshops) specifically to build networks and introductory knowledge around health and safety assessment and treatment services. These were held over 2009 to 2014, mainly at organizational and managerial levels rather than front-line services.

This study focused on current policies and service provision for work-related health and safety at selected PCUs in several provinces that had been in the above pilot training schemes. Even though, there was some research on models for providing occupational health care services in PCUs or training health service delivery personnel at that level, few studies had explored whether PCU staff provided the services or not [6-8].

Materials and Methods

Study design and setting

This was a multi-method study using questionnaires, in-depth interviews (IDI) and focus group discussions (FGD). It was conducted in ten PCUs in four North-eastern Thailand provinces, namely Roi-et, Kalasin, Mahasarakham and Khon Kaen, the North-eastern pilot provinces for the nationally funded training programs described above. Data was collected between October 2014 to July 2015, at least one year after the pilot training workshops [9,10].

Participant recruitment

Multistage random sampling was used to recruit 111 PCU community nurses and public health personnel responsible for providing worker care and 326 community group members (LAO members, community leaders, village health volunteers [VHVs] and informal sector worker leaders) [11]. In addition, 5 executive staff at provincial administrative level and 20 members of health services contracting units (CUP) were purposively recruited from within the 111 health workers.

*Corresponding author: Kessarawan Nilvarangkul, Director of Research and Training Center for Enhancing Quality of Life of Working-Age People, Khon Kaen University, Khon Kaen 40002, Thailand, Email: kessa_ni@kku.ac.th, kessarawan2559@gmail.com

Research instruments

A survey questionnaire was developed to collect demographic data and occupational health and safety knowledge levels from health personnel and community group members. The health personnel questionnaire had 20 and the community group 15 items respectively. Scores were considered high if over 80% correct, average if 60-79.99% correct and poor if lower than 60%.Three occupational health experts reviewed the questionnaire for content validity and their feedback contributed to the final draft [12,13]. The questionnaire was pretested with 30 health personnel and 30 community group members in Khon Kaen Province. Reliability was assessed using K-R 20, yielding scores of 0.80 and 0.82 which were judged acceptable [14].

Semi structured interview guides probing a range of issues around policies; service provision and financial and human resources support were used in the FGDs and in the IDIs to collect qualitative data.

Data collection

Data collection took place in the community or at participants' workplaces. Quantitative data, using the individual questionnaires, was collected from 111 PCU community nurses and public health personnel and the 326-strong community group members.

Qualitative data were collected using five IDIs with the executive staff to collect information related to existing policies and their understanding of their responsibility to provide work-related health promotion and safety services for informal sector workers in PCUs. Two FGDs were used to gather information from the 20 CUP members related to budget and organizational support for encouraging PCUs to provide health promotion and safety services for the workers. Eight FGDs were used to collect data from 80 PCU community nurses, public health personnel and community group members about policies and provision of health promotion and work and safety health services for informal sector workers. Each IDI or FGD took from one to one and half hours. All IDIs and FGDs were audio recorded and transcribed verbatim by researchers.

Lincoln and Guba's four criteria, creditability, transferability, dependability and confirmability, were used to test the scientific rigor of the study [15].

Data analysis

Questionnaire data were validated and coded. Descriptive statistics were used to display health personnel and community group member's demographic and occupational health policies and practice knowledge. The IDI and FGD data was analysed using content analysis. Data was read through until researchers were fully familiar with it, then open coding, item grouping and categorization into themes was used [16].

Research ethics

This study was reviewed and approved by Khon Kaen University's Human Ethics Committee (HE 572126).

Results

Demographic details

There were 4 females and one male in the executive staff of the provincial administrative sample. Four had bachelor's degrees and one had completed a PhD. The 20 CUP committee members included 16 males, and four females. Nineteen had completed bachelor's degrees and one had a master's degree.

Among the 111 health services personnel, 67.6% were female, average age was 40.47 years (S.D.=9.64) years 70.3% were married and 70.3% had bachelor's degrees 70.3%.

Of the 326 community group members67% were female, average age was 48.36 years (S.D.=9.80) and 92.6% were married. Almost 40 percent had finished primary school and 35.9% had completed secondary school.

Policy and service provision

Data on primary occupational health care services (POHCS) are reported in 3 broad topic areas: policy support, networking and training and PHC service provision.

Policy support for POHCS

Four provinces were found not to have any formal policies to support POHCS. Only one province had established cholinesterase blood checks for farmers as a key performance index for health personnel, but even then it was not compulsory. The CUPs which were responsible for annual health services budget allocation in their district had neither policy requirements nor budget provision for providing primary occupational care for informal sector workers. The CUP focused on chronic illnesses such as diabetes mellitus and hypertension. One CUP committee said "The chair of our CUP committee provided budget for chronic illness following the government policy. He did not support budget for primary occupational health services" (Male 50 year old).

In addition, most members of LAOs, local politicians responsible for financial support for sub-district level health care services, did not support budget for such services. One health worker suggested "It was difficult to gain final support from the local politician since they wanted to use money for chronic illness and materials rather than support PCU to provide primary occupational health for informal sector workers" (female 45 years old").

Training and network building for providing POHCS

The pilot training had provided strategies and knowledge for health staff and community group members about occupational health care needs. VHVs, LAO members, and informal sector workers leaders had learned about occupational health and safety issues such as, agricultural chemical toxicity and how to self-protect from toxicity, and how to work with good posture. Health staff was also encouraged to establish data bases related to work safety and risk of the illness. From the survey questionnaires the majority of health staff had high levels of knowledge related to providing PHC occupational health services (87.4%) with only 12.6 percent having average knowledge levels.

Health personnel had also built networks with VHVs, LAO member and community leaders to help them to provide the services. Community group members' questionnaire data showed high levels of knowledge for POHCS needs (46.3%), average knowledge levels (46.9%), with a very small number having low level knowledge (6.8%).

Providing POHCS

From IDIs and FGD data it was clear that most PCUs did not provide occupational health services for informal sector workers. Even though health workers had good knowledge they did not provide services mainly as there was no government policy or budget support to provide these services. Some PCUs provided cholinesterase blood checks for farmers, but only sporadically, dependent on budget allocations. As a result, they focused on PHC mandated and budgeted chronic illness care. One health personal reflected "We did not receive any support, such as financial, from our CUP or government to provide the services" (male 25 year old). Another said "Therefore, for informal sector (workers) we could check only cholinesterase in their blood but not regularly and could check only some farmers not all who were at risk by contact with agricultural chemical" (female 48 years old). A CUP member said "Most PCU health staff thought that to provide primary occupational health services was not their responsibility since the ministry of public health focused on chronic illness rather than work-related diseases. They also did not have financial support to provide the services" (male 56 years old). Most of PCUs did not have occupational health-related data based. A community nurse said "My PCU does not record diseases related to work and surveillance illness related to work" (female 40 years old).

Almost none of the community group members e.g. VHVs, who worked with PCU health workers provided any occupational health care services. Some felt they did not have enough knowledge and did not feel confident to offer advice to the workers. Furthermore, most PCU health personnel did not provide work-related services accept a few blood cholinesterase checks if their budget allowed. Few made suggestions related to agricultural chemical toxicity. One VHV said "I had never provided any suggestion related to primary occupational health to informal sector workers. I suggested them about how to care for themselves to prevent diabetes mellitus (female 50 years old). A community leader reflected "Health personnel did not give me any leaflet to provide health education or over the broadcasting tower (village public address system) related to work and safety but they did give leaflet on how to prevent dengue haemorrhagic fever in rainy season" (male 35 years old).

Although most PCUs had never provided occupational health care services to informal sector workers, two PCU were found that provided such services, both via outreach and within the PCU. Community group members helped PCU health staff to provide outreach services, e.g. health education related to preventing musculoskeletal disorder, to avoid agricultural chemical toxicity, and investigate work accidents and injury and work environments. They also monitored workers' adherence to occupational health and safety advice by visiting them at their work places. Additionally, they provided health screening and basic work-related care. One CPU health personal said "Our PCU collaborated with local politicians, VHVs, community leaders and leaders or representative of the informal sector workers in our responsible area to provide education related to occupational health and safety and care for the workers...also provide basic cure for them" (health personal 43 years old). This PCU was able to provide occupational health services because it had a close working relationship with its LAO and community. As a result, they gained financial support from the LAO and good collaboration from community leaders, VHVs and workers. Further, the health personnel were local people and had a sense of community commitment. A health personal reflected "I am local person and love people in my village. I do not want them to have illness related to work since the disease related to work I can prevent. I am also familiar with members of LAO. I am also able to work with them and ask support such as financial support or workforce support." (Female 48 years old). Another member of LAO said "We are local people. We love our people and want to help them. We have to help each other and care for our villagers. Our chief executive of LAO also gives financial support to the health personnel's project to provide occupational health and work safety for the workers" (female 35 years old). However, one PCU had problems related to on-going financial support when local politicians changed—they are elected every four years by community vote.

Discussion

Despite specific central-government pilot funding for training to improve PCU-level occupational health and safety knowledge and services, we found only two of our 10 selected PCUs provided such care. Most considered such services outside their responsibility with neither budget provision, nor formal policy requirements to do so. Some PCUs did provide occasional blood cholinesterase level checks for farmers, dependent on budgets. Even though we found PCU health workers occupational health knowledge levels were relatively high, other reasons suggested for lack of service provision included, limited numbers of health personnel expert in occupational care and heavy non-worker related workloads, as also noted earlier by Office of Disease Prevention and Control, Region 4 [17].

In contrast, all PCUs and CUP contracting units focused on chronic diseases such as diabetes and hypertension in line with mandated services policies and budget provision. These two successful PCUs had clear distinguishing features. Their personnel were local, strongly committed to their communities and had good collaborative working relationships with other stakeholders, both, throughout the community via village health volunteers and informal sector worker leaders, and also within elected community leadership and formal sub-district LAO administrative structures. These interlocking collaborative layers between the elected leadership decision-making infrastructure and the community reflect a sense of joint ownership of health service processes and priorities and community empowerment considered crucial for fostering their organizational and practical implementation [10,18,19]. The above are positive PCU service examples; however, the role of local elected officials in decentralized health service decision-making and management structures is a potentially significant destabilizer for sustainable services. Successful health decentralization assumes the existence of appropriate levels of local expertise and capacity and stable on-going political will for sustainable services. This is often not the case; see examples from, Thailand, Philippines, Ghana, Zambia and Uganda [9].

Conclusion

Our study revealed that despite specific formal training initiatives to improve PCU occupational health care services, service provision remained limited. The two successful units showed PCU personnel and services well valued and embedded in their local communities. They also had strong working relationships with members of LAOs and elected officials who supported and facilitated occupational health service activities without any central policy directives or budget allocation to do so. However, this level of infrastructure functionality and community engagement and motivation typically needs to be developed rather than assumed. We recommend that future efforts to enhance PCU occupational health and safety services must include new policy priorities and organizational/managerial infrastructure development. Just enhancing specific work-related health service knowledge and skills at the PCU level without strengthening policy and infrastructure support is unlikely to be successful. Future policy development and implementation should also be integrated with research strategies to develop effective occupational health and safety services for this worker group.

Acknowledgement

The authors are grateful thank to health personnel and community group members who participate in the study. They also would like to thank you National Health Security Office region 7 and Research and Training Center for Enhancing Quality of Life of Working Age People for financial support. The author(s) declared the receipt of the following financial support for the research, authorship, and/or publication of this article: This study was funded by the National Health Security Office region 7 of Thailand and Research and Training Center for Enhancing Quality of Life of Working Age People, Khon Kaen University, Thailand.

References

1. Institute for Population and Social Research (2016) Thai population 2016. Mahidol Population Gazette 25:1-2.

2. National Statistical Office. The informal employment survey 2015.

3. Nilvarangkul K, Adler-Collins J, Thawenongiew K (2009) Community participation in health service system for informal sector workers in primary care units: A case study of sugarcane farmers. Khon Kaen: Klangnanavittaya Press.

4. Thai Health Committee. Thai Health 2012: Food security-the illusion of money vs. the reality of food.

5. Nilvarangkul K, Wongprom J, Tumnong C (2006) Strengthening the self-care of women working in the informal sector: Local fabric weaving in Khon Kaen, Thailand (Phase I). Industrial Health 44: 101-107.

6. Wittayapun Y, Lagampan S, Kalampakorn S, Rogers B, Vorapongsathorn T (2008) Application of the occupational health services model in Thai primary care units. AAOHN Journal 56: 197-205.

7. Thai Bureau of Occupational and Environmental Diseases (2010) Occupational health services in public health services for informal sector workers (2008-2009). Bangkok: Thailand: Thai health promotion foundation.

8. Nilvarangkul K, Arphorn S, Kessomboon N (2016) Action research to develop occupational health services in primary care units for informal sector workers in Thailand. Action Research 14: 113-131.

9. Wongthanvasu S, Sudhipongpracha T (2013) Analysis of the capacity and preparedness of local administrative organizations in health management. Nonthaburi: Health System Research Institute.

10. Sudhipongpracha T (2013) Measuring community empowerment as a process and an outcome: Preliminary evaluation of the decentralized primary health care programs in northeast Thailand. Community Development 44: 551-566.

11. Polit DF, Beck CT (2008) Nursing research: Generating and assign evidence for nursing practice. 8th ed. Philadelphia, PA: Lippincott.

12. Lobiondo-Wood G, Haber J (2010) Nursing research: Methods and critical appraisal for evaluation-base practice. 7th ed. Louis: Mosby.

13. Lincoln YS, Guba EG (1985) Naturalistic inquiry. Newbury Park, CA: Sage.

14. Elo J, Kyngas H (2008) The qualitative content analysis process. JAN.

15. Office of Disease Prevention and Control, Region 4. Implementation report from experience of developing occupational health services in public services for informal sector worker during 2008-2009 in central region. Bangkok: Thailand Health Promotion Foundation, 2009.

16. Pretty J (1995) The many Interpretation of Participation. In Focus 16: 4-5.

17. Honey A (1999) Empowerment versus power: Consumer participation in mental health service. Occupational Therapy International 6: 257-276.

18. Bossert TJ, Beauvais JC (2002) Decentralization of health system in Ghana, Zambia, Uganda and the Philippines: A comparative analysis of decision space. Health Policy and Planning 17: 14-31.

19. Tae-Arak P (2010) Synthesis of health service decentralization approaches. Nonthaburi: Health System Research Institute.

13

Fruit and Vegetable Consumption in Rural Victorian School Children

Ervin K[1]*, Dalle Nogare N[2], Orr J[3], Soutter E[2,4] and Spiller R[2]

[1]*University of Melbourne, Department of Rural Health, Shepparton, Australia*
[2]*Goulburn Valley Primary Care Partnership, Shepparton, Australia*
[3]*Goulburn Valley Health, Shepparton, Australia*
[4]*Numurkah District Health Service, Numurkah, Australia*

Abstract

Fruit and vegetable consumption is accepted as the cornerstone of healthy eating practices. In turn, healthy eating is linked to the prevention of a number of chronic diseases. Healthy eating practices should begin in early childhood and continue throughout life. This study aimed to determine fruit and vegetable consumption in children aged 6-12 years in three local government areas in rural Australia, and examines the factors which influence consumption, such as access, cost and parental education and behaviours.

Parents of school children in grades one and three from 41 schools completed a survey regarding fruit and vegetable consumption, and associated factors, for their child. Five hundred and forty four surveys were completed and returned. The results showed that while fruit consumption was within the recommended guidelines for 97% of children, only 12% ate the recommended serves of vegetables for this age group. The results did not vary between the age and gender of children nor parental income or education. Parental sources of knowledge for healthy eating was reported as predominantly family and friends as well as newspapers, internet and magazines.

Examining fruit and vegetable consumption separately highlighted the need for a focused intervention on increasing vegetable consumption in the three local government areas. The sources of parental knowledge provided important information for health promotion activities.

Keywords: Fruit and vegetable consumption; Rural; Children; Survey; Local government area (LGA)

Introduction

Adequate fruit and vegetable consumption can be linked to the prevention of a number of chronic conditions such as cardiovascular disease, diabetes, obesity and some cancers [1,2]. Healthy eating includes a dietary intake of a variety of fruit and vegetables which contributes to better overall health by providing a range of nutrients and dietary fiber [2,3].

In 2012, healthy eating was identified as a priority area by agencies funded for Integrated Health Promotion in the Goulburn Valley Primary Care Partnership (GVPCP) catchment area. Three Victorian local government areas (LGA) comprise the catchment: Greater Shepparton, Moira and Strathbogie Shire. They are geographically diverse areas, with varying population sizes (from 63,000 in Greater Shepparton to 10,000 in Strathbogie) and various primary industries. Heavily influenced by agriculture, the catchment is widely recognized as the 'food bowl' of Australia.

The percentage of adults meeting fruit and vegetable dietary guidelines was known to be low in the GVPCP catchment. Fifty five percent in Moira Shire, 53.9% in Greater Shepparton and 50.7% in Strathbogie were not meeting the recommended daily intake of fruit and vegetables [4-6]. The current Australian recommended daily intake for adults is two serves of fruit and five serves of vegetables [7].

The Australian Guide to Healthy Eating sets out specific recommended serves of fruit and vegetables for children aged 4-8 and 9-11 years [8]. One and a half servings of fruit and four and a half servings of vegetables are recommended for children aged four to eight years. Two serves of fruit and five serves of vegetables are recommended for children aged nine to eleven years. Serving sizes are specified as half a cup [8].

This study targeted school children aged six to ten years in Greater Shepparton, Moira and Strathbogie Shires. It was already known that 66.9% of children aged 4-12 years in the Hume Region (where these

LGAs are located) did not meet the daily recommended intake for fruit and vegetables [9]. No local government area data was available and all available regional data combined fruit and vegetable consumption as one measure. This study intended to identify consumption rates of fruit and vegetables separately at a local level to give more meaningful data. As well as providing an accurate baseline, the information would assist local organizations to tailor potential health promotion interventions that aim to increase consumption as well as measure the effect of any introduced interventions.

Parents influence children's consumption of food through modeling, purchasing and preparing food for their children [10]. There is a great deal of evidence from previous studies regarding the parental influence on children's fruit and vegetable consumption, thus parental behaviours, attitudes and beliefs are also important to capture [11-14].

Given parental influence on children's eating patterns, the secondary aim of the survey was to identify parents' sources of nutritional knowledge and perceived barriers to fruit and vegetable consumption. Proxy measures of childhood fruit and vegetable consumption, such as parental reporting, are common and were utilised for this survey.

Methods

Survey tool

The survey was developed over a period of four months by a project

***Corresponding author:** Kaye Ervin, University of Melbourne, Department of Rural Health, Graham St, Shepparton, Australia, E-mail: ervink@humehealth.org.au*

team comprised of two dietitians, four health promotion workers, a local government community wellbeing officer and a research academic. There were three iterations of the survey after trialing it twice to determine participant understanding and reliability. The survey was also informed by a rigorous literature review which had earlier been undertaken by the project team [15].

The survey included questions on demographic characteristics of the child and their parent/career; the child's intake of fruit and vegetables; barriers and enablers to fruit and vegetable intake; and types of resources parents use to access nutrition information. Parent/career demographic questions also included the highest level of education achieved; respondent's relationship to the child; and possession of a health care card. For the sake of brevity, other questions not reported included: cultural groups; healthy eating messages; other influences on family eating patterns; shopping habits and frequency; the structure of family meals; take away food consumption; and types of fluids consumed by children.

To measure intake of fruit and vegetable foods, the food record method was employed in the form of a matrix table that represented a typical day. Vegetable intake included fresh, frozen, cooked, raw and baked beans. Fruit intake included fresh, dried and tinned but excluded fruit juice. Respondents were given a page of food photographs that demonstrated standard serve sizes [16]. Examples of one serve were also described in the matrix, such as ½ cup of cooked vegetables, 1 cup of salad. The weight of the serve was not included in the descriptor. In the matrix table, respondents were then asked to select how many daily serves their child ate from the following: none, 1, 2, 3, 4, 5 or more or do not know.

To measure barriers and enablers to fruit and vegetable intake a matrix table was again employed. Respondents were asked to agree or disagree with a range of statements relating to: perceived access and perceived cost of fruit and vegetables; ability to make healthy meals and snacks; self-perception of healthy food knowledge; child's food preference; importance of the child eating fruit and vegetables; preparation time of healthy meals; and rewarding with lollies or treats.

A collectively exhaustive multiple response questions were included to determine where parents and guardians usually get information and advice about healthy eating for his or her child. Responses included: family, friends, internet, TV, radio, doctor, maternal and child health nurse, dietitian, books or brochures, newspapers or magazines, library, own knowledge, parents with children of the same age, teachers or school and pharmacist. Respondents were also provided with a space to write other sources they used to access information.

Procedure

The study population was grade one and three students who attend primary schools in the three local government areas of Greater Shepparton, Moira and Strathbogie Shire in North East Victoria. Parents and guardians were invited to complete the survey about their child. No other inclusion or exclusion criteria were set, however the survey was only provided in English language.

Approval to conduct the study was granted by the Goulburn Valley Health Human Research Ethics Committee and the Department of Education and Early Childhood Development. Primary school principals were contacted directly by the research team by phone or email to provide information about the study and obtain consent to participate. The surveys, with a plain language statement were delivered to schools that consented. Teachers of grades one and three distributed the surveys to their students to take home to their parent/guardians to complete. A collection box was placed at each school administration office for two weeks for participants to return completed surveys, as instructed in the plain language statement.

Statistical analysis

Data analysis was undertaken using SPSS (Statistical Package for Social Sciences) version 21 (IBM, Ireland). Descriptive statistics were generated for the demographic characteristics, food intake and sources of knowledge. Age groups of children were combined into 6-7 years and 8-10 years to allow further analysis with acceptable numbers in age categories. Pearson's Chi-Square tests were used to compare gender and age of children with vegetable intake. In addition, Pearson's Chi-Square tests were used to analyses relationships between child vegetable consumption and parental age, education level and health care card status as well as local government area. Pearson product-moment correlation coefficient and Spearman's rho were used to investigate the relationship between the perceived cost of fruit and vegetables and children's consumption of both. Median results are reported where distribution of scores was skewed, either positively or negatively.

Results

Response rate

Sixty primary schools from the three local government areas were invited to participate in the survey, with 41 schools (68.3%) consenting to being involved. Almost half (48.8%, n=20) of the schools were located in Greater Shepparton, with a further 41.5% (n=17) located in Moira, and 9.8% (n=4) in Strathbogie. A total of 556 surveys were completed out of 1933 surveys distributed, providing an overall response rate of 28.5%. Non responders were not asked the reason for non-response, as the researchers did not directly recruit, but relied on teachers to distribute the surveys via the children, who in turn gave them to parents. This chain increased the chances of non-response.

Response rates across local government areas varied, with Strathbogie producing the highest rate of 40.9% (n=58), Moira received 32.2% (n=233), and Greater Shepparton had a response rate of 24.4% (n=256).

Participants' characteristics

Participants in the study were parents or carers of school children in grades one and three of primary schools consenting to be surveyed.

Demographic information about the participants and their child is shown in Table 1. The majority (n=498) of parent/carer respondents identified as the mother of child, with 30 fathers also completing the survey. Of those who responded, the parents/carers listed first were mostly mothers (92.1%) and those listed second were mostly fathers (50%). The majority of respondents had completed tertiary level education (including Technical and Further Education); 60.2% (n=331) for parent/carer one and 46.6% (n=256) for parent/carer two.

Almost a third of overall respondents held a Health Care Card (HCC) (32.0%, n=173). The proportion of Health Care Card holders was slightly higher in Greater Shepparton (34.8%, n=89) and Moira (31.3%, n=73), in comparison with Strathbogie (25.0%, n=14).

The gender of children reported in the study showed an even representation of males (49%) and females (51%). The ages of children ranged from 6-10 years, with a median age of 7.5 years. There were 297 (54%) in the 6-7 year age group and 250 (46%) in the 8-10 year age group.

Eleven percent (n=61) of the sample met both the recommended guidelines for fruit and vegetable intake, with 2.7% (n=14) of the sample meeting neither guidelines. Children from the sample were reported as eating a median of 2.3 serves of fruit and two serves of

vegetables per day. Twelve precent (n=67) of sample were within the recommended four and a half to five serves of vegetables, with the majority (87.5%, n=476) not meeting the recommended guidelines for vegetable intake. A small proportion of children (3%, n=17) was not meeting the recommended guidelines of one and a half to two serves of fruit.

Because consumption of fruit met or exceeded the guidelines for 97% of children, further analysis focused on vegetable consumption, with the exception of cost. In addition, smaller numbers in the 6 year age group (n=54), 8 year age group (n=57), and 10 year age group (n=10), meant that ages 6-7 (n=297) were combined, as were ages 8-10 (n= 250) to undertake further analysis.

In Figure 1, there were equivalent numbers from both genders who did not meet the recommended guidelines for vegetable intake. A Pearson's Chi-Square test identified no significant difference between males (n=226, 42%) and females (n=240, 45%) not meeting the recommended four and a half to five serves of vegetables, $p=0.087$.

There was no relationship between the age of the child and vegetable consumption. A Pearson's Chi Square test revealed no significant differences between children in 6-7 year age group (n=253, 54%) and those in the 8-10 year age group (n=215, 46%) not meeting the vegetable guidelines, $p=0.858$.

Although the number of children who did not meet the recommended vegetable consumption was slighter higher in Shepparton (n=228, 92%) compared to Strathbogie (n=50, 86%) and Moira (n=190, 83%), this was not statistically significant, $p=0.012$. (Figure 1).

Differences in vegetable consumption between children with parent/guardians who were HCC holders, and those who were not, was further analysed and is (Figure 1). There was no significant difference between children not meeting the recommended vegetable intake of parents who were HCC holders (n=145, 86%) and those without a HCC (n=309, 88%), $p=0.637$. Similarly, the age of the parent/carer had no relationship to vegetable consumption in children, $p=0.335$.

Parental/carer education and vegetable consumption was further

Characteristic	Subcategory	Total sample (n=541)	
		n	%
Relationship to child	Mother	498	92.1
	Father	30	5.5
	Grandparent	4	0.7
	Guardian	5	0.9
	Other	4	0.7
		Carer 1	
Health Care Card	Yes	173	32.5
	No	359	67.5
	Median (IQR)	**Range**	
Age (years)	39.2 (35,43)	23-73	
Carer 2			
		(n=470) 164 missing	
Relationship to child	Mother	20	3.6
	Father	275	50
	Grandparent	5	0.9
	Guardian	1	0.2
	Other	5	0.9
	Median (IQR)	**Range**	
Age (years)	40.9 (37,44)	20-70	
Children			
Characteristic	Subcategory	(n=548)	
		n	%
Gender	Males	270	49
	Females	278	51
	Median (IQR)	**Range**	
Age (years) **Age groups (years)**	7.5 (7,9) 6-7	6-10 8-10	

Table 1: Parent/guardian's and children's characteristics.

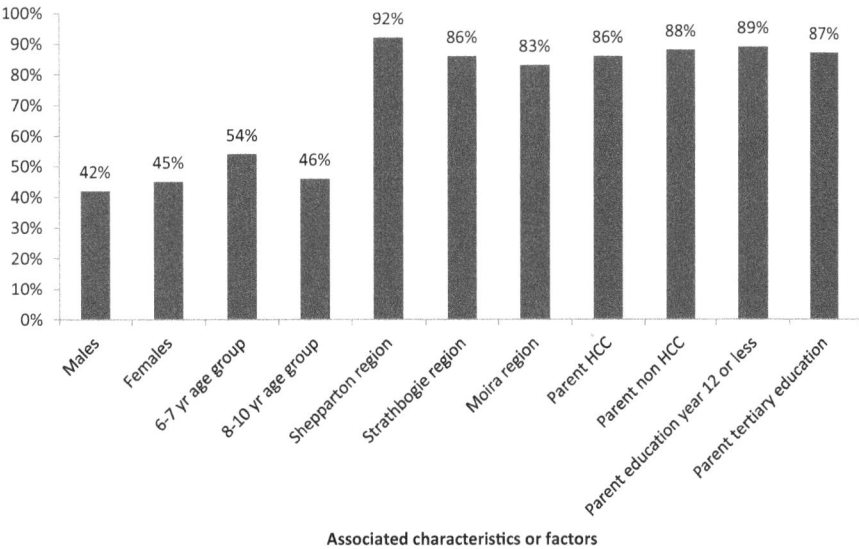

Figure 1: Percentage of children not meeting the recommended guidelines for vegetable intake and associated characteristics and factors.

explored. When considering the sample that did not meet vegetable guidelines, the number of parents/carers who had completed year 12 or less (n=175, 89%) was not significantly higher than those who had achieved a tertiary education (n=281, 87%), p=0.351. Figure 1 also shows the percentage of children who did not meet the guidelines broken down by parental education levels.

Barriers to fruit and vegetable consumption and healthy eating

Respondents were asked whether they agreed or disagreed with a series of statements relating to barriers to healthy eating. The statements and response rates are shown in Table 2.

Knowledge indicators produced a high level of agreement overall, whereby 95.8% (n=527) of respondents agreed to the statement 'I know how to make healthy meals for my child'. Access did not appear to be a barrier for the majority of the sample; 94.5% (n=520) agreed to the statement 'It is easy to get fresh fruit and vegetables'.

Forty percent (n=220) agreed to the statement 'Fruit costs too much' and 36.7% (n=202) agreed to the statement 'Vegetables cost too much'.

Child's food preferences were also explored as potential barriers to healthy food consumption, with particular focus on fruit and vegetables. Almost a fifth (n=99) of respondents agreed to the statement 'My child doesn't like vegetables'. A smaller proportion of respondents (6.7%, n=37) agreed to the statement 'My child does not like fruit'.

There was no statistically significant correlation between children's consumption of vegetables and parents/carers who reported that vegetables cost too much (r=-0.05). Similarly, there was no statistically significant correlation between children of parents/carers who reported that fruit costs too much and their consumption of fruit (r=0.01). Both relationships were investigated using Pearson product-moment correlation and Spearman's rho.

Sources of healthy eating knowledge

Survey participants were asked to report their main sources of information for healthy eating, using predetermined categories. Respondents were invited to select as many applicable categories as they liked. The major sources of information identified were: Family (57.8%, n=318); Friends (50.9%, n=280); Newspapers/magazines (49.8%, n=274); Internet (46.2%, n=254); and Book/brochures (39.8%, n=219).

Discussion

Only twelve percent of school children in this study were reported to be eating the recommended amount of fruits and vegetables. Although only a small proportion (3%) did not meet the recommended intake of fruit, 87.5% did not consume the daily recommended serves of vegetables. Analysis showed no relationships between the gender of the child; the local government area; or the age of the child or their parent and fruit and vegetable servings eaten. Although some survey respondents cited fruit and vegetables as being costly (40% for fruit and 36.7% for vegetables), this did not influence their children's rates of consumption compared to the rest of the sample. The parents/carers in the study perceived that they had knowledge of preparing healthy food (95.8%). Sources of knowledge for healthy eating varied, the highest being family (57.8%), friends (50.9%) and all popular media.

The high proportion of children meeting the recommended fruit intake, but low proportion meeting vegetables highlighted the potential for greater impact with an intervention that focuses on vegetable consumption.

Parents/guardians indicated that their child was more likely to dislike vegetables compared with fruit. Previous qualitative studies provide hypotheses to explain children's preference to eat fruit, rather than vegetables. Children perceive fruit to be sweet, juicy and fun to eat, while vegetables can be linked with negative sensory experiences [17-19].

This study found no significant difference between vegetable consumption and the child's gender, the results being similar for males and females, in contrast to other studies [18,20]. For adults, males are less likely to consume adequate quantities of fruit and vegetables than females [21]. The age of the children in this study was younger than those in other studies. Thus, the differences in preferences by gender may emerge with age, accounting for the lack of significance between genders in this study.

HCC status was asked in the survey as a proxy measure of income. To qualify for a HCC income must not exceed $913 (AUD) per week for couples or single parents [22]. Slightly more than 31% of respondents were HCC holders. The results showed no correlation between vegetable consumption levels for children and parents who were HCC holders, compared to those who were not. This result may be explained by lower income in rural areas overall compared to urban areas, so the differences between those on a HCC and those not, do not have a marked difference in income in rural Australia [23].

Positive statements	Disagree		Agree	
	n	%	n	%
It is easy to get fresh fruit and vegetables	20	3.6	520	94.5
I know how to make healthy meals for my child	18	3.3	527	95.8
I know how to make healthy snacks for my child	23	4.2	512	93.1
It is important for my child to eat fruit and vegetables	4	0.7	540	99.1
Negative statements	Disagree		Agree	
	n	%	n	%
Fruit costs too much	304	55.3	220	40.0
Vegetables cost too much	327	59.5	202	36.7
I'm not sure what healthy foods are	538	97.8	9	1.6
My child doesn't like fruit	507	92.2	37	6.7
My child doesn't like vegetables	443	80.5	99	18.0
Healthy meals take too long to prepare	497	90.4	34	6.2
Sometimes it seems like the only way to get my child to behave is to promise lollies or other treats	487	88.5	52	9.5

Table 2: Responses to positive and negative statements about healthy eating.

There is evidence that children living in households with an income of less than $40,000 (AUD) in rural Victoria are more likely to not meet the recommended guidelines for fruit and vegetable consumption [24]. In addition, previous studies show that adults who are unemployed or who have low annual household income are more likely to have inadequate consumption of fruit and vegetables [21].

Surprisingly given the rurality of respondents and limited transport in some of the local government areas, physical access to fruit and vegetables did not appear to be a barrier for the majority of survey respondents, which is consistent with previous studies [25] When asked about affordability, an alternate determinant of access, some respondents perceived fruit and vegetables to cost too much. One previous study [26] found that healthy foods were more expensive in rural areas, compared with metropolitan areas. There is limited data comparing rural and metropolitan healthy food prices. In this study, when comparing consumption of fruit and vegetables with the perception that fruit and vegetables cost too much, no differences were observed. Dibsdall, Lambert, Bobbin and Frewer, (2002) proposed that lack of money may be identified as the barrier to fruit and vegetable intake when there could actually be other, more complex causes.

Respondents reported good levels of knowledge of healthy foods and preparing healthy meals and snacks. A high proportion of parents/carers indicated that they knew how to make healthy meals for their child; however this did not translate into children meeting the recommended serves of vegetables. The low consumption of vegetables may indicate a discrepancy in perceived knowledge compared to actual knowledge. Dibsdall et al. (2002) reported that low-income participants in their study believed they were already eating healthy irrespective of their low consumption levels of fruit and vegetable. The alternative explanation for this discrepancy is the inability to translate nutrition and food preparation knowledge into healthy eating behaviours in their children. Previous studies [18] also highlighted that knowledge in itself is unlikely to bring about healthy eating behaviour change. Several other extrinsic and intrinsic factors influence the ability to make changes. In Dibsdall et al's (2002) study, motivation and lifestyle factors in particular were raised as barriers to healthy eating.

The sizeable proportion of respondents who identified that family and friends were their main sources of healthy eating information underscores the influence that informal social networks can have on eating habits and the importance of considering this when planning health promotion interventions. Other major identified sources of nutrition information, such as Newspapers/magazines, Internet and Books/brochures could be media of choice when planning social marketing strategies.

Limitations

The study utilised a non-validated, self-developed tool which the authors acknowledge has limitations. Also, due to the non-random sampling method applied, results from the study cannot be generalised to the broader population.

Parental knowledge of recommended serves of fruit and vegetables was not tested in this study, due to national advertising campaigns and easy access to the information. The study focused on actual consumption and potential barriers.

Because parental knowledge of recommended consumption of fruit and vegetables was not tested, the study did not determine if the barriers to consumption were linked to poor knowledge or simply lack of knowledge translation into practice, behaviour, or both.

Social desirability bias may have influenced estimates of fruit and vegetable intake, meaning that consumption may be even lower than reported. Knowledge of preparing healthy meals may also be affected by social desirability bias – parents wish to appear adequate.

Although the response rate of 28.5% could be considered low, a study of response rates of six well regarded journals found that the average response rate was below 40% [27] it is unwise to define a level above which a response rate is acceptable, as this depends on many local factors [28]. While it is acknowledged that non-response bias represents a significant threat to validity, high response rates are also found to contain bias [29].

Conclusion

This study gathered local government area level fruit and vegetable consumption data for children, which was previously not available.

The study confirmed the need for nutrition intervention in the Goulburn Valley catchment area. It further identified that vegetable consumption should be the focus of future interventions, rather than fruit and vegetables together.

Results highlight the complexity of influences on fruit and vegetable consumption. Determinants of consumption of fruit and vegetables are widely documented in the literature and include price, access, attitudes and knowledge. A series of attitudinal statements in the survey were intended provide insight into the obstacles faced by parents and identify where strategies may be implemented. Study findings were consistent with broader literature that found discrepancies between parental knowledge of healthy foods and adequate consumption of vegetables in children. Strength of the study was provision of photographic page of serving sizes which allowed more accurate measurement of actual consumption. No information was provided on recommended guidelines to avoid socially desirable responses.

Recommendation

Education interventions alone that are aimed at individuals are unlikely to bring about changes to behaviour. A socio-ecological approach to healthy eating is recommended which considers multiple spheres of influence [30] such an approach acknowledges broader impacts on children's eating habits beyond the individual and family context. Environmental influences where children live learn and play has an important role in determining what types of foods are available and accessible to children. Policy initiatives that focus on ensuring children's environments are supportive of healthy eating culture include interventions such as Health Promoting Schools, a settings-based initiative that encourages healthy school food policies and role modelling by staff [31]. Education settings have frequently been used as the target for health promotion interventions aimed at children. Schools and early childhood centres are embedded in broader communities and thus interventions must be designed to work with and meet the distinct local needs of these communities, in order to have long-term sustainable impacts.

With the common goal to increase vegetable consumption across the catchment, a coordinated approach using a mutually reinforcing plan across the three LGAs would optimise collective impact. A practice framework that allows for differentiated activities in each LGA that contribute to achieving one common goal is required. Healthy Food Connect [32], a model that addresses local food system change has been identified through an extensive systematic selection process, to be suitable for nutrition intervention across the Goulburn Valley catchment. The model aims to identify possible activities, strategies and policy changes that will create supportive environments to ensure that healthy eating choices are the easy and preferred choices for children, families and communities overall.

References

1. Australian Institute of Health and Welfare (AIHW) (2000) Australia's Health.

2. World Health Organization (WHO) (2002) Diet, nutrition and the prevention of chronic diseases: Report of a joint WHO/FAO expert consultation. WHO technical report series: 916.

3. Australian Institute of Health and Welfare (2010) premature mortality from chronic disease. AIHW, Canberra 84: 133.

4. Department of Health Victoria (2013) Greater Shepparton Population Health Profile.

5. Department of Health Victoria (2013) Moira Population Health Profile.

6. Department of Health Victoria (2013) Strathbogie Population Health Profile Population-Health-Profile.

7. National Health and Medical Research Council (2013) Eat for Health: Providing the scientific evidence for healthier Australian diets. Australian Dietary Guidelines Canberra: National Health and Medical Research Council.

8. National Health and Medical Research Council (2013) Australian Guidelines for healthy eating.

9. Department of Education and Early Childhood Development (2010) Early Childhood Community Profile Hume Region.

10. Birch L, Fisher J (1998) Development of Eating Behaviours of Children and Adolescents 101: 539-49.

11. Oosthuizen D, Oldewage-Theron, Napier C (2011) The impact of a nutrition programme on the dietary intake patterns of primary school children. South African Journal of Clinical Nutrition 24: 75-81.

12. Sirikulchayanonta C, Iedsee K, Shuaytong P, Srisorrachatr S (2010) Using food experience, multimedia and role models for promoting fruit and vegetable consumption in Bangkok kindergarten children. Nutrition and Dietetics 67: 97-101.

13. Cade J, Frear L, Greenwood D (2006) Assessment of diet in young children with an emphasis on fruit and vegetable intake: using CADET - Child and Diet Evaluation Tool. Public Health Nutr 9: 501-508.

14. Prelip M, Thai C, Erausquin J, Slusser W (2011) Improving low-income parents' fruit and vegetable intake and their potential to impact children's nutrition. Health Education 111: 391-411.

15. Spiller R, Orr J, Mills H, Ervin K (2014) Measurement of Fruit and Vegetable Consumption: Research Informing Practice. Health Care 2: 41-6.

16. World Health Organization (WHO) (2008) Collaborating Centre on Obesity Prevention and Related Research and Training Eating and Physical Activity Questionnaire (EPAQ).

17. Krolner R, Rasmussen M, Brug J, Klepp K, Wind M, et al. (2011)Determinants of fruit and vegetable consumption among children and adolescents: A review of the literature. International Journal of Behavioral Nutrition and Physical Activity 8: 112.

18. Brug J, Tak NI, te Velde SJ, Bere E, de Bourdeaudhij I, et al.(2008) Taste preferences, liking and other factors related to fruit and vegetable intakes among schoolchildren: Results from observational studies. Br J Nutr 1: s7-s14.

19. Glasson C, Chapman K, James E (2011) Fruit and vegetables should be targeted separately in health promotion programmes: differences in consumption levels, barriers, knowledge and stages of readiness for change. Public Health Nutr 4: 694-701.

20. Rasmussen M, Krolner R, Klepp K, Lytle L, Brug J, et al. (2006) Determinants of fruit and vegetable consumption among children and adolescents: A review of the literature. International Journal of Behavioral Nutrition and Physical Activity 3: 22.

21. Department of Health. Victorian Population Health Survey 2011–12, Survey findings. State Government of Victoria, Melbourne 2014.

22. Australian Government (2015) Eligibility for a health care card - Department of Human Services.

23. Australian Bureau of Statistics. Household Income and Income Distribution, Australia 2011-12.

24. Department of Education and Early Childhood Development. The state of Victoria's children report (2011) A report on how children and young people in rural and regional Victoria are faring.

25. Dibsdall L, Lambert N, Bobbin R, Frewer L (2002) Low-income consumers' attitudes and behaviour towards access, availability and motivation to eat fruit and vegetables. Public Health Nutr 6:159-168.

26. Ward P, Coveney J, Verity F, Carter P, Schilling M, et al. (2012) Cost and affordability of healthy food in rural South Australia. Rural and Remote Health 12: 1938.

27. Sivo S, Saunders C, Chang Q, Jiang J (2006) How Low Should You Go? Low Response Rates and the Validity of Inference in IS Questionnaire Research Journal of the Association for Information Systems 7: 351-414.

28. Kelley K, Clark B, Brown V, Sitzia J (2003) Good practice in the conduct and reporting of survey research. Int J Qual Health Care 15: 261-266.

29. Kelly B, Fraze T, Hornik R (2010) Response rates to a mailed survey of a representative sample of cancer patients randomly drawn from the Pennsylvania Cancer Registry: A randomized trial of incentive and length effects. BMC Medical Research Methodology 10: 65.

30. Kamphuis C, Giskes K, de Bruijn G, Wendel-Vos W, Brug J, et al. (2006) Environmental determinants of fruit and vegetable consumption among adults: a systematic review. British Journal of Nutrition 96: 620-635.

31. World Health Organisation (1998) Health Promoting Schools: a healthy setting for living, learning and working.

32. Australian Government (2014) Healthy Food Connect: A-support-resource.

14

Gender, Grade and Personality Differences in Internet Addiction and Positive Psychological Health among Chinese College Students

Qian Dai*

Department of Centre for Psychological Health and Education, Sichuan University, China

Abstract

The purpose of this research is to investigate the prevalence of internet addiction and positive psychological health among Chinese college students and to explore the relationship of positive psychological health and internet addiction. A total number of 811 university students (the mean age: 19.70 years) who completed a on line survey that included the Internet Addiction Test (IAT) and PERMA scale. According to results, internet addiction was different between grade and personality and psychological health was different in gender and personality. Students with higher levels of internet addiction are more likely to be low in positive psychological health. The results indicated that positive psychological health was affected by Internet addiction negatively; and provided a better understanding on the positive psychological interventions in reduce internet addiction among Chinese college students.

Keywords: Positive psychological health; Internet addiction; College students

Introduction

Internet services as a technological advancement tool, which offers several direct benefits in our daily life. Internet delivers some practical purpose such as on-line shopping, business transaction, communication, social sharing and entertainment [1-3]. Despite those inherent advantages, many studies showed excessive internet use attribute negative effects to people's physical, social and psychological health, such as tiredness depression; loneness lower self-esteem [4-7]. Moreover, some studies found that excessive internet use affects students' educational performance, such as decrease in academic performance; wasting of time; problem in communication with peers [8-10].

Internet addiction

There are different terminologies in define excessive use of internet. The concept of internet addiction was first introduced by Young, and it appeared to be the most frequently used term in the literature [11,12]. Internet addiction has been considered as an impulse control disorder, which does not involve an intoxicant [1]. It is appeared to be a kind of technology addiction and a behavioral addiction similar to a gambling habit [9]. Internet addiction has been coined as "pathological Internet use (PIU)" and "problematic Internet use" [13,14]. Although there is still lack of a consensual definition of internet addiction, many scholars have agreed that internet addiction is a maladaptive pattern of internet use [15,16]. It does not only time-consuming, but also lead to clinically significant impairment, and negative, behavioral, psychological and physical consequences [17,18].

Increasing attention has focused on internet addiction as it has become a universal problem, particularly has negative influence to young people. Research showed adolescents is more easily to be influenced by internet addiction [19,20]. Internet addiction is very prevalent among secondary school and university students [21]. Identified 10.6% of Chinese college students are internet addicted. Noticeably, the research showed excessive or pathological use of internet is visible to different cultures [22,23]. Research with European adolescents identified poor sleeping problems and risk-behaviors were strongly associated with their internet addiction [24]. By using a national representative dataset, Ha and Hwang's study found that internet addiction was prevalent among Korean adolescents. After control for gender, internet addiction has showed negative correlation to adolescents' physical well-being and

subjective happiness [25]. Based those research evidences, it is plausible to say that internet addiction is a problem that has been observed in both Eastern and Western culture and it is particularly cause psychological distress to adolescents.

Positive psychological well-being

Positive psychology in recent years has been one of the rapidly expanding subfields in psychology that has potential contributions to the field of internet addiction. Positive psychology seeks to explore factors and develop methods to help individuals find paths to thriving and flourishing; it is the study of the human strengths and virtues that make people feel good about lives. Based on its tenets, positive psychology has been utilized to the workings of positive experiences and positive personality traits that enable people to find lives of happiness, fulfillment and meaning and in turn to reach their full potential [2]. Decades of research in the discipline have shown the value in studying people's positive psychological character that shape healthy well-being and demonstrated the effects of positive traits as buffers, helping people, for example, cope with stress in life and fix psychological disorders [26,27].

One of the prominent models in the field of positive psychology is PERMA (Positive emotions, Engagement, Relationships, Meaning and Accomplishment). PERMA was developed by the co-founder, Martin Seligman, of positive psychology as a conceptual model to help people flourish [2]. Positive emotions as the first aspect of the PERMA model are believed to be able to broaden one's awareness, stimulate one's innovative thoughts and develop one's skills for future actions [28]. Engagement refers to individuals who are absorbed by the activity and concentrate on the tasks without the awareness of the time

---

*Corresponding author: Qian Dai, Department of Center for Psychological Health and Education, Sichuan University, China, E-mail: daiqian_1111@hotmail.com

[29,30]. Positive relationships emphasize the importance of individuals integrated themselves to society or community, been cared by important others and established one's social network [31]. Positive relationships are associated to decreased depressive symptoms and increased health outcomes [32]. Meaning refers to having a purpose and direction in life [2]. Although meaningful does not necessarily mean happy life, individuals who reported to have meaningful life were associated to wellbeing [33]. Accomplishment can be perceived as someone who is motived to achieve, to master and to competence in his best possible [2].

As the increasing research evidence has acknowledged that well-being can not only help to decrease stress and depression, it is also help individuals to become more productive, initiative and enable to build better relationship with others [34,35]. Therefore, the current study hypothesized that positive psychological health is negatively correlated to internet addiction. The people who are more addicted to internet may have lower grade of positive psychological health. In the present study, the researcher conducted an on-line survey to college-level students in China to explore their positive psychological health and internet addiction.

There are four research questions formulated in the study

1. Whether internet addiction is different between gender, grade and self-reported personality type? It is hypothesized that the level of internet addition will different between gender, grade and self-reported personality type. The extrovert students will feel less addicted to internet that introverts students.

2. Whether positive psychological health is different between gender, grade and self-reported personality type? It is hypothesized that positive psychological health is different in gender, grade and self-reported personality type. Students with extrovert personalities will score higher in positive psychological health.

3. Is there any relationship between internet addiction and positive psychological health? It is hypothesized that internet addiction is negatively correlated to positive psychological health.

4. Is there psychological health differ among different severity internet addicts? It is hypothesized that students who have better positive psychological health will have lower levels of internet addition.

Materials and Methods

Participants

There is a total number of 811 university students participated in the on line survey (Mean age=19.70, SD=1.40). Of the participants, 406 (50.1%) were freshmen, 254 (31.3%) were second-year students, 111 (13.7%) were third-year students and 40 (4.9%) were fourth-year students. The participants were composed of 345 (42.5%) male students and 466 (57.5%) female students.

The investigator designed background information to investigate the questions on the time spending on internet, purpose of using internet, and self-reported personality. Average daily hours of Internet use were 5.75 hours for the whole sample. There were no significant gender differences in spending the time on internet (Male: M=5.57, SD=4.21; Female: M=5.85, SD=3.42). Regarding to main purpose of using internet, free responses to the question have been content analyzed into four categories: on line gaming (38.6%), communication tools (32.4%), searching information (21.3%), entertainment (27.5%), assistant tool with studies (19.8%). In terms of personality type, 111 (13.7%) students classified themselves as introvert personality, 158

(19.5%) of them were extrovert personality, 526 (64.9%) of them were combined personality (both introvert and extrovert) and 16 (2.0%) of them perceived their personality as others (including very hard to describe, very strange, I do not know).

Measurements

The internet addiction test (IAT): IAT test is developed from Internet Addiction Diagnostic Questionnaire (IADQ) [1,11]. It is composed of 20 items with 6 point scale, range from "rarely" coded 1 to "always' coded 5 and the other response option is "does not apply" coded as 0 [36,37]. The total score of IAT ranged from 0-100, with higher scores reflecting a greater tendency toward internet addiction. In addition, IAT differentiate the extent of internet using by setting up cut-off scores: normal Internet users (score range 0–30); mild internet user (score range 31–49); moderate internet user (score range 50–79) and severe internet user (score range 80–100). IAT test was translated into Mandarin Chinese and back translated into English by two researchers from Psychology field who are blind to the purpose of the study. After translation of the questionnaire, internal coefficients of consistence of scale was tested, the Cronbach Alpha was calculated as 0.924.

Perma scale: Perma scale constructed by Seligman was used in measure psychological wellbeing [2]. This scale consisted of 23 items, and results in six different dimensions: positive emotion, engagement, meaning, positive relationships, accomplishment and over all wellbeing. It used a 10-point likert scale range from "not at all" (coded 0) to "all the time" (coded 10). Similar to IAT test, the translation and back translation procedure was applied to PERMA Scale. The Cronbach's alpha was 0.902.

Procedure

Convenience sampling was the method used while recruiting the participants. The investigator sent the online questionnaire link to contacts in universities' student associations located at Beijing (northern China), Chongqing (Southwestern China), Chengdu (Southwestern China), Shanghai (Eastern China). The snowballing process was used to recruit participants. The instruction of completing the online questionnaire reminded all the participants that this questionnaire was anonymous, and all their answers were for the use of research only and would be confidential. Subjects were free to withdraw from the study at any stage.

Results

Comparison of interest addiction by grade, gender and personality

One way ANOVA was used to analysis the differences of internet addiction in different grade. The results showed the there was a significant differences of internet addiction across the different grade of university students: $F(3,807)=5.82$, $p<0.001$. Post hoc analysis showed the differences were between first year (M=29.75, SD=17.22) and second year university students (M=24.56, SD=15.47) and between second year (M=24.56, SD=15.47) and fourth year university student (M=31.38, SD=19.26). The study indicated that the first year and the fourth year University students were more addicted to internet than the second year of University students.

One way ANOVA was used to analysis the differences of personalities in internet addiction. The results revealed the significant differences of internet addiction in personality: $F(3,807)=3.19$, $p<0.05$. Post hoc analysis showed the significant differences were between adolescents' reported their personality as others (M=39.00, SD=27.65) and all the other three types of personalities (introvert: M=29,22, SD=18.11; extrovert: M=26.18, SD=16.98; combination: M=27.70, SD=15.76) (p<0.01). However, the scores regarding internet addiction did not differ between genders (p>0.05).

Comparison of positive psychological health by grade, gender and personality

One way ANOVA was used to analysis the differences of personality in psychological health. The results showed there was significant difference of personality on psychological health (Table 1). In positive emotion, individuals with extrovert personality have significantly higher level of positive emotions than people with introvert, combination and others personality (p<0.01). Individuals have combination personality has significantly higher positive emotions than people with introvert personality (p<0.01).

In engagement, extrovert personality types showed more engagement than people with introvert and other personality (p<0.01). Combination personality showed significantly higher level of engagement than that of introvert and other personality type (p<0.05).

In relationship, people with extrovert personality scored significantly higher in relationship than people with introvert (p<0.001), combination (p<0.01) and others personality (p<0.05). Individuals with combination personality scored significantly higher in relationship than people with introvert personality (p<0.05).

In meaning of life, people with extrovert personality has scored significantly higher than people with introvert (p<0.001), combination (p<0.01) and others personality people (p<0.05). Individuals have combination personality has score significantly higher than people with introvert personality (p<0.001).

In accomplishment, people with extrovert personality scored

higher in accomplishment than people with introvert (p<0.001) and combination personality (p<0.05). People with combination personality scored higher than introvert personality (p<0.001).

In overall wellbeing, people with extrovert personality scored higher than people with other three types of personality (p<0.01). People with combination personality scored higher than people in introvert personality (p<0.001).

In terms of examining gender differences in positive psychological health, T-test revealed female students showed more positive emotion, relationship, and overall wellbeing than male students: positive emotion, t=-2.39, df=809, p<0.05, (Female: M=6.47, SD=1.76; Male: M=6.16, SD=1.88), relationships, t=-3.37 df=809, p<0.001, (Female: M=6.49, SD=1.71; Male=6.05, SD=1.96) and overall wellbeing, t=-1.97 df=809, p<0.05, (Female: M=6.16, SD=1.46; Male=5.95, SD=1.59). However, no significant differences were found among grade in positive psychological health.

Comparison of severity of internet addiction in positive psychological health

According to cut off scores in IAT, scores in IAT have been divided into four groups (normal, mild, moderate and severe) depending on their severity of using internet [1]. One-way ANOVA was used to examine the different level of using internet in positive psychological health. Except engagement, there were significant differences of positive psychological health score in different level of internet addicts (Table 2). In positive emotion, there was no significant different of positive emotions between severe and moderate internet users. Except that, positive emotion score was decreasing with the severity of internet using was increased. Regarding to relationship, meaning and accomplishment and overall wellbeing, the differences were existed between normal internet user and other three levels of internet addicts (p<0.001).

		N	Mean	SD	Sig
Positive emotion	Introvert	111	5.57	1.57	F(3,807)=12.73, p<0.001
	Extrovert	158	6.87	1.96	
	Combination	526	6.36	1.74	
	Others	16	5.52	2.27	
Engagement	Introvert	111	5.43	1.63	F(3,807)=4.14, p<0.01
	Extrovert	158	5.97	1.92	
	Combination	526	5.86	1.58	
	Others	16	4.90	2.24	
Relationships	Introvert	111	5.81	1.78	F(3,807)=6.43, p<0.001
	Extrovert	158	6.73	1.99	
	Combination	526	6.30	1.74	
	Others	16	5.63	2.48	
Meaning	Introvert	111	5.33	1.92	F(3,807)=7.67, p<0.001
	Extrovert	158	6.41	2.00	
	Combination	526	5.96	1.84	
	Others	16	5.33	2.17	
Accomplishment	Introvert	111	5.22	1.73	F(3,807)=7.59, p<0.001
	Extrovert	158	6.20	1.86	
	Combination	526	5.80	1.63	
	Others	16	5.33	2.09	
Overall well-being	Introvert	111	5.50	1.37	F(3,807)=10.72, p<0.001
	Extrovert	158	6.48	1.69	
	Combination	526	6.09	1.43	
	Others	16	5.36	2.07	

Table 1: Scores of psychological well-being in different personality types (Number, Mean, SD, Sig).

		N	Mean	Std. Deviation	Sig
Positive emotion	Normal	499	6.60	1.87	F(3,807)=13.80, p<0.001
	Mild	227	6.12	1.66	
	Moderate	81	5.42	1.40	
	Severe	4	4.25	2.28	
Engagement	Normal	499	5.87	1.75	F(3,807)=1.44, p>0.05
	Mild	227	5.77	1.52	
	Moderate	81	5.61	1.63	
	Severe	4	4.50	2.89	
Relationships	Normal	499	6.55	1.92	F(3,807)=9.82, p<0.001
	Mild	227	6.01	1.62	
	Moderate	81	5.71	1.52	
	Severe	4	4.25	2.32	
Meaning	Normal	499	6.27	2.015	F(3,807)=13.59, p<0.001
	Mild	227	5.54	1.65	
	Moderate	81	5.18	1.46	
	Severe	4	5.00	1.19	
Accomplishment	Normal	499	6.08	1.81	F(3,807)=15.10, p<0.001
	Mild	227	5.46	1.46	
	Moderate	81	5.00	1.26	
	Severe	4	4.25	2.60	
Overall well-being	Normal	499	6.31	1.60	F(3,807)=13.72, p<0.001
	Mild	227	5.81	1.34	
	Moderate	81	5.42	1.04	
	Severe	4	4.39	2.11	

Table 2: Scores of psychological well-being in different severity of internet addiction (Number, Mean, SD, Sig).

Correlation between internet addiction and positive psychological health

The correlation test was used to analysis the relationship between internet addiction and positive psychological health. The results showed there was a significant negative correlation between internet addiction and positive emotion (r=-0.228, N=811, p<0.001); between internet addiction and relationships (r=-0.202, N=811, p<0.001); between internet addiction and meaning (r=-0.259, N=811, p<0.001); between internet addiction and accomplishment (r=-0.242, N=811, p<0.001), between internet addiction and overall-wellbeing (r=-0.236, N=811, p<0.001). There was no significant correlation between internet addiction and engagement (r=-0.044, N=811, p>0.05).

Discussion

The aim of this study was to investigate the internet addiction and psychological health among Chinese college students. The results showed significant grade differences of internet addiction among university students. First-year and fourth-year university students were more addicted to internet than the second-year of university students. The first year and the fourth year of university students were more prone to addicted to internet may due to they have more free time and less academic pressure than second year of University students. This finding was not completed agreed with the previous studies which showed senior grade students exhibited more internet addiction than those in junior classes due to the fact that senior grade students may use internet for academic activities. In the current study, the most senior and the most junior year of university students showed more addiction to internet than students in the middle year of the university.

In addition, personality showed significant influence in internet addition and positive psychological health. Individuals reported themselves to have "others" personality was more addicted to internet than those with three other personality types (introvert, extrovert and combination). This finding suggested that internet addiction were more sever in ones who have no clue of their personality looks like. However, people with extrovert, introvert and combination personality have no differ in internet addiction. This is consistent with the previous study which showed after controlled by age and gender, individual differences in personality were not significantly related to internet addition [38].

In terms of personality differences in positive psychological health, the current study showed individuals reported themselves as extrovert personalities showed more positive emotion, more engagement, better relationships, more meaning in life, better accomplishment and overall wellbeing than people with introvert and combinations personalities. Individuals with combination of both introvert and extrovert personalities have better psychological health than people with introvert personalities. This is in line with the previous study in which suggested personality dispositions such as extraversion, neuroticism, and self-esteem can markedly influence levels of subjective wellbeing [39].

Gender was not found differ in internet addition in the current study. It is in line with Beranuy et al.'s study that there were no gender differences in internet addition [40]. However, it is disagreed with other studies pointed male college students were more likely to addicted to internet than female students [41,42]. In terms of psychological health, female students scored higher in positive emotion, relationship and over all wellbeing than male students. This is consistent with previous studies that women in general are more willing to express and share positive emotions than men as well as more attuned to create and sustain meaningful social relationships [43].

The study revealed normal internet user has better positive psychological health than mild, moderate and severe internet users. Individuals with more positive emotions related to less severity of internet addition. A large number of research evidences have suggested internet addiction hindering people's emotional problems, such as anxiety, depression, as well as social skills [1]. Within the framework of the body of research on internet addition and wellbeing, negative effect of internet addiction and subjective wellbeing, as illustrated by the present study [44].

The final research question examined the relationships between internet addiction and positive psychological health. Mainly, as hypothesized, internet addiction has negatively correlated with positive psychological health (positive emotion, relationships, meaning, accomplishment and overall-wellbeing) among college students. The finding supported previous study in which stated individual's subjective health was negatively related to internet addiction. In Diener's study, subjective well-being encompasses satisfaction with life, self-perceptions of well-being, satisfying relationships and positive emotions [45,46]. The present findings connoting that, internet addiction was negatively associated with psychological well-being is consistent with previous research. In return, it appears that if individuals can enhance their positive psychological health, they may decrease their internet addiction [47].

Conclusion

The study discussed the recent research in internet addiction and positive psychological health, gathered empirical data from college students through on line survey. The study found that internet addiction is different in grade and personalities, whereas positive psychological health was different in personalities and gender among Chinese college students. Although the internet provides advantageous and convenience in adolescent's life, the normal internet users showed much more positive psychological health than mild, moderate and severe internet users indicated that internet addiction function negatively to college students' health and wellbeing. The strong correlation was observed between internet addiction and psychological well-being, underlines the importance of enhance positive psychological interventions in higher education, treating or preventing the internet addiction in adolescents.

References

1. Young KS (1998) Caught in the net: How to recognize internet addiction and a winning strategy for recovery. John Wiley and Sons, New York.

2. Seligman MEP (2011) Learned optimism: How to change our mind and your life. Vintage: Knopf Doubleday Publishing Group.

3. Bradley K (2005) Internet lives: Social context and moral domain in adolescent development. New Directions for Youth Development 108: 57–76.

4. Akin A, Iskender M (2011) Internet addiction and depression, anxiety and stress. International Online Journal of Educational Sciences 3: 138–148.

5. Yen JY, Ko CH, Yen CF, Wu HY, Yang MJ (2007) The Comorbid psychiatric symptoms of internet addiction: attention deficit and hyperactivity disorder (ADHD), depression, social phobia and hostility. J Adolesc Health 41: 93–98.

6. Morahan-Martin J, Schumacher P (2003) Incidence and correlates of pathological internet use among college students. Comput Human Behav 16: 13–29.

7. Aydin B, San S.V (2011) 3rd world conference on educational sciences – 2011 internet addiction among adolescents: The role of self-esteem. Procedia - Social and Behavioral Sciences 15: 3500–3505.

8. Aboujaoude E (2010) Problematic internet use: an overview. World Psychiatry 9: 85–90.

9. Griffiths M (2000) Does internet and computer "addiction" exist? Some case study evidence. Cyber Psychology & Behavior 3: 211–218.

10. Gross EF, Juvonen J, Gable S.L (2002) Internet use and well-being in adolescence. J Soc Issues 58: 75–90.

11. Young KS (1996) Internet addiction: The emergence of a new clinical disorder. Presented at the 104th annual meeting of the American psychological association, Toronto, Canada.

12. Lai CM, Mak KK, Watanabe H, Ang RP, Pang JS, et al. (2013) Psychometric properties of the internet addiction test in Chinese adolescents. J Pediatr Psychol 38: 794–807.

13. Young KS (2004) Internet addiction a new clinical phenomenon and its consequences. Am J Health Behav 48: 402–415.

14. Kaltiala-Heino R, Lintonen T, Rimpelä A (2004) Internet addiction? Potentially problematic use of the internet in a population of 12–18 year old adolescents. Addiction Research & Theory 12: 89–96.

15. Spada MM (2014) An overview of problematic Internet use. Addict Behav 39: 3–6.

16. Laconi S, Rodgers RF, Chabrol H (2014) The measurement of internet addiction: A critical review of existing scales and their psychometric properties. Comput Human Behav 41: 190–202.

17. Weinstein A, Lejoyeux M (2010) Internet addiction or excessive internet use. Am J Drug Alcohol Abuse, pp: 277-283.

18. Wallace BE, Masiak J (2011) A review of internet addiction with regards to assessment method design and the limited parameters examined. Current Problems of Psychiatry 12: 558–561.

19. Mossbarger B (2008) Is "Internet addiction" addressed in the classroom? A survey of psychology textbooks. Comput Human Behav 24:468–474.

20. Yen JY, Ko CH, Yen CF, Chen SH, Chung WL, et al. (2008) Psychiatric symptoms in adolescents with Internet addiction: comparison with substance use. Psychiatry Clin Neurosci 62: 9–16.

21. Lin SSJ, Tsai CC (2002) Sensation seeking and internet dependence of Taiwanese high school adolescents. Comput Human Behav 18: 411–426.

22. Wu HR, Zhu KJ (2004a) Path analysis on related factors causing internet addiction disorder in college students. Chinese Journal of Public Health 20: 1363–1366.

23. Cao F, Su L (2007) Internet addiction among Chinese adolescents: Prevalence and psychological features. Child: Care, Health and Development 33: 275–281.

24. Durkee T, Carli V, Floderus B, Wasserman C, Sarchiapone M, et al. (2016) Pathological internet use and risk-behaviors among european adolescents. Int J Environ Res Public Health 13: 294.

25. Ha YM, Hwang WJ (2014) Gender differences in internet addiction associated with psychological health indicators among adolescents using a national web-based survey. Int J Ment Health Addict12: 660–669.

26. Masten AS, Coatsworth JD (1998) The development of competence in favorable and unfavorable environments: Lessons from research on successful children. Am Psychol 53: 205.

27. Seligman MEP, Csikszentmihalyi M (2000) Special issue on happiness, excellence and optimal human functioning. Am Psychol 55: 5–183.

28. Fredrickson BL (2001) The role of positive emotions in positive psychology: The broaden-and-build theory of positive emotions. Am Psychol 56: 218.

29. Csikszentmihalyi M (1990) Flow: The psychology of optimal experience. New York: Plenum.

30. Csikszentmihalyi M (1997) Finding flow. New York: Basic Books.

31. Khaw D, Kern M (2014) A cross-cultural comparison of the PERMA model of well-being. At Berkeley, p: 10.

32. Perissinotto CM, Cenzer IS, Covinsky KE (2012) Loneliness in older persons: A predictor of functional decline and death. Arch Intern Med 172: 1078–1084.

33. Baumeister RF, Vohs KD, Aaker JL, Garbinsky EN (2013) Some key differences between a happy life and a meaningful life. J Posit Psychol 8: 505–516.

34. Wood AM, Joseph S (2010) The absence of positive psychological (eudemonic) well-being as a risk factor for depression: A ten year cohort study. J Affect Disord 122: 213–217.

35. Achor S (2012) Positive intelligence. Harvard Business Review 90: 100–102.

36. Young KS, de Abreu (2010) Internet addiction: A handbook and guide to evaluation and treatment. John Wiley & Sons.

37. Young KS, Rogers RC (2009) The relationship between depression and internet addiction. Cyber Psychology & Behavior 1: 25–28.

38. Hills P, Argyle M (2003) Uses of the internet and their relationships with individual differences in personality. Comput Human Behav 19: 59–70.

39. Diener E, Oishi S, Lucas RE (2003) Personality, culture and subjective well-Being: Emotional and cognitive evaluations of life. Ann Rev Psychol 54:403-425.

40. Beranuy M, Oberst U, Carbonell X, Chamarro A (2009) Problematic internet and mobile phone use and clinical symptoms in college students: The role of emotional intelligence. Comput Human Behav 25:1182–1187.

41. Gnisci A, Perugini M, Pedone R, Di Conza A (2011) Construct validation of the use, abuse and dependence on the internet inventory. Comput Human Behav 27: 240–247.

42. Wu HR, Zhu KJ (2004b) Path analysis on related factors causing internet addiction disorder in college students. Chinese Journal of Public Health 20: 1363–1364.

43. Kashdan TB, Mishra A, Breen WE, Froh JJ (2009) Gender differences in gratitude: Examining appraisals, narratives, the willingness to express emotions and changes in psychological needs. J Pers 77: 691–730.

44. Akın A (2012) The relationships between internet addiction, subjective vitality and subjective happiness. Cyber Psychology & Behavior 15: 404–410.

45. Diener E (2000) Subjective well-being: The science of happiness and a proposal for a national index. Am Psychol 55: 34-43.

46. Diener E, Seligman M.E.P (2002) Very happy people. Psychol Sci 13: 81–84.

47. Lyubomirsky S (2001) Why are some people happier than others? The role of cognitive and motivational processes in well-being. Am Psychol 56: 239–249.

15

Analysis of Healthy Lifestlye Behaviours of Hypertensive Patients

Mukadder Mollaoglu* and Gurcan Solmaz

Faculty of Health Sciences, Cumhuriyet University, Turkey

Abstract

Objective: The present study was conducted with the aim of determining the healthy lifestyle behaviours and affecting factors in hyptertensive patients.

Method: This descriptive study was carried out with 155 patients who were hospitalized at Internal Medicine and Endocrinology Clinics of Cumhuriyet University Hospital. Data were obtained using Personal Information Form (PIF) and Healthy Lifestyle Behaviours Scale (HLBS) and evaluated with number, percent, Mann Whitney U test, Kruskal-Wallis test and qui square test.

Results: While the highest HLBS subscale scores were obtained from self-actualization, health responsibility, interpersonal relationships, stress management, the lowest scores were obtained from nutrition and physical activity subscales. Officers, married subjects and subjects with low income obtained high scores in self-actualization subscale; subjects who were 55 years old or above, graduates of intermediate school obtained high scores in health responsibility subscale; graduates of elemantary school and married subjects obtained high scores in physical activity subscale; male and married subjects obtained high scores in nutritional habits subscale and retired patients obtained high scores in total scale score ($p<0.05$).

Conclusion: This research indicates that hypertensive patients do not follow healthy nutritional and physical activity principles and personal characteristics of patients affect healthy lifestyle behaviours.

Keywords: Hypertensive; Healthy lifestyle; Chronic diseases; Statistical

Introduction

Chronic diseases is the first leading cause of deaths worldwide. World Health Organization (WHO) stated in 2005 that chronic diseases is a neglected health problem which concern all humans. Hyptertension is the most common chronic disease [1]. Approximately 31.8% of Turkish population is known to have hyptertension [2]. Although there are approximately 70 million hyptertensive patients in USA, approximately half of the patients have a hyptertension under control [3]. According to three large scale studies conducted in our country, hyptertension prevalence was detected as 33.7%, 31.8% and 41.7% [2,4,5]. Ratio of the patients whose hyptertension is under control is about 30% and this ratio is under 10% in places where health services are not satisfactory [4]. However hyptertension is a preventable and controllable disease. Therefore hypertension development must be tried to be prevented with measures taken beginning from childhood [2]. Studies toward lifestyle changes and education programs should be performed. Giving instructions to the patients considering their sociodemographic features and disease- related features may create awareness and helps controlling the disease [6]. Blood pressure control and education for healthy lifestyle behaviours positively affect disease control [7,8]. Hypertensive patients should be instructed by health professionals in order to develop Healthy Lifestyle Behaviours (HLSB). Almost all of the patients (92.5%) included in the study of Topuzoglu et al. were found not to be educated about hypertension [9]. Living conditions are as important as education about hypertension. In the research of Nidal and Eshah, working under heavy conditions, low income, living out of the city center were found to negatively affect health lifestyle behaviours [10]. Developing healthy lifestyle conditions is of great importance in chronic diseases like hypertension. This study was conducted with the aim of determining Healthy Lifestyle Behaviours (HLB) of hypertensive patients and affecting factors.

Materials and Methods

Study universe was composed of all hypetensive patients hospitalized at Internal Medicine and Endocrinology Clinics of Cumhuriyet University Universty Hospital. Sample was composed of 155 patients above 18 years who had been diagnosed with hypertension at least three months ago , who did not have disorders or disturbances which could affect cognitive functions and who were volunteer for participation.

Personal Information Form (PIF), Healthy Lifestyle Behaviours Scale (HLSBS) were used for data collection. Data were collected with face to face interview method after required explanation had been made by the researcher and through reviewing patient files.

Personal Information Form (PIF): This form which was prepared by the researchers under the light of literature [11-13] data included 35 questions about age, gender, marital status, sociodemographic features of the patient, disease and treatment and the clinic he was being hospitalized.

Healthy Life-Style Behaviour Scale (HLSBS)

HLSBS was developed by Walker, Sechrist and Pender in 1987 [14]. A study for the validity and reliability of the scale was made by Esin in 1997 [15] in Turkey and Cronbach Alpha value was found as 0.91. Questions in the scale are used to measure an individual's health-promoting behaviours in relation to his/her healthy life-style. Consisting of 48 items, the scale has 6 subgroups. Each subgroup may be used on its own independently. Subgroups include self-realization,

*Corresponding author: Mukadder Mollaoglu, Cumhuriyet University,Faculty of Health Sciences, 58140 Sivas, Turkey, E-mail: mollaoglumukadder@gmail.com

health responsibility, exercise, nutrition, interpersonal support and stress management. Self-realization consists of 13 items with the lowest possible score of 13 and highest score of 52. Health responsibility consists of 10 items, with the lowest possible score of 10 and the highest score of 40. Exercise consists of 5 items, with the lowest possible score of 5 and the highest score of 20. Nutrition consists of 6 items, with the lowest possible score of 6 and the highest score of 24. Interpersonal support consists of 7 items, with the lowest possible score of 7 and the highest score of 28. Stress management consists of 7 items, with the lowest possible score of 7 and the highest score of 28. The total score of the scale constitutes HLSB total point.

All items of the HLSB are positive. Marking is made on a 4- point Likert scale. 1 point is assigned to the answer "never", 2 points are assigned to the answer "sometimes", 3 points are assigned to the answer "frequently" and 4 points are assigned to the answer "regularly". The lowest score for the whole scale is 48 and the highest score is 192. Higher scores obtained in the scale indicate that the individual applies stated health behaviours at a high level [14,15].

Ethical Considerations

Institutional approval was obtained from Cumhuriyet University Medical Sciences Ethical Committee. Study aims, plans and benefits were explained to patients who met the study criteria. Patients were asked if they would voluntarily participate in the study and their written/oral consents were obtained. Confidentiality was maintained at all times.

Data Analysis

The research data were loaded on the Statistical Package for the Social Sciences (SPSS) for Windows program, version 14.0. Percentage calculation, mean, test of significance between two means, qui-square test, one way analysis of variance, Mann-Whitney -U test and Kruskal Wallis test were used in the analysis of the data. The data were evaluated in tables taking arithmetic means and standard deviation at 0.05.

Results

While mean age of the patients is $56{,}45 \pm 7{,}98$ years, 72.3% of the patients are women, more than half (58.1%) are housewives, 27.7% are retired, remaining are unemployed and officers, 59.4% are married, 53.5% are only literate, 77.4% have low income. Mean duration of disease was found as 3.73 years (SD:1.07) (Table 1). When patients were questioned about controls of blood pressure and hypertension treatment, 78.1% of the patients stated that they did not go controls for blood pressure and hypertension treatment. When the habit of eating salt was analysed, almost all of them stated that they ate their meals with litte salt or normal amount of salt. When patients were questioned about alternative ways for treatment, 75.5% stated that they consumed lemon for reduction of blood pressure. More than half of the patients stated that they did not do physical exercises.

When patients were analysed for HLSB subscale scores , the highest scores were seen to be obtained from self actualization, health responsibility, interpersonal relationships, stress management subscales and the lowest score was seen to be obtained from nutritional habits and physical activity subscale (Table 2).

Health responsibility subscale score of the patients 55 years and above was found to be greater than that of the patients 55 years and

Gender	n %
Male	43 (27.7)
Female	112 (72.3)
Age (years)	
<55	66 (42.6)
≥55	89 (57.4)
X ± SS	56,45 ± 7.98
Min- max	39-78
Occupation Housewifes	90 (58.1)
Retired	43 (27.7)
Unemployed	15 (9.7)
Officer	7 (4.5)
Marital status	
Married	92 (59.4)
Single	63 (40.6)
Education level	
Literate	83 (53.5)
Elementary	50 (32.3)
Junior high school	22 (14.2)
Income level	
Low	120 (77.4)
High	35 (22.6)
Controls for blood pressure and hypertension treatment	
Yes	34 (21.9)
No	121 (78.1)
The habit of eating salt	
Litte salt or normal amount of salt	153 (98.7)
Very salt	2 (1.3)
Alternative methods are used for lowering blood pressure Consuming garlic	38 (24.5)
Consuming lemon	117 (75.5)
Making physical activity status	
No	92 (59.4)
Yes	63 (40.6)

Table 1: Patients Characteristics.

HLSB subgroup scores	X ± SS	Min-Max Values
Self-realization	37.43 ± 7.13	13.00-52.00
Health responsibility	28.83 ± 5.40	10.00-40.00
Exercise	15.55 ± 2.01	5.00-20.00
Nutrition	17.81 ± 2.50	6.00-24.00
Interpersonal support	19.43 ± 2.96	7.00-28.00
Stress management	19.08 ± 3.46	7.00-28.00
HLSB Total	137.59 ± 11.94	48.00-192.00

Table 2: Distribution of the mean scores of the patients HLSB.

below ($p<0.05$). Nutritional habits subscale score of male patients was found to be greater than that of females. While self-actualization, physical activity, nutritional habits subscale scores and total scale scores of married patients were found to be greater than those of singles, health responsbility and interpersonal relationships subscale scores of singles were found to be greater. While health responsibility subscale score of gradutaes of intermediate school was found to be greater than that of graduates of elemantary school and literates, physical activity subscale score of graduates of elemantary school was found to be greater than that of graduates of intermediate school and literates. While self-actualization subscale score of officers was found to be greater than that

	Self-realization	Health responsibility	Exercise	Nutrition	Interpersoal support	Stress management	HLSB Total Score
Age <55	38.20 ± 7.51	28.74 ± 6.37	15.77 ± 2.14	17.98 ± 2.62	19.23 ± 3.19	19.11 ± 3.84	137.91 ± 12.72
≥55	36.85 ± 6.82 p>0.05	28.89 ± 4.58 **p<0.05**	15.38 ± 1.91 p>0.05	17.69 ± 2.42 p>0.05	19.57 ± 2.78 p>0.05	19.06 ± 3.19 p>0.05	137.36 ± 11.45 p>0.05
Gender							
Male	39.63 ± 6.64	30.51 ± 4.27	16.07 ± 1.94	17.91 ± 2.74	19.60 ± 2.70	19.21 ± 3.09	142.56 ± 12.35
Female	36.58 ± 7.16 p>0.05	28.18 ± 5.66 p>0.05	15.35 ± 2.01 p>0.05	17.78 ± 2.42 **p<0.05**	19.36 ± 3.06 p>0.05	19.03 ± 3.62 p>0.05	135.69 ± 11.31 **p<0.05**
Marital status							
Married	37.59 ± 6.79	28.78 ± 5.38	15.71 ± 1.97	17.91 ± 2.39	19.24 ± 3.00	18.79 ± 3.55	137.77 ± 11.42
Single	37.19 ± 7.65 p>0.05	28.89 ± 5.47 p>0.05	15.32 ± 2.07 p>0.05	17.67 ± 2.68 p>0.05	19.70 ± 2.89 p>0.05	19.49 ± 3.34 p>0.05	137.33 ± 12.81 p>0.05
Education level							
Literate	37.11 ± 6.63	28.67 ± 5.20	15.07 ± 1.89	17.51 ± 2.33	19.71 ± 2.95	19.22 ± 3.39	137.00 ± 10.75
Elementary	37.64 ± 7.10	27.84 ± 5.49	16.12 ± 1.97	18.42 ± 2.58	19.04 ± 3.06	18.80 ± 3.68	137.28 ± 12.27
Junior high school	38.14 ± 9.07 p>0.05	31.64 ± 5.19 **p<0.05**	15.55 ± 2.01 **p<0.05**	17.59 ± 2.84 p>0.05	19.23 ± 2.75 p>0.05	19.08 ± 3.47 p>0.05	140.55 ± 15.40 p>0.05
Occupation							
Housewifes	36.26 ± 7.00	28.54 ± 5.49	15.27 ± 1.97	17.68 ± 2.32	19.23 ± 3.10	19.22 ± 3.41	135.68 ± 10.68
Retired	39.77 ± 7.27	30.23 ± 4.82	16.14 ± 2.07	18.19 ± 2.80	19.72 ± 2.52	19.37 ± 3.18	142.81 ± 12.19
Officer	40.29 ± 7.25	29.57 ± 1.98	15.43 ± 2.29	17.00 ± 2.30	21.86 ± 2.19	19.29 ± 5.05	142.00 ± 16.72
Unemployed	36.40 ± 5.96 **p<0.05**	26.13 ± 6.54 p>0.05	15.60 ± 1.72 p>0.05	17.93 ± 2.86 p>0.05	18.60 ± 3.13 p>0.05	17.27 ± 3.63 p>0.05	132.07 ± 11.67 **p<0.05**
Income level							
Low	39.32 ± 5.82	28.88 ± 4.96	15.49 ± 1.79	17.76 ± 2.71	19.51 ± 3.35	18.93 ± 3.63	139.29 ± 12.17
High	36.75 ± 7.45 **p<0.05**	28.81 ± 5.57 p>0.05	15.57 ± 2.09 p>0.05	17.83 ± 2.44 p>0.05	19.39 ± 2.82 p>0.05	19.13 ± 3.43 p>0.05	136.98 ± 11.89 p>0.05

Table 3: Comparison of average score of HLSB Subgroups according to personal characteristics of patients.

of housewives, retired patients and unemployed patients, total score of retired patients was found to be greater than that of other occupational groups. Self-actualization subscale score of patients with low income was found to be greater than that of high income (Table 3).

Discussion

Mean HLBS score of hypertensive patients is 137,59 ± 11,94 and this value is above the mean score. This condition indicates that hypertensive patients adopt health promotion behaviours. Similar results were obtained also from another study [6].

While the highest scores were obtained from self-actualization, health responsibility, interpersonal relationships and stress management, the lowest parameters were found to be nutrition and physical activity. The lowest mean score was found to belong to physical activity in the study conducted with patients with heart diseases and health professionals [6,13,16,17]. These findings suggest that physical activity habit is low in our country. On the other hand, hypertension development risk is 20-50% greater among individuals who live a sedentary life compared to the ones who do regular physical activity. Systolic blood pressure declines 4-8 mmHg in hypertensive patients who regularly do physical activity [18]. Risk facors for heart diseases were analysed in Turkey and Germany in EUROASPIRE III trial. The most important risk factor was found as sedentary lifestyle in both countries [19].

Health responsibility which implies one's being responsible for his health and admitting to health professionals when required was found greater in advanced age patients compared to the younger. Health promotion behaviours included in health promotion model are affected from situational factors [20]. Environment of the individual and share with people may influence health promotion. Advanced aged people's

frequently sharing their life experiences may probably enable increased awareness about diseases. In a study investigating social relations of individuals living in nursing home , friend support and sharing life experience were found greater than other social support fields [21].

In our study, male patients were found to have more healthier eating habits than females. This result is considered to be related with male patients' having a higher educational level. Therefore influence of healthy nutrition on healthy life style should be addressed in education programs especially toward women. In the study of Vançelik et al. carried out with university students, mean score of eating habit was found statistically significantly greater in males than females [22]. Similar results were also obtained in another study [6].

In the study, marital status was found to be another factor affecting HLBS. Married patients were found to have healthier lifestyle behaviours than singles. They were found to be better especially in self-actualization, physical activity, eating habits. It is reported that married people's having a regular lifestyle, being supported financially and morally help them to gain healthy lifestyle behaviours [13].

While health responsibility subscale score of graduates of intermediate school was found to be greater than that of literates, physical activity subscale score of graduates of elementary school was found to be greater than that of graduates of intermediate school and literates. In previous studies, health responsibility subscale score was seen to increase as education level increased [13,16,23]. On the other hand, it is striking to find that physical activity subscale score of graduates of elementary school is grater than that of graduates of intermediate school while it is expected to find it greater than that of literates. Most of the women enrolled in the study are graduates of elementary school, housewives and unemployed and the results may be related with their having more time for physical activity.

Self-actualization levels of officers were found greater than those of members of other occupational groups. Workig environment enables one's self-actualization. However retired patients' having healthier lifestyle behaviours is considered to be related with individuals' who are not in work life being able to spare time for themselves and easily change lifestyle.

Self-actualization subscale score of patients with low income was found greater than those with high income. In the study of Johansson et al. HLBS scores were found to increase as socioeconomic status improved and this is conflicting with the results of our study [24]. Self-actualization is related with feeling morally good and sense of spirituality [12]. Therefore this is considered to be resulted from sociocultural characteristics of participants.

In conclusion, HLBS score of hypertensive patients is moderate and scores of physical activity and eating habits were found low. Officers, married patients and patients wth low income obtained high scores in self-actualization subscale; patients 55 years and above , graduates of intermediate school obtained high scores in health responsibility subscale; graduates of elemantary school, married patients obtained high scores in physical activity subscale; male and married patients obtained high scores in eating habits subscale and retired patients obtained high scores in total scale. According to these data, it may be recommended to arrange educations about the importance of healthy lifestyle behaviours, mainly nutrition and physical activity, on controlling hyptertension, to prepare and present programs toward changing knowledge, attitudes and skills of hypertensive patients who are in risk group but not having healthy life style behaviours.

Acknowledgement

We thank Dr. Ziynet Çınar, Department of Biostatistics, Cumhuriyet University for her help in analyzing the data.

References

1. World Health Organization (WHO) (2005) Preventing Chronic Diseases: A Vital Investment: Who Global Report. Geneva Switzerland.

2. Altun B, Arici M, NergizoAYlu G, Derici U, Karatan O, et al. (2005) Prevalence, awareness, treatment and control of hypertension in Turkey (the Patent study) in 2003. J Hypertens 23: 1817-1823.

3. Centers for Disease Control and Prevention (CDC) (2012) Vital signs: awareness and treatment of uncontrolled hypertension among adults--United States, 2003-2010. MMWR Morb Mortal Wkly Rep 61: 703-709.

4. Ongen Z (2005) Çözümü zor bir toplumsal sorun: hipertansiyon. Klinik Gelisim 18: 4-7.

5. Soydan I (2003) Hipertansiyon ile ilgili TEKHARF çalismasi verileri ve yorumu. In: Onat A Türk Eriskinlerde Kalp Sagligi (TEKHARF).Istanbul: Argos iletisim.

6. Küçükberber N, Ozdilli K, Yorulmaz H (2011) [Evaluation of factors affecting healthy life style behaviors and quality of life in patients with heart disease]. Anadolu Kardiyol Derg 11: 619-626.

7. Bell RA, Kravitz RL (2008) Physician counseling for hypertension: what do doctors really do? Patient Educ Couns 72: 115-121.

8. Dickson BK, Blackledge J, Hajjar IM (2006) The impact of lifestyle behavior on hypertension awareness, treatment, and control in a southeastern population. Am J Med Sci 332: 211-215.

9. Topuzoglu A, Hidiroglu S, Önsüz MF, Polat G (2011) Istanbul'da Bir Birinci Basamak Saglik Kurulusunda Kronik Hastaliklardan Korunmada Kaçirilmis Firsatlar. TSK Koruyucu Hekimlik Bülteni;10: 665-674.

10. Nidal F, Eshah NF (2011) Lifestyle And Health Promoting Behaviours In Jordanian Subjects Without Prior History Of Coronary Heart Disease. International Journal of Nursing Practice 17: 27–35.

11. Özkan S, Yilmaz E (2008) Hastanede Çalisan Hemsirelerin Saglikli Yasam Biçimi Davranislari. Firat Saglik Hizmetleri Dergisi 3: 89-104.

12. Tuygar SF (2009) Bagimlilarda Saglikli Yasam Biçimi Davranisi Gelistirme Egitiminin Beden Kitle Indeksi Üzerine Etkisi. Yüksek Lisans Tezi, Ege Üniversitesi Saglik Bilimleri Enstitüsü Psikiyatri Anabilim Dali Bagimlilik Danismanligi Programi, Izmir: 128-162.

13. Türkol E, Günes G (2012) Inönü Üniversitesi Tip Fakültesi Hastanesinde İhtisas Yapan Asistanlarin Saglikli Yasam Biçimi Davranislari Inönü Üniversitesi Tip Fakültesi Dergisi 19: 159-166.

14. Walker SN, Sechrist KR, Pender NJ(1987) The Health Promoting Lifestyle Profile Development And Psychometric Characteristics. Nursing Research 36: 76-80.

15. EsinN (1997) Healthy lifestyle behaviors scale of adopted Turkish. Nursing Bulletin.

16. Özkan S, Yilmaz E (2008) Hastanede Çalisan Hemsirelerin Saglikli Yasam Biçimi Davranislari. Firat Saglik Hizmetleri Dergisi;3: 89-104.

17. Yalçinkaya M, Özer FG, Karamanoglu AY (2007) Saglik Çalisanlarinda Saglikli Yasam Biçimi Davranislarinin Degerlendirilmesi. TSK Koruyucu Hekimlik Bülteni 6: 409-420.

18. Öksüz E (2004) Hipertansiyonda Klinik Degerlendirme Ve Ilaç Disi Tedavi Degerlendirme Formu. Sürekli Tip Egitim Dergisi 13: 100-104

19. TokgÄzoÄŸlu L, Kaya EB, Erol C, Ergene O; EUROASPIRE III Turkey Study Group (2010) [EUROASPIRE III: a comparison between Turkey and Europe]. Turk Kardiyol Dern Ars 38: 164-172.

20. Palank CL (1991) Determinants of health-promotive behavior. A review of current research. Nurs Clin North Am 26: 815-832.

21. Aksüllü N, Dogan S (2004) Huzurevinde Ve Evde Yasayan Yaslilarda Algilanan Sosyal Destek Etkenleri Ile Depresyon Arasindaki Iliski. Anadolu Psikiyatri Dergisi

22. Vançelik S, Önal SG, Güraksin A, Beyhun E (2007) Üniversite Ögrencilerinin Beslenme Bilgi Ve Aliskanliklari Ile Iliskili Faktörler TSK Koruyucu Hekimlik Bülteni 6: 242-248

23. Westin L, Carlsson R, Erhardt L, Cantor-Graae E, McNeil T (1999) Differences in quality of life in men and women with ischemic heart disease. A prospective controlled study. Scand Cardiovasc J 33: 160-165.

24. Johansson P, Dahlström U, Broström A (2006) Factors and interventions influencing health-related quality of life in patients with heart failure: a review of the literature. Eur J Cardiovasc Nurs 5: 5-15.

16

Impact of Symptoms Duration in Chronic Obstructive Pulmonary Disease is there Any Meaningful Link?

Khalid A. Ansari[1]*, Niall P. Keaney[2] and Hajed M. Al. Otaibi[1]

[1]University of Dammam, Department of Respiratory Care, Dammam, Saudi Arabia
[2]Royal Hospital, Sunderland, Sunderland, Tyne & Wear, UK

Abstract

Aim: To examine the relationship of duration of symptoms with the disease outcomes in patients with COPD.

Background: COPD patients have varying degree of symptoms. We hypothesized that duration of symptoms may be useful to understand the disease progression.

Methods: This observational study carried out in England. The patients were recruited and followed up between September 1999 and December 2002 and then 2007-2008, respectively. Patient's demographics were recorded. Medical Research Council Dyspnoea (D) score were used to measure degree of breathlessness and spirometry were utilized to evaluate the severity of disease. Patients were asked about the COPD symptoms and for how long they have these symptoms including shortness of breath, cough, and the duration of their symptoms.

Results: A total of 269 subjects were recruited. Of those 227 were with the diagnosis of COPD and 42 as non COPD or control group. The data is normally distributed. The study results show that there is a strong correlation between duration of symptoms and physiological variables both at baseline and at follow up. These include age (p=0.04), pack years (p=0.02), MRC score (p=0.04) and FEV_1 (p<0.001).When GOLD stages of severity were used to explore the relationship; it becomes evident that patients with higher GOLD stage had longer duration of symptoms.

Conclusion: These findings indicate the possible role of considering duration of symptoms as a useful marker of disease progression and its relationship with other disease outcomes in chronic obstructive pulmonary disease patients.

Keywords: COPD; Duration of symptoms; GOLD

Introduction

To date COPD is often undiagnosed or misdiagnosed until it gets advanced [1]. Earlier diagnosis is therefore essential to control or reduce systemic manifestations, comorbidity, and improve health status [2]. Spirometry is considered the gold standard to establishing a diagnosis of COPD alongside patient's symptoms, age and smoking status. Additional measurements and tools may be helpful in the differentiating between COPD and asthma [3-7]. Key areas for improvement include enhanced case identification, improved quality and interpretation of findings on spirometry, and increased use of tools such as differential diagnosis questionnaires and in order to achieve optimal outcomes. There is also a need to explore every aspect of the disease, duration of symptoms of duration, for example, to establish a firm diagnosis.

Symptom is a subjective representation of a disease. There are two types of symptoms. A sudden onset and short duration "acute" and a gradual onset and long standing "chronic" symptoms. Acute symptoms commonly occur in cases such as cholecystitis, appendicitis or acute gout that required immediate therapeutic or surgical intervention. On the other hand, chronic symptoms are common in conditions such as rheumatoid arthritis, osteoarthritis and COPD that require long term treatment and management plan, regular monitoring to minimize disease progression and control patients' symptoms and their negative impacts on patients' life which makes the condition even worse. In very severe cases, surgical intervention may be applied.

Literature review suggests that "symptoms" of patient with COPD and its relationship with other COPD outcomes have not been fully understood [8-12]. Therefore, the present study aimed to explore and examine the role of duration of symptoms in diagnosing and managing patients with COPD and its link with other prognostic indicators [13,14].

Furthermore, COPD guidelines classify severity with FEV_1 alone, though impairment correlates poorly with symptoms and disability. Previous study and the more recent BOD scores showing a 4 year and 10 year mortality and found that lower BODE and BOD scores survived longer than the worst quartile [14,15]. The BODE index is now considered useful in assessing patients progression and the present study also investigated the relationship of BODE index with duration of symptoms in patients with COPD.

Methods and Materials

Study design

This is a retrospective and prospective study carried out in Northeast of England. The patients were recruited and followed up between September 1999 and December 2002 and 2007-2008, respectively. The data were collected from patients attending Chest Clinics in general practice in Sunderland who were suspected to have COPD according to GOLD criteria.

Data collection

Spirometry was carried out to confirm the diagnosis. The spirometry was done according to BTS guidelines [16]. Patients were classified as COPD if the FEV_1/FVC ratio was less the 0.70. Those who did not meet the criteria but have some symptoms were classified as non COPD

*Corresponding author: Khalid Ansari, University of Dammam, Department of Respiratory Care, Dammam, Saudi Arabia, E-mail: Kaansari@uod.edu.sa

(control group). Other measurement include demographics, present symptoms, duration of symptoms; smoking history (pack-years), hand grip strength using hand dynamometer, co-morbidities (using Charlson Index), dyspnoea status using Medical Research Council Dyspnoea. Also, Pre- and post-bronchodilator spirometric data were obtained. All-cause mortality data for the cohort was collected from the UK Registrar General's mortality returns to December 2010 giving a median follow up period of 10 years.

To identify the duration of symptoms in patients with COPD, the question asked was "For how many years you have symptoms of your breathlessness/lung problem including cough (with or without phlegm), shortness of breath, wheezing or any other complaint?"

The total number of years was recorded in a Patient Report Form. The duration of symptoms at baseline (1999-2002 cohorts) were determined by subtracting number of years when the patient was first seen (between 1999-2002).

Sample size calculation

The sample size calculation was estimated based on previous data as well as the available database of patients who fulfil the inclusion criteria for this study.

Data analysis

Data for continuous variables are presented as mean ± standard deviation or number (%) The normality of the datasets was checked via the Kolmogorov-Smirnov test. Baseline differences between COPD and Non COPD were analyzed. For continuous variables, the Mann-Whitney U test and student t-test was employed for non-parametric and parametric data respectively. Chi-square was used for comparison of nominal variables. Data are presented as mean ± SD unless otherwise stated.

Results

The baseline demographic is presented in Table 1. The mean is 65.90 ± 9.71 in COPD 60.86 ± 11.10 in control group. The study cohort (n=227) the symptoms duration in years ranges from 0-40 years with a mean duration of 22 years in COPD. The symptoms mainly include cough, sputum production, wheeze, breathlessness which are predominant in COPD group. Pack year history is also high in COPD patients (37.37 ± 17.67 vs. 25.40 ± 17.30). The FEV_1 was 54.60 ± 16.70 vs. 95.71 ± 11.95 in two groups.

Definition of abbreviations- BMI: Body Mass Index; FEV_1 (% Predicted): Forced Expiratory Volume in 1 s Predicted for Age and Sex;

Baseline N=341	COPD N=227
Age (years)	65.90 ± 9.71
Duration of symptoms (years) (n=227)	22.70 ± 16.80
Cough Sputum Wheeze Breathlessness No symptoms	n=64 (28%) n=58 (25%) n=12 (5%) n=41 (18%) n=52 (28%)
Comorbidity Score	0.66 ± 0.95
Pack year	37.37 ± 17.67
BMI (kg/m²)	25.60 ± 5.33
FEV_1 % Pred	54.60 ± 16.70
MRC (1-5)	2.55 ± 1.00

Table 1: Baseline demographics of COPD and controls in the study.

MRC: Medical Research Council Dyspnoea Score; Dyspnoea Score by MRC Scale compared with patients who completed follow up (t test) (Figure 1).

Figure 1 indicates that there are subjects in non COPD group control group with range of symptoms indicating a group of people who are at risk of developing COPD (Stage I of GOLD). In addition, there are patients who were diagnosed to have COPD (GOLD guidelines) but with no clinical symptoms of COPD what so ever (Tables 2 and 3).

Correlations of duration of symptoms with COPD measurements at baseline

The correlations of symptoms durations with other COPD markers are presented in Tables 2 and 3 at baseline and on follow up respectively. The Table 2 shows that age, pack year, MRC and FEV_1% predicted were significantly associated with duration of symptoms at baseline. Age and MRC are positively correlated with duration of symptoms in years whereas pack years and FEV_1% predicted were negatively correlated.

At follow up (2007-2008) few additional measurements were done in addition to the baseline measurements including exercise testing (to calculate BODE Scores) and hand grip strength. The findings demonstrate that the relationship of symptoms duration was consistent

1999-2002	Correlation Coefficient	p value
Age	0.17	0.04
Pack year	-0.20	0.02
MRC	0.17	0.04
FEV_1 (% Predicted)	-0.28	<0.001

Table 2: Correlations of duration of symptoms with COPD measurements at baseline.

2007-2008	Correlation Coefficient	p value
BOD	0.64	<0.001
BODE	0.19	0.04
FEV_1 (% Predicted)	-0.24	0.004
MRC	0.47	0.04
Hand Grip Strength (% Predicted)	-0.25	0.002

Table 3: Correlations of duration of symptoms with COPD measurements on follow-up.

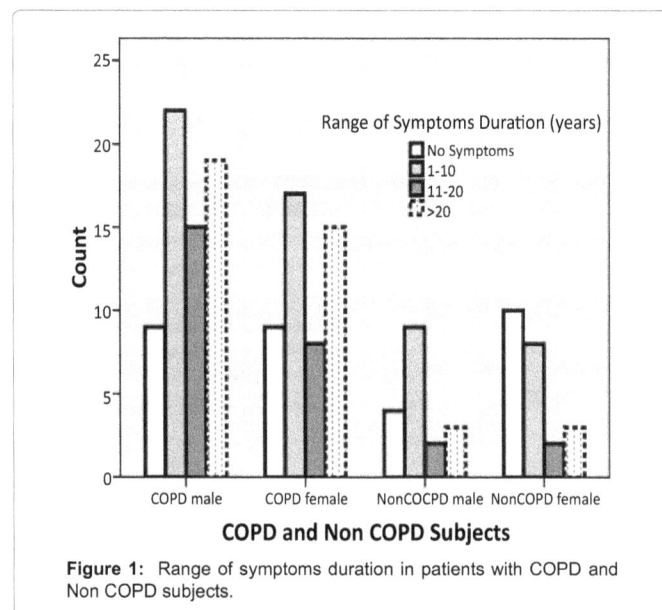

Figure 1: Range of symptoms duration in patients with COPD and Non COPD subjects.

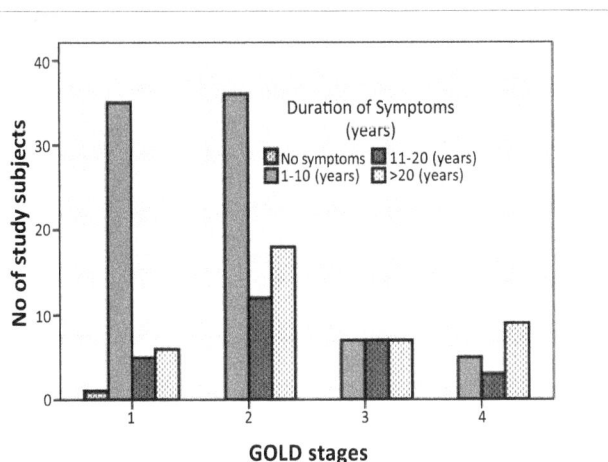

Figure 2: Distribution of duration of symptoms in different GOLD stages.

with BODE and FEV$_1$% predicted whereas as seen at baseline correlations; age, pack year history and MRC were no longer associated with duration of symptoms. Additionally two new measurements that were carried out on follow up visits only, i.e., BODE and hand grip strength were also correlated significantly with duration of symptoms (Figure 2).

Figure 2 shows the distribution of duration of symptoms in different stages of severity of COPD as measured by GOLD. The distribution clearly indicates that most of COPD patients have symptoms duration from 0-10 years particularly in stage 1 and 2. However some of the patients even in stage I (mild COPD) have symptoms duration of more than 20 years.

Discussion

The new Global Initiative for Chronic Obstructive Lung Disease update has moved the principles of treatment in stable COPD patient forward by including the concepts of symptom [17]. This study highlight the importance of determining the duration of symptoms in patients with COPD as it may provide clinically useful information about disease development, progression and outcomes. It also suggests that the duration of symptoms COPD Patients would be a potential marker that can be utilized to understand the disease. This might improve clinical management.

The present data suggests one of the potential phenotypes of COPD patients is the one who exhibit no symptoms even in presence of severe airflow obstruction as measured by spirometry [18,19]. On contrary, there is another group of potential phenotype that have more than 20 years of symptoms without clinically significant airflow obstruction.

Another important finding is the relationship between symptoms duration with other prognostic and physiological indicators of COPD such body mass index, MRC scores and BODE index [20].

The association of duration of symptoms with hand grip strength and FEV$_1$% suggests that the duration of symptoms can be utilised to reduce the occurrence of any future disability in patients who have longer duration of symptoms [21-23]. In such cases, early pulmonary rehabilitation program may be helpful to minimize and reduce the chances of disability in patients with COPD. However, more research is needed to examine this relationship.

There are some limitations in this study. As duration of symptoms have

not been studied in relation to COPD outcomes, there is no standard method and/or tool for accurate measure of duration of symptoms and therefore there is a strong chances of bias as consider the age group for COPD cohort, patient may not be able to remind and recall their onset of symptoms accurately. However, the author tried best to minimize chances of bias by asking patients about the duration of symptoms on two different occasions (one year apart) and there was no difference found in patient's response with respect to their recall about the history of onset of their symptoms. Second limitation is the data about the handgrip strength and BODE which was measured once, only on follow ups (between 2007-2008). The BODE was not considered as a part of measurement at baseline as it was published in 2004. The addition of handgrip in follow-up visit was to evaluate if these patient have any disability after 7-8 years as handgrip strength is known to be a predictor of disability in patients with long standing disease. Furthermore, more follow up studies are needed in order to make any firm conclusion regarding duration of symptoms and its importance and utilisation in identifying and assessing these patients.

Further researches will be needed to explore the under-studied and under-estimated use of duration of symptoms in patients with COPD. There is also a need of developing a structured and validated tool to get this information accurately irrespective of spirometric confirmation in these patients that potentially play a critical role in managing disease in these patients.

Conclusion

These findings indicate the possible role of considering duration of symptoms as a useful marker of disease progression and its relationship with other disease outcomes in chronic obstructive pulmonary disease patients.   •

Funding

The study has supported by Higher Education Commission, Pakistan (Grant Number: .1-6/HEC/HRD/2006) and Sunderland Royal Hospital Research and Development Research Grant (Grant Number: 390593B/2009).

References

1. Bednarek M, Maciejewski J, Wozniak M, Kuca P, Zielinski J (2008) Prevalence, severity and under-diagnosis of COPD in primary care setting. Thorax 63: 402-407.

2. Price D, Freeman D, Cleland J, Kaplan A, Cerasoli F (2011) Earlier diagnosis and earlier treatment of COPD in primary care. Prim Care Respir J 20:15-22.

3. Global Initiative for Chronic Obstructive Lung Disease.

4. Puhan MA, Garcia-Aymerich J, Frey M, ter Riet G, Antó JM, et al. (2009) Expansion of the prognostic assessment of patients with chronic obstructive pulmonary disease: The updated BODE index and the ADO index. Lancet 374: 704-711.

5. Jones RC, Donaldson GC, Chavannes NH, Kida K, Dickson-Spillmann M, et al. (2009) Derivation and validation of a composite index of severity in chronic obstructive pulmonary disease - the dose index. Am J Respir Crit Care Med 180: 1189-1195.

6. Chang J, Mosenifar Z (2007) Differentiating COPD from asthma in clinical practice. J Intensive Care Med 22: 300-309.

7. Cosgrove JBR (1955) An evaluation of the importance of symptoms, signs and spinal fluid findings in the diagnosis of poliomyelitis in the absence of paralysis. Can Med Assoc J 72: 808-811.

8. Han MK, Agusti A, Calverley PM, Celli BR, Criner G, et al. (2010) Chronic obstructive pulmonary disease phenotypes. The future of COPD. Am J Respir Crit Care Med 182: 598-604.

9. Calle Rubio M, Rodríguez-Hermosa JL, Ortega González A, et al. (2007) Fenotipos de la enfermedad pulmonar obstructiva crónica. Med Clin Monogr 8: 22.

10. Garcia-Aymerich J, Agustí A, Barberà JA (2009) La heterogeneidad fenotípica de la EPOC. Arch Bronconeumol 45: 129-138.

11. Soriano JB, Davis KJ, Coleman B, Visick G, Mannino D, et al. (2003) The proportional Venn diagram of obstructive lung disease. Chest 124: 474-481.

12. Rennard SI, Vestbo J (2008) The many small COPDs: COPD should be an orphan disease. Chest 134: 623-627.

13. Bartolome RC, Claudia GC, Jose MM, Ciro C, Maria Md, et al. (2004) The body-mass index, airflow obstruction, dyspnoea and exercise capacity index in chronic obstructive pulmonary disease. N Engl J Med 350: 205-212.

14. Keaney NP, Ansari K, Kay AD (2012) Multidimensional index BOD predicts ten year mortality for COPD in primary care. International Primary Care Respiratory Group 216 (A).

15. Ansari K, Keaney N, Kay A, Price M, Munby J, Billett A, et al. (2016) Body mass index, airflow obstruction and dyspnea and body mass index, airflow obstruction, dyspnea scores, age and pack years-predictive properties of new multidimensional prognostic indices of chronic obstructive pulmonary disease in primary care. Ann Thorac Med 11: 261–268.

16. The British Thoracic Society Standards of Care Committee (1997) BTS Guidelines on the management of COPD. Thorax, p: 52.

17. Global Initiative for chronic obstructive lung disease (2011) Global strategy for the diagnosis, management and prevention of COPD.

18. Han MK, Agusti A, Calverley PM, Celli BR, Criner G, et al. (2010) Chronic obstructive pulmonary disease phenotypes: The future of COPD. Am J Respir Crit Care Med 182: 598-604.

19. Miravitlles M, Soler Cataluna J, Calle M, Soriano J (2013) Treatment of COPD by clinical phenotypes: putting old evidence into clinical practice. ERJ 41: 1252-1256.

20. Bestall J, Paul E, Garrod R, Garnham R, Jones P, et al. (1999) Usefulness of the Medical Research Council (MRC) dyspnoea scale as a measure of disability in patients with chronic obstructive pulmonary disease. Thorax 54: 581-586.

21. Sunnerhagen KS, Hedberg M, Henning GB, Cider A, Svantesson U, et al. (2000) Muscle performance in an urban population sample of 40 to 79 year old men and women. Scandinavian Journal of Rehabilitation Medicine 32:159-167.

22. Rantanen T, Masaki K, Foley D, Izmirlian G, White L, et al. (1985) Grip strength changes over 27 year in Japanese-American men. J Appl Physiol 85: 2047-2053.

23. Rantanen T, Volpato S, Ferrucci L, Heikkinen E, Fried LP, et al. (2003) Hand grip strength and cause of total mortality in older disable women. J Am Geriatr Soc 51: 636-641.

17

Implementation of Patient Safety in Obstetric Primary Care Health Center Padang based Malcolm Baldrige Performance Excellence

Dien Gusta Anggraini N[1,2]*, Rizanda M[1], Eryati D[1] and Nana M[3]

[1]*Faculty of Medicine, Andalas University, Padang, Indonesia*
[2]*Faculty of Public Health, Andalas University, Padang, Indonesia*
[3]*Ministry of Health, Andalas University, Padang, Indonesia*

Abstract

Background: A high number of adverse event based on the data from Minister of Health in Indonesia showed that patient safety still not going well, while patient safety is a measure of the quality of health services in Indonesia.

Objective: The purpose of this study is to determine the implementation of the seven patient safety standard as the basic of patient safety model development based on Malcolm Baldrige in BEmONC Health Center of Padang.

Methods: This study uses a qualitative research method. The number of informant is 25 from Department of Health of West Sumatera, Department of Health of Padang, the Head, health care workers and patients of BEmONC Health Center.

Result: There is no guidelines about patient safety from Department of Health of West Sumatera to the BEmONC Health Center, it is also obtained that the patient safety incident that occurs is in the form of patient falls, diagnostic errors and drug delivery personally without reporting to the Department of Health.

Conclusion: The standard of patient safety hasn't been completely implemented, so it is necessary to do a socialization about patient safety to the health care workers and also from a Malcolm Baldrige-based patient safety model.

Keywords: Patient safety; Obstetric primary care; MBNQA

Introduction

WHO had identified the risk of adverse event in health services which are serious and threaten the safety of patients globally? [1]. Risks detected since the report of the Institute of Medicine (IOM), reported adverse events on the hospital in Utah and Colorado by 2.9% which 6.6% of them died, and the New York Hospital by 3.7% with the mortality rate is 13.6% of them [2-5]. The report of adverse event in Indonesia from the Ministry of Health is quite high. Until February 2016, it is reached 289 reports. The type of adverse event consists of 69 events of near miss (43.67%) in the form of medication errors (29.2%), patient falls (23.4%), canceled operations (14.3%), diagnosis errors (11%), incorrect laboratory tests (8.4%) and incorrect roentgen (5.2%) [6].

Since the implementation of JKN in 2012, PT BPJS as the executor of JKN adjust a procedure starting from the first level of health care. To reduce maternal and infants mortality rate in Indonesia was done by the availability of BEOC-CHC in each district as a gate keeper for the safety of mothers and children. BEOC-CHC will improve access to maternal and neonatal to cope with obstetric and neonatal emergency cases which is the largest contributor to maternal and child mortality rate [7]. The aspects of patient safety in the primary health centers appears as the part of the Regulation of Ministry of Health number 75 of 2014, but still no clear guidelines for its implementation [8,9].

There isn't much information about adverse event in primary care [10]. Based on some research, it is in the form of missed or delayed diagnosis and medication management, medication and diagnosis errors, failures communication between the human resources [11,12]. Teamwork, management support, communication, staff and the value of patient safety the lack of guidance, ineffective communication, lack of knowledge and lack of quality assurance mechanisms [13-15].

To provide a high quality health services and be able to compete in the global marketplace, it can be used the Malcolm Baldrige Criteria for Performance Healthcare (MBHCP). The advantages of MBHCP are its ability to provide a comprehensive and integrated assessment. MBHCP is used because of its ability to identify the strengths and opportunities for improvements, provide a framework to improve performance advantages by giving liberties to the management to implement its management strategies. An integrated management framework includes every factor that defines the organization, operational processes and a clear and measurable work, increases the process speed and quality of work, building a high work system, translating the vision and mission into strategy and builds the loyalty of patients. The purpose of this study is to determine the implementation of the seven standards of patient safety as the basic of patient safety model development based on Malcolm Baldrige in BEOC-CHC of Padang as the implementation of maternal and child safety [16].

Materials and Methods

This study uses a descriptive exploratory study with a qualitative design. The study was held in Department of Health of West Sumatera as the policies holder, Department of Health of Padang as the direct supervisor and BEOC-CHC. The study was conducted from January to August 2016.

The number of informants is 25 which are the Head of Health Registry Section, Accreditation and Sertification of Department of Health of West Sumatera, the Head of Health Services of Department of Health of Padang, the Head of Lubuk Buaya and Seberang Padang

---

*Corresponding author: Dien Gusta Anggraini N, Faculty of Public Health, Andalas University, Padang, Indonesia, E-mail: diennursal@gmail.com

BEOC-CHC. All informants got in-depth interview. Six health personnel from Lubuk Buaya BEOC-CHC, nine health personnel Seberang Padang BEOC-CHC, and also 12 patients got focus group discussion (FGD). Informants get asked about the implementation of the seven standards of patient safety based on a system approach in terms of input, process and output using the guidelines which are derived from the hospital patient safety guidelines which were modified and adjusted based on research purposes.

The result of in-depth interviews and FGD will be written in the field notes, personal documents, official documents, drawings and photographs. Furthermore, the result would be read and analyzed. The analyzed was done by interpret and dechiper the data that has been acquired into a substantive theory. The data that had been required were analyzed descriptively, summarized and presented.

Results

Based on the 25 informants in this study, the average age of the respondents is 39 years old, with the youngest is 25 and the oldest is 52 years old. The average length of work is 13 years, the longest is 22 years and the shortest is 2 years. For almost all patients were housewives.

Based on the results, the adverse event was found last year in BEOC-CHC is medication errors and patient falls out of the bed. This adverse event was completed amicably between health centers and patient's family. Incidents didn't report in writing to the Department of Health of Padang because there are no guidelines and reporting format for adverse events. Until now there are still no guidelines for patient safety from Department of Health of West Sumatra, Department of Health of Padang and BEOC-CHC in Padang about the implementation of patient safety in the BEOC-CHC (Figure 1).

Patient rights

There are no guidelines to fulfill the patient rights on BEOC-CHC yet. The doctor in charge of service making plans of service and done assessment of patients. Medical records and informant consent as the document of services planning and implementations. In the implementation process, information provide and explanations to the patients and their families about plans and results are not always given, but for every services performed is always preceded by the signing of informed consent. Patients or family explained about the services that will be given but without being informed about the result of services, the further services plans and the likelihood of adverse events. The output has not been running well. Patients have not been informed about the results of the services given and the possibility of adverse events.

Educate patients and their families

There are no specific plans to educate the patients and their families about patient safety at BEOC-CHC. The health guidance and promotion about the maternal and child safety limitary given only to the mother through maternal classes every month, without educate the patient's

family. The implementation of giving right information, transparent and honest to patients was not done yet but patients have already know their obligations and responsibilities, patients understand and accept the consequences of services, also patients and families fulfill their financial obligations. The output has not been accomplished too.

Patient safety and continual care

Planning of the patient flow from registered until finish was conduct through the workshops in BEOC-CHC every month. Every health personnel in charge from patients register until the medication and patient go home. Standard Operational Procedures (SOP) for each supporting facilities and the flowchart of patient services flows has been displayed on the walls of health centers. The coordination of services started from the patient registered until going home accordingly to the patient needs, but sometimes constrained due to the limitations of doctors, sometimes patients were examined and given a prescription not by doctor. The improvements of communications and transfer communication among health personnel running well. The output already performing well.

The use of improvement methods of performances to evaluate and improve patient safety

Planning in the input by conducted performance assessment for health personnel is carried through the accreditation process of BEOC-CHC. All heath personnel of BEOC-CHC will empowered all health personnel. Lubuk Buaya BEOC-CHC is one of the best CHC in Padang which already have an ISO 9001 certificate. Implementation of patient safety not done yet. There is no designing plan of improvement with the 7 standards patient safety, accumulation of data, such as incident reports, risk management and audit quality of health services. Likewise, there has been no intensive evaluation of adverse events and proactively evaluate the high-risk cases, because there are no result of data analysis, thus the change of system have not been implemented. The output has not accomplished.

The role of leadership to improve patient safety

For input, the planning has not specifically for patient safety. The head of BEOC-CHC has not appointed a specialized team. There are no guidelines and documents about patient safety in the health center yet because the patient safety issue is still a new issue for the health center. The implementation is also has not been done yet, no interdisciplinary team, no risk identification, no mechanism of work, no responsive procedure towards incidents, no internal and external reporting mechanisms, no mechanism to handle incidents, no open collaboration and communication between units, no resource and information system, no measurable targets. The output has not been accomplished too.

Educate the personnels about patient safety

Plans for training and orientation process about patient safety

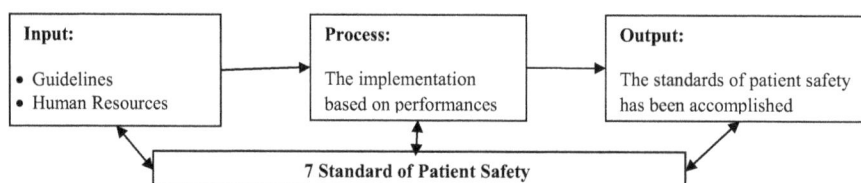

Figure 1: Thinking flow of the implementation of patient safety standard in BEOC health centers.

which adjusted based on the decision from the Department of Health of Padang as the direct supervisor of BEOC-CHC. There are no guidelines and documents about patient safety. There are no integrating patient safety topics in every in-service training activities and also providing a clear guidance about reporting incidents yet, but there are trainings about teamwork to support interdisciplinary approach and collaboration in serving patients. Based on the output, education and training programs and orientation about patient safety for new health personnels in accordance with their respective duties has not yet accomplished.

Comunication is the key to the personnels to achieve a patient safety

There is no specific planning about comunicating about patient safety. There are no guidelines and documents about patient safety in BEOC-CHC yet because the patient safety issue is still a new issue. For process, no budget available to plan and design data processing to obtain data and information that is related to patient safety. For the output the implementation of data transmission still is not clear and the information still is not timely and accurate yet.

Discussion

Based on the research, it is obtained that the adverse event occurred at BEOC-CHC at the last year. The implementation of patient safety in BEOC-CHC had been varied because no specific guidelines available yet [4].

In Indonesia, the regulation about the accreditation of primary health centers just had been declared recently on Permenkes number 75 of 2014, the implication in the health centers is not clear yet [8]. The risk management which is the core of the implementation of patient safety in the BEOC-CHC has not been running yet. And the adverse event still is the fault of the individual because 'blaming culture' still is applied [17,18].

The implementations of the 7 standards of patient safety at BEOC-CHC are reviewed with the system approach of input, process and output. Almost at all standards about patient safety (input, process and output) is not accomplished yet. Only the third standard about patient safety and continual care are systematically goes well. Changes happen in health care providers, now patient is an important aspect of the design of the health care and improving the quality of health services (patient centered care) [19]. Patients have an important role in helping to achieve an accurate diagnosis, in deciding on the appropriate treatment, in choosing an experienced and secured provider, in ensuring that the right treatment is given, monitored and adhered to, and in identifying the side effects and take appropriate action [19-21]. Therefore, it is important to fulfill patients' rights and educating patients and families. Communication between health personnel in the unit are good but between units still worse. Worse communication can lead to adverse event. Good communication between heath personnel and with patient and family it's important for patient safety [22,23].

Performance assessment in BEOC-CHC all this time based on health personnel attendances. Planning performance assessments in BEOC-CHC can be carried through the accreditation process of CHC. Good health personnel performance can improve patient safety through fix inadequate work space, fulfil incomplete equipment, given adequate information from the health personnel, and fix busy and disorganized working environment is busy and disorganized [24]. Such as strong, unwavering leadership and open communication and action can improve patient safety with encourage and ensure the implementation

of the patient safety program through the implementation of "7 Steps to the Hospital Patient Safety" [25].

Health personnel as the practitioner must understand about patient safety. Educate the health personnel about patient safety was the sixth standard of patient safety, done by planning training and orientation process about patient safety [16-18]. Since training of health personnel is determined by the Department of Health of Padang as the direct supervisor of BEOC-CHC, it is necessary to planning about training health all personnel about patient safety in BEOC-CHC. Comunication was the key to the health personnel to achieve a patient safety. Good communication between health personnel, between health personnel and patients can reduce adverse event. Open communication is necesarry too, open communication would make good patient safety culture. To make good patient safety culture it is necessary to develop a model thats fit to patient safety in BEOC-CHC which can be develop bases malcom baldridge performance.

Conclusion

In general it can be seen that out of the 7 standards of patient safety based on patient safety guidelines by KPPRS, only the third standard about patient safety and continuous care that has been running systematically, started from input, process until its output, while the patient safety standard number 1, 2, 4, 5, 6 and 7 had not been accomplished yet. It is required a patient safety system that matches the conditions of the BEOC-CHC based on Malcolm Baldridge performance as the standard of the performance of the organization which is applied on the patient safety performance.

Acknowledgement

This Research is a part of Competitive Professor Grant Andalas University number 81/UN.16/HKRGB/LPPM/2016. Researchers would like to thanks to dr. Adang Bachtiar DSc, Prof. Dr. Herkutanto SpF SH LLM FACLM, Prof. Dr. Nur Indrawati Liputo SpGK PhD, Nilda Tri Putri ST, MT PhD. BEOC-CHC Seberang Padang and Lubuk Buaya, Department of Health Sumatera Barat and Padang, and Andalas University.

References

1. Varnam R (2012) Institute for innovation and improvement.

2. Findyartini A, Mustika R, Felaza E, Herqutanto, Wardhani ESK, et al. (2015) Modul Pelatihan untuk Pelatih Keselamatan Pasien: Kolaborasi Bidang Pendidikan Proyek P4K-RSP.

3. Kohn LT, Corrigan J, Donaldson M (2000) To err is human: Building a safer health system. Washington: National Academy Press.

4. Marchon SG, Mendes Junior WV (2014) Patient safety in primary health care: A systematic review. Cadernos de saúde pública 30:1815-1835.

5. Varnam R (2012) Patient Safety: A Primary Concern? In Institute for Innovation and Improvement.

6. Subdit Pelayanan Medis dan Keperawatan (2016) Evaluasi pelaporan E-Reporting Pelaporan Insiden Keselamatan Pasien RS Sampai. In: RS SKKP, editor. Workshop Keselamatan Pasien di Hotel Horizon Bogor 2-4 Maret 2016; Bogor.

7. Rahmanita DRP, Bachtiar A (2014) Penilaian Kinerja Pelayanan Obstetri Neonatal Emergensi Dasar di Puskesmas Poned Tanah Sareal Kota Bogor dengan Pendekatan Balanced Scorecard tahun 2014. Fakultas Kesehatan Masyarakat UI.

8. Peraturan Menteri Kesehatan Republik Indonesia No 75 Tahun 2014 tentang Pusat Kesehatan Masyarakat (2014).

9. Peraturan Menteri Kesehatan Republik Indonesia Nomor 46 Tahun 2015 tentang Akreditasi Puskesmas, Klinik Pertama, Tempat Praktik Mandiri Dokter, dan Tempat Praktik Mandiri Doketr Gigi, (2015).

10. Kingston-Riechers J, Ospina M, Jonsson E, Childs P, McLeod L, et al. (2010) Patient safety in primary care. Edmonton AB: Canadian Patient Safety Institute and BC Patient Safety and Quality Council.

11. O'Rourke M (2007) The Australian Commission on safety and quality in health care agenda for improvement and implementation. Asia Pacific Journal of Health Management 2: 21.

12. Marchon SG, Junior WVM (2014) Patient safety in primary health care: A systematic review. Cad Saude Publica 30: 1815-1835.

13. Molloy PA (2012) Examining the relationship between work climate and patient safety among nurses in acute care settings.

14. Walston SL, Al-Omar BA, Al-Mutari FA (2010) Factors affecting the climate of hospital patient safety: A study of hospitals in Saudi Arabia. Int J Health Care Qual Assur 3: 35-50.

15. Pettker CM, Thung SF, Norwitz ER, Buhimschi CS, Raab CA, et al. (2009) Impact of a comprehensive patient safety strategy on obstetric adverse events. Am J Obstet Gynecol 200: 492e1-e8.

16. Sadikin I (2010) Malcom Baldrodge National Quality Award (MBNQA). Surabaya: Lembayung Central Indonesia.

17. Chassin MR (2016) The need for a paradigm shift in healthcare culture: Old versus new. High Reliability Organizations: A Healthcare Handbook for Patient Safety and Quality: 3.

18. Nieva V, Sorra J (2003) Safety culture assessment: A tool for improving patient safety in healthcare organizations. Qual Saf Health Care 12: ii17-ii23.

19. Johnson B, Abraham M, Conway J, Simmons L, Edgman-Levitan S, et al. (2008) Partnering with patients and families to design a patient-and family-centered health care system. Bethesda MD: Institute for Family-Centered Care.

20. Vincent CA, Coulter A (2002) Patient safety: What about the patient? Quality and Safety in Health Care 11: 76-80.

21. Davis RE, Jacklin R, Sevdalis N, Vincent CA (2007) Patient involvement in patient safety: What factors influence patient participation and engagement? Health Expectations 10: 259-267.

22. Top M, Tekingündüz S (2015) Patient safety culture in a Turkish public hospital: A study of nurses' perceptions about patient safety. Syst Pract Action Res 28: 87-110.

23. Bishop AC, Cregan BR (2015) Patient safety culture: Finding meaning in patient experiences. Int J Health Care Qual Assur 28: 595-610.

24. Gurses AP (2005) Performance obstacles and facilitators, workload, quality of working life and quality and safety of care among intensive care nurses. Ann Arbor: The University of Wisconsin – Madison.

25. Bagian JP (2005) Patient safety: What is really at issue? Frontiers of Health Services Management 22: 3-16.

18

Improving Maternal Health in the Volta Region of Ghana: Development Action Plan from a Baseline Assessment using 5As Framework

Sarita Dhakal[1,2,3], Eun Woo Nam[1,2,3]*, Young Suk Jun[4], Ha Yun Kim[1,2], Festus Adams[5] and Jin Sung Song[1,2]

[1]Yonsei Global Health Center, Yonsei University, Wonju, Korea
[2]Department of Health Administration, Graduate School, Yonsei University, Korea
[3]Institute of Poverty Allivaiton and International Development, Yonsei University, Wonju, Korea
[4]West Africa Team, Korea International Cooperation Agency, Headquater, Korea
[5]Ministry of Health, Ghana

Abstract

Introduction: KOICA and the Yonsei Global Health Center of Yonsei University finalized a baseline survey for the development of a maternal health program in the Volta Region of Ghana. Community, Health facility and health care provider surveys were conducted in the Region (Keta Municipality, Ketu North and South District) to evaluate the accessibility of essential reproductive health care, especially maternity services. Access to quality maternal health care is essential to reduce maternal mortality.

Objective: To assess the strength and weakness of maternal health service and develop an action plan according to the problems to strengthen maternal health and reduce maternal mortality ratio in the Volta Region

Method: Access to maternal health service had been categorized into five dimensions: availability, accessibility, affordability, accommodation and acceptability. 5As framework was used to assess the strength and weakness to the improvement of the maternal health.

Results: Bested on the result it was found that, many obstacles to achieving every "A", excluding acceptability and problems include; insufficient health personnel, inadequate knowledge in health service provider and inadequate instruments in health facilities.

Conclusion: Based on the survey, training of service providers, regular supply of essential medicine and equipment and strengthening basic unit of the health service are recommended to improve access to maternal health care in the Volta Region, Ghana.

Keywords: Maternal health; Access to maternal health care; Ghana; KOICA

Background

The West African country of Ghana has a population of 24,658,823 according to the Population and Housing Census (PHC) report of 2010. The country has ten administrative regions and 170 districts. Ghana has one of the highest gross domestic products (GDP) per capita in West Africa and is ranked as a Lower-Middle Income Economy by the World Bank. The country has a diverse and rich resource base, with foreign trade in gold, cocoa, timber, diamond, bauxite, and manganese.

Globally, maternal death has dropped 45% between 1990 and 2013 [1]. While considerable progress has been achieved in almost all regions, many countries, particularly Sub-Saharan Africa, have fallen short of Millennium Development Goal 5, i.e., improve maternal health. In fact, among all Millennium Development Goals (MDGs), the least progress has been made in maternal health [2,3]. The maternal mortality rate in Ghana was 350 per 100,000 live births in 2012.

The Korea International Cooperation Agency (KOICA) is the governmental organization for Official Development Assistance (ODA) charged with enhancing the effectiveness of the Republic of Korea's grant aid for developing countries by implementing development program and coordinating aid. At the request of the government of Ghana, a Maternal and Child Health (MCH) project was conducted in Ghana in collaboration with KOICA and Yonsei University; Yonsei Global Health Center did a baseline survey of the Volta region [4]. One goal of the baseline survey was to evaluate community health.

The 5As of Access framework was used to identify problems related to maternal health care in the Volta region, using the categories of availability, accessibility, affordability, accommodation and acceptability [5,6]. Access is the opportunity to identify health care needs, to seek health care service to reach or use the service to fulfil the need of the health service [7]. The more accessible a system is, the more people utilize health service to improve their health [8]. The access can be measured by developing indicator, both objective and subjective indicator. Objective indicators are the observable facts and figure like the availability of the service in the health facilities, a number of health care provider, service cost, etc. and subjective indicators are normally derived from people's perception and satisfaction level [9].

The objective of this study was to assess the strength and weakness of maternal health service and develop an action plan according to the problems to strengthen maternal health and reduce Maternal Mortality Ratio (MMR) in the Volta Region.

Methodology

This study applied two methodologies. The first one was baseline survey and the baseline survey had 3 line surveys (community, facility

*Corresponding author: Eun Woo Nam, Yonseidae- gil, Wonju City, Ganwon-do 220-710, Republic of Korea, E-mail: ewnam@yonsei.ac.kr

and provider survey). The second method was 5As (availability, accessibility, affordability, accommodation and acceptability) framework as shown in Table 1.

Baseline survey

The study design was a cross sectional descriptive survey. The survey was conducted at the level of the community, facility and health care provider in Keta Municipality, Keta North and South District in the Volta Region.

Community survey

A structured questionnaire was administered to the women of the reproductive age (WRA) 15-49 years who were pregnant or had children under 5 years old in order to ascertain knowledge, attitudes and opinions about maternal, neonatal and child health services in the community. The information on demographic characteristics, economic status, knowledge, attitude and practice (KAP) about nutrition, health and illness, maternal, neonatal and child health service delivery, environmental health conditions and perceived health care needs was gathered.

Selection of communities and households

The EPI "30 x 7" cluster sampling was method developed by the World Health Organization (WHO) with the aim of calculating the prevalence of immunized children was used to select communities for the survey. The design was adopted for other purposes such as rapid needs assessment with no modification. This sampling method is thought to be sufficient for most sampling of community health factors. The clusters were selected at the district using enumeration areas (EAs) developed for use by the Ghana Statistical Service in the 2010 Population and Housing Census. An EA is defined as a community cluster in an urban area and a village, and part of a village or a group of villages in the rural areas; each EA has approximately 200 households.

A sampling of "30 × 7" means that 30 EAs were randomly selected from a list of all the EAs in the district, and 7 households per EA were selected. EAs were selected in stage one through a method known as probability proportional to population size.

The sample size (n=30 × 7) per each district was 210 households. Since three districts were included, the total sample size [N=3 (30 × 7)] was 610 households/respondents.

Enumeration Areas (EAs) for each of the districts were listed by Ghana Statistical Services. The EAs within Ketu North, Ketu South and Keta Municipal were stratified into Rural and Urban EAs. Within each stratum, a Simple Random Sampling based on the Probability Proportional to Size was used to select the required number of both Rural and Urban EAs in the selected districts. Rural EAs made up 0% of the total, with the remaining 40% consisting of urban EAs. The total number of Enumeration Areas for the 2010 Population and Housing Census was used. All EAs were given an equal chance to be selected (Table 2).

The following attributes were used:

N=N1+N2=Total number of Urban or Rural EAs within Ketu South, Ketu North and Keta Municipal

n=n1+n2=required number of Rural or Urban EAs within the selected district

SI=Sample Interval (i.e., N/n)

rn=Random Number Generated

(SI*rn=k)=Random Start (The first EA to be selected), (K+SI)=the next EA to be selected

5 A's of Access category	Definition of the 5 A's of access	Items for the assessment of the access
Availability	The relationship of the volume and type of existing services (and resources) to the clients' volume and types of needs. It refers to the adequacy of the supply of physicians, dentists and other providers; of facilities such as clinics and hospitals; and specialized programs and services such as mental health and emergency care.	The total number of services in which user makes a choice and availability of the service providers and equipment.
Accessibility	The relationship between the location of supply and the location of clients, taking account of client transportation resources and travel time, distance and cost.	Travel time or distance between location of user and service (nearest health facilities).
Affordability	The relationship of prices of services and providers' insurance or deposit requirements to the clients' income, ability to pay and existing health insurance. The clients' perception of worth relative to total cost is a concern here, as is their knowledge of prices, total cost and possible credit arrangements.	The direct cost (doctor's fee) and indirect cost (travel and medication cost).
Accommodation	The relationship between the manner in which the supply resources are organized to accept clients (including appointment systems, hours of operation, walk-in facilities, telephone services) and the clients' ability to accommodate to these factors and their perception of their appropriateness.	Quality of service provided and personal treatment by the provider.
Acceptability	The relationship of clients' attitudes about personal and practice characteristics of providers to the actual characteristics of existing providers, as well as to provider attitudes about acceptable personal characteristics of clients. In the literature, the term appears to be used most often to refer to the specific consumer reaction to such provider attributes as age, sex, ethnicity, type of facility, neighborhood of the facility, or religious affiliation of the facility or provider. In turn, providers have attitudes about the preferred attributes of clients or their financing mechanisms. Providers either may be unwilling to serve certain types of clients (e.g. Welfare patients) or, through accommodation, may make themselves more or less available.	Belief and expectation of different groups of people/ cultural and religious factor.

Source: Penchansky R, Thomas JW, 1981. The concept of access, definition and relationship to consumer satisfaction. Medical Care, 19 (2): 127–140.

Table 1: 5 A's framework.

Region (Volta)	Total EAs (N)	Urban EAs (N$_1$)	Rural EAs (N$_2$)	Total EAs Sampled (n)	Urban EAs Sampled (n$_1$)	Rural EAs Sampled (n$_2$)
Ketu North	175	57	118	30	10	20
Ketu South	230	80	150	30	12	18
Keta Municipal	219	101	118	30	14	16
Volta	3,609	1,068	2,541			

Table 2: Total number of enumeration areas for selected districts.

Enumeration Area maps for each of the selected EAs generated by Ghana Statistical Services were used to identify each EA's demarcation. With the selected EAs, a modified random walk method was used to select the households in the study.

To avoid redundancy, improve sample distribution and reduce design defects, the sample was restricted to one eligible respondent per household, in essence making the household the sample unit.

Data Collection Process

Data collection instruments

The research team worked in close collaboration with the KOICA team and Ministry of Health (MOH), Policy, planning , monitoring and evaluation to develop the questionnaire to interview community members, as users of Maternal child Health and Nutrition (MCHN) services are interviewed at the community level. The unit of analysis for the study was a client.

Field work

A total of seven research assistants from the three study districts (Keta Municipality, Ketu North and South districts) was selected, orientated to the project and trained to use the baseline data collection tools. Facilitated by staff from Research and Development Division (RDD) of Ghana Health Service in Keta over five days, the training enabled the trainees to: a) Understand and describe the background, purpose and basic methodological approach of the study; b) Discuss the role of the interviewers in the data collection process; c) Review the purpose, principles and techniques of interviewing; d) Apply interview techniques in pre-testing the questionnaire in the classroom situation through role plays; e) Conduct field pre-tests and assist in finalized the instruments in preparation for data collection; and f) Develop a detailed plan of data collection.

Three field work teams were formed, one per each district. The teams were made of non-health workers. A supervisor was appointed to each of the three districts. The data collectors met with their supervisors to review the tools for completeness and accuracy in the field. The coordinator closely monitored the initial fieldwork and assist in harmonizing the data collection. At the end of data collection, the coordinator met with the supervisors for a wrap up meeting. Field notes were prepared and compiled in separated field reports. The data collection was done from the 8th to the 17th of April 2013.

Facility and provider survey

The study design was a cross sectional descriptive survey. Two main data collection techniques were used: in-depth interviews with health providers and a facility inventory using a checklist.

Facility inventory

Twenty selected health facilities in the three study districts were visited. The facilities included 3 District Hospitals (DH), 9 Health Centers (HC) and 8 Community-based Health Planning (CHPs) zones that were selected in consultation with the regional research coordinator to reflect the diversity of public health facilities in the three districts. The facility inventory retrospectively examined facility health records to collect information on the utilization of maternal, neonatal and child health services.

Health providers

Respondents were purposefully selected based on the ability to provide the necessary information. Health providers who were providing maternal and child health care during the time of the visit to the facility and were available to participate were interviewed.

Data collection process:

Data collection instruments: The research team worked in close collaboration with the KOICA team and MOH PPME to develop three study data collection instruments: 1) Inventory of facilities available and services provided at the service delivery point; 2) Health provider assessment guide; and 3) Community survey questionnaire. The units of analysis for the study were service delivery facilities and providers.

These tools were designed to be used as follows: a) Take an inventory of services, equipment and supplies at selected service delivery sites; b) Obtain service statistics, where available, recorded for the past 12 months; c) Interview MCNH service providers to self-assess their capabilities of providing maternal, newborn and child health services.

Field work

One research assistant (practicing midwife) from each of the three study districts (Keta Municipality, Ketu North and South districts) was selected, provided orientation of the project and trained to use the data collection tools. The training, facilitated by staff from Research and Development Division (RDD) of Ghana Health Service for over five days, enabled the interviewers to: a) Understand and describe the background, purpose and the basic methodological approach of the study; b) Discuss the role of the interviewers in the data collection process; c) Review the purpose, principles and techniques of interviewing; d) Apply interview techniques in pre-testing the questionnaire in the classroom situation through role plays; e) Conduct field pre-tests and assist in finalizing the instruments in preparation for data collection; and f) Develop a detailed plan of data collection.

A supervisor was appointed to monitor the research assistants. The data collectors met with their supervisor to review the tools for completeness and accuracy in the field. The coordinator closely monitored the initial fieldwork and assisted in harmonizing the data collection. Data collection was done in 25th to 30th of March, 2013.

Data processing and analysis

The completed questionnaires were processed at the Resilient Distributed Datasets (RDD) data processing unit using Epi data and analyzed using Stata software.

Measuring the dimensions of access

Depending on the nature of the developed indicators, each dimension of access to health service was measured and compared using descriptive statistics. Access is defined as the opportunity to reach and obtain appropriate health care service in situations when the need for care is identified [10-13]. Access can be measured subjectively and objectively; measurement of access in terms of the client's satisfaction level is a subjective measure and that concerned with various utilization rates falls under objective measure [14]. In the health system there is a supplier or provider side, demand or receiver side and a process which link the supply and demand. The factor which contains in the process to link the supply and demand side, access can be identified. In this process; the ability to perceive health literacy, health beliefs, trust and expectation, ability to seek, ability to reach, ability to pay and ability to engage are included.

Results

Descriptive statistics for availability of service

To reduce maternal mortality, the United Nations (UN) recommends that 100% of women with obstetric complications be treated in Comprehensive Emergency Obstetric Care (EmOC) facilities. However, EmOC was available in 66.67% of hospitals and 22.22% of health centers (HCs). Comprehensive emergency obstetric care can be provided only through hospital level. In the study area, 66.67% hospitals were providing Basic Emergency Obstetric Care (BEmOC). Remaining all services; Ante Natal Care (ANC), delivery service, postnatal care, family planning (FP) and post abortion service were continually provided from the hospitals. All 9 health centers were providing ANC and FP services, 7 centres were providing delivery and postnatal care services, 3 centers were providing post abortion care and 2 centers were providing BEmOC services. CHPs zones are the basic structure of the health service in Ghana. Among the 8 CHPs zones, 4, 2 and all 8 zones were providing ANC, postnatal care and FP services, respectively (Table 3 and 4).

The availability of FP services is an important factor in reducing maternal mortality. Only 66.6% of surveyed hospitals provided FP, and none offered vasectomy service. All (100%) of the health centers provided contraception in the form of condoms, pills and injections. Only 44% of HCs provided long term FP methods. Of the CHPs, 87.5% provided condoms and 100% provided pills and injectable contraceptives. Only 12.5% provided Norplant, a long term FP method.

As expected, the hospitals were better equipped than the HCs and CHPs zones. All twenty facilities had Sphygmomanometers and stethoscopes in the ANC departments. However, on average, only one of each was in good condition and almost two needed replacements. Only two out of the eight CHPs zones had an emergency vaginal examination tray at the antenatal clinic. Equipment for infant resuscitation was lacking, particularly at the HCs and CHPs levels. No CHPs zones had oxygen or suction machines. Even though two CHPs zones had infant weighing scales, all needed to be replaced. Items such as clocks, examination tables, cupboards for storing medications and beds were largely available, but most of them needed replacement. Availability refers to the physical existence of health resources with sufficient capacity to provide service [15]. The survey results suggested that the equipment that is necessary to reduce MMR is insufficient in the Volta region. Overall, inadequate services, insufficient staffs, inadequate equipment and medicines in the surveyed facilities were found.

Descriptive statistics for Accessibility

Accessibility was measured in terms of travel time or distance between the location of the user and the service (distance from the household to the nearest health facilities). Distance was classified into 4 categories: very far, far, close and very close. Among respondents, 7.1 % ranked their nearest facility is very far away, 33.3% said they are far, 51.6% said they are close and 8% said that they are very close to the nearest facility (Table 5). Accessibility refers to the fact of people facing the problem health need due to geography [16]. Identified problem is the nearest facilities are far from the client location.

Maternal health services availability	Hospital n (%)	Health Center n (%)	CHPs n (%)	Total n (%)
	N=3	N=9	N=8	N=20
ANC	3 (100.0)	9 (100.0)	4 (50.0)	16 (80.0)
Delivery	3 (100.0)	7 (77.77)	0	10 (50.0)
Basic emergency obstetric care	2 (66.67)	2 (22.22)	0	4 (20.0)
Comprehensive emergency obstetric care	2 (66.67)	0	0	2 (10.0)
Post natal care	3 (100.0)	7 (77.77)	2 (25.0)	12 (60.0)
Family planning	3 (100.0)	9 (100.0)	8 (100.0)	20 (100.0)
Post abortion care	3 (100.0)	3 (33.34)	0	6 (30.0)

Table 3: Availability of maternal health service by facility.

Area	Essential MCH services	Very well	Well	Moderate	Little	None	Total
Pre-pregnancy	Family planning	17	6	5	3	-	31
	Antenatal care	15	12	2	2	-	31
Pregnancy	Prevention of mother to child transmission of HIV	10	11	8	2	-	31
	Intermittent preventive treatment of malaria for pregnant women	18	11	-	1	1	31
	Neonatal care	21	5	5	-	-	31
Birth	Skilled attendant at birth	15	2	5	8	1	31
Postnatal	Postpartum care	15	6	3	3	4	31
	Early initiation of breastfeeding	25	5	1	-	-	31

Table 4: Provider's self-assessment of knowledge of maternal health services.

Indicator	Keta Municipal n (%)	Ketu North n (%)	Ketu South n (%)	Total n (%)
	Distance from household to the nearest health facility			
Very far	20 (9.5)	6 (2.8)	19 (9.0)	45 (7.1)
Far	92 (43.8)	55 (26.2)	63 (30.0)	210 (33.3)
Close	93 (44.3)	127 (60.5)	105 (50.0)	325 (51.6)
Very close	5 (2.4)	22 (10.5)	23 (11.0)	50 (8.0)
Total	210 (100.0)	210 (100.0)	210 (100.0)	630 (100)

Table 5: Self-reported distance from household to the nearest health facility.

Descriptive statistics for affordability

Affordability was measured by both the direct costs (doctor's fee) and indirect costs (travel and medications) of care. Our study indicated that 90.3% of surveyed people had utilized treatment services of health facilities. Social demographics indicated that 43.2% held income-generating jobs, leaving the remaining 56.8% with a job status of unemployed including housewife, farmer and student. Emergencies and unexpected complications may be especially difficult for low socioeconomic status individuals. In addition, 40.4 % live far from the nearest health facility. Affordability reflects the economic capacity of the people to spend for the health service utilization. A low socioeconomic status of the people was found in the region.

Descriptive statistics for accommodation

Accommodation/adequacy was measured by the quality of service provided and personal treatment by the provider. Respondents reported that 39% of deliveries occurred at home and of them, 39.2% were conducted by an untrained person. Adequate knowledge is essential for providers to be able to provide quality service. Accommodation is related with quality care, the clients' ability to accommodate to these factors and their perception of their appropriateness. There is a lack of service provider and lack of sufficient room in the health institution. So, difficulty in providing timely treatment and maintaining privacy were identified problems.

Descriptive statistics for acceptability

For the acceptability check, number of individuals who received antenatal, delivery and postnatal services were evaluated. A 94.8%, 60.1% and 76.1% of respondents, respectively, replied that they received antenatal, delivery and the postnatal service. Factors like preference towards the gender of medical personnel, physical appearance of the facility, hours of operation, and trust in medical ability were not observed in the study area. Of total, 91.4% respondents were satisfied with the available service in the study area. Acceptability related to cultural and social factors determining the possibility for people to accept the service and to seek service were not found in the Volta region, indicating no any problem on the acceptability.

Action Plan

KOICA and Yonsei Global Health Center developed an action plan through baseline survey, utilizing 5As framework. Seven problems related to availability, accessibility and accommodation was identified and the enhancement activities are being implemented in the study area as shown in Figure 1.

To overcome the current maternal health care problems of the Volta region, various health interventions were recommended. For the accessibility, inadequate service, inadequate service providers' knowledge, insufficient staffs, inadequate equipment and medicine in the facility were identified. Training programs are conducted to enhance knowledge. In order to solve the problem of the scarcity of the service provider, midwifery school is constructed in that region and essential medicine and equipment is provided. Previous study shows that strengthening midwife training and improving availability, training to health care providers can improve the maternal health [17,18]. For the accessibility, the nearest facilities are found far from the client location.

Previous study provided strong evidence of improved physical access to health care services for women who live within one hour of the health facility [19]. Therefore, it was felt necessary to improve awareness of maternal and child health service among local residents, enhance the capabilities of CHPs, community level workers play a important role to enhance maternal health [20,21], enhance the skills of maternal and child health service providers, upgrade the quality of public maternal and child health service. Also, the improvement of public transport facilities/access, establishment of a midwifery training school and opening of a post basic midwifery training course were recommended in the region. For the accommodation, training course for midwife and capacity enhancement was conducted. Due to poor quality service such as lack of service provider and lack of sufficient rooms in the health institution, providing timely treatment and maintaining privacy was difficult. One study suggests that staff attitude, provision of respectful and supportive care have a considerable impact on the choice of health facilities [22].

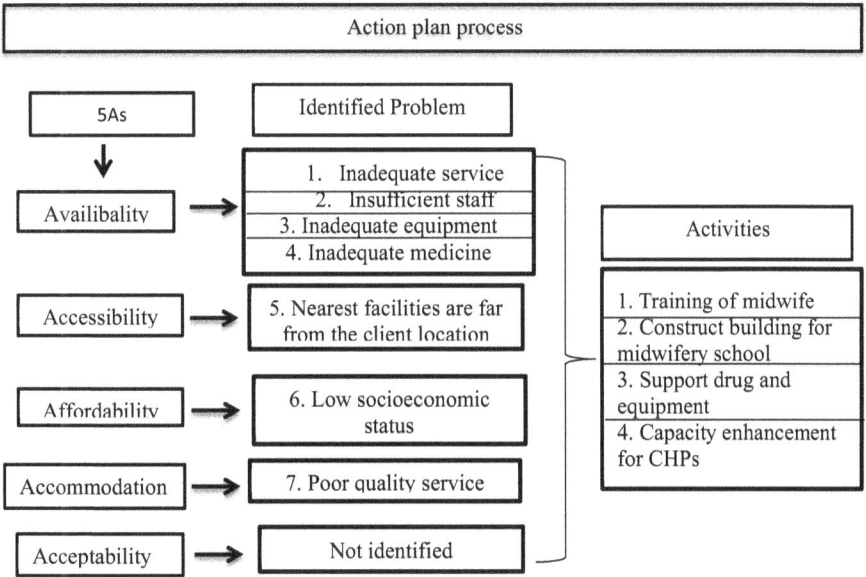

Figure 1: Action plan for improving maternal and child health care in the Volta region.

Discussion

An estimated 28,900 women died due to complications in pregnancy and childbirth globally in 2013. Nearly all of these deaths could be prevented. Among them only 2,300 occurred in a developed region and the remaining 28,600 occurred in the developing region [23]. At least 12 million women suffered severe maternal complications in 2012 [24]. The rate of death is higher in poor countries [25]. Developing countries have been challenged by the overall capacity of weak health systems. The health care system of the developing countries is suffering from a lack of leadership and management skills, improper staffing, inadequate or improper supplies of essential medications and tools, inadequate financing and budget allocations, inadequate water and sanitation, poor health care-related infrastructures, poor or unmanaged information systems, and poor data management systems or a lack of data for policy formulation and implementation. Considerable progress towards MDG 5 has been made as various health survey results indicate a decline in regional average MMR from 740 per 100,000 live births in 1990 to 380 per 100,000 live births in 2014. However, improvements are not on track to achieve MDG 5 in 2015 [24].

Providing proper access to health care could be a major achievement for a community. Even developed countries find it difficult to achieve the goal of providing universal and equitable quality care [26]. Obviously, the challenge for developing countries is a lack of access to health care [27]. Improving access to health service providers would concentrate on a key factor influencing access to health care, which is commonly defined as utilization [4,7,28,29].

The distance to the nearest medical facilities influence postpartum checkup. More PNC is utilized if the respondent lives nearby medical facility than far distance. Because of the distance, respondents usually underutilized PNC service. It is necessary to expand the medical facility in the community level to increase the postpartum checkup [30].

KOICA and the Yonsei Global Health Center conducted a baseline survey, identified problems and developed an action plan in collaboration with the Government of Ghana. A 5As framework was used to identify barriers to health care utilization. Inadequate service, inadequate service providers, insufficient equipment and medicine, poor geographic access to health facilities, and insufficient knowledge in service provider were the most commonly identified barriers. Maternal health condition in the study area can be improved by addressing above identified weakness of maternal health service. It is recommended that an Overseas Development Aid Project of KOICA in cooperation with the Ghana Ministry of Health will follow the findings to strengthen maternal health in the study area.

Conclusion

A collaboration program between KOICA and Ghana Government was developed to improve maternal and child health care services and reduce maternal mortality rate in the Volta Region. An action plan was developed from the baseline survey and they were gradually implemented for improvement of maternity care services in the region. This study was primarily concerned with the evaluation of access to maternal health care in the Volta region, Ghana (Keta municipality, Ketu North and South District) and considered various physical, financial, institutional and social factors contributing to maternal healthcare in the Volta Region through a baseline study. We used a 5As framework of availability, accessibility, affordability, accommodation/adequacy and acceptability. We found insufficient midwife, inadequate equipment and medicine, health facilities that were far away from their client, poor and low socioeconomic status and lack of knowledge in

health service providers and midwife. To overcome these problems KOICA and Yonsei Global Health Center suggests implementation of the action plan, including training for midwife and service providers, construction of a Midwifery school, supplying essential medicine and equipment, capacity enhancement, and strengthening the basic unit of the health service (i.e., CHPs) in the Volta Region of Ghana.

Acknowledgement

We would like to gratefully acknowledge to the Korea International Cooperation Agency (KOICA) and National Research Foundation of Korea Grant by Korean Government (NRF-2013S1A01055336) for the support of this study.

References

1. UNICEF (2014) Trends in Maternal Mortality: 1990-2013.

2. The Millennium Development Goals Report, 2014, United Nations, New York.

3. World Health Organization, Ghana Health Profile.

4. Korea International Cooperation Agency, Yonsei University, Project for improving maternal, newborn and child health care in Volta region of Ghana Basic Design Study. Yonsei Healthy City Research Center, July 2013.

5. Penchansky R, Thomas JW (1981) The concept of access: Definition and relationship to consumer satisfaction. Med Care 19: 127-140.

6. Andersen RM (1995) Revisiting the behavioral model and access to medical care: Does it matter? J Health Aoc Behav 36: 1-10.

7. Levesque JF, Harris MF, Russell G (2013) Patient-centred access to health care: Conceptualizing access at the interface of health systems and populations. Int J Equity Health 12: 18.

8. Kerssens JJ, Groenewegen PP, Sixma HJ, Boerma WG, van der Eijk I (2004) Comparison of patient evaluations of health care quality in relation to WHO measures of achievement in 12 European countries. Bull World Health Organ 82: 106-114.

9. Lee T, Marans RW (1980) Objective and subjective indicator: Effects of scale discordance of interrelationship. Social indicator research 8: 4 7-6 4.

10. Waters HR (2000) Measuring equity in access to health care. Soc Sci Med 51: 599-612.

11. Goddard M, Smith P (2001) Equity of access to health care services: Theory and evidence from the UK. Soc Sci Med 53: 1149-1162.

12. Oliver A, Mossialos E (2004) Equity of access to health care: Outlining the foundations for action. J Epidemiol Community Health 58: 655-658.

13. Peters DH, Garg A, Bloom G, Walker DG, Brieger WR, et al. (2008) Poverty and access to health care in developing countries. Ann N Y Acad Sci 1136: 161-171.

14. Daniels N (1982) Equity of access to health care: some conceptual and ethical issues. Milbank Mem Fund Q Health Soc 60: 51-81.

15. Gage AJ, Guirlène Calixte M (2006) Effects of the physical accessibility of maternal health services on their use in rural Haiti. Population studies 60: 271-288.

16. Grzybowski S, Stoll K, Kornelsen J (2011) Distance matters: a population based study examining access to maternity services for rural women. BMC Health Serv Res 11: 147.

17. Van Lerberghe W, Matthews Z, Achadi E, Ancona C, Campbell J, et al. (2014) Country experience with strengthening of health systems and deployment of midwives in countries with high maternal mortality. Lancet 384: 1215-1225.

18. Woods J, Gagliardi L, Nara S, Phally S, Varang O, et al. (2015) An innovative approach to in-service training of maternal health staff in Cambodian hospitals. Int J Gynaecol Obstet 129: 178-183.

19. Hotchkiss DR (2001) Expansion of rural health care and the use of maternal services in Nepal. Health Place 7: 39-45.

20. Abosede, Sholeye (2014) Strengthening the Foundation for Sustainable Primary Health Care Services in Nigeria. Primary Health Care 4:167. doi: 10.4172/2167-1079.1000167

21. Mane Abhay B, Khandekar Sanjay V (2014) Strengthening Primary Health Care through Asha Workers: A Novel Approach in India. Primary Health Care 4:149. doi: 10.4172/2167-1079.1000149

22. Ith P, Dawson A, Homer CS (2013) Women's perspective of maternity care in Cambodia. Women Birth 26: 71-75.

23. Moyer CA, McLaren ZM, Adanu RM, Lantz PM (2013) Understanding the relationship between access to care and facility-based delivery through analysis of the 2008 Ghana Demographic Health Survey. Int J Gynaecol Obstet 122: 224-229.

24. WHO, UNICEF, UNFPA, The World Bank, United Nations, 1990–2013, Population Division. Trends in Maternal Mortality. May 2014. Geneva: WHO

25. USAID (2014) Ending preventable maternal mortality: USAID maternal health vision for action.

26. Stanton ME, Brandes N (2012) A new perspective on maternal ill-health and its consequences. J Health Popul Nutr 30: 121-123.

27. Oliver A, Mossialos E (2004) Equity of access to health care: Outlining the foundations for action. J Epidemiol Community Health 58: 655-658.

28. Gwatkin DR (2001) The need for equity-oriented health sector reforms. Int J Epidemiol 30: 720-723.

29. Fiedler JL (1981) A review of the literature on access and utilization of medical care with special emphasis on rural primary care. Soc Sci Med C 15: 129-142.

30. Nam EW, Song YLA, Cho KG (2013) Factors Associated with Postpartum Maternal Health Check in Volta Region of Ghana. Korea Association of International Development and Cooperation 5: 37-57 (In Korean)

19

Incidence of Patients Diagnosed with Acute Cystitis in Nuuk, Greenland Management in the Primary Health Care Setting

Marie-Louise Mariager Pedersen[1]* and Michael Lynge Pedersen[1,2]

1Queen Ingrid Primary Health Care Center, Nuuk, Greenland, Denmark
[2]Greenland Center for Health Research, Institute of Nursing and Health Science, University of Greenland, Denmark

Abstract

Objective: To estimate the incidence of adult patients diagnosed with acute cystitis and evaluate the assessment and treatment of acute cystitis in Nuuk, Greenland.

Study design: Retrospective follow-up study including all adult patients diagnosed with acute cystitis at Queen Ingrid Primary Health Care Center within a fourteen-day long observation period.

Methods: Patients diagnosed with acute cystitis were identified using the electronical medical record (EMR). From EMR information about age, gender, diagnose, examinations, treatment and medical history was obtained.

Results: A total of 66 patients (7 males and 59 females) diagnosed with acute cystitis were identified. Out of the 66 patients, 34 patients were classified with uncomplicated acute cystitis, while the other 32 patients were classified with complicated acute cystitis. The overall incidence rate among female patients was 189/1,000 person-years (95 % CI 181-198) and 20/1,000 person-years (95% CI 17-23) among male patients. A urine dipstick was performed in 53.0 % of the cases while a urine culture was performed in 39.4 % of the cases. Escherichia coli was the most common uropathogen found in the urine cultures (42.3% of the cases). In 34.6 % of the cases, no bacteria were found in the urine cultures. The majority of patients (98.5%) were treated with antibiotics, almost exclusively Sulfamethizole or Pivmecillinam (92.3 % of patients treated with antibiotics).

Conclusion: Acute cystitis is a common diagnosis among adult women in Nuuk, Greenland, with *E. coli* as the most common uropathogen. The majority of patients are treated with the recommended antibiotics.

Keywords: Cystitis, Inuit; Greenland; Primary health care

Introduction

Lower urinary tract infections (acute cystitis) are a common infection in women and account for a substantial financial burden on society [1-3]. In Denmark, patients with symptoms of urinary tract infections account for 2-5% of all contacts in general practice [1]. Antibiotic resistance among common uropathogens is increasing in many countries and this causes concern [4-7]. In Denmark, the official recommendations regarding assessment and treatment of urinary tract infections are provided by the Institute of Rational Pharmacotherapy, a partly independent institute under the Danish Health and Medicines Authority [8]. According to their latest recommendations from 2007, general practitioners should distinguish between an uncomplicated acute cystitis and a complicated acute cystitis when making decisions on assessment and treatment. Empirical treatment with either Sulfamethizole or Pivmecillinam is recommended for treatment of uncomplicated acute cystitis, while decisions regarding choice of antibiotics for complicated acute cystitis should be based on urine culture. These recommendations are in line with the European Association of Urology 2010 guidelines on urological infections [9]. Greenland is part of the Danish Realm and the health care system in Greenland is widely inspired by the Danish health care system, although major logistic differences exist. Similiarly, Danish treatment guidelines are widely used in Greenland. Thus, treatment with Sulfamethizol or Pivmecillinam is recommended as first choice at Queen Ingrid Health Care Center in Nuuk. However, both incidence and management of patients diagnosed with acute cystitis in the population of Greenland remain unknown. The aim of this study was to determine the incidence of patients diagnosed with acute cystitis and to evaluate the assessment and treatment of acute cystitis in Nuuk, Greenland.

Material and Methods

This study was carried out as a Retrospective follow-up study including all patients diagnosed with acute cystitis at Queen Ingrid Primary Health Care Center from 27th January to 9th February 2014, both days included.

Setting

The whole population of Greenland by January 1st 2014 was 56,282 people [10]. They live in the 18 towns and 60 settlements spread along the coastline of Greenland. The health care system in Greenland provides free health care service to all people with a permanent address in Greenland. In Nuuk, Queen Ingrid Primary Health Care Center exclusively provides primary care service for all people living in the Nuuk district, including the two minor settlements Kapisillit and Qerqerarsuatsiaat. All contact with patients is registered in the electronic medical record system (EMR). In addition, all prescriptions are handled electronically in EMR. The population of Nuuk district was by January 1st 2014 17,085 people [11] which constitutes around one third of the overall population of Greenland.

Study population

All adult patients (minimum18 years of age) with a permanent address in the Nuuk district treated for acute cystitis at Queen Ingrid Primary Health Care Center within the study period were included. First, all patients treated with a relevant antibiotics were identified in EMR (Sulfamethizole (J01EB02), Pivmecillinam (J01CA08), Nitrofurantoine (J01XE01), Pondocilline (J01CA02), Ciprofloxacin

*Corresponding author: Marie-Louise Mariager Pedersen, Queen Ingrid Primary Health Care Center, Nuuk, Greenland, Denmark, E-mail:maloumape@yahoo.dk

(J01MA02) and Trimethoprim (J01EA01)). Second, the medical records of these patients were reviewed to identify the patients treated for acute cystitis. Furthermore, all patient contact headlines in the timetable of EMR were reviewed to identify any additional patients diagnosed with acute cystitis who had not been treated with antibiotics. Patients diagnosed with acute cystitis who were not associated with Queen Ingrid Primary Health Care Center were not included in the study. In the fourteen-day period after the initial diagnosis of acute cystitis, patients were observed in order to monitor any further contact they might have had with Queen Ingrid Primary Health Care Center. From EMR information about age, gender, diagnose, examinations, treatment and medical history was obtained. Urine dipsticks were performed at Queen Ingrid Primary Health Care Center while urine cultures were performed at the Central laboratory of Queen Ingrid Hospital.

Variables

In this study, an uncomplicated acute cystitis was defined as an acute cystitis in otherwise healthy, non-pregnant women up to 65 years old who have not received antibiotics for an acute cystitis within the last three months and who have not received any kind of antibiotics within the last 2 weeks. All other cases of acute cystitis including acute cystitis in men and women older than 65 years were defined as complicated acute cystitis [8-9,12].

Statistics

Age and gender specific incidence rates were calculated using the Nuuk population per January 1st 2014 as background population. Estimates are calculated with 95% confidence intervals. Chi-square test was used to compare frequencies. P-value at 0.05 was used as level of significance. The ethics committee for medical research in Greenland approved the study.

Results

One hundred and three patients who had received a prescription for at least one of the included antibiotics from Queen Ingrid Primary Health Care Center in the period from 27th January to 9th February 2014 were identified. Of these, 71 patients were diagnosed with acute cystitis. Thirty-two patients were excluded due to other diagnoses. By reviewing the electronic timetable in EMR, four additional patients diagnosed with acute cystitis were identified. Of those, two had a permanent address in Nuuk and were included in the study population. Seven patients were excluded due to age below 18 years. Thus, in total 66 patients diagnosed with acute cystitis were included in the study. Of these, 34 patients were classified with uncomplicated acute cystitis, whereas 32 patients were classified with complicated acute cystitis. The reasons for the classification of complicated acute cystitis were male gender (n=7), chronic diseases (n=6), use of immuno suppressive drugs (n=1), urological disease (n=14), use of prophylactic antibiotics for chronic cystitis (n=4), antibiotic treatment for acute cystitis within 3 months (n=22), any antibiotic treatment within 2 weeks (n=3) or a combination of the above-mentioned reasons.

Incidence rates and annual incidence proportions

Incidence rates for uncomplicated and complicated acute cystitis are shown in Table 1. The overall incidence rate of patients diagnosed with acute cystitis at Queen Ingrid Primary Health Care Center in the period from 27th January to 9th February 2014 was 101/1,000 person-years (95% CI 96-105). Age and gender specific incidence rates and gender specific annual incidence proportions are shown in Table 2. The highest incidence rate observed was 542/1,000 person-years in the 60-

	Uncomplicated		Complicated		Total	
	n	%	n	%	n	%
Study Population	34	51.5	32	48.5	66	100.0
Gender						
-Female	34	100.0	25	78.1	59	89.4
-Male	-	-	7	21.9	7	10.6
Assesment						
Diagnosis based solely on patienthistory	21	31.8	5	7.6	26	39.4
Urine dipstick	13	38.2	22	68.8	35	53.0
-leucocyte positive	11	84.6	11	50.0	22	62.9
-Nitrite positive	0	0.0	3	13.6	3	8.6
-Leucocyte and nitrite positive	1	7.7	3	13.6	4	11.4
-Negative	1	7.7	5	22.7	6	17.1
Urine culture	4	11.8	22	68.8	26	39.4
Escherichia coli	1	25.0	10	45.5	11	42.3
Enterococcus	0	0.0	3	13.6	3	11.5
klebsiella	0	0.0	2	9.1	2	7.7
Aerococcus	0	0.0	1	4.5	1	3.8
-Mixed florae	0	0.0	0	0.0	0	0.0
-Negative	3	75.0	6	27.3	9	34.6
Antibiotic treatment	34	100.0	31	96.9	65	98.5
Pivmecillinam	10	29.4	13	41.9	23	35.4
Sulfametizole	24	70.6	13	41.9	37	56.9
Ciprofloxacine	0	0.0	1	3.2	1	1.5
Nitrofurantoine	0	0.0	0	0.0	0	0.0
Nitrolurantoin	0	0.0	2	6.5	2	3.1
Trimethoprim	0	0.0	2	6.5	2	3.1
Patients with no further contact*	30/34	88.2	27/32	84.4	57/66	86.4
		95 %CI		95 %CI		95 % CI
Incidence rate (n/1,000 person-years)	52	(49-55)	49	(46-52)	101	(96-105)

*Patients with no further contact with Queen Ingrid primary health care center within the 14 day observation period.

Table 1: Characteristics of Greenlandic acute cystitis from Queen Ingrid primary health care center from (27th of January to 9th of February 2014).

Age	Women Incidence/1,000 person fears (95 %0I)	n/N	Men Incidence/1,000 person-years (95 %, CI)	n/N
20-29	212 (191-233)	12/1477	19 (12-26)	1/1392
30-39	214 (191-237)	10/1218	0(0-0)	0/1351
40-49	293 (269-318)	15/1333	0 (0-0)	0/1544
50-59	146(127466)	7/1246	17 (11-24)	1/1508
60-69	542(497-587)	10/481	117 (92-141)	3/671
70+	343(281-405)	3/228	223 (170-276)	2/234
Overall	189(181-198)	59/8124	20 (17-23)	7/8958
Annual incidence proportion (%)	17.25		2.02	

Table 2: age and gender specific incidence rates, gender specific annual incidence proportions and relative risk of acute cystitis among patients from Queen Ingrid primary health care center from (27th of January to 9th of February 2014).

69 years age group of female patients (95 % CI 497-587). The overall incidence rate among female patients was 189/1,000 person-years (95% CI 181-198) and 20/1,000 person-years (95% CI 17-23) among male patients. These incidence rates correspond to an annual incidence proportion of 17.25% and 2.02% respectively.

Population characteristics and management

Characteristics and examination results are summarized in Table 1. The diagnosis was based solely on the history of symptoms in 39.4 % cases while a urine dipstick was performed in 53.0% of cases and a urine culture was performed in 39.4 % of cases. Escherichia coli were the most common uropathogen found in the urine cultures and was found in 42.3 % of the cases (Table 1). In 34.6 % of the cases, no bacteria were found in the urine cultures. Almost all patients (98.5 %) were treated with antibiotics. The majority (56.9%) of patients were treated with Sulfamethizole. Pivmecillinam was the second most common drug used in 35.4% of the cases. Overall, 92.3% (60/65) of patients diagnosed with acute cystitis and treated with antibiotics were treated with either Sulfamethizole or Pivmecillinam in accordance with the recommendation of first choice. No additional contact to Queen Ingrid Health Care Center within the fourteen-day observation period after initial treatment was observed for 86.4 % of the patients.

Discussion

In this study, we found an overall incidence rate of 189/1,000 person-years among women and 20/1,000 person-years among men in Nuuk, Greenland. Furthermore, the majority of patients were treated with antibiotics in line with official recommendations. Among women, we found an equitable distribution of uncomplicated and complicated acute cystitis. The majority of acute cystitis cases was classified as complicated due to prior treatment of acute cystitis within 3 months. Among patients diagnosed with complicated acute cystitis, the majority was examined with a urine dipstick and/or a urine culture before initiation of treatment.

Other studies

The data from our study are in line with data from other studies. First of all, the incidence rate of patients diagnosed with acute cystitis was found to be high among women and low among men. In 2014, Foxman B. reports of similar results regarding the incidence of acute cystitis among US/canadian men and women.[3]. Secondly, because of the anatomical differences between men and women, acute cystitis is known to primarily affect women Many studies, consistent with our study, confirm this [2,3,13-15]. Thirdly, E. coli was found to be the most common uropathogen that is also consistent with other studies [6].

In the vast majority of cases, the treatment guidelines were followed. In addition, no further contact within the fourteen-day observation period was observed in 86.4 % of the cases. This may indicate a generally effective assessment and treatment procedure. However, in nearly 35 % of urine cultures no bacteria were found. A certain proportion of negative urine cultures is expected. Even though, this does suggest some over diagnosis. Furthermore, a relatively large proportion of female patients were diagnosed and classified with complicated acute cystitis due to prior antibiotic treatment of acute cystitis within the last 3 months. This also points towards some over diagnosis. In Nuuk, Greenland, the incidence rates of sexually transmitted diseases (Chlamydia and Gonnorhea) are known to be very high [16]. Therefore, the possibility that some of these patients did not in fact have an acute cystitis but instead had a sexually transmitted disease must be considered. So far, patients presenting symptoms of acute cystitis at Queen Ingrid Primary Health Care Center are not routinely checked for sexually transmitted diseases. In light of the known high incidence rates of sexually transmitted diseases, and in order to limit the use of antibiotics, routine checks for sexually transmitted diseases should be considered for future patients presenting symptoms of complicated acute cystitis before

initiating antibiotics. Especially those patients recently treated with antibiotics. In addition, focus on awareness of preventive initiatives among patients with acute cystitis could be considered in order to reduce incidence and need for antibiotic treatment.

Strengths and limitations

This study is the first to estimate the incidence of patients diagnosed with acute cystitis in Nuuk, Greenland. The major strength of this study is that all patients in Nuuk district are included, that is 17,085 people, constituting approximately 30.4% of the overall population of Greenland. In Nuuk district, Queen Ingrid Primary Health Care Center exclusively provides primary health care service. Therefore, this study is expected to include all patients diagnosed with acute cystitis where there has been a need of medical advice or treatment. However, there are several limitations. The study period was relatively short and there are reservations with regard to the relatively small figures. Season variability with a peak during summer, cannot be excluded and this consequently leads to underestimation of the true annual incidence. On the other hand, since diagnosis was made on the history of symptoms in 39.4% of the cases without urine tests, some kind of overdiagnosis must have occurred leading to an overestimation of the true incidence of acute cystitis. Furthermore, it must be expected that some patients with an acute cystitis during the registration period did not seek medical aid. Thus, the percentage of a self-limiting number of acute cystitis remains unknown. This would underestimate the true incidence. However, primary health care is free to everyone and quite accessible [17]. Therefore, the vast majority of patients with acute cystitis are expected to have been in contact with Queen Ingrid's Health Care Center. Detailed information about urinary irritative symptoms, absence of vaginal/urethral discharge or vaginal irritation would have strengthened the diagnostic classification. A urinary dipstick or microscopy to indicate inflammation in all cases of suspected acute cystitis would also have strengthened the diagnostic classification. However, this information was only accessible in some cases. Thus, this study describes the group of patients actually given the diagnosis of acute cystitis rather than an ideal population of known cases of acute cystitis. Finally, the short observation period after initial treatment limits the possibility to evaluate whether or not the initial treatment was a success.

Conclusion

In conclusion, acute cystitis is a common diagnosis in Nuuk, Greenland and it primarily affects women with E. coli as the most common uropathogen as seen in other populations. The majority of patients are treated with the recommended antibiotics. Performing a urine sample for sexually transmitted diseases in addition to a conventional urine culture in complicated cases should be considered. Preventive procedures among patients with acute cystitis should be explored.

References

1. Bjerrum LG, Højbjerg P, Diagnostik T (2012) af urinvejsinfektion i almen praksis. Maanedsskrift for Praktisk Laegegerning. 90:134-45.

2. Foxman B (2003) Epidemiology of urinary tract infections: incidence, morbidity, and economic costs. Disease-a-month.DM. 49:53-70.

3. Foxman B (2014) Urinary tract infection syndromes: occurrence, recurrence, bacteriology, risk factors, and disease burden. Infectious disease clinics of North America. 28:1-13.

4. Kahlmeter G (2003) Prevalence and antimicrobial susceptibility of pathogens in uncomplicated cystitis in Europe. The ECO.SENS study. Int J Antimicrob Agents. 2:49-52.

5. Kahlmeter G (2003) An international survey of the antimicrobial susceptibility of

pathogens from uncomplicated urinary tract infections: the ECO.SENS Project. J Antimicrob Chemother 51:69-76.

6. Kahlmeter G, Poulsen HO (2012) Antimicrobial susceptibility of Escherichia coli from community-acquired urinary tract infections in Europe: the ECO.SENS study revisited. Int J Antimicrob Agents. 39:45-51.

7. Kamenski G, Wagner G, Zehetmayer S, Fink W, Spiegel W, et al.(2012) Antibacterial resistances in uncomplicated urinary tract infections in women: ECO.SENS II data from primary health care in Austria. BMC Infect Dis 12:222.

8. Stenvang Pedersen SG-H (2007) Antibiotikavejledningtil almen praksis. Rationel Farmakoterapi 4.

9. Grabe MB-J, Botto TE, Cek H, Naber M, Tenke K, et al. (2010) Guidelines on Urological Infections. Eur Urol 11-67.

10. http://undesadspd.org/indigenouspeoples/seconddecade.aspx

11. http://bank.stat.gl/Dialog/varval.asp?ma=BEEST3&path=../Database/ Greenland/Population/Population%20in%20Greenland/&lang=1:%20 Statistics%20Greenland;%202014.

12. Bjerrum L, Gahrn-Hansen B, Grinsted P (2009) Pivmecillinam versus sulfamethizole for short-term treatment of uncomplicated acute cystitis in general practice: a randomized controlled trial. Scand J Prim Health Care 27:6-11.

13. ACOG Practice Bulletin No. 91(2008) Treatment of urinary tract infections in nonpregnant women. Obstet Gynecol Int 111:785-94.

14. Foster RT, Sr (2008) Uncomplicated urinary tract infections in women. Obstet Gynecol Clin North Am 35:235-48.

15. Foxman B, Barlow R, D'Arcy H, Gillespie B, Sobel JD (2000) Urinary tract infection: self-reported incidence and associated costs. Ann Epidemiol 10:509-15.

16. Law DGR, Mulvad E,.Koch G (2008) Sexual Health and Sexually Transmitted Infections in the North American Arctic. Emerg Infect Dis 1:4-9.

17. Pedersen ML, Rolskov A, Jacobsen JL, Lynge AR (2012) Frequent use of primary health care service in Greenland: an opportunity for undiagnosed disease case-finding. Int J Circumpolar Health 71:18431.

20

Incomplete Immunization Coverage in Delhi: Reasons and Solutions

Shantanu Sharma[1]*, Charu Kohli[1], Nandini Sharma[1] and Devika Mehra[2]

[1]*Department of Community Medicine, Maulana Azad Medical College, India*
[2]*Department of Public Health, Sweden*

Abstract

Background: Immunization is considered as a cost-effective public health intervention to reduce the morbidity and mortality associated with infectious diseases. This study was planned with an objective to find the reasons for defaulters of immunization in an urban resettlement area in Delhi.

Methods: The study was conducted over a period of 6 months in four blocks of an urban resettlement colony in Delhi. Children who were not completely immunized as per records were tracked by the research team and caretakers were interviewed to find reasons for incomplete immunization, using a semi structured, pre tested questionnaire.

Results: Out of 87 incompletely immunized children, only 44 could be traced. The reasons reported were non availability of vaccine at the centre, long waiting time and poor awareness of parents about importance of immunization despite the fact that most of the parents were literate and employed. However 22.7% were wrongly classified as their immunization was not recorded by the health worker in the centre.

Conclusion: Sustained efforts are required to raise the awareness of community about importance of immunization. Workers need to be trained about need for maintaining appropriate records and use the MCTS system.

Keywords: Defaulters; Immunization; Delhi

Introduction

Preventing under-5 mortality is one of the key focus areas of policy makers nationally and internationally. The Sustainable Development Goals' target 3.2 in alignment with WHO global strategy for mother and child 2016-2030 aims to achieve reduction of under-5 mortality to less than 25 per 1000 live births in every country [1,2]. The Government of India 12th five year plan and also the reproductive, maternal, newborn, child and adolescent health (RMNCH+A) strategy 2013 focuses on bringing down under 5 mortality rate [3]. About 25%, of under-5 mortality is due to vaccine-preventable diseases globally [4]. Vaccine preventable diseases put a huge financial and social burden on individuals, families and society. Children who contract these preventable diseases usually suffer from impaired physical growth, cognitive development, emotional development, and social skills [5]. In India, vaccine-preventable mortality was estimated to be that of the 826,000 deaths in under-5 children, almost 604,000 deaths were due to vaccine-preventable diseases including diarrhea, pertussis, measles, meningitis, and pneumonia [6]. Immunization is considered as a cost-effective public health intervention to reduce the morbidity and mortality associated with infectious diseases. As per estimates, over two million deaths are delayed through immunization each year worldwide [7]. Within SEARO region, India has the lowest immunization coverage of 70% whereas in every other country like Bangldesh (85%); Indonesia (83%); Nepal (79%), Mynannmar (82%), etc. the coverage is more than India [8].

India's immunization programme, launched in 1985, is one of the largest health programmes of its kind in the world catering to a birth cohort of 27 million children annually. The programme targets immunization against seven vaccine preventable diseases (diphtheria, whooping cough, tetanus, polio, tuberculosis, measles and hepatitis B) in the country. The programme has been operational for over 30 years and yet only 65% children in India received all vaccines during infancy. It has been calculated that over 89 lakh children in the country do not receive all vaccines that are available under the immunization programme which is highest compared to other countries in the world [9].

To improve the rate of full immunization coverage, it is important

to investigate the reasons for incomplete immunization. This will help to frame future policies to improve immunization services and involve all stakeholders in the planning process. Keeping the above points in view, this study was planned with an objective to find the reasons for defaulters of immunization in an urban resettlement area in Delhi.

Methodology

The study was conducted over a period of 6 months in four blocks of an urban resettlement colony in Delhi which were catered by one Urban Health Centre (UHC). The UHC in the area offers multiple services including general OPD, ante natal and post natal care, immunization, breastfeeding counseling and growth monitoring. It caters primarily to 4 blocks of the Gokulpuri (urban resettlement colony) with adjoining slums. The centre is also teaching centre for interns and post graduates from Maulana Azad Medical College. The centre has two medical officers, 2 Lady Health visitors, ANMs, social worker and other staff. A total of 790 under 2 years old children were registered in UHC from all 4 blocks. First, a list of all the defaulters (child missing any vaccine) was prepared by the Auxiliary Nurse Midwife (ANM) from the records in immunization register at the UHC. From the list, all defaulters were then segregated block wise. A team of two field investigators, ANM responsible for that block and a field supervisor was constituted under the guidance of medical officer in charge of the centre. Before starting survey, all team members were trained and explained about the purpose of the survey, data collection and interviewing techniques so as to minimize interviewer bias. At the end of the day, all the data collected through questionnaires was analyzed by a senior supervisor. A semi

*Corresponding author: Shantanu Sharma, Department of Community Medicine, Maulana Azad Medical College, India, E-mail: shantanusharma145@gmail.com

structured, pre tested questionnaire was prepared in local language consisting of items on socio demographic profile like age, gender of the child, education and occupation status of parents. Details of the immunization of the children were assessed. The information was cross checked with immunization card available with the family. All efforts were made to interview mothers as they are the primary caregiver at home. In case, the mother was not available at the time of visit, repeat visits were made later. However, those defaulter families' which were reported to be shifted out of the area were not visited again. At the end of the interview, the mother was explained about the importance of the immunization and was counseled to complete the immunization of her child as soon as possible. The data were fed into Excel sheet and analyzed using SPSS version17 (USA II Chicago). Errors while entering data and analyzing were minimized by cross checking by the senior supervisor of the team. The study is approved by institutional ethical committee. Informed verbal consent was obtained from all the subjects before the start of interview. The subjects were assured about the anonymity of the data and voluntary participation in the study.

Results

There were a total of 87 defaulters as per records available (11%). Immunization coverage is the area is 89%. Out of 87, only 44 families could be traced, the remaining families could not be traced due to a number of reasons. For 26 families, wrong addresses were found written on records while surveying and rest 17 families were found to have left the areas.

Table 1 shows socio demographic characteristics of study subjects. A majority of families were Hindu (95.5%) and non migrant (97.7%). Most of the parents were literate and were employed (Table 1).

Immunization status of children

The number of defaulters approached and interviewed was 44. The investigators went out in the community to survey the defaulters. Out of 44 defaulters, 14 (31.8%) were found to be completely immunized. The reason for misclassification of 10 out of 14 defaulters by ANM was incomplete entry on records or registers. They were completely immunized with correct and complete entry on immunization cards with them. This could be due to the fact that the Mother and Child Tracking System system was operated by a NHRM data entry operator who came on alternate days and the Public Health Nurse at the centre did not inform nor updated the records. In the rest 4 out of 14 defaulters,

Characteristic	Frequency (N=44)	Percentage
Religion		
Hindu	42	95.5
Muslim	2	4.5
Education of mother		
Illiterate	3	6.8
Literate	41	93.2
Education of father		
Illiterate	2	4.5
Literate	42	95.5
Occupation		
Unemployed	1	2.3
Employed	43	97.7
Migration status		
Non migrant	43	97.7
Migrant	1	2.3

Table 1: Demographic characteristics of study subjects.

Reason	Frequency (n=30)	Percentage
No need of vaccination	1	3.3
Vaccine not available	3	10.0
Time is not convenient	2	6.67
Long waiting time	1	3.3
Will get the vaccination later	4	13.3
Weather was not good so didn't go and then forgot	1	3.3
Do not know what vaccines are needed and when	6	20
No time to take child for immunization	3	10.0
Do not know where to take child for immunization	1	3.3
Fear of side effects	2	6.67
Services not available when required	6	20

Table 2: Reason for incomplete immunization.

entry was not being made into the card for the vaccine which the mother claimed to have been given to child. The reasons were enquired regarding the card being partially filled. The reasons for card being incompletely filled were non entry by health staff (5.9%) or mistake of not carrying the card along on the day of receipt of vaccination (5.9%).

Only 30 (68.2%) children were found to have incomplete immunization. Table 2 shows reasons for incomplete vaccination in study subjects. Factors/ reasons for incomplete (partial) immunization of the children were also assessed (Table 2).

Although all the 44 children surveyed had ever received immunization from the urban health centre (UHC), 7 had received some of the vaccines from other government and private hospitals as well, whereas 37 had entire immunization from UHC only. Twenty two (50%) subjects reported that they paid more visits than recommended for vaccination. Most common reason for same was non availability of vaccines (27.5%). Other cited reasons were long waiting queue (18.2%) and non availability of service providers (4.5%).

Beneficiary satisfaction level

Data were collected regarding the beneficiary satisfaction levels and also about the immunization services provided in UHC. Thirty six (81.8%) were satisfied by services provided there while 7 (15.9%) were dissatisfied from the same and 1 (2.3%) said "cannot say". The reasons for dissatisfaction were also assessed. Long queue and long waiting period (2), insufficient vaccines which finish off before their turn (2) and rough attitude of the staff (3) were reported reasons.

Counseling services were also provided in UHC. Subjects were asked about their perception of counseling services. Forty (90.9%) admitted that side effects of vaccination and their management was explained to them when they went for services. Next visit for immunization was also reported and instruction to bring immunization card in next visit was told to 41 (93.2%).

About frequency of visits of health workers to the community, it was reported that mostly health workers used to pay visit monthly (36.4%) followed by 2-3 times in a month (22.7%), weekly (15.9%), once in a quarter (4.5%), sometimes (11.4%) and never by (9.1%) subjects. On non-reporting at scheduled time for immunization of child, it was revealed by only 21 (47.7%) subjects that health workers paid home visit.

Various sources of information about immunization services were assessed. Anganwadi workers (50%) were the most common sources of information (Table 3).

Source	Frequency (n=44)	Percentage (%)
Health worker staff		
1) ANM	6	13.6
2) ASHA	7	16
3) AWW	22	50
4) Doctors in government settings	16	36.3
5) Doctors in private hospitals	1	2.27
Newspaper	1	2.27
Self from hoardings or boards	3	7

Table 3: Sources of information about immunization.

Discussion

The present study showed that majority of subjects were Hindu, non migrant with literate and employed parents. Immunization coverage is 89% in the area which is much above then that reported in CES 2009 (71%) for Delhi [10]. Reasons for incomplete immunization were related to both health system and social factors. Non entry by health staff in immunization card on the day of vaccination was found. Such misclassification by health centre staff was an important area which should be improved because it will spuriously gives impression of poor immunization coverage. Health centre staff should be sensitized and trained about the importance of accurate record keeping and records should be cross checked by Medical Officer In charge. Similar findings have been previously reported by other authors as well [11]. Other health system related reasons cited were non availability of vaccine at the centre and long waiting time. Convenience of immunization services are known factor which improves immunization coverage as stated by Mohammed et al [12]. Similar findings were reported by a study conducted by Lim et al where some of the reasons for refusal for immunization of children were long waiting time and unsatisfactory services at the clinic [13]. In another study by Gupta et al from Lucknow, most common reason for partial or non-immunization cited were family problems (24%) of the respondents followed by unawareness of immunization (20%) and fear of side effects (16%) [14]. Other reasons were child too young for immunization, illness of child and parents have no faith in immunization (12%). All efforts should be taken to improve vaccine constant availability at the health canters.

According to CES 2009, reasons for complete immunization were, 28.2% families didn't feel the need, 26.3% were not aware of vaccine, 10.8% were unaware of where to go for immunization, 8.9% didn't find time convenient and 8.1% were afraid of side effects. Awareness of parents about importance of immunization was found to be inadequate. Parent's lack of awareness about need of timely immunization, place to go for vaccination and fear of side effects were found. These are consistent with results from a study conducted in Aurangabad where lack of motivation and information about immunization were reported [15]. Counselling services provided at the health centre at the time of vaccination should focus on such issues so as to allay the anxiety of parents about side effects of vaccines and importance, place and date of next visit for immunization. Health staff should be trained in counselling to improve the effectiveness. Health workers should approach the families as soon as the child don not turn up for vaccination at due date to ask he reasons for not bringing the child. Most common source of information about immunization services was Anganwadi workers followed by doctors. They should be involved actively in ensuring complete immunization of the children in their area by keeping the record of immunization and bringing them to the health centre for immunization. WHO world immunization week was held in April 2016 with the aim to promote the use of vaccines to protect people of all ages against diseases.

Conclusion

The reasons for incomplete immunization were mainly lack of awareness of parents and health care system flaws. All efforts should be taken to raise the awareness of community about importance of immunization along with providing complete information about the immunization services being available to them. Intersectoral coordination should be strengthened by participation of Anganwadi workers in providing immunization services. Workers need to be trained about need for maintaining appropriate records and use the MCTS system. Proper data recording and management would reduce these errors and help policy makers designing progammes based on true data.

References

1. UN. Transforming our world: The 2030 Agenda for Sustainable Development.
2. Every Woman Every Child. The Global Strategy for Women's, Children's and Adolescents' Health (2016–2030) Survive, Thrive, Transform 2015.
3. Ministry of health and family welfare, Government of India.
4. Kalaivani K, Mathiyazhagan T, Patro BC (2006) Editorial. News Lett Nat Inst Hlth Fam Welfare 8: 1–2.
5. Belli PC, Bustreo F, Preker A (2005) Investing in children's health: What are the economic benefits? Bull World Health Organ 83: 777-784.
6. Black RE, Cousens S, Johnson HL, Lawn JE, Rudan I, et al. (2010) Global, regional and national causes of child mortality in 2008: A systematic analysis. Lancet 375: 1969–1987.
7. World Health Organization (WHO) Immunization.
8. World health Organization (2010) World health statistics, WHO.
9. NHM (2015) Mission Indradhanush Operational Guidelines.
10. Coverage evaluation survey 2009 report. UNICEF.
11. Singh A (2006) Record-Based Immunization coverage assessment in rural north India. Internet J Third World Med 4:1-6.
12. Mohammed H, Atomsa A (2013) Assessment of child immunization coverage and associated factors in oromia regional state, eastern Ethiopia. SciTechnol Arts Res J 2: 36-41.
13. Lim WY, Singh A, Jeganathan N, Rahmat H, Mustafa NA, et al. (2016) Exploring immunisation refusal by parents in the Malaysian context. Cogent Med 3:1142410.
14. Gupta P, Prakash D, Srivastava JP (2015) Determinants of immunization coverage in Lucknow District. N Am J Med Sci 7: 36-40.
15. Ingale A, Dixit JV, Deshpande D (2013) Reasons behind incomplete immunization: A cross sectional study at urban health centre of government medical college, Aurangabad. Natl J Comm Med 4:253-336.

21

Individual Risk Factors Contributing to the Prevalence of Teenage Pregnancy among Teenagers at Naguru Teenage Centre Kampala, Uganda

Akanbi F[1], Afolabi KK[2*] and Aremu AB[3]

[1]Department of Nursing, International Health Science University, Uganda
[2]Department of Public Health, Cavendish University, Uganda
[3]Department of Community Medicine, Islamic University, Uganda

Abstract

Introduction: Teenage pregnancy and its effects on teen motherhood are among the major societal challenges of the teenagers in the contemporary global community. In a 30 million population 25 percent pregnancy rate among adolescents is an issue of great concern to the government and the whole of Uganda.

Objective: This study identifies and analyses the individual factors contributing to the prevalence of teenage pregnancy among teenagers assessing Naguru teenage centre.

Methodology: A cross sectional study design was used employing both quantitative and qualitative approaches using 384 population sample size among teenagers assessing Naguru teenage centre. A consecutive sampling technique with structured questionnaire was used to identify the individual factors contributing to teenage pregnancy. Data were statistically analysed using SPSS for the relationship between the variables.

Results: The result shows that 4 in every 10 teenagers accessing Naguru teenage centre were pregnant. Individual risk factors found to be associated with teenage pregnancy were educational level (P=0.024, X^2=7.452), age at the start of contraceptives (P=0.049, X^2=7.852), siblings are sexually active (X^2=12.727, P=0.005) and siblings ever got pregnant (X^2=15.214, P<0.001). Teenagers that were not educated (OR=3.437, CI=6.906-1.711) were more likely to be pregnant. Teenagers who start the use of contraceptives at the age of 13years and above were more likely to get pregnant (OR=2.484, CI=4.938-1.25). Teenagers whose siblings were sexually active (OR=5.308, CI=11.295-2.494) were more likely to get pregnant. Teenagers whose siblings ever got pregnant were more likely to get pregnant (OR=2.575, CI=4.642-1.428).

Conclusion: The study concluded that the prevalence of teenage pregnancy among teenager accessing Naguru teenage centre is moderately high. Risk factors for teenage pregnancy were educational level, age at the start of contraceptives, sibling sexually active and siblings ever got pregnant.

Recommendation: Government, Stakeholders, community leaders, teachers and parents have more efforts such as sensitization, monitoring, counseling, etc to intensify on various means of reducing teenager's pregnancy.

Keywords: Teenage pregnancy; Contraceptives; Risk factors

Introduction

Teenage pregnancy remains a perturbing issue which requires urgent intervention worldwide [1]. Globally, the prevalence of teenage pregnancy was reported to be about 16 million girls aged 15 to 19 year and mostly one million girls fewer than 15 years yearly in low- and middle-income countries [2]. Also, childbirth complications during pregnancy are the second cause of death for 15-19 year old girls [2]. An approximate of 95% of teenage pregnancies occurs in developing countries with 36.4 million female becoming mothers before the age of 18years [1].

Sub-Saharan Africa recorded the highest prevalence of teenage pregnancy in the world in 2013 [1]. Teenage births accounted for more than half of all the births in this region: an estimated 101 births per 1000 women aged 15 to 19 (ibid). Sub-Saharan Africa consists of countries with prevalence of teenage pregnancy above 30% [3]. Government and non-governmental organizations (NGOs) have decided to address this issue through policies and other initiatives. In spite of the huge investments and modification of concerned policies and interventions, teenage pregnancy still persists to the extent of reaching crisis proportions in most African countries [4]. In a study conducted in Soweto South Africa, it was found that 23% of pregnancies were carried by 13—16 year old young women and 49% of which falls between 17-19 year ages ended in abortion [5].

In Uganda evidence suggests that the proportion of teenagers who have started childbearing has declined over time, from 43 per cent in the 1995 UDHS, to 31 per cent in the UDHS 2006 and finally, to 24 percent in 2011 [6]. The factors associated with childbearing in Uganda are intriguing and important for both health, economic and social concerns; Maternity registry statistics specifically reveal significantly high numbers of teenagers passing through Naguru Teenage Centre in Kampala. In a study by Matteo et al., Physicians, care managers, and patients displayed general agreement concerning the positive impacts on patient health and self-management, and attributed the outcomes to the strong "partnership" between the care manager and the patient [7]. This was a major thrust of this study which prompts the study to explore individual factors contributing to teenage pregnancy among teenagers assessing Naguru teenage centre in Kampala.

Methods and Materials

Study area

This study was carried out at Naguru teenage and information

*Corresponding author: Afolabi KK, Department of Public health, Cavendish Univeristy Uganda, Uganda, E-mail: khamaphor@gmail.com

health centre. Naguru teenage information and health centre is a pioneer program which provides friendly Adolescent sexual reproductive health services.

Sample size and population

This study targeted teenagers in Kampala which was accessed at Naguru teenage centre only. The sample size used was 384, which was determined using Kishi and Leslie formula.

Sampling procedure

A consecutive sampling method was adopted. Teenagers were enrolled consecutively into this study at Naguru teenage centre until the desired sample size was achieved

Procedure for data collection

Questionnaire: Data were collected using structured questionnaire which was administered to the respondents. The questionnaires contain questions to determine individual risk factors and prevalence of teenage pregnancy.

Pre testing: Pre-testing was done using 10 respondents at Kisugu health centre in Namuwongo Kampala district. This was done to ensure clarity and to make necessary adjustment based on the outcome of the results.

Research assistant: Research assistants were trained on the objectives of the study and the research assistants selected were nurses working at Naguru health centers.

Data analysis

The coded data were double entered in Statistical Package for Social Sciences (SPSS). The same Statistical Package for Social Sciences (SPSS) was used for data processing, analysis and manipulation. Descriptive analysis of background variables was used to analyse the proportion of exposed and unexposed teenagers. The teenage pregnancy risk associated with the exposure was estimated using the chi-square method, i.e., checking the strength of association between suspected predisposing factor to sex (exposure) and pregnancy with the p value as the guide. Multivariate regression analysis was done to determine the role of confounding factors on final results.

Ethical considerations

Permission was obtained from the director of Medical Services (DMS) in Naguru Health canters to carry out this study. The purpose of the study was explained to participants by means of information sheet. The participants were assured of strict confidentiality of any information they will provide. Each participant was required to fill an informed written consent letter. The entire participants were treated with dignity and respect. Anonymity was assured to the participant by using codes for identification instead of their names. The participants were informed that taking part in this study is completely of your own choice; any attempts to opt out of this exercise will not stop you from receiving all services that you normally get from this canter.

Study limitations

The study design cannot be used to analyse behaviour over a period to time. The data were collected at once; we are unable to study the respondent for a long period of time which may limit the information extracted.

The use of questionnaire only as the tool for data collection limit

the exploration in this study, as qualitative data were not captured to validate the quantitative data collected.

Considering the sampling techniques used (convenience sampling) which is the best means that can be used to get the data from the centre because the teenagers were only visiting the hospital not hospitalized, the degree of generalizability is questionable. Respondents were interviewed based on the availability not randomized.

Results

Socio-demographic characteristics

The study captured the demographic characteristics of the teenagers attending Naguru teenage centre. The key background characteristics here explained in the Table 1 below;

From the table above, the study found the majority of the respondents to be within the age range of 17-18 years with total number 132 (42%) out of 315 respondent. The least age range of the respondent were those that falls between 13-14 years with 31 (9.9%) out of 315 respondents. The majority of the respondents practiced catholic religion with a total number of 119 (37.8%) respondents while the least religion group that responded falls under other religion such as Seventh day, born-again and so on with 32 (10.2%) respondents out of 315 respondents.

The respondents with no formal education are 25 in number accounting for 8% of the respondent with the least number of respondents, primary education have 93 respondents (29.6%) and secondary education have the highest number of the respondents with 196 (62.4%) out of 315 respondents.

Prevalence of teenage pregnancy

The chart below shows the prevalence of teenage pregnancy among teenagers attending Naguru teenage centre with almost 39.7% of the respondents were pregnant before and the remaining 60.30% of the respondents were not pregnant.

Individual factors influencing the prevalence of teenage pregnancy

The individual factors found to be associated with teenage pregnancy among teenagers attending Naguru teenage centre were educational level (P=0.024, X^2=7.452), age at the start of contraceptives (P=0.049, X^2=7.852), sibling who are sexually active (X^2=12.727, P=0.005) and siblings ever got pregnant (X^2=15.214, P<0.001) as indicated in Table 2 below.

Teenagers that were not educated (OR=3.437, CI=6.906-1.711)

Variable	Category	N	Percent
Age	13-14	31	9.9
	15-16	91	29.1
	17-18	132	42.2
	19-20	59	18.8
Religion	Moslem	88	27.9
	Protestant	76	24.1
	Catholic	119	37.8
	Others	32	10.2
Education level	None	25	8
	Primary	93	29.6
	Secondary	196	62.4

Table 1: Socio-demographic characteristics of Adolescents in Naguru Teenager centre.

Prevalence of pregnancy					
Variable	Yes (%)	No (%)	χ^2	p-value	Odd ratio
Age					
13-14	8 (6.5)	23 (12.1)	4.221	0.239	
15-16	34 (27.6)	57 (30.0)			
17-18	59 (48.0)	73 (38.4)			
19-20	22 (17.9)	37 (19.5)			
Religion					
Moslem	37 (29.6)	51 (26.8)	0.949	0.814	
Protestant	28 (22.4)	48 (25.3)			
Catholic	49 (39.2)	70 (36.8)			
Others	11 (8.8)	21 (11.1)			
Education level					
None	4 (3.2)	21 (11.1)	7.452	**0.024**	3.437 (6.906-0.711)
Primary	35 (28.0)	58 (30.7)			2.468 (5.180-1.176)
Secondary	86 (68.8)	110 (58.2)			1
Age of menarche					
≤ 9 years	1 (0.8)	2 (1.1)	0.051	0.975	
10-13 years	45 (36.0)	68 (35.8)			
>13 years	79 (63.2)	120 (63.2)			
Age at 1st sexual intercourse					
≤ 9 years	2 (1.7)	11 (6.2)	3.871	0.144	
10-13 years	32 (26.4)	40 (22.5)			
>13 years	87 (71.9)	127 (71.3)			
Ever used contraceptives					
Yes	62 (49.6)	100 (53.8)	3.115	0.211	
No	58 (46.4)	84 (45.2)			
Aware of safe sex					
Yes	98 (87.5)	150 (79.4)	5.413	0.067	
No	12 (10.7)	38 (20.1)			
Age at start of contraceptives					
≤ 9 years	7 (8.0)	6 (4.7)	7.852	**0.049**	0.738 (1.717-0.317)
10-13 years	17 (19.3)	45 (34.9)			1
>13 years	63 (71.6)	78 (60.5)			2.484 (4.938-1.250)
Sibling sexually active					
Yes	69 (56.1)	65 (35.7)			5.308 (11.295-2.494)
No	13 (10.6)	25 (13.7)			1
I don't know/NA	41 (33.3)	92 (50.5)			1.210 (2.299-0.637)
Receive sexual education					
Yes	87 (69.6)	126 (68.1)	1.751	0.417	
No	37 (29.6)	57 (30.8)			
Drink alcohol					
Yes	54 (43.9)	75 (39.7)	15.214	**<0.001**	
No	69 (56.1)	112 (59.3)			
Sibling ever pregnant					
Yes	91 (75.2)	97 (53.0)			2.575 (4.642-1.428)
No	30 (24.8)	86 (47.0)			1

Table 2: Individual factors associated with teenage pregnancy among teenagers in Naguru centre.

were more likely to be pregnant followed by those with primary school education level (OR=2.468, CI=5.180-1.178). Teenagers who started the use of contraceptives at the age of 13 years and above were more likely to get pregnant (OR=2.484, CI=4.938-1.25). Teenagers whose siblings were sexually active (OR=5.308, CI=11.295-2.494) were more likely to get pregnant followed by teenagers who didn't know maybe their siblings were sexually active (OR=1.210, CI=2.299-0.637). Teenagers whose siblings ever got pregnant were more likely to get pregnant (OR=2.575, CI=4.642-1.428).

Discussion

Prevalence of pregnancy

The prevalence of teenage pregnancy at Naguru teenage centre shows that four in every ten teenagers attending Naguru teenage center were pregnant. The prevalence is moderately high; this may be due to early sexual exposure, poverty, family background, traditional and cultural norms etc. Considering the socio-economic situation of Uganda, it is obvious that the poverty rate is high which has been a long time predictor of teenage pregnancy; so also several studies have discovered the impact of early exposure to sex, family influences and cultural norms as contributing factors to the high prevalence of teenage pregnancy. This result is in close conformity with a study that found eight in every ten pregnant women attending antenatal care in Butaleja district were teenagers [8]. This observation peculiarly exposed the high prevalence of teenage pregnancy, for the population of pregnant teenagers to outweigh the population of the pregnant adults at the antenatal care. According to the figures from Uganda demographic health survey 2011, 24% of all female teenagers are either pregnant or have given birth already [9,10]. More so, a close proximity in the results obtained was observed with the regional demographic and health survey that shows that in central Uganda, 3 out of every 10 teenagers are pregnant [11]. This confirmed and validates the study because Naguru teenage centre is located at the central Uganda. The implications of high prevalence of teenage pregnancy are overpopulation, economic burden, increase in poverty rate, increase in maternal and child health challenges etc. If teenage pregnancy persists the population will grow in multitudes till it get beyond the normal growth rate which will posed a great burden to the economic development of the country resulting into high crime rate, ecology imbalance, severity of health challenges etc. High poverty rate which has been a revolving predictor for teenage pregnancy will continue to increase as the population grows, increase in population and high poverty rate are two factors that accompany each other all around. So also, the psychosocial trauma teenagers go through after pregnancy is indescribable, teenagers who got pregnant by accident or unwanted pregnancy in most cases have the probability

of marriage instability. Clinically, high prevalence of teenage pregnancy may result into various cases of birth complications such as still birth, miscarriage, cervical cancer etc. All these complications have a great burden on the economical situation of the country as high financial expenditure is required to overcome them.

Individual factors influencing the prevalence of teenage pregnancy

The individual factors associated with teenage pregnancy among teenagers attending Naguru teenage centre shows educational level to be significantly associated with the prevalence of teenage pregnancy. Teenagers that were not educated and those with primary school education were more likely to be pregnant. The result from this study is in line with the findings of Uganda bureau of statistics which said 2 out of every 10 adolescents who are able to complete secondary school were pregnant, this tend to reflect low pregnancy rates among secondary school students compared to the proportion among adolescents who dropped out or have no secondary education which is 5 out of every 10 adolescence [12]. The findings maybe as a result of exposure and peer influences, because at secondary school level most females have their prime exposure to sex and several factors will be attracting them to it such as poverty, hormonal development, peer group influences etc. So also, teenagers who dropped out or have no secondary education are susceptible to teenage pregnancy too due to poverty level, idleness, social strives etc. High school dropout rate may be the resulting effects of teenage pregnancy which will increase poverty, truancy, reduced productivity of the community and country etc. Several births complications will be recorded as well.

Age at the start of contraceptives use have a meaningful relationship with teenage pregnancy. Teenagers who started the use of contraceptives at the age of 13years and above were more likely to get pregnant. This study indicated that the use of contraceptives is high but still yet teenage pregnancy is high, this shows that teenagers may sometimes be feed up of using the common contraceptives such as condom and tends to explore sexual activities more which placed them at higher risk of pregnancy. This is in line with a study which stated that conscious use of contraceptives appeared to be the main difference between pregnant and never pregnant among teenagers in Uganda; however there was a lack of knowledge and/or misconception about family planning methods other than condoms in Uganda [13]. Obviously, this will place the community at risk of overpopulation and associated effects. Several cases of births complications will be recorded as well.

Siblings are sexually active has a strong relationship with prevalence of teenage pregnancy. Teenagers whose siblings were sexually active and teenagers who didn't know maybe their siblings were sexually active were more likely to get pregnant. Sexual activities of siblings will surely influence each other, as most siblings see their elderly ones as role model and follow their steps always. This is in line with a study that said sexual behavior of younger siblings is affected by exposure to a sibling teen pregnancy [14]. This will leads to a recurrent of teenage pregnancy within the same households which can lead to overpopulation couple with poverty. Several cases of births complications can be recorded as well.

Siblings ever got pregnant have significant relationship with prevalence of teenage pregnancy. Teenagers whose siblings ever got pregnant were more likely to get pregnant. The pregnancy of a siblings will definitely influences others because the entire family may see as a norms and careless about the implication, which will be reoccurring within the household. Which is in line with a study which stated

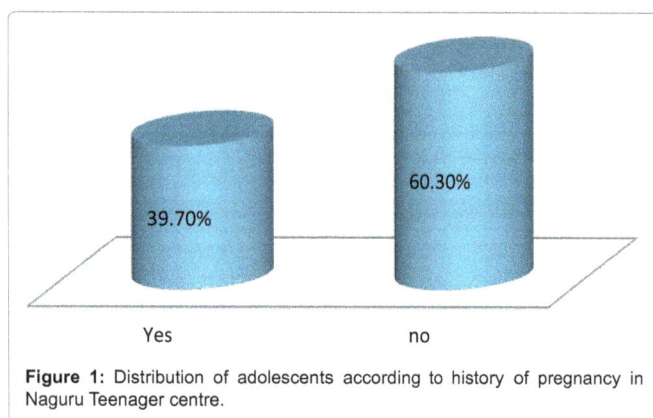

Figure 1: Distribution of adolescents according to history of pregnancy in Naguru Teenager centre.

that after an older siblings teen pregnancy, younger siblings are more sexually active, have more sexual partners and are more likely to have a teen pregnancy themselves [14,15]. Increases in poverty rate, school dropout, frustrations are the likely implication of consistence teenage pregnancy in the community and entire country.

Conclusion

The prevalence of teenage pregnancy was found to be moderately high accounting for four in every ten teenagers attending Naguru teenage center. Educational level, age at the start of contraceptives, siblings sexually active and siblings ever got pregnant were Individual factors found to have influence on prevalence of teenage pregnancy.

Recommendation

Government should channel an effective law enforcing agent to properly cater for teenage pregnancy, because it is a criminal offence to impregnate a girl under the age of 18 but the major shortcomings of Uganda's health policies is the lack of full and proper implementation of the laws.

Much effort should be intensified on sex education in various institute of learning, sex education should be regarded as a core course to learn, so as to make sex education easy for teenagers to acquire.

Teenager's empowerment model or framework should be designed which will considers the teenager as one of the most important member of the community. The model should give teenagers the power as a major not minor, in order for them to see the need for personal protection, advancement and advocacy. This will enhance and support services to the teenagers provided by primary health care system.

References

1. United Nations Population Fund (2013) Motherhood in childhood: Facing the challenges of adolescent pregnancy, New York: UNFPA.
2. World Health Organization (2014) Adolescent pregnancy.
3. Loaiza E, Liang M (2013) Adolescence Pregnancy: A review of evidence, New York: United Nation Population Fund.
4. United Nations Population Fund (2010) Motherhood in childhood: Facing the challenges of adolescent pregnancy, New York: UNFPA.
5. Buchmann EJ, MensabK, Pillay P (2002) Legal termination of pregnancy among teenagers and older women in Soweto, 1999-2001. S Afr Med J 92: 729-731.
6. Uganda Bureau of Statistics (UBOS) 2013.
7. Marco MC, Ambrogio A, Francesca C, Pietro S, Marco S (2010) Feasibility and effectiveness of a disease and care management model in the primary health care system for patients with heart failure and diabetes (Project Leonardo). Vasc Health Risk Manag 6: 297–305.
8. Kalende H (2008) Prevalence and factors associated with teenage pregnancy among prime gravidas in Butaleja district, Uganda.
9. UBOS and ICE international (2011) The Uganda demographic and health survey 2011. Kampala, Uganda.
10. Uganda Demography Health Survey 2011.
11. Uganda Demography Health Survey (2000-2001).
12. UBOS and ICF International (2011) Kampala, Uganda.
13. YRWPS (2008) Outcomes for teenage child bearing: What does data Show.
14. Anand P, Lissa BK (2013) The effects of teen pregnancy on siblings sexual behaviours.
15. Uganda Bureau of Statistics (UBOS) and ORC Macro 2001.

22

Knowledge, Attitude and Practice on HIV/AIDS Prevention among Batu Terara Preparatory School Students in Goba Town, Bale Zone, Southeast Ethiopia

Ahmed Yasin Mohammed[1]*, Tomas Benti Tefera[2] and Muktar Beshir Ahmed[2]

[1]*Department of Public Health, College of Medicine and Health Science, Madawalabu University, Bale Goba, Ethiopia*
[2]*Department of Nursing, College of Medicine and Health Science, Madawalabu University, Bale Goba, Ethiopi*

Abstract

Introduction: There are 11.8 million HIV infected youth worldwide African youth face growing rates of infection with HIV/AIDS and STI. In this region most new HIV infection occur among people ages 15-24 and are sexually acquired .The highest prevalence of HIV is seen in the group of 15-24 years. The knowledge, attitude and practice study that was done in Ethiopia in 1997 on high school student's show that students have good knowledge about HIV/AIDS prevention.

Objectives: To assess knowledge, attitude and practice on HIV/AIDS prevention among preparatory school students.

Methods: A cross sectional study design was conducted between April 2-5, 2013 in Goba Batu Preparatory school students. Data was collected by using self-administered questionnaire through and analyzed using scientific calculator which was presented by using tables.

Result: Almost all of students in study area had heard at least one HIV prevention method. Knowledge on some aspect of the disease is quite low in the study group. About 53% of respondents had positive attitude toward using condom. 62.1% and 67.8% of respondents had positive attitude towards abstinence and being faithful with friends respectively. About 54.1% of respondents were used condom and 38.5% of them used nothing.

Conclusion: There were low recognition in condom usage & some misconceptions on way of HIV/AIDS transition.

Recommendation: Our investigation call for continued and strengthened health education to bring change in knowledge in regard to misconceptions of HIV/AIDS transmission ways & Promoting condoms as one of the strategies of HIV/AIDS prevention process . We recommend this for the word's health bureau and Madawalabu University College of medicine & health science.

Keywords: HIV virus; AIDS; Preparatory school

Abbreviations: HIV: Human Immunodeficiency syndrome; AIDS: Acquired immunodeficiency syndrome.

Background

Human immunodeficiency virus/Acquired immunodeficiency syndrome is a chronic infections disease caused by HIV virus is characterized by spectrum starting from primary infection with or without the acute syndrome by relatively long period of asymptomatic stage after which in most patients progress to advanced and life threatening disease. The major mode of transmission of HIV/AIDS worldwide is heterosexual contacts particularly in developing countries other routes of transmission include transfusion of infected blood and blood products, occupational transmission, prenatal transfusion and others. The two most important risk of HIV infection are having sexual contact with many partners and having STDS [1-3].

AIDS was 1st recognized in USA in 1981 among homo sexual males: pneumocystic carnie pneumonia was seen among 5(five) homo sexual and Kaposi sarcoma was diagnosed in 26 homosexuals with the virus. HIV virus was isolated from patients with lymphadenopathy in 1983 and on 1984. The virus was clearly demonstrated to be the causative agent for AIDS [1].

There are 11.8 million HIV infected youth worldwide African youth face fast growing rates of infection with HIV and STIS. In this region most new HIV infection occurs among people ages 15-24 and are sexually acquired [1].

In 1983, AIDS was diagnosed for the first time in two patients. In South Africa, the first recorded death owing to AIDS occurred in 1983. By 1986, there were 46 recorded AIDS diagnosis. Estimates from 2000 indicated that 5% of actual infection and only 1% of actual death due to AIDS among homosexual people were reported prior to 1990. AIDS infection started reaching pandemic proportional around 1995 [2].

In Ethiopia, the first how zero- positive cases were reported in 1984 from Addis Ababa, the capital city and the two AIDS cased were reported a couple of years later. Since then a growing number of cases from different areas of the country was reported. According to MOH, the total number of adults and children living with HIV/AIDS in 2001 was estimated to be 2.2 million of which children comprised 200,000. Both men and women were equally affected [3].

Youth(15-24) is the period between the onset of puberty to the complication of 24 years of age which is characterized by when he/she attains maturity, gets employed , get married, develops financial and psychological autonomy stability , integrity and compassion [4].

*Corresponding author: Ahmed Yasin Mohammed,Department of Public Health, College of Medicine and Health Science,Madawalabu University, Bale Goba, Ethiopia¬¬, E-mail: ahmedyassinmoha@yahoo.com

Statement of the Problem:

The HIV/AIDS pandemic is the worst health crisis in history. It is clearly moved beyond being HIV primarily a health and psychosocial issue to economic and developmental crisis. Over 65 million people have been infected with HIV to date and AIDS has killed more than 25 million people since it was first recognized in 1981. Moreover in many region of the world, new infections are highly concentrated among young people (15-24) years of age [5].

According to UN AIDS report at the end of 2000 about 39.5 million people were living with HIV/AIDS, out of which 2.3 million were children and 17.7 million were women. There were 4.3 million new infection out of which 530,000 were children <15 years. There were about 2.9 million death out of which 380,000 were children [3].

Sub-Sahara Africa is by far the worst affected by pandemic with 25.7 million living with HIV/AIDS. Out of which 2.1 million are children<15 years. The overall adult prevalence in this region is 5.9%. There were about 2.1 million deaths due to HIV/AIDS in 2006 [5].

High prevalence countries are experiencing dramatic drops in life expectancy, the ill and the dying are overwhelming. The already strained public health services and millions of children being orphaned often without adequate social safety nets, HIV/AIDS deepens household poverty, threatens development, social cohesion , political stability, food security and life expectancy and imposes devastating economic burden. Without effective reduction of its spread and impact, the epidemic will slash human and economic development on the continent and under the separations expressed in the millennium development goals and by the new partnership for African development (NEPAD) to value Africa forward into a renaissance of development and reduced poverty. In East Africa in 2001, rates were at or over five [5] percent in Uganda, Ethiopia, Tanzania, Congo, Burundi and Rwanda and at fifteen percent in Kenya [6].

Ethiopia has the 16th highest HIV/AIDS prevalence rate and the third largest population living with HIV/AIDS (PLWHA). According to UNAIDS the infection rate rises quickly from an estimate of 2.2 million Ethiopian adults and about 1,200,000 children are orphan due to AIDS and according to MOH, the prevalence rat is estimated to be 6.6% with urban HIV prevalence estimated reaching as high as 13.7% and that of rural as low as 3.7%. The highest prevalence of HIV is seen in group of 15-24 years, Ethiopians effort to decrease poverty is systematically hindered by AIDS. This pandemic is significantly affecting the Ethiopian education sector with doubled face. It affects the demand of education by reducing the number of students attending education and it also affects supply of education due to increased death and sickness of teacher or instructors. A lack of information continues to be a primary stumbling which together with several other factors limits the effectiveness of effort to counter the spread and impact of the disease. This factor includes stigma, discrimination, silence and develop about the disease, poverty, inequality, gender inequality, war, conflict and STDs [5].

The social cost of HIV/AIDS to individual people, to families and to the whole country of Ethiopia cannot be underestimated in Ethiopia AIDS is the leading cause of death in 15-49 age group. This has enormous implications for the encouraging of the region because so many of the working populations are affected by the disease almost 72,000 people in Ethiopia died of AIDS in 2007 [8].

The devastating effect of HIV/AIDS in Ethiopia has become male and more visible over time and life expectancy is estimated to have fallen from 50 years to 42 years. Today 42 percent of the hospital bed in the country is estimated to be AIDS patients, draining the scarce resource allocated to the health sector [8].

Significance of the Study

The continued spread of HIV/AIDS despite aggressive prevention programs and wide spread public awareness presents a public health issue.

This study has a significance use by identifying knowledge, attitude and practice of HIV/AIDS prevention among preparatory school students, which clearly show the gap and help all concerning body give consideration to reduce the mortality and prevalence of highly active age groups due to HIV/AIDS disease.

Therefore, the study will helpful in providing information about knowledge, attitude and practice of HIV/AIDS prevention among Batu Terara preparatory school students. Thisin turn will help as baseline date for policy makers and concerned bodies related to health to design strategy.

Literature Review

In the countries of East Africa, HIV prevalence began declining about a decade ago and has remained stable in many countries. The HIV prevalence in Kenya fell from 14% in 1990 to 6% in 2006. Uganda prevalence has remained between 6 percent and 7 percent. Similarly in Ruanda, HIV prevalence has remained the same, however the HIV prevalence in Rwanda is over three times higher in urban areas than rural areas. Prevalence in Kenya, Tanzania and Uganda exceeds 5 percent (6.3 percent, 5.6 percent and 5.4 percent respectively [9].

The study conducted at East Africa Tanzania in 2005 show that 93.7% of students knew how HIV is transmitted and 86.6% knew faithfulness to one partners as best methods for HIV prevention. Despite of the knowledge they have, very few students reported to have use condom in their last sexual contacts [10].

Young people in Malawi become sexually active at an early age. Almost 60% of secondary school student's interview by Band Aiwa and faster in 1996 said that they were sexually active with a mean age of first intercourse being 15 years. While there is little good quality evidence it also seems that adolescents in Malawi are becoming sexually active younger. Male focus group discussion in Malawi indicated that there was strong poor pressure to become sexually active:

The guys who have girlfriends are seen as hero as "However less than one quarter of sexually active adolescents consistently used condom [11].

A number of studies on knowledge attitude and practice of HIV/AIDS were done in our country. According to BSS in 2002, about 98% of the study population where aware of HIV/AIDS. Almost all groups knew at least one prevention method. The study show that significant proportion of the population was at increased risk of HIV infections despite high level of knowledge. Similar observations were found in other studies, Awareness of HIV/AIDS among worker in the informal sectors in Addis Ababa was found to be 96.3%. This study also revealed that there was a 34.1 of misconception rate on the way of transmission of HIV/AIDS [12,13]. The KAP study that was done in 1997 on high school students show that the students have good knowledge about the HIV/AIDS although found to be have risky sexual behavior [14].

The study conducted in Gondar in 2007 show that, the majority (97.5) of the participants responded that HIV/AIDS is an etiologic agent for AIDS. Unprotected sex, unsafe blood transfusion, contaminated needles and mother to child transmission were reported by 84.6%, 64.2%, 78.8% and 69% of the students respectively as the common ways of HIV transmission [15].

Only 3.6% reported mosquito bite (2.5%), shaking hands (0.7%) and eating and drinking with infected individual (0.4%) as mode of HIV transmission. Abstinence, faithfulness to one's partner and use of condom as a means to prevent transmission on HIV was responded by 84.1%, 60.4% and 41.8% of student respectively. Avoiding social life with AIDS patients was reported by 1.8% of the respondents as way to prevent transmission of HIV infection [16].

The study done in Gondar, Ethiopia, in 2009 shows that, all students had heard about HIV/AIDS before the interview. The sources of information were radio (50%), Television (46.7%), newspaper (33.3%), teacher (25%), parents (21.7), Health workers (13.3%) and youth club (11.7). Where more than one source were common .About (34%) of the students(respondents) had negative attitude towards HIV, AIDS patients and other STDs. 40% of sexually active respondents had multiple sexual partners including commercial sex workers (CSWS) indicates that such rising behavior can predispose the students to the accusation of STDs [16].

More than 30% of the students associated AIDS with an immoral lifestyle and even recommended isolation of AIDS patients. Half of the students favored for screening of HIV/STIs. However one third of the students were not willing to visit infection control clinic following acquisitions of STDs other than HIV/AIDS [17].

According to the BSS (2005) report in Ethiopia, only 9.3% and 13% of the in-school youth and the out-school youth had undergone HIV test respectively. Studies undertaken in Ethiopia and other countries have shown that having stigmatizing attitude towards people living with AIDS (PLWHA) was associated with lower likelihood of HIV testing while being female or married were associated with higher odds of HIV testing. Various studies had shown that having had sex with multiple sexual partners, are those at risk and neighborhood knowledge of a test were associated with increased previous HIV testing [18].

The study conducted in Awassa in 1995 shows that 93.8% of those who responded to have heard about HIV/AIDS remembered up to three mode of disease transmission. Among these, some had wrong conceptions and speculation about HIV/AIDS transmission, such as kissing and saliva by 5.3%, body contact by 4.8% and air droplet by 1.5%. The three major risk factors perceived to expose a person for HIV infection were sexual promiscuity, taking injections , using unsterile needles and frequent sexual contact with commercial sex workers in that respective order [19].

Study done in Jimma on high school students show that about 100% of the respondents know or heard about HIV/AIDS. Radio and television is the main source of information (97.4%) and include other sources. However, only 53% rely on radio/television only. Only 39.5 got information from religious institution. About 10.5% of the subjects had undergone HIV testing and counseling. Only 57.9% of the students would change their behavior to avoid contracting HIV/AIDS. About 21.1% of the respondents don't know if a person looks healthy is infected with HIV or not [20-22]. The study that conducted in Jima zone Agaro town in 2001 indicates 40% of males and 7.5% females reported to have 2-5 and more than 5 partners respectively. Among 90 students sexual exposure 54.4% of them use condom at least once. Of those 55.7% were males and 50% were females. Among those who had used condom, 46.9 % used always and 38.8% used occasionally [21].

Objective

General Objective:

To assess the level of knowledge, attitude and practice of HIV/AIDS prevention among Batu Terara preparatory school students.

Specific Objectives

1. To assess level of knowledge on HIV/AIDS prevention method in Batu Terara preparatory school students.

2. To assess attitude towards HIV/AIDS prevention method among Batu Terara preparatory school students.

3. To assess HIV/AIDS prevention method utilization among Batu Terara preparatory school students.

Methodology

Study area and Period:

The study was conducted among Batu Terara preparatory school students in Goba town, Bale zone, Oromia from April 2-5. Batu Terara preparatory school is a governmental which was established in 1995. The school is located South East Goba town 445km far from Addis Ababa. The altitude is between 2400 to 3200 meters above sea level with a weather condition of Daga. There were 493 male and 333 female students with 826 total numbers of students in the school.

Study design

Institutional based cross sectional study design was conducted.

Source population:

All Batu Terara preparatory school students during study period.

Study population:

Sample students from Batu Terara preparatory school students.

Inclusive criteria:

All regular students.

Exclusive criteria:

All night students.

Sample size determination

Sample size was calculated from the source population using single population formula.

With the following assumptions

p= proportional=0.5 or 50%

z= standard normal distribution (1.96)

d= Margin of error (accepted error) =0.05

n= $Z_{a/2}$ P (1-P)/d²= (1.96)2(0.5) (1-0.5)/ (0.05)2=382

Considering 10% non-respondents rate =383+10%=422. A total of 422 were selected.

Sampling Technique

There were total of 826 students (Grade 11 and 12) in Batu Terara preparatory school during the study period (April 2-5) distributed in to 14 sections. In each class there were 58-60 students. 422 students were selected from all classby using systematic random sampling from student's rosters.

Study Variables

Dependent variables

-Knowledge of HIV prevention

-Attitude of HIV prevention

-Practice of HIV prevention methods

Independent variables

-Age

-Sex

-Marital status

-Peer pressure

-Religion

-Ethnicity

-Health extension workers

-Health professions

-Family educational status

-Health service accessibility

-Accessibility to different Medias like radio, TV...

-Residence

-Teachers

Data collection

The study instrument was a self-administered questionnaire which comprised of 4 parts, Part one questions related to socio-demographic status, part two questions related to knowledge on HIV prevention methods, part three questions on attitude towards HIV prevention methods and part four questions related to practice on HIV prevention methods.

Data analysis and processing

Data was processed and analyses using tally sheets and manual scientific calculator. Finally the result presented using tables based on finding then discussion, conclusion and recommendation was given depending on the result.

Data quality management

Pre-tested questionnaire was used before the actual data collection done to increase the quality of data. The questionnaire was translated to the local language to check its consistency & we returned tothe respondents for our data completeness.

Operational definitions

Knowledge: In this research paper, those who were respond-correctly 5 or less questions (<50%) out of knowledge questions will be rated as having poor knowledge while those who answered correctly 6 or more questions (60-100%) was categorized as having good knowledge.

Attitude: A tendency of mind or of relatively constant feeling of the respondent towards HIV prevention method. In this research paper

those who responded more than half of the attitude questions were recognized as having positive attitude.

Practice: Is defined as a health behavior that may promote Heath or prevent disease or opposite, what the individual have been doing regarding HIV prevention.

Method: Is measure taken by person to prevent HIV transmission.

Ethical consideration

The study proposal was first submitted to Department of public health for approval. Then supportive letters was obtained from Madawalabu University ethical committee and similarly permission from Batu Terara preparatory school administrative office also obtained. The privacy right of the respondents was respected. Data collection in Batu Terara preparatory school was conducted without disrupting the learning teaching process.

Dissemination of the result

The study shall be prepared in hard and soft copy and distributed in MWU, faculty of education and Madawalabu CBE coordinator.

Result

Socio-Demographic characteristics of Respondent

Two hundred twenty two (52.6%) of the respondents were males and two hundred (47.5%) were female students. Themean age of the respondents was 18. (1.32 ± SD). .We have 244 (57.9%) respondents from grade 11 and 178 (42.1%) from grade 12 and the majority of the respondents 390 (92.4%) were single and 32 (7.5%)have been married. Majority of the respondents were Orthodox Christian 310(74.1%) in Religion followed by Muslim 59(13.9%). The distribution of the respondents by their ethnicity indicated that about 64.7% were from the Oromo and 25.3% from Amhara. 253 (60%) of students were from urban and 169 (40%) were come from rural (Table 1).

Their family educational status were highest in the number from grade (1-8th) were their fathers were 143 (33.9%) and mothers 111(26.3%) and they involved on farming activity were the father 180 (43%) and the mother 117 (28%) .With regarding to their socio-economic 34 (8.1%) is fall in ≤500birr/month and the rest were fall in ≥500 birr/month.279 (66.1%) of the students were live with their parents and the remaining 56 (13.2%), 72 (17%) and 15 (3.6%) were lived alone, with friends and others respectively (Table 1).

Knowledge of HIV prevention

Almost all of the students in our study are had heard at least one of HIV/AIDS preventive methods. Abstinence, faithfulness to one's partner and usage of condom as a means of HIV/AIDS prevention methods were responded by 394 (93.4%), 355 (84.1%), 199 (47.1%) of students respectively. Unsafe sex (96.7%), sharing sharp material (90%), unsafe blood transfusion (96.5%) and mother to child transmission were reported by students. Only (12.6%) reported mosquito bite, (10.7%) eating raw meat, prepared by HIV infected person, (8.76%) sharing toilet, (9%) sharing public swimming and (10.4%) shaking hands with infected person as a mode of transmission. 64% of students were respond as a pregnant woman can transmit HIV to her unborn child and 73.9% reported that mother can transmit HIV/AIDS to her child during breast feeding (Table 2).

Result on Attitude towards HIV/AIDS prevention

About 224 (53%) of respondents were interested to use condom

Variables		Frequency	Percentage
Sex	Male	222	52.6
	Female	200	47.4
Age	15-19	368	87.1
	20-24	54	12.9
Grade	11th	244	57.8
	12th	178	42.2
Your Marital status	Single	390	92.4
	Married	32	7.6
Your Religion	Orthodox	310	73.4
	Muslim	59	13.98
	Protestant	40	9.5
	Catholic	3	0.7
	Other	10	2.3
Ethnicity	Oromo	273	64.7
	Amhara	107	25.3
	Gurage	8	2
	Tigre	13	3
	Other*	21	5
Residence	Urban	253	60
	Rural	169	40
Father's educational status	Unable to read	37	8.7
	Only read and write	64	15.1
	1-8th grade	143	33.9
	9-10th grade	48	11.3
	11th-12 grade	59	13.9
	Certificate and above	57	16.8
Mother's educational status	Unable to read	34	8
	Only read and write	77	18.2
	1-8th grade	111	16.3
	9-10th grade	56	13.2
	11th-12 grade	56	13.2
	Certificate and above	88	20.8
Father's occupational status	Employee	91	22
	Farmer	180	43
	Merchant	72	17.1
	Daily laborer	9	2.1
	Other	70	17
Mother's occupational status	Employee	81	19.2
	Farmer	117	28
	Merchant	102	24.2
	Daily laborer	52	42.3
	Other	70	17
Family income	‹500 birr/month	34	8.1
	≥500 birr/month	388	91.9
Living with	Parents	279	66.2
	Alone	56	13.2
	Friends	72	17
	Other	15	3.6

Table 1: Socio-demographic distribution of marital status, residence and with whom they living of BatuTerara preparatory students, Bale zone, Oromia regional state, south east Ethiopia, June, 2013.

and 283 (67.1%) were voluntary to give advice to use condom for someone who is sexually active. 262(62.1) of students were agreed to stay abstinence until marriage.67.8% of the students were agreed to be faithful with one friends (Table 3).

Result of Practice on HIV/Aids Prevention

122 (28.9%) of the respondents were sexually active and the majority 75 (61.1 %) of them started at the age of (15) to (19). 54.1% of them used condom and 38.5% of them use nothing. 81 (66.4%) of the respondents had reported to had constant sexual partner. From 258 (61%) of students who know the presence of anti-HIV/AIDS club in their school 102 (39.5%) were participated in the anti-HIV/AIDS club. Three hundred (71.9%) of students reported that they were tested for HIV and the rest 122 (28.9%) are not tested for HIV/AIDS, from this where the majority (27.6%) who were not tested are because of fear of the result (Table 4).

Conclusion and Recommendation

Conclusion:

In our cross-sectional survey of preparatory school students in Goba, almost all students, had heard at least one HIV/AIDS prevention method and mode of transmission, where as there is low recognition in condom usage and some misconception on HIV/AIDS transmission way through mosquito bites, eating raw meat prepared by infected person and sharing public swimming and also there is negative attitude towards condom usage and practice.

Recommendation

Our investigation call for continued and strengthened health

Knowledge		Frequency	Percentage
Heard about HIV/AIDS prevention		418	99.1
Means of HIV transmission prevention they know	Abstinence	394	93.4
	Be faithful	355	84.1
	Condom	93	47.1
Way of transmission	Unsafe sex	408	96.7
	Sharing sharp material	381	90.5
	Blood transfusion	407	96.5
	Mother to child transmission	369	87.5
	Mosquito bite	53	12.6
	Eating raw meat prepared by infected person	45	10.7
	pregnant women to her unborn child	272	64
	Through breast feeding	312	73.9
	Sharing toilet	370	8.76
	Sharing public swimming	40	9
	Shaking hand	44	10.4

Table 2: Percentage distribution of result of respondents by the knowledge on HIV/ AIDS Prevention Goba, Bale zone Oromia, June 2013.

Attitude		Frequency (%)
Interests to use condom	YES	224(53%)
	No	198(47%)
Giving advice to somebody to use condom	Yes	283(67.1%)
	No	139(32.9%)
Stay abstinence until marry	Agree	262(62.1%)
	Neutral	73(17.3%)
	Disagree	87(20.6%)
Be faithful with one friend	Agree	286(67.8%)
	Neutral	59(14%)
	Disagree	77(17.4%)

Table 3: Percentage distribution result of respondents by their attitude towards HIV/AIDS prevention, Goba Bale zone, Oromia, June, 2013.

Practice		Frequency	percent
Have you ever had sex?	Yes	122	28.9
	No	300	71.1
For "yes" Q no 1	Age		
	15-19	75	61.1
	20-24	47	38.9
Used prevention method	Condom	66	54.1
	Nothing	47	38.5
	Non-respondent	9	7.4
Constant sexual partner	Yes	81	66.4
	No	41	33.6
Know ant-HIV in their school	Yes	258	61.1
	No	164	38.9
For "yes" Q above who participate	Yes	102	39.5
	No	156	60.5

Table 4: Percentage distribution of result of respondent s by their on HIV/AIDS prevention, in Goba, Bale zone, Oromia, June 2013.

education to bring change in knowledge in regard to misconceptions of HIV/AIDS transmission ways & Promoting condoms as one of the strategies of HIV/AIDS prevention process . We recommend this for the word's health bureau and Madawalabu University College of medicine & health science.

The local and school community should be thought of the importance of discussing about knowledge, attitude and practice which their children and students.

The influential people to adolescents must be parts of the education process.

References

1. Lissan S (2004) Sociodemographic and clinical profile of AIDS patients in Jimma Referral Hospital, South West Ethiopia, Eth.j.H. Dev't 18:203-207.

2. Encyclopedia Wikipedia, estimated HIV infection in south Africa, 2007.

3. Getachew T , Taddese A (2005) Lecture note of internal medicine for health science students, Jimma University :79-130.

4. Molla T. Prevalence of risk of sexual behavior and associated predisposing factor to STI/HIV/AIDS infection among in school and out school youth in Gondar North West Ethiopia.

5. Madawalabu University, on policy and strategy on HIV/AIDS. November 2010.

6. Berhanu L (2009) Editorial of public health digest magazine focuses on HIV/ AIDS, STI'S and Tuberculosis. EPH and sponsored quarterly PH Digest magazine 4:1-2 Editorial .

7. Ndgwa, Wangechi Ik, Makoha A, Kijungo (2008) Knowledge, Attitude and practice towards HIV/AIDS among students and Teachers.

8. MOH (2000) Disease prevention and control programm, MOH third edition AIDS in Ethiopia, Addis Ababa Ethiopia.

9. National institute of statistics of Rwanda (NISR), Ministry of health (MOH) Rwanda and ICF international, Rwanda Demographic health survey 2010.

10. Kemala B, Abouds (2005) Knowledge, Attitude and practice on HIV prevention Among secondary school students in Bukoba Rural, KAGERA region, TANZANIA .

11. Planning, Monitoring, Evaluation and research response progress report: Malawi country report for 2010 and 2011.67.

12. Degu (2002) Knowledge and practice of condom in preventing HIV/AIDS infection among commercial sex workers in 3 small towns of North Western Ethiopia. Ethiopia. J Health Development 16:277-286.

13. Woldemeskel Y,chekola A,Negaw (1997) Preminaly report of knowledge, attitude and behavior of high school students in Gambella town.

14. MOH (2002) AIDS in Ethiopia, 4th edition, disease prevention and control department.

15. Abera z (2003) knowledge, Attitude and behavioral on HIV/AIDS/STDs among workers in the informal sectors in Addis Abeba Ethiopia .J Health Development 17:53-62.

16. Gashaw A, Afework k, Feleke M, Yigzaw k, Molla G, et al. (2007) Solomon A. low prevalence of HIV infection and knowledge, Attitude and practice on HIV/ AIDS among high school students in Gondar North west Ethiopia.

17. Yitayl Sh, Agersaw A, Amanuel G (2009) Assessment of knowledge, attitude and risk behaviors towards HIV/AIDS and STI among preparatory school students of Gondar town Northwest Ethiopia.

18. Nibiyo H (2006) Assessment of factors affecting HIV voluntary and testing uptake among behavior university students, behavior town EPHA sponsored master's thesis extracts on HIV/AIDS in Southern Ethiopia.

19. Nigussie T (2006) Sexual activity of our school youth and their knowledge and attitude about STDs and HIV/AIDS in Southern Ethiopia.

20. Bazzeew B, Ascheneke B (2012) Assessment of HIV/AIDS awareness among grade nine (9) and ten (10) students: case study of Jimma university community high school.

21. Belayneh G, Demeke A, Kora T (2005) on Determinant of Condom use among Agaro high school students using behavioral models .

22. Yaleyeh N, Bête Mariam G, Mebratu B (2003) Knowledge, Attitude and Practice study on HIV/AIDS in Gambela town, Western Ethiopia. J Health Dev 17.

23

Knowledge, Attitude and Practice regarding Lifestyle Modification of Hypertensive Patients at Jimma University Specialized Hospital, Ethiopia

Shibiru Tesema[1]*, Bayeta Disasa[1], Selamu Kebamo[2] and Eliyas Kadi[1]

[1]Department of Pharmacy, college of health sciences, Jimma University, Jimma, Ethiopia
[2]Department of pharmacy, college of medical and health sciences, Wollega University, Ethiopia

Abstract

Introduction: Hypertension is an overwhelming global challenge. Appropriate lifestyle changes are the cornerstone for the prevention of hypertension. They are also important for its treatment; although they should never delay the initiation of drug therapy in patients at a high level of risk. The study was conducted to assess the knowledge, attitude and practices of hypertensive patients on life style modification to control hypertension at JUSH.

Methods: A prospective cross sectional descriptive study design was used to determine the knowledge, attitudes and practices of hypertensive patients with respect to importance of lifestyle modification in the management of hypertension. 130 patients with hypertension were identified and interviewed using questionnaire.

Results: Out of the 130 participants, majority (57.7%) were females. 80% of participants said they avoid salt in their diet and 15% 0f them drink alcohol. 59.2% know the ideal BP and 67.7% believe the fact that exercise reduces BP. Only 1.5% of them were smoking and large majority (94.6%) were having salt restriction. Majority (90.7%) of them reported that health care provider taught them about danger of too much salt.

Conclusion: The results of this study indicates that although patients do receive advice on lifestyle modification, it was not enough and effective in changing patient behavior, knowledge and practice. Therefore, clinicians should give adequate time to provide relevant information on the value of life style modification in the control of their blood pressure.

Keywords: Attitude; Hypertension; Knowledge; Life style; Practice

Introduction

Hypertension remains as one of the most important public health challenges world wide because of the associated morbidity, mortality, and the cost to the society [1]. It is one of the most significant risk factors for cardiovascular (CV) morbidity and mortality resulting from target-organ damage to blood vessels in the heart, brain, kidney, and eyes [2,3]. Hypertension causes 7.1 million premature deaths each year worldwide and accounts for 13% of all deaths, globally [4].

Analysis of the global burden of hypertension revealed that over 25% of the world's adult population had hypertension in 2000, and the proportion is expected to increase to 29% by 2025 [1,2]. According to some estimates, the larger proportion of the world's hypertensive population will be in economically developing countries by the year 2025 owing to their larger population proportion, a change in life style and sedentary life [5].

In Africa, 15% of the population has hypertension [2,3]. Although there is shortage of extensive data, 6% of the Ethiopian population has been estimated to have hypertension. Approximately 30% of adults in Addis Ababa have hypertension above 140/90 mmHg or reported use of anti-hypertensive medication [3]. Prevalence of hypertension was 13.2% in 2013 in Jimma [1].

Despite the availability of safe and effective antihypertensive medications and the existence of clear treatment guidelines, hyperstension is still inadequately controlled in a large proportion of patients worldwide [6]. Unawareness of lifestyle modifications, and failure to apply these were one of the identified patient- related barriers to blood pressure control [7].

It is possible to prevent the development of hypertension and to lower blood pressure levels by simply adopting a healthy lifestyle. The recommended lifestyle measures that have been shown to be capable of reducing blood pressure include: (i) salt restriction, (ii) moderation of alcohol consumption, (iii) high consumption of vegetables and fruits and low-fat and other types of diet, (iv) weight reduction and maintenance and (v) regular physical exercise. In addition, insistence on cessation of smoking should be part of any comprehensive lifestyle modification plan to reduce the risk of high blood pressure and cardiovascular disease [8,9]. Hypertensive patients irrespective of their stage or grade should be motivated to adopt these measures. Motivating patients to implement lifestyle changes is probably one of the most difficult aspects of managing hypertension.

Various studies have been conducted in different countries on awareness regarding hypertension, compliance with antihypertensive treatment, prevalence of hypertension, and awareness of hypertensive patients regarding lifestyle modifications[1-3,5,6,10-14]. However; there is no study that has comprehensively assessed hypertensive patient's knowledge, attitudes and practices on the importance of lifestyle modification in controlling hypertension at the study site. Therefore, this study was aimed to assess knowledge, attitude and practice and life style changes for blood pressure control among the patients with hypertension in JUSH.

Methods and Material

A cross-sectional descriptive study design was used to assess hypertensive patients' knowledge, attitude and practice of lifestyle

---

*Corresponding author: Shibiru Tesema, Department of Pharmacy, College of Health sciences, Jimma University, Jimma, Ethiopia, E-mail: shibtesema007@yahoo.com

modifications in Jimma University specialized hospital (JUSH), from February 9 to 20, 2015. Currently, JUSH is the only teaching and referral Hospital in South-western Ethiopia. Geographically, it is located in Jimma town 346 km southwest of the capiatal city, Addis Ababa. There are currently 1694 hypertensive patients on follow-up at the chronic clinic of the Hospital.

Hypertensive patients who came to JUSH chronic clinic for follow up during the data collection time were included in the study. Hypertensive patients with mental illnesses, e.g. delirium, dementia, psychosis, schizophrenia etc, were prevented from participating in the study. A pretested structured questionnaire was administered through face-to-face interview to 130 patients who participated in the study. Data regarding knowledge, attitude and practices related to life style modification, and socio-demographic variables such as age, sex, marital status, education, occupation, ethnicity, duration of HTN, duration of treatment, co morbidity was collected.

Ethical clearance

Ethical approval was obtained from ethical review board of college of health sciences, Jimma University. The reason why the data will be collected from the patient was explained to them by the data collector before the interview. Informed verbal consent was obtained from all patients included in the study in order to protect patient's rights of privacy and confidentiality.

Result

From the total of 130 patients, the majority (57.7%) were females. The largest number, 73(56.2%), of respondents fell in the 45-60 years age group. On the basis of ethnic composition, the majority of the interviewed respondents belonged to Oromo ethnic group (63.8%), followed by SNNP (20%). A large majority, 26 (43.3%), of the respondents had schooling below high school level; with only 10% having received high school education and 28.3% had either Diploma or Degree while 18.3% were not educated (Table 1).

Assessment of the level of patient physical activity revealed that 10.2% of the patients reported to practice "little or no activity", 32.0% reported occasional activity, 41.8% walked briskly or run and only 14 percent claimed doing regular physical activity.

The participants daily activity distribution shows that most of the

participants involved in walking (43.1%), heavy labor (27%) and 18.5% pass most of their daily activity by sitting. (Table 2)

Diet habit of the respondents

Majority (34%) of the respondents didn't eat diet like cheese and eggs at all, only 7% ate them rarely, and 3.3% regularly. A vast majority (95%) didn't get fish at all. Some (5.4%) of the participants ate cooked food with salt on a regular basis while 94.6% avoided adding salt to their food. The alcohol intake result indicated that 15% of respondents drank alcohol, with 20% having 1-2 drinks per day (Table 3).

As indicated in Table 3 below, most respondents had no co morbid condition (63.9%) and the duration since became hypertensive was less than five years (86.2%). Most (96.15%) of them know their BP readings.

The respondents were also asked about their weight, and current medications. Eighty six percent of the respondents were found to know their weight in Kg correctly, but about 93% don't know their current medication. ACE inhibitors (43%) and Hydrochlorothiazide (31%) were the most prescribed drugs. These drugs were prescribed either alone or in combination.

Out of the total participants, 59.2% of them knew the ideal BP and 67.7% of them believe the fact that exercise reduces BP (Table 4).

Patients	Daily activity primarily involves				Total
	Sitting N (%)	Standing N (%)	Walking or other exercise N (%)	Heavy labor N (%)	
Male	17(13.1)	11 (8.5)	37 (28.5)	23(17.7)	88(68)
Female	7(5.4)	4 (3)	19(14.6)	12 (9.3)	42 (32)
Total	24(18.5)	15(11.5)	56 (43.1)	35(27)	130 (100)

Table 2: Daily activities of the patients.

Questions		Frequency	Percent (n=130)
Is there other chronic disease you suffer?	Yes	47	36.1
	No	83	63.9
Duration since hypertensive	0-5 year	112	86.2
	6-10 year	11	8.4
	>10 year	7	5.4
What's your current BP reading?	Pre-hypertensive	6	4.6
	Stage1	104	80
	Stage 2	13	10
	Urgency	2	1.55
	I don't know	5	3.85

Table 3: Co-morbid disease, duration since became hypertensive and current BP readings of the patients.

Questions		Frequency and % (n=130)
What's your ideal BP?	Correct	77(59.2)
	Incorrect	35(26.91)
	I don't know	18(13.8)
Who advised on how to exercise?	No one	26(20)
	Doctor	96(73.8)
	Experience	8(6.2)
Believe whether exercise reduce BP	Yes	88(67.7)
	No	3(2.3)
	I don't know	39(30)
Time spent by HP to advice patient	None	20(15.4)
	<5 minute	93(71.5)
	5-10 minute	8(6.2)
	>10 minute	9(6.9)

Table 4: Knowledge and attitude of the patients about BP and exercises.

Patient information		Frequency and percent (n=130)
Sex	Female	75(57.7)
	Male	55(42.3)
Age in years	<18	3(2.3)
	18-30	13(10)
	31-45	23(18)
	46-60	73(56,2)
	>60	18(13.8)
Ethnicity	Oromo	83(63.8)
	Amhara	15(11.6)
	Tigre	2(1.5)
	SNNP	26(20)
	Other	4(3.1)
Educational level	No education	49(37.7)
	Grade 1-8	42(32.3)
	Grade 9-12	25(19.2)
	Diploma	10(7.7)
	Degree or more	4(3.1)

Table 1: Socio-demographicic characteristics of the patients.

Questions		Frequency and percent (n=130)
Do you think adding salt affects BP?	Yes	123(94.6)
	No	2(1.54)
	I don't know	4(3.07)
Did HP teach you about the dangers of too much salt?	Yes	118(90.7)
	No	12(9.3)
Do you think alcohol affect BP?	Yes	109(83.8)
	No	8(6.2)
	I don't know	14(10)
Did HP teach you about too much alcohol?	Yes	98(75.4)
	No	32(24.6)
Do you think smoking affect BP?	Yes	74(56.9)
	No	17(13.1)
	I don't know	39(30)
Did HP teach you about the dangers of smoking?	Yes	105(80.7)
	No	25(19.3)
Do you smoke?	Yes	2(1.5)
	No	128(98.5)

Table 5: KAP of the patients on salt, alcohol and smoking.

The participants' knowledge regarding balanced diet is that 39% of them knows benefits of balanced diet in the management of HTN and 65.4%, 56.2% of them haven't eaten balanced diet and didn't taught by health professionals respectively.

Only 1.5% of the participants were smokers, and 94.6% said they were avoiding salt in their food. HP had thought 90.7% of them about danger of too much salt (Table 5).

Discussion

Good knowledge about salt, alcohol and smoking effect is an essential part of successful treatment of hypertension. Out of 130 of participants, 94.6%, 83.8%, and 59.9% participants had knowledge of the danger of salt, alcohol and smoking on hypertension management, respectively. Eighty percent, 85% and 98.5% of the participants avoid adding salt in their food, drinking alcohol and smoking, respectively. The number of participants with knowledge about salt restriction and avoiding smoking are more than the findings in a research done in Ghana, (60%) and (38%), respectively. Regarding the knowledge about the balanced diet, only 39.2% know the importance of balanced diet and this finding is low when compared with research done in Ghana (59%) [12].

The patient's knowledge on blood pressure and exercise was 59.2% and 67.7%, respectively. The attitude toward exercise is good when compared with the result of a research done in Ghana (60%) [12]. On the contrary, knowledge about hypertension is low when compared with a research done in Kinondoni Municipality, Dar es Salaam (66.8%) [14].

The attitude of the patients in avoiding salt intake and smoking cigarette was 94.6% and 98.5%. These findings are higher when compared with a study conducted last year at the same place, 45.2% and 95.5% avoided salt intake and smoking cigarette, respectively [10]. This may be due to the improvement of the knowledge of the patients towards these habits relative to last year. The common reasons given by respondents for not avoiding this practice completely were that they could not avoid salt intake and quit salt intake and some new participants do not know the danger of these practices.

Assessment of the level of patient physical activity revealed that 10.2% of the patients reported to practice "little or no activity", 32.0% reported occasional activity, 41.8% walked briskly or run and only 14% claimed doing regular physical activity. The number of patients who did vigorous physical activity (regular physical activity) and walked briskly or run is low when compared with a study done in Nairobi, Kenya 75.7% and 77.4% respectively [11].

Furthermore, the number of patients who walk briskly is low when compared with the finding in Nigeria (99.3%) [13]. This may be due to poor knowledge on the importance of physical activity in management of hypertension. The patient's daily activity among study participants as measured in this study was, sitting 18.5%, standing 11.5%, walking 43.1% and heavy labour 27%. The number of patients whose daily activity include sitting was lower when compared with the study done in Nigeria (29%) [13]. The difference may be because of the fact that participants are engaged in different activity to get their daily food and most of them do not have care givers.

Generally, practice of the participants and their knowledge toward life style modification in management of hypertension is not as required. This may be because of the poor knowledge and poor adherence to the practices. In addition, health professional might not be counseling their clients by giving adequate time regarding the importance of the lifestyle in the management of hypertension and its cost effectiveness.

Conclusion and Recommendation

The study found inadequate levels of knowledge and practice of non-drug control of hypertension. Furthermore, this study showed that the desired level of changes in the attitude of patients was not attained merely because of inadequate level of advice provided to them by the physicians. Patients should be educated on the components and application of life style modification for better control and prevention of their BP. The health care providers should motivate and enable the patients to control their BP by giving consistent advices on the life style modification. The public authority, NGOs and other interested bodies in health services should promote and where necessary enforce the implementation of life style modification to control patient's BP.

Acknowledgement

The authors are grateful to Jimma University for financial support provided to conduct the research.

References

1. Esayas k, Yadani M, Sahilu A (2013) Prevalence of hypertension and its risk factors in southwest Ethiopia: a hospital-based cross-sectional survey. Integr Blood Press Control 6: 111-117.

2. Khan MU, Shah S, Hameed T (2014) Barriers to and determinants of medication adherence among hypertensive patients attended National Health Service Hospital, Sunderland. J Pharm Bioallied Sci 6: 104-108.

3. Vrijens B, Vincze G, Kristanto P, Burnier M (2008) Adherence to prescribed antihypertensive drug treatments: longitudinal study of electronically compiled dosing histories. BMJ 336: 1114-7.

4. Lawes CM, Vander Hoorn S, Rodgers A (2008) International Society of Hypertension. Global burden of blood-pressure-related disease, 2001. Lancet 371: 1513–1518.

5. Habtamu A, Mesfin A, Tadese A (2013) Assessments of adherence to hypertension managements and its influencing factors among hypertensive patients attending black lion hospital chronic follow up unit, Addis Ababa, Ethiopia. IJPSR 4: 1086-1095.

6. Anthony H, Valinsky L, Inbar Z, Gabriel C, Varda S (2012) Perceptions of hypertension treatment among patients with and without diabetes. BMC Family Practice 13: 24.

7. Okwuonu CG, Ojimadu NE, Okaka EI, Akemokwe FM (2014) Patient-related barriers to hypertension control in a Nigerian population. Int J Gen Med 7: 345-353.

8. Appel LJ (2003) Lifestyle Modification as a Means to Prevent and Treat High Blood Pressure. J Am Soc Nephrol 14: S99-S102.

9. Wexler R, Aukerman G (2006) Nonpharmacologic Strategies for Managing Hypertension. Am Fam Physician 73: 1953-1956.

10. Girma F, Emishaw S, Alemseged F, Mekonnen A (2014) Compliance with Anti-Hypertensive Treatment and Associated Factors among Hypertensive Patients on Follow-Up in Jimma University Specialized Hospital, Jimma, South West Ethiopia: A Quantitative Cross-Sectional Study. J Hypertens 3: 174.

11. Joshi MD, Ayah R, Njau EK, Wanjiru R, Kayima JK, et al. (2014) Prevalence of hypertension and associated cardiovascular risk factors in an urban slum in Nairobi, Kenya: A population-based survey. BMC Public Health 14: 1177.

12. Marfo AF, Owusu-Daaku FT, Addo MO, Saana II (2014) Ghanaian hypertensive patients understanding of their medicines and life style modification for managing hypertension. Int J Pharm Pharm Sci 6: 165-170.

13. Awotidebe, Adedoyin T, Rasaq R, Adeyeye W, Mbada V, Akinola C, Otwombe O (2014) Knowledge, attitude and Practice of Exercise for blood pressure control: A cross-sectional survey. Journal of Exercise Science and Physiotherapy 10: 1-10.

14. Linda M (2007) Knowledge, Attitude and Practices towards Risk Factors for Hypertension in Kinondoni Municipality, Dar es Salaam. DMSJ 14: 59-62.

24

Level of Institutional Delivery Service Utilization and Associated Factors among Women who Gave Birth in the Last One Year in Gonji Kollela District, Amhara Region, Ethiopia

Tsegahun Worku Brhanie[1]* and Habtamu Alemay Anteneh[2]

[1]Department of Public health, College of Medicine and Health Sciences, Bahir Dar University, Ethiopia
[2]Federal Ministry of Health, Ethiopia

Abstract

Background: Institutional delivery is giving birth in health institution under the Overall supervision of trained health professional. Proper care during pregnancy and delivery is important for the health of both the mother and the baby.

Methods: Collected questionnaires were checked for completeness coded and entered into SPSS version 16.0 software package. The strength of association of predictor variables with institutional delivery service utilization was assessed using odds ratio with 95% confidence interval.

Results: From a total of 573 respondents, only 97 (16.9%) of them gave birth at health facilities and majority of them (83.1%) delivered at home. Regarding preference of the mothers about delivery place during their last pregnancy, 310 (54.1%) preferred to deliver at home, 148 (25.8%) preferred to give birth in health facilities with the assistance of skilled professionals and 20.1% of the mothers preferred to deliver in their mother's home. Most of the respondents 315 (55%) of mothers prefer to be attended by their mothers and relatives and 190 (34%) preferred traditional (untrained) birth attendants.

Conclusion: Low utilization of institutional delivery service and low antenatal care visit in their last pregnancy. Mothers who gave birth at home without a skilled attendant were account the large proportion. Educational status, monthly incomes, ANC visit, distance of health institute, gravidity and abortion experience were significantly associated with the utilization of institutional delivery service.

Keywords: Institution; Delivery; Home; Utilization; Birth; Gravidity

Introduction

A woman requires special attention during 15-44 years of her life since she gets matured sexually and socially, gets married, conceives and gives birth to children during this phase [1]. If proper care is not taken during this childbearing process, then it affects the overall health especially the reproductive health of the woman as well as the health and wellbeing of the new-born child [2]. Access to proper medical attention and hygienic conditions during delivery can reduce the risk of complications and infections that may lead to death or serious illness for the mother and/or baby [3,4].

Ethiopia agreed to decrease maternal mortality by 75% from 1990 to 2015. But still the expected level is not achieved. Assessment of Institutional delivery in Gonji Kollela District is not previously done. Therefore the purpose of this study is assessing the institutional delivery and the hindering factors to take appropriate intervention in order to improve the institutional delivery service in the District.

Methods

Study area

The study was conducted in Gonji Kollela District which is located 70 km to the south east of Bihar Dar, the capital city of Amhara region .The District has 26 kebeles (the smallest administrative unite of district). The total population is estimated to be 103,554 Women with reproductive age accounts for 27,742. The District has 6 public (Government) health center and 10 private clinics.

Measurements

Community based cross sectional study was conducted. Sample size was determined by the formula for single population proportion.

$$n = \frac{(Za/2)^2 \times P\left(1-P\right)}{w^2}$$

CI=95% and p=10%, w=3.5%

n=(1.96 × 1.96) × 0.1 × 0.9/(0.035)²=283.

Since it is multistage 283*2=566

For non-respondents were account for 10% then, n=622.

Sampling procedure

Multistage sampling technique was used during sampling. In sampling process first six kebeles were selected by lottery method. From the selected kebeles eligible mothers in the selected kebeles were registered and there were 686 mothers who deliver in the last one year during data registration. Six hundred twenty two participant mothers were selected by proportional allocation to each Kebele.

Data collection procedure

The data were collected using face to face interview by the trained interviewers using the prepared structured questionnaire. The questionnaires are designed in such a way that the necessary variables (questions) would be answered. Therefore the data about socio demographic characteristics, obstetrics characteristics were collected.

*Corresponding author: Tsegahun Worku Brhanie, Department of Public Health, College of Medicine and Health Sciences, BahirDar University, Ethiopia, E-mail: tsegahunw73@gmail.com

Quality assurance

In order to get the quality data during data collection, the data collectors were trained first and then the supervisors also were trained. There was daily follow up and check-up of the collected data.

Data analysis

Collected questionnaires were checked for completeness, coded and entered into SPSS version 16.0 software package. Binary logistic regressions and multiple logistic were run to assess the associations of various factors with institutional delivery service utilization. The strength of association of predictor variables with institutional delivery service utilization was assessed using odds ratio with 95% confidence interval.

Results

A total of 573 mothers were interviewed; from these the majority 456 (79.6%) were married while 78 (13.6%) and 39(6.8%) of them were separated and divorced, respectively. One hundred forty (24.4%) of the mothers were in the age range of 20–24 years and 136 (23.7%) were in the age range of 25-29. 44 (7.7%) of the mothers attended primary and 32 (5.6%) attended secondary education while 424 (74%) of the mothers were unable to read and write.

From a total of 573 respondents 456 (60.6%) of mothers were housewives. Thirty one (5.4%) of mothers was government employed mothers. Three hundred seventeen (57.5%) of the husbands were unable to read and write, 83 (15.1%) and 36 (6.6%) attended primary and secondary education and 115 of them were able to read and write. As to the husband's occupational status, the majority 311 (56.4%) were farmers. Economically, 132 (23%) of the households had net monthly income of less than $20US and 202 (35.1%) had $20-$33US monthly income. Concerning the time they travelled by bare foot to reach the nearby health center, 343 (60.7%) of them took less than 1 h, 144 (25%) took between one to two hours and 86 (15.3%) took more than 2 h. 426 (74.3%) of mothers had family size of 2–4 and 147 (25.7%) had more than five individuals within the house hold (Tables 1 and 2).

Socio-demographic variables	Frequency	Percent
Age of mothers at interview		
15-19	78	(13.6)
20-24	140	(24.4)
25-29	136	(23.7)
30-34	79	(13.8)
35-39	87	(15.2)
40-44	41	(7.2)
45-49	12	(2.1)
Marital status		
Married	456	(79.6)
Separated	78	(13.6)
Divorced	39	(6.8)
Educational status of mothers		
Not read and write	424	(74)
Read and write	73	(12.7)
Primary education	44	(7.7)
Secondary education and above	32	(5.6)
Educational status of husband		
Not read and	317	(57.5)
Read and write	115	(20.8)
Primary education	83	(15.1)
Secondary education and above	36	(6.6)

Table 1: Socio-demographic characteristics of mothers in Gonji Kollela District, Ethiopia, 2013.

Socio-demographic variables	Frequency	Percent
Occupational status of mother		
House wife	371	(64.7)
Merchant	147	(25.7)
Government employee	31	(5.4)
Others	24	(4.2)
Occupational status of husband		
Farmer	311	(56.4)
Government employ	185	(33.6)
Merchant	49	(8.9)
Others	6	(1.1)
Number of family		
2-4	426	(74.3)
>=5	147	(25.7)

Table 2: Socio-demographic characteristics of mothers in Gonji Kollela District, Ethiopia.

Variables	Frequency	Percent
Age at first marriage		
<15	244	(42.6)
15-19	244	(42.6)
20-24	76	(13.3)
25-29	8	(1.4)
>30	1	(0.2)
Age at first pregnancy		
<20	328	(57.2)
>=20	245	(42.8)
Gravidity		
1	198	(34.5)
2-4	288	(50.3)
>=5	87	(15.2)
Parity		
1	218	(38)
2-4	298	(53.6)
>=5	57	(9.9)
Institutional delivery		
Yes	97	(16.9)
No	476	(83.1)

Table 3: Obstetric characteristics of mothers in Gonji Kollela Woreda, District, Ethiopia.

488 (85.2%) of the respondents were married before the age of 20 years. 288 (50.3%) of the mothers were gravid two to four and 87 (15.2%) of them were gravid five and above. 218 (38%) were para one and more than half of the respondents 298 (52.0%) were between para two and four while 57 (9.9%) were para five and above (Tables 3 and 4).

One hundred seventy 176 (30.7%) of the respondents had visited health facilities during last pregnancy for ANC purposes. Among the mothers who attended ANC 25 (14.2%), 91 (51.7%), 60 (34.1%) of them visited health facilities once, two to three times and more than four time respectively. 89 (15.5%) of the mothers had abortion experience in their life time.

From those who deliver at home the majority; 259 (51%) were attended by untrained birth attendants.

Institutional delivery service utilization

From a total of 573 respondents, only 97 (16.9%) of them deliver

Variables	Frequency	Percent
Abortion experience in life		
Yes	89	(15.5)
No	484	(84.5)
ANC visit in the last pregnancies		
Yes	176	(30.7)
No	415	(72.3)
Number of ANC visits during last pregnancy		
One	25	(14.2)
Two to three	91	(51.7)
Four and above	60	(34.1)
ANC visit in the previous pregnancies		
Yes	183	(32)
No		
Assistant during last Delivery at home		
My mother and Family member	161	(32)
TBA (Untrained)	239	(51)
One/Myself	76	(16.2)

Table 4: Obstetric characteristics of the respondents in Gonji Kolela district.

Variables	Frequency	Percent
Preference of the mother about delivery place		
Health facility	148	(25.8)
My home	310	(54.1)
My mother's home	115	(20.1)
Preference of the mother about delivery attendants		
SBAs	46	(8)
TBAs	190	(33.2)
My mother and relatives	315	(55)

Abbreviations: SBAs: Skilled Birth Attendants, TBAS: Traditional Birth Attendants

Table 5: Preference of the respondents about place of delivery and delivery attendants during their last pregnancy in Gonji Kollela, district.

in the health facilities and majority of them (83.1%) delivered at their home. Regarding preference of the mothers about delivery place during their last pregnancy, 310 (54.1%) preferred to deliver at home, 148 (25.8%) preferred to give birth in health facilities with the assistance of skilled health professionals, and 20.1% of the mothers preferred to deliver in their mother's home. Most of the respondents 315 (55%) of mothers prefer to be attended by their mothers and relatives and 190 (34%) preferred traditional (untrained) birth attendants.

The common reasons for home delivery were distance of health facilities, home delivery is usual practice, fear of mothers, husband's influence and closer attention from families and relatives (Table 5).

Factors associated with institutional delivery service utilization

Binary logistic regression analysis shows; distance from health facility, monthly income, gravidity, ANC visit during last pregnancy, abortion experience of women, educational status of women and their husbands were the factors significantly associated with institutional delivery service utilization. ANC visit during last pregnancy was also a strong predictor of institutional delivery service utilization. Mothers who had ANC visit during pregnancy were 4 times more likely to deliver in health facilities than those who did not ANC visit during last pregnancy (95% CI=(2.206, 5.418). Mothers with educational level of secondary and above were about 2 times more likely to give birth in health facilities than those with primary education and below (95% CI=(2.4, 8.8) and 6 times more likely than who do not read and write.

Distance of health facility is also another factor for the utilization of institutional delivery service.

Mothers' monthly income was another significant factor associated to the utilization of institutional delivery service which showed that women with the house hold income of greater than \$47US were about 2 times more likely to deliver in the health facility than women with monthly income of \$33-\$47US. Occupational status of the mother also significant factor for place of delivery (Tables 5 and 6).

Multi variant analysis shows; educational status of husbands did not show significant association with the utilization of institutional delivery service. Educational status of mothers, distance of the nearby health center, monthly income, gravidity and ANC visit in the last pregnancy had significance association with the utilization of institutional delivery service. Those who attended primary education were 2 times more likely to delivery at health institute than who did not read and write. The women who travel 1-2 h to reach the nearby health institute were more than 5 less likely to deliver at health institute than who travel less than1 hour. Women who had abortion experience were 3 times more likely to give birth at the health facilities than who did not (Tables 7-9).

Discussion

The study results showed that institutional delivery service utilization was 16.9% in the District and the majority of mothers (83.1%) gave birth at home. This study finding was higher than National EDHS result of 2011 and the study done in Sekela District in 2012 which was 10% and 12.3% respectively; this might be due to the time gap, i.e., since 2011 there could be improvement in accessing and utilizing the service and probably due to relatively good commitment of the district health office and health professionals working there [5,6].

This study was in line with the findings of Magnitude and Factors Affecting Safe Delivery Service Utilization done in Gedio Zone 18.2% [7]. But the finding was lower than the report of ministry of health in Ethiopia nationally 20% [8]. The difference probably my study was done in rural district.

Variables	Utilization of institution delivery service		COR	
	Yes	No	(95% CI)	P-value
Income in month				
≤ \$20	7	125	1.00	0.003
\$20-\$33	15	187	1.4 (1.2, 3.6)	
\$33-\$47	31	102	5.4 (2.02, 11.0)	
>\$47	44	62	12.6 (7.4, 28.9)	
Time taking to reach health Center				
>1 h	89	254	9.69 (1.0-28.9)	0.000
1-2 h	5	139	0.995 (0.234-4.314)	
>2 h	3	83		
Gravidity				
1	62	136	9.5 (3.5-28.1)	0.000
2-4	31	257	2.503 (1.37-12.65)	
≥ 5	4	83	1.00	
Educational status of mothers				
Not read and write	49	375	1.00	0.001
Read and write	17	56	2.32 (1.8, 4.54)	
Primary education	17	27	4.82 (3.46, 9.707)	
Secondary education and above	14	18	6.56 (4, 11.2)	

Table 6: Binary logistic regression analysis of factors associated with institutional delivery service utilization among mothers in Gonji Kollela district.

ANC visit in last pregnancy	Utilization of institution delivery service		COR	
	Yes	No	(95% CI)	P-value
Yes	53	123	3.457 (2.206-5.418)	0.032
No	44	371	1.00	
No of ANC visit				
One	9	10	1.895 (0.611-2.524)	0.3234
Two to three	30	68	0.95 (0.184-1.513)	
Four and above	19	40	1.00	
Educational status of husband				
Not read and write	24	293	1.00	0.030
Read and write	20	95	2.5 (1.63, 4.21)	
Primary education	29	54	6.5 (3.03, 11.3)	
Secondary Education and above	17	19	10.9 (5.3, 15.3)	
Occupational status of women				
House wife	46	323	1.00	0.003
Merchant	37	110	2.36 (1.2, 3.9)	
Government employed	10	20	3.5 (6, 11.2)	
Others *	4	20	1.04 (0.78, 3.54)	

* Daily Labors, Tala Sellers, No Job at All and Family Dependent

Table 7: Binary logistic regression analysis of factors associated with institutional delivery service utilization among mothers in Gonji Kollela district, Ethiopia.

Variables	Utilization of institutional delivery service			AOR (95% CI)	P value
	Yes	No	COR		
ANC					
yes	53	123	3.457 (2.2, 5.4)	2.2 (1.2, 4.1)	0.001
No	44	353	1.00	1.00	
Gravidity					
1	62	136	13.4 (3.5, 28.1)	5.4 (2.9, 8.4)	0.02
2-4	30	258	3.26 (1.37, 11.65)	1.8 (1.2, 3.6)	
>=5	3	84	1.00 (2.202, 5.418)	1.00	
Abortion					
Yes	37	52	5.02 (3.047, 8.3)	3.1 (1.23, 5.7)	
No	60	424	1	1.00	
Educational status					
Not read and write	49	375	1.00	1.00	0.001
Read and write	17	56	2.32 (1.8, 4.54)	1.03 (0.81, 2.3)	
Primary Education	17	27	4.82 (3.46, 9.707)	2.4 (0.9, 6.7)	
Secondary Education and above	14	18	6.56 (4, 11.2)	4.51 (1.89, 8.2)	
Educational status of husband					
Not read and write	24	293	1.00	1.00	0.000
Read and write	20	95	2.5 (1.63, 4.21)	1.5 (1.03, 3.6)	
Primary education	29	54	6.5 (3.03, 11.3)	3.4 (2.1, 4.8)	
Secondary Education and above	17	19	10.9 (5.3, 15.3)	4.82 (3.02, 7.2)	

Table 8: Multi variant analysis of factors associated with institutional delivery Service utilization among mothers in Gonji Kollela district, Ethiopia.

Variables	Utilization of institutional delivery service			AOR (95% CI)	P value
	Yes	No	COR		
Occupational status of women					
House wife	46	323	1.00	1.00	0.003
Merchant	37	110	2.36 (1.2, 3.9)	1.8 (0.4, 1.2)	
Government employed	10	23	3.5 (6, 11.2)	2.3 (2.6, 4.9)	
Others *	4	20	1.04 (0.78, 3.54)	0.94 (1.0, 2.12)	
Distance of health Institute					
<1 h	89	254	9.69 (2.1, 28.9)	5.2 (2.8, 12.3)	0.032
1-2 h	5	139	0.995 (0.23, 4.3)	0.97 (0.56, 2.31)	
>2 h	3	83	1.00	1.00	
Income in month					
≤ 408 birr	7	125	1.00	1.00	0.000
409-693 birr	15	187	1.4 (1.2, 3.6)	1.2 (1.01, 2.5)	
694-987 birr	31	102	5.4 (2.02, 11.0)	2.8 (2.1, 4.9)	
>988 birr	44	62	12.6 (7.4, 28.9)	5.4 (3.2, 11.4)	

Table 9: Multi variant analysis of factors associated with institutional delivery service utilization among mothers in Gonji Kollela district, Ethiopia.

Women who attended secondary education and above were about 2.2 times more likely to deliver at the health institution when compared to women who attended primary education and below. This finding was similar to the study conducted in Sekela district on the utilization of institutional delivery service which showed that Mothers who attended secondary education and above were 12 times more likely to utilize delivery service than those mothers who had primary education and below. Other finding of the study conducted in North Gondar, Ethiopia indicated that mothers with educational status of secondary and above were 2.3 times more likely to delivery in health facilities than mothers with lower educational level [9,10].

Monthly income of the house hold was strongly associated with the utilization of institutional delivery service. Mothers whose monthly income is greater than $47US were about 5.4 times more likely to give birth at the health institution than women with the house hold income of less than $20 US. This finding was similar to the finding of the study conducted in Ghana on Expectant Mothers and the Demand for Institutional Delivery [11].

The time taking to reach health facilities was another factor for the utilization of institutional delivery service. Mothers who travel less than one hour by bare foot to reach to the nearby health institute were 5 times more likely to give birth in the health institution than mothers who travel more than 2 h and those who travel 1-2 times were 7 times more likely to delivery in the health institution than those mothers who travel more than 2 h.

This study also revealed that mothers who visited ANC during last pregnancy were about 2 times more likely to deliver in health facilities than mothers who did not visit ANC which was Similar to studies conducted in north Gondar, Sekela district and in Metekel Zone [6-8].

Conclusion

From the result of this study we conclude the low utilization of institutional delivery service and low anti natal care visit in their last pregnancy. Mothers who gave birth at home without a skilled attendant were account the large proportion.

Educational status, monthly incomes, ANC visit, distance of health institute, gravidity and abortion experience were factors associated with the low utilization of institutional delivery service. Closer care by families and relatives and fear to assist by unknown persons were major reasons for home delivery.

Communities' awareness creation on institutional delivery service should be done cooperatively by all sector institutes. More over the District Health Office should plan and implement in such a way that health education programs will address all women and do not wait pregnant mothers to come to the health institution. They should give health information about the service.

Authors' Contributions

Tsegahun W and Habtamu A were done all activities of the research and contributed for the final outcome of the research. Both authors write and edit and approved the final manuscript.

Acknowledgement

We like to acknowledge Bahir Dar University for giving this opportunity and also we like to thank Gongi Kolela district health office and health extension workers for their cooperation during data collection.

References

1. Global Maternal Mortality Fact Sheet.

2. USAID (2007) Mothers in the Middle: Potential for Integrated Programs in Maternal Health. Bangkok 3-8.

3. Fedral Ministry of Health (2009) UNICEF, UNFPA, WHO and AMDD national base line assessment for emergency obstetric and new born care. ETHIOPIA 3.

4. UNFPA (2005) Ethiopian Society of Population Studies. Maternal mortality findings from EDHS 2005: In-depth Analysis of the Ethiopian Demographic and Health Survey. Addis Ababa, Ethiopia.

5. Ethiopian Demographic and Health Survey (2011) Preliminary Report. Central Statistica Agency Addis Ababa, Ethiopia.

6. Teferra S (2012) Institutional delivery service utilization and associated factors: A community cross-sectional study among mothers who gave birth in the last 12 months in Sekela District, North West of Ethiopia. A community-based cross sectional study. BMC Pregnancy and Childbirth 12.

7. Bisrat A (2012) Magnitude and factors affecting safe delivery service utilization in Bule Woreda, Gedeo Zone, SNNPR, Ethiopia. Harar Bulletin of Health Sciences.

8. Ethiopian (2009) Journal of Reproductive Health 3.

9. Nigussie M (2004) Safe delivery service utilization: A cross sectional study among women of child bearing age in north Gondar Zone, North West Ethiopia. Ethiopian J Health Dev 18:145-152.

10. Edward N (2009) Expectant Mothers and the Demand for Institutional Delivery: Some insight from Ghana. Europian Journal of Social Sciences 8.

11. Gurmesa T (2008) Safe delivery service utilization: A cross sectional study in Metekel Zone, North West Ethiopia. Ethiopian J Health Sci 17: 217.

25

Measuring the Percentage of Consanguinity in Sickle Cell Patients and its Effect on the Prognosis of the Disease

Hassan MB*, Hammam NA, Fuad AR, Bakr HA and Abdulrhman Ahmed G

Department of Medicine, Taibah University, Saudi Arabia

Abstract

SCD is one of the major health problems in Saudi Arabia, especially in Southern, Western and Eastern areas where the gene frequency of this disease is quite prevalent. Many studies were carried out in these areas. There is a lack of studies of the effect of consanguinity on disease outcome and prognosis. We did this study in western area in Almadinah Almunawarah. We determined the effect of consanguinity on the disease by three factors. These factors are (Blood Transfusion, First complain and complications).

In this study, we carried out a retrograde analysis of patients' files, and found that 44% of the patients were products of consanguineous marriages. But the research concluded that there was no clear increase in complications caused by the state of consanguinity of the patient's parents, although patients on consanguineous parents have had slightly more incidences of vaso-oclusive crisis.

Keywords: Anemia; Consanguinity; Sickle cell disease; Sickle cell prognosis

Introduction

Sickle cell disease (SCD) and its variants are genetic disorders resulting from the presence of a mutated form of hemoglobin, hemoglobin S (HbS). The most common form of SCD found in North America is homozygous HbS disease (HbSS), an autosomal recessive disorder first described by Herrick in 1910. SCD causes significant morbidity and mortality, particularly in people of African and Mediterranean ancestry.

Sickle cell disease (SCD) usually manifests early in childhood. Complaints may include, Acute and chronic pain in any body part: The most common clinical manifestation of SCD is vaso-occlusive crisis. Anemia: Universally present, chronic, and hemolytic in nature aplastic crisis: Serious complication due to infection with B19V. Splenic sequestration: Characterized by the onset of life-threatening anemia with rapid enlargement of the spleen and high reticulocyte count. Infection: Organisms that pose the greatest danger include encapsulated respiratory bacteria, particularly Streptococcus pneumonia; adult infections are predominately with gram-negative organisms, especially Salmonella. Growth retardation, delayed sexual maturation, being underweight. Hand-foot syndrome: This is a dactylitis presenting as bilateral painful and swollen hands and/or feet in children. Acute chest syndrome: Young children present with chest pain, fever, cough, tachypnea, leukocytosis, and pulmonary infiltrates in the upper lobes; adults are usually afebrile, dyspneic with severe chest pain, with multilobar/lower lobe disease.

Pulmonary hypertension: Increasingly recognized as a serious complication of SCD. Avascular necrosis of the femoral or humeral head: This is due to vascular occlusion. CNS involvement: Most severe manifestation is stroke Ophthalmologic involvement: Ptosis, retinal vascular changes, proliferative retinitis. Cardiac involvement: Dilation of both ventricles and the left atrium. GI involvement: Cholelithiasis is common in children; liver may become involved. GU involvement: Kidneys lose concentrating capacity; priapism is a well-recognized complication of SCD. Dermatologic involvement: Leg ulcers are a chronic painful problem [1].

Methods and Materials

Litreature review

Sickle cell disease (SCD) is one of the most important single gene

disorders of human beings. In the United States, SCD affects about 72 000 people and 2 million are carriers [2].

In Africa, more than 200 000 infants are born yearly with SCD [3]. In the United States, mortality has decreased dramatically with new-born screening and better comprehensive care. The median age of death in patients with SCD in the United States is now 53 years for men and 58 years for women. However, SCD patients are still hospitalized frequently and by the fifth decade of life, 48% of surviving patients have documented irreversible organ damage.

SCD in Saudi Arabia was first reported in the Eastern province in the 1960s [4]. This led to the initiation of multiple regional and national screening studies to determine the clinical characteristics and frequency of SCD genes in different regions of Saudi Arabia. Sickle cell disease was detected in 108 of 45,682 children and adolescents with a prevalence of 24 per 10,000. The regional distribution of sickle cell disease showed eastern region dominance with a prevalence of 145 per 10,000, followed by the southern region with a prevalence of 24 per 10,000, western region 12 per 10,000, and central region with 6 per 10,000. No cases were found in the northern regions. The male to female ratio was approximately 1:1 of a total of 488,315 individuals screened, 4.20% had sickle cell trait, 0.26% had sickle cell disease, 3.22% had thalassemia trait, and 0.07% had thalassemia disease [5]. Both the diseases were focused mainly in the eastern, western and south-western parts of the country. Among the 207,333 couples who were issued certificates for matching, 2.14% were declared high risk. Among the 2,375 high-risk couples contacted by telephone, 89.6% married each other, despite the known high-risk status [6].

Comprehensive national survey of the distribution of the sickle-

*Corresponding author: Hassan MB, Department of Medicine, Taibah University, Saudi Arabia, E-mail: haslberw@icloud.com

cell (Hb S) gene and thalassemia genes was initiated in 1982, with more than 30,055 blood samples collected. The Hb S, alpha- and beta-thalassemia gene frequency range was 0.005-0.145, 0.01-0.40 and 0.01-0.15, respectively in various areas of Saudi Arabia. We present here an appraisal of sickle-cell and thalassemia gene occurrence in the Saudi population, based on our studies conducted over 10 years in different regions of Saudi Arabia [7]. During the two year study period (2004-2005), 11 554 of 11 874 (97%) mothers answered the question on consanguinity, and 6470 of 11 554 (56%) were consanguineous. there was no significant association with either sickle cell disease (P=0.97) or glucose-6-phosphate dehydrogenase deficiency (P=0.67) for first-cousin consanguinity [8].

Methodology

The study was conducted in Maternity and Children Hospital, Madinah, Saudi Arabia.

Data was obtained from the medical records by data collection sheets. The data collection sheet was built partially on previous studies on clinical presentations of sickle cell disease. The data collection sheet included the following variables: socio-demographic variables (Age, sex, residency, nationality…), first clinical presentation of the disease (Main complain, clinical sign and investigations), age at diagnosis, duration of illness, type of Sickle Cell anemia, electrophoresis, number and causes of following admissions(acute infections, fever, Splenic Sequestration, painful crisis, stroke, priapism…), blood transfusions, surgical procedures, use of hydroxyurea medication, presence of Dactylitis, vaccination, family pedigree, age and cause of death (if deceased) and other complications that are attributed to the disease. Coding of the data was be carried out by the investigators. A total of 120 samples were collected, varying in age from 6 months to 18 years. There was no documentation of mortality due to the lack of a system that shares medical records across all hospitals.

Data management and analysis

Data was analyzed through the Statistical Package for the Social Sciences (SPSS). Descriptive analysis has been used for categorical variables and chi-square test was applied to identify the main factors under study by using the statistical significance. Backward logistic regression was also used to find the association between related factors.

Results

During the period of this study, which was conducted on a sample size of 120 patients, we have found out that the incidence of sickle cell disease in children of Almadinah Almunawarah city is 1.2:100000. The prevalence of sickle cell disease in children of Almadinah Almunawarah city is 38:100000. We also found out that 44% of the patients were products of consanguineous relationships. Although both consanguineous and non-consanguineous groups suffered from complications, however, consanguineous group were more likely to suffer from more serious complications like vaso-occlusive crisis, and they were more likely to undergo splenectomy because of complications from SCD (Tables 1-10) (Figures 1-5).

The study participant's Demographic analysis: This is shown in Tables 1-4 and Figures 1-5. Table 5 shows significance of the relation between the incidence of SCD and consanguinity and from Table 6, we can say that there is no significance of consanguinity in sickle cell anemia incidence.

The effect of consanguinity on disease outcome and prognosis by

Variable		Frequency	Percent
Age	Younger than 5	29	24.2
	Older than 5 and younger than 10	52	43.3
	Older than 10	39	32.5
	Total	120	100.0

Table 1: Shows age group distribution.

Variable		Frequency	Percent
Gender	Male	69	57.5
	Female	51	42.5
	Total	120	100.0

Table 2: Shows gender distribution.

Variable		Frequency	Percent
Nationality	Saudi	88	73.3
	Non-Saudi	32	26.7
	Total	120	100.0

Table 3: Shows nationalities.

Variable		Frequency	Percent
Consanguinity	Yes	53	44
	No	67	56
	Total	120	100.0

Table 4: Shows consanguinity.

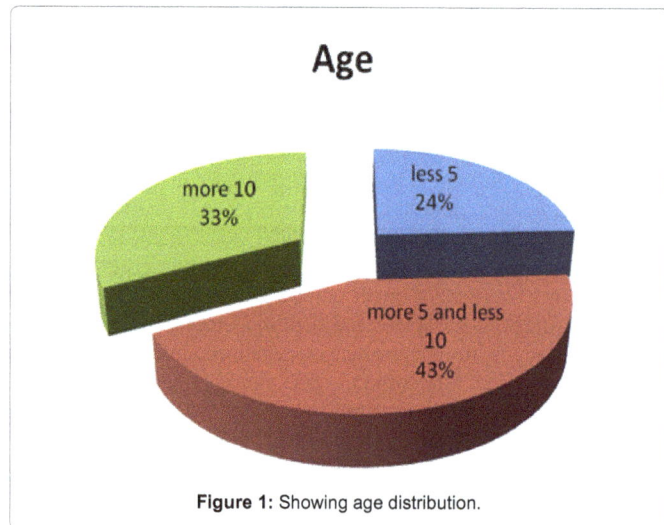

Figure 1: Showing age distribution.

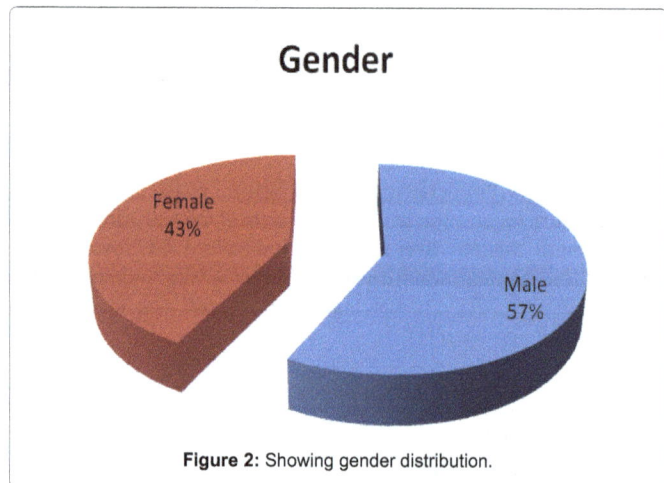

Figure 2: Showing gender distribution.

Nationality

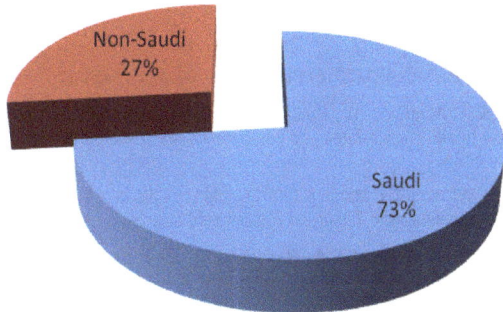

Figure 3: Showing nationality distribution.

Consanguinity

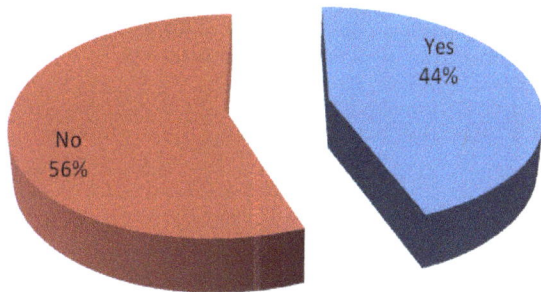

Figure 4: Showing rate of consanguinity.

Time of diagnosis

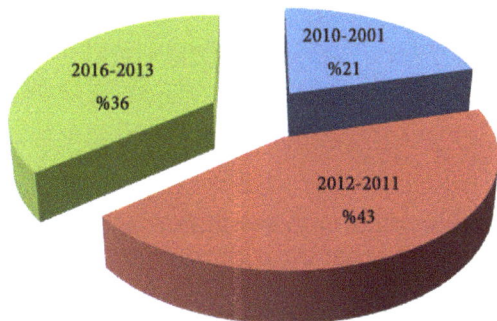

Figure 5: Show distribution of the participants by date of diagnosis.

(Blood Transfusion, First complain and complications are mentioned in Tables 7-9, whereas, Table 10 shows that all chi tests are not significant and that there is no correlation of the mentioned variables to consanguinity.

Discussion

SCD is one of the major health problems in Saudi Arabia, especially in Southern, Western and Eastern areas where the gene frequency of this disease is quite prevalent. Many studies were carried out in these areas. There is lack of study in effect of consanguinity on disease outcome and prognosis. We inducted this study in western area in Almadinah Almunawarah. We determined the effect of consanguinity on disease by three factors according to pediatric hematological physician. These factor are (Blood Transfusion, First complain, and complications).

Variable		Frequency	Percent
Date of Diagnosis	2001-2010	25	21
	2011-2012	52	43
	2013-2016	43	36
	Total	120	100.0

Table 5: Shows the time of diagnosis.

	Correlation	Chi test	df	Sig
Pearson Chi-Square	0.043	12.136	5	0.033
N of Valid Cases	120			

Table 6: We can say that there is no sign of consanguinity in sickle cell anemia incidence.

Complications	Consanguinity		Total
	Yes	No	
Vaso-oclussive crisis	6	3	9
Infection	3	5	8
Stroke	2	3	5
Anemia	1	0	1
Hand foot syndrome	0	2	2
Hepatitis	6	1	7
Acute chest syndrome	15	24	39
Splenomegaly	10	14	24
Pain crisis	10	15	25

Table 7: Distribution and rate of complications.

Complications	Consanguinity		Total
	Yes	No	
Vaso-oclussive crisis	6	3	9
Infection	3	5	8
Stroke	2	3	5
Anemia	1	0	1
Hand foot syndrome	0	2	2
Hepatitis	6	1	7
Acute chest syndrome	15	24	39
Splenomegaly	10	14	24
Pain crisis	10	15	25

Table 8: First complain.

First Complain	Consanguinity		Total
	Yes	No	Yes
Pain crisis	12	19	31
Anemia	7	11	18
Infection	2	5	7
others	32	32	64
Total	53	67	120

Table 9: Surgical procedures.

		Correlation	Chi test	df	Sig.
Blood transfusion	Pearson Chi-Square	0.085	0.862	1	0.353
	N of Valid Cases	120			
First complain	Pearson Chi-Square	-0.104	2.15	3	0.542
	N of Valid Cases	120			
complications	Pearson Chi-Square	0.158	17.333	9	0.044
	N of Valid Cases	120			

Table 10: Significance of data.

There was lack of mortality data, due to this we didn't put in in the study.

We also determine the percent of consanguinity in compared to non- consanguinity. Consanguinity was 44% and non-consanguinity 56%. This high percent of consanguinity is due to our tribal culture and lack of community education about this disease. We will educate our community by publishing our study in form of posters. In consanguinity group the percent of blood transfusion was 68%. In non-consanguinity group the percent of blood transfusion was 59%. The first presenting complaint presented in table.

Conclusion

We have found in our study that the non-consanguineous patients suffer from more complications (this may due to decreased awareness in less educated families and noncompliance to medication). However, the consanguineous group are more likely to develop more serious complication (vaso-oculusive criss) and they are more likely to undergo surgical procedures (splenectomy and cholecystectomy).

We would like to conduct further research in the future with a larger sample size to improve the significance and have a clearer results and correlations.

References

1. Maakaron JE, Besa EC (2016) Sickle cell anemia. Medscape.

2. Creary M, Williamson W, Kulkarni R (2007) Sickle cell disease: Current activities, health implications, and future directions. J Womens Health (Larchmt) 16: 575–582.

3. Makani J, Williams TN, Marsh K (2007) Sickle cell disease in Africa: Burden and research priorities. Ann Trop Med Parasitol 101: 3–14.

4. Powars DR, Chan LS, Hiti A, Ramicone E, Johnson C (2005) Outcome of sickle cell anemia: A 4 decade observational study of 1056 patients. Medicine (Baltimore) 84: 363–376.

5. Al-Qurashi MM, El-Mouzan MI, Al-Herbish AS, Al-Salloum AA, Al-Omar AA (2008) The prevalence of sickle cell disease in Saudi children and adolescents. A community-based survey. Saudi Med J. 29: 1480–1483.

6. AlHamdan NA, AlMazrou YY, AlSwaidi FM, Choudhry AJ (2007) Premarital screening for thalassemia and sickle cell disease in Saudi Arabia. Genet Med 9: 372–377.

7. El-Hazmi MA, Warsy AS (1999) Appraisal of sickle-cell and thalassemia genes in Saudi Arabia. East Mediterr Health J 5:1147–1153.

8. El Mouzan MI1, Al Salloum AA, Al Herbish AS, Qurachi MM, Al Omar AA (2008) Consanguinity and major genetic disorders in Saudi children: A community-based cross-sectional study. Ann Saudi Med 28:169-173.

26

Neuropsychological Functioning of Children and Youth with Acquired Brain Injury 2 Years after Onset

Inge M Verhoeven[1,2], Marjan J Klippel[1], Monique A M Berger[1], Frederike van Markus[3] and Arend J de Kloet[1,3]*

[1]The Hague University of Applied Sciences, Johanna Westerdijkplein 75, 2521 EN The Hague, The Netherlands
[2]Technical University, Jaffalaan 9, 2628 BX Delft, The Netherlands
[3]Sophia Rehabilitation, Vrederustlaan 180, 2543 SW The Hague, The Netherlands

Abstract

Background: Neurocognitive deficits following pediatric acquired brain injury (ABI) often remain under reported, whereas these sequalae impact several domains of activities and participation.

Objective: To screen neurocognitive consequences of pediatric ABI in a hospital-based cohort using both a professional and parent reported screening tool.

Methods: Follow-up study including children with a hospital-based diagnosis, aged 4-20 years at onset of ABI, using the Processing Speed and Attention subtests of the Amsterdamse Neuropsychological Tasks (ANT) and the parent reported Brain Injury Alert (BIA). Age, type and severity of injury were used in analysis as associated factors.

Results: 103 children, aged 4 up to 20 years (median 13y) at onset of ABI, were assessed 2 years later. 89 (86%) on injuries were classified as mild and 80 (78%) had a traumatic cause (TBI). The study cohort responded more accurate (accuracy 29.4-30.4%, >1 SD) and slow (inhibition speed 25.5-38.2%, >1 SD) on the ANT tasks compared to the norm group without neurocognitive deficits. One or more cognitive problems were reported by 62 (65%) of the parents, 1 or more social emotional problems by 66 (69%) and 1 or more cognitive and social emotional problem by 70 (77%). Type (NTBI) and severity (moderate/severe) of injury were associated with worse neurocognitive outcome in both professional (ANT) and parent reported (BIA) outcome, whereas age (younger age group) was only associated with parent (BIA) outcome.

Conclusion: Neurocognitive problems were found in this hospital-based cohort of children with ABI, especially in the older age and NTBI group, with parents reporting strikingly more problems than professionals.

Keywords: Traumatic brain injury; Non traumatic brain injury; Cognitive functioning; Emotional functioning; Social functioning; Behaviour; Young adults

Introduction

Acquired Brain Injury (ABI) in children young adults (25 years), refers to any damage to the brain that occurs after birth and may result from events with an external cause (Traumatic Brain Injury, TBI) or internal cause (Non-Traumatic Brain Injury, NTBI) such as brain tumor, stroke or infections such as meningitis or encephalitis [1,2]. With ABI, depending on its nature and severity, multiple neural systems may be involved, resulting in a large variety in combinations of potential neurocognitive and emotional-behavioral consequences [3,4]. The course of outcome after ABI is highly variable, ranging from full recovery, persisting and severe impairment, absence of impairment initially, with emerging problems over time to early slowed development, with catch-up over time [5,6].

Patients with ABI and caregivers experience neurocognitive limitations as major, chronic and most disabling problems. The most common functional neurocognitive outcomes following brain injury reported, in mild as well as moderate and severe ABI, are impairments of attention, memory, processing speed and executive dysfunction, reciprocal influencing in problems in problemes fatigue or sleep rhytm [7-15]. These acquired neurocognitive consequences adversely affect activities of daily living and social and societal participation [16].

Injury characteristics severity (moderate/severe>mild) and type (NTBI>TBI), age at onset (younger>older), environmental factors and interventions have been identified as being associated with negative and long-term neurocognitive impairments [17-19]. The developmental stage of the brain at onset of the injury is also crucial: growth, maturation and development of the brain interact with injury parameters and impact on acquisition and modification of knowledge, competences and skills and executive functions (e.g. in transitions to higher levels of education, work, social intimacy or living independently) [20-23]. This cumulative phenomenon, the interaction between growth, maturation and ABI, is called 'growing into deficit' [20,24,25].

However, literature on neurocognitive outcomes in children and young adults with ABI shows inconsistent results, due to differences in definitions and methodology, especially regarding classification, variety in age at inclusion, age range, time since onset of injury, follow-uptime [26-29]. Moreover, the vast majority of research was focussed on TBI. Although it is suggested that the consequences of NTBI are often similar to those of TBI, due to differences in their causes and nature the outcome after a TBI cannot be extrapolated to the various aetiologies of NTBI [25].

The importance of screening and monitoring consequences of pediatric ABI are broadly supported, with a longer follow up than 6-12 months after onset, to enable interventions for the child and family and school support [8,19]. In the assessment of neurocognitive consequensces of pediatric ABI it is recommended to merge different

---

*Corresponding author: Arend J de Kloet, The Hague University of Applied Sciences, Johanna Westerdijkplein 75, 2521 EN, The Hague, The Netherlands, E-mail: a.j.dekloet@hhs.nl

perspectives to get a more complete and ecological valid impression of the Childs' neurocognitive functioning and activities and participation [26], ideally these assessments should be based on different perspectives: i.e., child, parents and professional [27-30].

Therefore the aim of our study was to assess neurocognitive problems in a hospital-based cohort of children with ABI, 2 years after onset, using a parent and professional reported screening tool.

Our 1st hypothesis was, that type (NTBI>TBI) and severity (moderate/severe>mild) of injury and age group (young>old) would be associated with worse results on the neuropsychological screening and the the parent's report. Our 2nd hypothesis was that parents report more neurocognitive problems than professionals.

Methods

Design and setting

This study on neurocognitive consequences was part of a larger cross-sectional two year follow-up study on outcome of ABI in children and youth aged 5-23 years living in the south-western part of the Netherlands [31-33]. A stratified sample was drawn from a multi-centre incidence cohort of 1892 patients with a diagnosis of ABI, year of onset 2008 or 2009, from large tertiary care hospitals in Rotterdam (Erasmus University Medical Centre, including Sophia Children's Hospital) and The Hague (Haga Hospital, including the Juliana Children's Hospital and Medical Centre Haaglanden). The sample was stratified for year of onset (2008; 2009), severity of injury (mild; moderate; severe) and age at onset (3-12 years; 13-21 years).

The classification of TBI was done during hospital admission, using The Glasgow Coma Scale (GCS). The GCS is a neurological scale which aims to give a reliable and objective way of recording the conscious state of a person for initial as well as subsequent assessment. A patient is assessed against the criteria of the 3 scales: Eye Response, Motor Response and Verbal Response, with the resulting points give a patient score between 3 (indicating deep unconsciousness) and 15. TBI was considered mild if the GCS was 13-15, moderate if the GCS was 9-12 or severe if the GCS was <9 [34]. The modified Ranking Scale (mRS) is a commonly used scale for measuring the degree of disability or dependence in the daily activities of people who have suffered a stroke or other causes of neurological disability (NTBI). The scale runs from 0-6, running from perfect health without symptoms to death. The severity of NTBI was determined at the time of discharge of the hospital: Mild injury (no limitations; mRS 0,1), moderate injury (mild motor impairments and/or mild problems with learning; mRS 2,3) and severe injury (severe motor impairments and/or severe problems with learning; mRS 4,5) [35].

Patients were first selected by age and subsequently a search in the patient files was performed using diagnosis codes and search terms related to ABI. Diagnosis codes are derived from the International Statistical Classification of Diseases and Related Health Problems (ICD-codes). The computer-based search strategy included the following terms: minor head injury, traumatic brain injury, concussion, skull/brain trauma, neurological trauma, epilepsy, brain tumour, stroke, infections (meningitis/encephalitis), post anoxia, ADEM (acute disseminated encephalo myelitis), MS (multiple sclerosis) or acute CNS (central nervous system) demyelinating disease and hypoxia-ischemia were labelled as NTBI. Participants were excluded if they were diagnosed with trauma capitis (minor head injury without brain symptoms).

The two year follow-up study was approved by the Medical Ethical Committee (METC) of the Erasmus University Medical Centre Rotterdam (METC-2009-440). All parents and patients, as required by law from 18 years, participating in the follow-up assessment gave written informed consent.

Participants

For the lager study patients were selected from the registries of the participating hospitals using the clinical diagnosis as mentioned above. Inclusion criteria for the follow-up study were: age at onset ABI (3-21 years) and parents' ability to understand and complete questionnaires in Dutch. Of all patients participating in the larger study, the age of onset, gender, type and severity were extracted from the medical records.

To select patients for the follow-up study the total group of participants was categorized by age (up to 14 years>older than 14 years), type of injury (TBI and NTBI) and severity of injury (mild-moderate/severe) (Figure 1) .

The patients in the stratified samples for 2008 and 2009 were invited, about 2 years (Figure 1) after onset of ABI, to participate in the study by sending the Patient Information Letter. Non responders were followed up after 2 weeks by a telephone call. After receiving the Patient Informed Consent an 'appointment assessment' was made for a consecutive neurological (60 min) and neuropsychological (60 min) screening. All neuropsychological testing was done according to the standard procedures for assessment. Parents also filled in the Dutch version of the BIA, a questionnaire about the cognitive and social emotional functioning of the child and give this to the neuropsychologist or returned it by post. Data were collected by two neuropsychologists under supervision of the principal investigator. Participants received a written report with results of the screening, integrated by the medical specialist. Participants were invited for a consult at the rehabilitation medical specialist if indicated by scores on medical and neuropsychological measures.

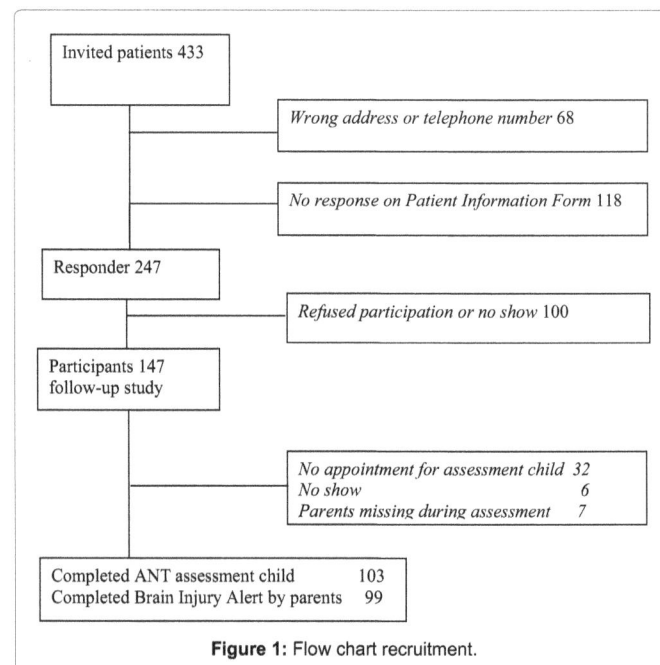

Figure 1: Flow chart recruitment.

Instruments

Neuropsychological measures

Cognitive functioning was measured with the Amsterdamse Neuropsychologische Tasks (ANT) program [36-38]. The ANT was found to be suitable to detect neuropsychological dysfunctions in patients with leukemia after chemotherapy and psychiatric conditions commonly associated with attention deficit disorders and behavior problems [39-42]. The ANT program evaluates various aspects of cognitive functioning. For this study the following two neuropsychological tests from the ANT were administered: Baseline Speed (BS) (test of attention) and Shifting Attentional Set – Visual (SSV) (test of response inhibition and flexibility), in order to screen most often occurring neuropsychological consequences of pediatric ABI [3,14,18,26,27].

1. Baseline Speed (BS), a test of attention (alertness) and speed (reaction time) involving minimal cognitive effort. The participant is required to press a mouse-key as quickly as possible when a fixation cross in the center of the computer screen changes into a white square (n=32 trials for left and right hand each). Main outcome parameters are the mean reaction time (in milli seconds, ms) of the dominant hand and the within-subject standard deviation of the reaction time (i.e., response speed stability) [43,44].

2. Shifting Attentional Set - Visual (SSV), a test of attentional flexibility, an important aspect of executive functioning. A colored square moves randomly to the right or to the left on a horizontal bar that is permanently present on the computer screen. The task consists of three parts. Depending on the color of the square, compatible responses (copying, part 1), or incompatible responses (mirroring, part 2) are required, by pressing the mouse-key on the same side as the direction of movement of the square (part 1), or on the side opposite to the direction of movement of the square (part 2). In these parts, the stimulus–response (SR) compatibility is fixed (either spatially compatible or incompatible). The incompatible condition requires inhibition of pre-potent responses. During part 3, the color of the moving square varies randomly, requiring attentional flexibility by continuously having to adjust response type (compatible/incompatible). It is expected that the incompatible (mirroring) responses will be executed slower than the compatible (copying) responses and that the reaction time in the third part of the task will be higher than those of part 1 and 2 because shifting attentional flexibility can be obtained by calculating the mean RT differences between compatible trials in the third part and compatible trials of the first part of the task with higher values indicating more difficulties with shifting attention. Discrepancy in reaction time (in ms) and accuracy (percentage/number of errors) between the third part and the first part of the task (flexibility) and of the second part and the first part (inhibition) were the outcome parameters and were included in statistical analyses [44,45]. Over the years, thousands of healthy children,adolescents, adults and elderly people were tested with the ANT. Based on these data nonlinear regression equations were derived by the reaction time/number of errors and the associated standard deviations described as a function of age. With these functions, the norm values with associated standard deviations, in an uninterrupted continuum age were published [36].

Questionaire

Parents were requested to administer the Brain Injury Alert (BIA). The Brian Injury Alert (BIA) was developed as a multidimensional screening tool, meant as a supportive aid in the clinical interview, of cognitive domains as well as of emotional and social consequences of paediatric TBI. The BIA was found to be a valid and reliable outcome measure in paediatric ABI [46,47].

The BIA consists of 10 items covering the cognitive domain and 9 covering the emotional and social domain. Each item contains a description of the problem in terms of "the child has difficulty with" illustrated with at least three examples of functioning in daily life. For each item the presence (scoring 1 or 0, respectively) can be indicated and the severity is scored (e.g. yes, the problem is present and it interferes with the development of the child; yes, the problem is present and but is not interfering with the development of the child; the problem is not present; or not sure whether there is an actual problem and there is some doubt. The leading rule for all items is that "the child has difficulty with… compared to age mates." For the purpose of this study both domains were included and the scores were dichotomized as 1 (problem present; either interference with development or not) and 0 (problem absent, either not present or doubtful). The results are presented as numbers (percentages) of problems present at this moment.

Statistical Analyses

All statistical analysis was conducted with SPSS 21.0 [48]. Participants were divided in groups according to age group (≤ 14 y vs. >14 y), type (TBI vs. NTBI) and severity (mild vs moderate/severe) of injury as independent variables. Dependent variables were a) Results of the Brain Injury Alert, reported in numbers and percentages; b) ANT measures of accuracy (error rate: misses+false alarms), information processing speed (reaction time of correct responses: mean of reaction time hits and reaction time correct rejections), and performance stability (SD of reaction time correct), reported in Z-scores. ANT-scores rangd of ≤ 1 SD below the mean (better performance), mean performance ≤ 1 Z>1 to ≥ 1 SD above the mean (worse performance) [38]. P-values were calculated with independent t-test, to compare the differences between subgroups.

Results

One hundred and three (103) participants completed the ANT assessment and 99 parents filled in the complete BI alert. They were part of a larger cross-sectional two-year follow-up study on outcome of ABI. Comparisons between participants in this follow-up study (n=147) and all invited patients (n=433) showed no significant differences regarding the distribution in age groups and types of injury. The number of BIA is lower, because some young adults arrived at the assessments without parents or did not give Informed Consent for administration of questionnaires by their parents.Comparisons between participants in the follow-up study (n=147) and all invited patients (n=433) showed no significant differences regarding the distribution in age groups and types of injury. The number of BIA is lower, because some young adults arrived at the assessments without parents or did not give Informed Consent for administration of questionnaires by their parents (Table 1).

Table 1 shows the characteristics of the 103 included participants with ABI and their parents. In the TBI group (78% of participants) the severity ratio mild versus moderate/severe was 78:22. In the NTBI group (22%) the severity ratio mild versus moderate/severe was 86:12, of 2 (2%) participants data about severity were missing in the medical file. In the total ABI group 23 cases (22%) reported pre-injury health problems versus 36 cases (35%) with health problems 2 years after onset of ABI. Parents reported a low educational level in 12 cases (12%) versus intermediate in 40 (39%) and high in 43 (42%) cases. Being a single parent household was reported by 30 (30%) parents (Table 2).

Table 2 shows the scores of the cohort on the 2 ANT tasks. Regarding Processing Speed age (older group>younger group), type (NTBI>TBI) and severity (moderate/severe>TBI) consistently determined worse results compared to the norm group without neurocognitive deficits. Between subgroups per category significant differences were found in type (NTBI<TBI) on reaction time and stability and in age (older<younger) on stability. In Attentional flexibility age (older group), type (NTBI) consistently determined worse speed (time) and accuracy (more errors) compared to the norm group without neurocognitive deficits. Between subgroups per category significant differences were found in age (older<younger) in required time. The cohort scored consistently better on accuracy (less errors) compared to the norm group without neurocognitive deficits, but needed more time (except for the younger group). Between subgroups per category significant differences were found in Inhibition time for age (older < younger) (Table 3)

Table 3 shows that between 49 and 87.3% of the group scored within 1 SD compared to the norm group without neurocognitive problems. On the Attentional tasks the study cohort responded relatively more accurate and slow. A significant proportion of the sampled population scored ≥ 1 SD above the mean (worse performance) compared to the norm group (Table 4).

On the BIA (see Table 4) 1 or more cognitive problems were reported by 62 (65%) of the parents, 1 or more social emotional problems by 66 (69%) and 1 or more cognitive and social emotional problem by 70 (77%). A higher percentage of parents endorsed cognitive, social emotional or cognitive and social emotional problems associated with age group (young>old), type (NTBI>TBI) and severity (moderate/severe>mild) of injury.

Discussion and Conclusion

Approximately 2 years after onset of ABI neurocognitive problems were assessed in a cohort of children and youth with a hospital-based diagnosis of ABI, aged 4 up to 20 years at onset of ABI, using the Amsterdamse Neuropsychological Tasks (ANT) and the parent reported Brain Injury Alert (BIA).

The cohort responded relatively more accurate and slow compared to the norm group without neurocognitive deficits. Scores on the ANT task Processing Speed varied strongly compared to the norm group

	Values N (%)	Missing values n (%)
Socio-demographic characteristics		
Age at onset in years; median (range)		0
≤ 14 y	60. (58.3)	
>14 y	43 (41.7)	
Gender		0
Boys	58 (56.3)	
Girls	45 (43.7)	
Type of injury		0
TBI total; number (% of total ABI)	80 (86.4)	
NTBI total; number (% of total ABI)	23 (22.3)	
Severity of injury[1]		2 (1.9)
Mild	89 (86,4)	
Moderate/severe	12 (11.7)	
Pre-injury problems in physical		5 (4.9)
or mental health	23 (22.3)	
Actual problems in physical		3 (2.9)
or mental health	36 (35.0)	
Educational level of parents; number (%)		8 (7.8)
Low[2]	12 (11.7)	
Intermediate	40 (38.8)	
High	43 (41.7)	
Single parent household; number (%)	30 (29.1)	7 (6.8)

y=years; TBI=Traumatic Brain Injury; NTBI=Non Traumatic Brain Injury
[1] Severity of TBI determined by means of the Glasgow Coma Scale (GCS) at hospital admission, severity of NTBI determined by means of a disability scale based on the Modified Rankin Scale (mRS) at hospital discharge
[2] Low (pre-vocational practical education or less), intermediate (pre-vocational theoretical education and upper secondary vocational education) or high (secondary education, higher education and/or university level education)

Table 1: Characteristics of the patients with acquired brain injury and their parents.

		Age group			Type of injury			Severity of injury		
		≤ 14 y n=59	>14y n=44	p	TBI n=80	NTBI n=23	p	Mild n=89	moderate/severe n=12	p
Processing Speed [3]	Simple reaction time M (SD)	-0.07[4] (1.58)	0.08 (1.09)	**0.04**	-0.19 (0.98)	0.63 (2.22)	**0.01**	-0.06 (1.44)	0.36 (1.01)	0.68
	Stability time M (SD)	-0.04 (1.15)	0.41 (0.89)	0.59	0.00 (0.80)	0.67 (1.63)	**0.01**	-0.12 (1.09)	0.26 (0.91)	0.34
Attention [5]	Flexibility time M (SD)	-0.45 (1.8)	0.76 (1.61)	**0.00**	-0.07 (1.67)	0.51 (2.25)	0.19	-0.08 (1.90)	-0.16 (1.31)	0.66
	Flexibility errors	-0.39 (2.3)	0.54 (4.28)	0.16	-0.14 (3.24)	0.54 (3.56)	0.39	-0.05 (3.51)	0.29 (1.72)	0.75
	Inhibition time M (SD)	-0.10 (1.23)	1.44 (1.63)	**0.00**	0.49 (1.67)	0.78 (1.33)	0.44	0.63 (1.66)	-0.01 (1.12)	0.20
	Inhibition errors	-0.10 (2.16)	-0.38 (2.80)	0.57	-0.17 (2.56)	-0.39 (1.96)	0.70	-0.16 (2.57)	-0.64 (1.25)	0.53

[1] a z-score is a measure of how many standard deviations below or above the population mean a raw score is.
[2] p-value calculated with independent t-test, to compare the differences between the groups.
[3] ANT subtask were completed using the dominant hand; Speed is simple reaction time in ms; Stability=within subject standard deviation on different tasks;
[4] Positive score meaning slower (time) or less accurate (errors) than norm group without neurocognitive problems; negative score meaning faster (time) or more accurate (errors) than norm group without neurocognitive problems
[5] Inhibition accuracy=percentage of errors; Flexibility accuracy=percentage of errors

Table 2: Z-scores[1] on 2 subtests of the Amsterdam Neuropsychological Tasks (ANT), related to age group, type and severity of injury.

n=103	≤ 1 SD (better)	-1 SD>Z<1 SD	≥ 1 SD (worse)
Attention Simple reaction time	16 (15.7%)	69 (69.6%)	15 (14.7%)
Stability	0 (0%)	89 (87.3%)	14 (12.7%)
Attention Flexibility speed	23 (22.5%)	53 (52%)	23.5 (25.5%)
Flexibility accuracy	30 (29.4%)	51 (49%)	22 (21.6%)
Inhibition speed	14 (13.7%)	55 (51.9%)	39 (38.2%)
Inhibition accuracy	31 (30.4%)	51 (49%)	21 (20.6%)

[1] Z-score is a measure of how many standard deviations below or above the population means a raw score is. Z-scores range from -3 standard deviations (SD) (which would fall to the far left of the normal distribution curve) to +3 SD (which would fall to the far right of the normal distribution curve).

Table 3: Z-scores[1] of the total cohort on 2 subtests of the Amsterdam Neuropsychological Tasks (ANT).

	Total n=99	Age group ≤ 14 y	>14 y	Severity of injury[1] Mild	Moderate Severe	Type of injury TBI	NTBI
Cognitive problems number (%)							
0	33 (34.7)	19 (33.9)	14 (35.9)	28 (34.6)	4 (33.3)	30 (41.7)	3 (13)
1	3 (3.2)	2 (3.6)	1 (2.6)	3 (3.7)		2 (2.8)	1 (4.3)
≥ 1	62 (65.3)	37 (66.1)	25 (64.1)	53 (65.4)	8 (66.7)	42 (58.3)	20 (87)
≥ 2	59 (62.1)	35 (62.5)	24 (61.5)	50 (61.7)	8 (66.7)	40 (55.5)	19 (82.7)
Emotional or social problems							
0	29 (31.2)	13 (24.1)	16 (41.0)	26 (32.5)	2 (18.2)	24 (34.4)	5 (21.7)
1	10 (10.8)	9 (16.7)	1 (2.6)	7 (8.8)	3 (27.3)	9 (12.9)	1 (4.3)
≥ 1	66 (68.8)	41 (75.9)		54 (67.5)	9 (81.8)		18 (78.3)
≥ 2	56 (58.1)	32 (59.2)	22 (56.4)	47 (58.7)	6 (54.5)	37 (52.8)	
Total cognitive and social emotional problems							
0	21 (23.1)	9 (17.0)	12 (31.6)	18 (23.1)	2 (18.2)	18 (26.5)	3 (13)
1	7 (7.7)	6 (11.3)	1 (2.6)	6 (7.7)	1 (9.1)	6 (8.8)	1 (4.3)
≥ 1	70 (76.9)		26 (68.4)	60 (76.9)	9 (81.8)	50 (73.5)	
≥ 2	63 (69.2)	38 (71.7)	25 (65.8)	54 (69.2)	8 (72.7)	44 (64.7)	19 (82.7)

[1] Severity of TBI determined by means of the Glasgow Coma Scale (GCS) at hospital admission, severity of NTBI determined by means of a disability scale based on the Modified Rankin Scale (mRS) at hospital discharge
[2] TBI=Traumatic Brain Injury; NTBI=Non Traumatic Brain Injury

Table 4: Parent reported problems on the brain injury alert, specified for age group, type and severity of injury.

without neurocognitive problems, worse results were associated with age (older group>younger group), type (NTBI>TBI) and severity (moderate/severe>TBI), with in subgroups significant differences in type (NTBI<TBI) on reaction time and stability and in age (older<younger) on stability. On the ANT task Attentional flexibility a large variation in scores was found as well compared with the norm group, worse results were associated with age (older<younger) and type (NTBI<TBI), with in subgroups significant differences in age (older<younger) in required time.

On the Attentional tasks the study cohort responded relatively more accurate (accuracy 29.4-30.4%, >1 SD) and slow (inhibition speed 25.5-38.2%, > 1 SD) compared to the norm group without neurocognitive deficits.

One or more cognitive problems were reported by 62 (65%) of the parents on the BIA, 1 or more social emotional problems by 66 (69%) and 1 or more cognitive and social emotional problem by 70 (77%), associated with age group (young>old), type (NTBI>TBI) and severity (moderate/severe>TBI).

The 1st hypothesis of this study, that type (NTBI versus TBI) and severity (moderate/severe versus mild) of injury would be associated with worse neurocognitive outcome were both confirmed in professional assessed (ANT) and parent reported (Brain Injury Alert) results. Lower age group (versus older age group) was associated with worse neurocognitive outcome was confirmed in the parent reported (BIA)

as well, but contradicted in the neuropsychologicaly assessed (ANT) results. The 2nd hypothesis, that parents report more neurocognitive problems than professionals, was confirmed as well.

The trend in the results of this study were similar with other studies according type and severity and age as associated with neurocognitive consequences following pediatric ABI [17-19,24,25]. Early detection of these neurocognitive problems IA important to enable child-based rehabilitation, school-based assistance and parent support, critical to optimize recovery and outcome for the injured child [19].

Several limitations of our study should be noted. First, the generalizability of the results is probably limited by the small number of participants and a relatively small number of children with moderate/severe ABI and with NTBI, the latter related to the selection of the cohort. Patient recruitment was done in hospitals and not in the rehabilitation setting. Therefore, the population of in particular patients with TBI consisted predominantly of patients with mild ABI, not requiring treatment. The results are therefore not generalizable to groups of patients with ABI who are currently treated for the consequences, for example in rehabilitation. According to literature approximately 20% of children with mild TBI is hindered by consequences after 3 months and 10% after 12 months, respectively [19]. Differences with other studies may be explained by these limitations.

Moreover, the relatively high number of non-responders may indicate the presence of selection bias; however, we did not systematically record the reasons for non-participation. Some of the non-response was due to wrong addresses, and is probably random. Although response bias cannot be excluded, the characteristics of the patients participating in the present follow-up study are fairly similar to those of the larger population, which was described in a previous publication [32,33]. Nevertheless, the relatively low response resulted in an overall small sample size, which may have limited the statistical power of the study. In addition, in future research yielding subgroups with sufficient sample sizes, more advanced statistical analyses could be employed to minimize non-response bias [49].

With regard to the parent reported neurocognitive functioning we used the BIA, which has only been found to be a reliable and valid measure in pediatric TBI, but not in NTBI. However, at the time the study was designed, it was considered the best available quantitative instrument in Dutch language, providing a parent report in all diagnosis groups. As well the ANT and BIA were originally developed in the Netherlands and hardly used in international studies. Therefore, the ANT and BIA results can not be compared with results in international studies. Another limitation of the BIA is that administration required average to higher Dutch language competencies, whereas some parents (about 10%) were not native Dutch speaking. When using the BIA as an interview instead of a questionnair, especially in this group with also parent who can't speak Dutch very well, will give the opportunity to ask more detailed about the problems wich are or are not experienced.

Another limitation of our study was that we did not gather information from school. In this cohort, with relatively many children without consequences after mild TBI and 2 years after onset, we concluded to avoid embaressment of parents due to the fear for stigmatisation and labeling by the teacher.

Furthermore, neurocognitive functioning is a complex construct with numerous interwoven determinants, many of which are likely influence the outcomes of interest in this study. In this study we focused on speed of information processing and attention and analysed the results of only 2 subtests of the ANT, possibly resulting in information bias.

To overcome these shortcomings, a larger scale and longitudinal study including sufficient numbers and proportions of children with mild, moderate and severe TBI and NTBI would be needed, using recommend outcome measures and measuring in 3 perspectives (parents, school, neuropsychologist) [50].

Conclusion

Neurocognitive problems were found in this hospital-based cohort of children with ABI, especially in the older age and NTBI group, with parents reporting strikingly more problems than professionals A multi perspective screening and assessment of neurocognitive conseuences of ABI is recommended to get a more complete and ecological valid impressions of the childs' functioning, activities and participation.

Acknowledgement

We are indebted to the children, young adults and their parents that participated in this study.

We are indebted to M. Roebroeck and S.Hilberink of Erasmus University Medical Center; C. Catsman-Berrevoets of Department of Paediatric Neurology, Sophia Children's hospital, Erasmus University Medical Center, Rotterdam; E. Peeters, Department of Paediatric Neurology, Haga Hospital and Medical Center Haaglanden, The Hague and T.P.M. Vliet Vlieland of Leiden University Medical Center for their contribution to the study. Furthermore to the medical specialists S. de Bruin, Neurologist, Haga Hospital, The Hague and P. Patka, Professor of Traumatology, Erasmus Medical Centre, Rotterdam and their secretaries to enable us to access medical records. We are also indebted to R.Wierenga, MSc neuro psychology, for collection data.

This study was financially supported by the Revalidatiefonds (project number 2010029), Johanna KinderFonds (0075-1403) and Stichting Kinderrevalidatie Fonds Adriaanstichting (0075-1403).

Declaration of Interest Statement

The authors report no conflicts of interest. The authors alone are responsible for the content and writing of the paper.

References

1. Greenwald BD, Burnett DM, Miller MA (2003) Congenital and acquired brain injury. Brain injury: Epidemiology and pathophysiology. Arch Phys Med Rehabil 84: S3-S7.

2. Giustini A, Pistarini C, Pisoni C (2013) Traumatic and non-traumatic brain injury. In: Barnes MP, Good DC (eds.). Neurological Rehabilitation: Handb Clin Neurol 110: 401-409.

3. Yeates KO (2010) Traumatic brain injury. In: Yeates KO, Ris MD, Taylor HG, Pennington BF (eds.). Pediatric Neuropsychology, research theory and practice, The Guilford Press, New York.

4. Tau GZ, Peterson BS (2010) Normal development of brain circuits. Neuropsychopharmacology 35: 147-168.

5. Anderson V, Godfrey C, Rosenfeld JV, Catroppa C (2012) Predictors of cognitive function and recovery 10 years after traumatic brain injury in young children. Pediatrics 129: e254-261.

6. Jonsson CA, Catroppa C, Godfrey C, Smedler A, Anderson V (2013) Cognitive recovery and development after traumatic brain injury in childhood: A person-oriented, longitudinal study.J Neurotrama 30: 76-83.

7. Anderson V, Catroppa C (2005) Recovery of executive skills following paediatric traumatic brain injury (TBI): A 2 year follow-up. Brain Inj 19: 459-470.

8. Muscara F, Catroppa C, Anderson V (2008) The impact of injury severity on executive function 7-10 years following pediatric traumatic brain injury. Dev Neuropsychol 33: 623-636.

9. Ewing-Cobbs L, Prasad MR, Kramer L, Cox CS, Baumgartner J, et al. (2006) Late intellectual and academic outcomes following traumatic brain injury sustained during early childhood. J Neurosurg 105: 287-296.

10. Taylor HG, Swartwout MD, Yeates KO, Walz NC, Stancin T, et al. (2008) Traumatic brain injury in young children: Post-acute effects on cognitive and school readiness skills. J Int Neuropsychol Soc 14:1-12.

11. Beebe DW, Krivitzky L, Wells CT, Wade SL, Taylor HG, et al. (2007) Brief report: Parental report of sleep behaviors following moderate or severe pediatric traumatic injury. J Pediatr Psychol 32: 845-850.

12. Tonks J, Slater A, Frampton I, Wall SE, Yates P, et al. (2009) The development of emotion and empathy skills after childhood brain injury. Dev Med Child Neurol 51: 8-16.

13. Blinman TA, Houseknecht E, Snyder C, Wiebe DJ, Nance L (2009) Post-concussive symptoms in hospitalized pediatric patients after mild traumatic brain injury. J Pediatr Surg 244: 1223-1228.

14. Crowe LM, Catroppa C, Bable FE, Anderson V (2012) Intellectual, behavioral and social outcomes of accidental traumatic brain injury in early childhood. Pediatrics 129: e262-268.

15. Tham SW, Palermo TM, Vavilala MS, Wang J, Jaffe KM, et al. (2012) The longitudinal course, risk factors and impact of sleep disturbances in children with traumatic brain injury. J Neurotrauma 29: 154-161.

16. Bedell G, Coster W, Law M, Liljenquist K, Kao YC, et al. (2013) Community participation, supports and barriers of school-age children with and without disabilities. Archives of Physical Medicine and Rehabilitation 94: 315-323.

17. Anderson V, Catroppa C, Morse S, Haritou F, Rosenfeld J (2001) Outcome from mild head injury in young children: A prospective study. J Clin Exp Neuropsychol 23: 705-717.

18. Babikian T, Asarnow R (2009) Neurocognitive outcomes and recovery after pediatric TBI: Meta-analytic review of the literature. Neuropsychology 23: 283-296.

19. Anderson V, Spencer-Smith M, Wood A (2011) Do children really recover better? Neurobehavioural plasticity after early brain insult. Brain 134: 2197-221.

20. Könings M, Heij HA, van der Sluijs JA, Vermeulen RJ, Goslings JC, et al. (2015) Pediatric traumatic brain injury and attention deficit. Pediatrics 136: 534-541.

21. Tagliaferri F, Compagnone C, Korsic M, Servadei F, Kraus J (2006) A systematic review of brain injury epidemiology in Europe. Acta Neurochir (Wien) 148: 255-268.

22. Ayr LK, Yeates KO, Taylor HG, Browne M (2009) Dimensions of post-concussive symptoms in children with mild traumatic brain injuries. J Int Neuropsychol Soc 15:19-30.

23. Ornstein TJ, Max JE, Schachar R, Dennis M, Barnes M, et al. (2013) Response inhibition in children with and without ADHD after traumatic brain injury. J Neuropsychol 7: 1-11.

24. Anderson V, Catroppa C, Morse S, Haritou F, Rosenfeld J (2005) Functional plasticity or vulnerability after early brain injury? Pediatrics 116: 1374-1382.

25. Dennis M, Yeates KO, Taylor HG (2013) Brain reserve capacity, cognitive reserve capacity, and age-based functional plasticity after congenital and acquired brain injury in children. In: Stern Y (ed.,). Cognitive reserve: Theory and Applications 4: 53-83.

26. Taylor HG, Dietrich A, Nuss K, Wright M, Rusin J, et al. (2010) Post-concussive symptoms in children with mild traumatic brain injury. Neuropsychology 24: 148-159.

27. Babikian L, Satz P, Zaucha K, Light R, Lewis RS, et al. (2011) The UCLA longitudinal study of neurocognitive outcomes following mild pediatric traumatic brain injury. J Int Neuropsychol Soc 17: 886-895.

28. Ross KA, Dorris L, McMillan T (2011) A systematic review of psychological interventions to alleviate cognitive and psychosocial problems in children with acquired brain injury. Dev Med Child Neurol 53: 692-701.

29. Trenchard SO, Rust S, Bunton P (2013) A systematic review of psychosocial outcomes within 2 years of paediatric traumatic brain injury in a school-aged population. Brain Inj 27: 1217-1237.

30. van Tol E, Gorter JW, DeMatteo C, Meester-Delver A (2011) Participation outcomes for children with acquired brain injury: A narrative review. Brain Inj 25: 1279-1287.

31. Van Pelt D, De Kloet AJ, Hilberink S, Lambregts S, Peeters E, et al. (2011) The incidence of traumatic brain injury in young people in the catchment area of the University Hospital Rotterdam, The Netherlands. Eur J Paediatr Neurol 15: 519-526.

32. de Kloet AJ, Hilberink SR, Roebroeck ME, Catsman-Berrevoets CE, Peeters E, et al. (2013) Youth with acquired brain injury in The Netherlands: A multi-centre study. Brain Inj 27: 843-849.

33. De Kloet AJ, Berger MAM, Bedell GM, Catsman-Berrevoets CE, Van Markus-Doornbosch F, et al. (2015) Psychometric evaluation of the Dutch language version of the child and family follow-up survey (CFFS). Dev Neurorehabil 24:1-8.

34. Teasdale G, Jennett B (1974) Assessment of coma and impaired consciousness. A practical scale. Lancet 2: 81-84.

35. Bonita R, Beaglehole R (1988) Recovery of motor function after stroke. Stroke 19: 1497-1500.

36. De Sonneville LMJ (1999) Amsterdam Neuropsychological Tasks: A computer-aided assessment program. In Den Brinker BPLM, Beek PJ, Brand AN, Maarse SJ, Mulder LJM (eds.,). Computers in Psychology: Vol. 6. Cognitive ergonomics, clinical assessment and computer-assisted learning. Lisse: Swets and Zeitlinger, The Netherlands.

37. De Sonneville LMJ (2005) Amsterdamse Neuropsychologische Taken: Wetenschappelijke en klinische toepassingen. Tijdschrift voor neuropsychologie 27-41.

38. De Sonneville LMJ (2014) Handboek Amsterdamse Neuropsychologische Taken. Amsterdam: Boom test uitgevers.

39. Buizer AI, De Sonneville LMJ, Van den Heuvel-Eibrink MM, Njiokiktjien C, Veerman AJP (2005) Visuomotor control in survivors of childhood acute lymphoblastic leukemia treated with chemotherapy only. J Int Neuropsychol Soc 11: 554-565.

40. Kalff AC, De Sonneville LMJ, Hurks PPM, Hendriksen JGM, Kroes M, et al. (2003) Low- and high-level controlled processing in executive motor control tasks in 5-6 year old children at risk of ADHD. J Child Psychol Psychiatry 44:1049-1057.

41. Slaats-Willemse D, Swaab-Barneveld H, De Sonneville L, Buitelaar J (2005) Familial clustering of executive functioning in affected sibling pair families with ADHD. J Am Acad Child Adolesc Psychiatry 44: 385-391.

42. Brunnekreef JA, De Sonneville LMJ, Althaus M, Minderaa RB, Oldehinkel AJ, et al. (2007) Information processing profiles of internalizing and external behavior problems: Evidence from a population-based sample of pre-adolescents. Journal of Child Psychology and Psychiatry 48: 185-193.

43. Huijbregts SCJ, De Sonneville LMJ, Van Spronsen FJ, Berends IE, Licht R, et al. (2003) Motor function under lower and higher controlled processing demands in early and continuously treated Phenylketonuria. Neuropsychology 17: 369-379.

44. Daams M, Schuitema I, Van Dijk B, Van Dulmen-den Broeder E, Veerman AJP, et al. (2012) Long-term effects of cranial irradiation and intrathecal chemotherapy in treatment of childhood leukemia: A MEG study of power spectrum and correlated cognitive dysfunction. BMC Neurol 12: 84.

45. Huijbregts SCJ, De Sonneville LMJ, Licht R, Sergeant JA, Van Spronsen F (2002) Inhibition of pre-potent responding and attentional flexibility in treated phenylketonuria. Dev Neuropsychol 22: 481-499.

46. Rasquin S, Van Heugten C, Winkens I, Ritzen W, Hendriksen J, et al. (2011) Development and validity of the Brain Injury Alert (BI Alert) screening tool for cognitive, emotional and social problems after paediatric acquired brain injury. Brain Injury 25: 777-786.

47. Van Heugten C, Rasquin S, Winkens I, Ritzen W (2009) De Brain Injury Alert: een signaleringsinstrument voor de onzichtbare gevolgen van verworven hersenletsel bij kinderen en jongeren. Revalidata 31: 2-5.

48. IBM SPSS Statistics for Windows (2012) Version 21.0. Armonk, New York: IBM Corp.

49. Little RJA (1993) Pattern-mixture models for multivariate incomplete data. Journal of the American Statistical Association 421: 125-134.

50. McCauley S, Wilde EA, Anderson VA, Bedell G, Beers SR, et al. (2012) Recommendations for the use of common outcome measures in pediatric traumatic brain injury research. J Neurotrauma 29: 678-705.

27

Obesity and Psychiatric Disorders in a Sample of Obese Candidates for Bariatric Surgery in Campania Region

Micanti F, Pecoraro G, Mosca P, Riccio F and Galletta D
Department of Psychiatry, Universita degli Studi di Napoli Federico II Naples, Italy

Abstract

Introduction: Obesity is now considered as pandemic. 40% of Italian population is overweight or obese. Many studies emphasize the association of obesity with mental disorders specifically depressive and anxiety disorders, substance use disorder, personality disorder. It has to be distinguished from the mental dimensions: impulsivity, mood, anxiety and body image connected to the emotional regulation system producing eating behaviors. Obesity subjects differ in eating behaviors: gorging, snacking, sweeteating, grazing and binge that are characterised by different level of psychopathology. Mental disorders are also associated to eating behaviors. Bariatric surgery is considered gold standard therapy for obesity. However, follow-up studies underline that the association obesity-mental disorders determines weight loss failure.

Methods: 2205 obese subjects underwent psychiatric assessment before bariatric surgery. Patients were divided into two groups as result of psychiatric assessment: 1392 obese subjects without association with mental disorders and 813 with mental disorders. These last (mean age 37,63 SD ± 12,07; 181 M, 632 W; mean body mass index (BMI), 45,16 SD ± 12,14) were enrolled in this study. Every patient underwent psychiatric evaluation. The absence of mental disorders was considered an exclusion criteria.

Results: In our sample, Binge Eating Disorder (BED) and Night Eating Syndrome (NES) have the major prevalence. General Anxiety Disorder (GAD) and Major Depressive Disorder (MDD) are also related to obesity. Educational level, in our sample, does not influence in a significant way the mental disorders. Age does not change the psychopathological frame.

Conclusion: This study emphasizes that the association between obesity and mental disorders is high among bariatric surgery candidates of our region. The relationship with eating behaviors is connected to the general features of the mental disorders but is not yet clear the reciprocal influences nor why some obese subjects suffer from both and some others does not.

Keywords: Obesity; Mental disorder; Psychopathology; Bariatric surgery; Weight loss

Introduction

Obesity is now considered as pandemic. All over the world obesity rates have increased. In Italy, the obesity adult rate is not so different from other European countries (approximately 10% of population). In 2014, Organization for Economic Co-operation and Development (OECD) study underlines that 40% of Italian population is overweight or obese and this data is consistent with the European rates. However, childhood obesity rates are considered one of the highest (36% for boys and 34% for girls) [1]. In addition, World Health Organization (WHO) projections forewarn that by 2030 disease prevalence rate will nearly double for the Italian community [2]. Obesity is a multifactorial chronic disease determined by genetic, metabolic and psychological factors. The obesity mental field is formed by the relationship between mental dimensions: impulsivity, mood, anxiety and body image connected to the emotional regulation system producing eating behaviors. Obesity subjects differ in eating behaviors: gorging, snacking, sweeteating, grazing and binge that are characterised by different levels of psychopathology related to the mental dimensions and the emotional regulation system [3-8]. The disorder of the mental dimensions should not be confused with the association of obesity with mental disorders. In this instance, obesity is a comorbidity and the relationship can be considered bi-directional. Many studies emphasize the association of obesity with mental disorders specifically depressive and anxiety disorders, substance use disorder and personality disorder connected to dysregulation of biological pathways [9,10]. Moreover, socio-economical and culture factors can be mediators between obesity and mental disorders. Depression and obesity have been well studied and researchers recognized a bi-directional pathway consequence of the interrelationship of brain anatomy and neuromodulation [11,12]. The association with anxiety disorders is more variable and not well

clarified even if obese females have a higher percentage than obese males [10]. Associations with bipolar disorder, psychosis, eating disorders: Binge Eating Disorder (BED) and Night Eating Syndrome (NES) are also described. The overall analysis of the literature highlights the relationship with mental disorders but it does not consider their relationship with eating behaviors that can worsen obesity or determine it. Obesity is a high cost and risk disease in time. Thus it is very important to apply preventing programs beginning with primary health care. Prevention is related to the primary ability to recognize every mental condition that can worsen or be determined by obesity [13]. Bariatric surgery is now the gold standard therapy for obesity and metabolic disease particularly for diabetes type 2. However, the American and European International guide lines, recognizing the importance of psychiatric/psychological factors contributing to obesity, stress the importance of a careful assessment before bariatric surgery [14,15]. Many mental disorders determine weight regain in short and long term or worsen after surgery [16,17]. This study shows the results of a sample of obese patients living in Campania, a region in the South of Italy, and stresses the prevalence of different mental disorders and their relationship with eating behaviors, considering each of them according to data literature and methods.

*Corresponding author: Micanti F, Department of Psychiatry, Universita degli Studi di Napoli Federico II Naples, Italy, E-mail: micanti@unina.it

The aim of this study is: 1) to describe the association and the prevalence of mental disorders and obesity in our sample; 2) to describe the association with eating behaviors demonstrating that they have different psychopathological traits related also to the specific mental disorders 3) to emphasize the importance of recognizing mental disorders which can determine failure in treatment of obesity surgery.

Materials and Methods

Recruitment

From January 2009 to December 2016, 2205 obese subjects underwent psychiatric assessment before bariatric surgery. The assessment is part of the multidisciplinary program for obesity treatment at Naples School of Medicine "Federico II" Department of Psychiatry: Eating Disorders and Obesity Unit. This Unit is a reference centre for psychiatric/psychological assessment before bariatric surgery of five bariatric surgery units with the highest numbers of operations in Campania region . These centres are Bariatric surgery General Surgery Department School of Medicine "Federico II", S.Giovanni Bosco Hospital, Cardarelli Hospital, General Surgery Department Second University of Naples. They are also reference centres for other regions in the South of Italy such as Molise, Calabria and Puglia.

813 obese outpatients (mean age 37,63 SD ± 12,07; 181 M, 632 W; mean body mass index (BMI), 45,16 SD ± 12,14) suffering from obesity and mental disorders were enrolled in this study. They were included after the psychiatric examination indicating the association

	SAMPLE pts. 813
SEX	
F	632 (77,73%)
M	181 (22,27%)
AGE, mean (SD)	37,63 (±12,07)
BMI, mean (SD)	45,16 (±12,14)
Educational level	
Low level	
F	371 (58,72%)
M	86 (47,45%)
Middle level	
F	224 (35,36%)
M	80 (44,44%)
High level	
F	37 (5,9%)
M	15 (8,1%)

Table 1: Demographic characteristics of the sample.

Mental Disorders	(%)
BED	24,1
NES	13,53
GAD	36,77
MDD	13,76
IND	4,42
PSYD	3,93
BD	4,54
BLPD	2,09
SUD	1,84
OTHERS	4,89

Table 2: Mental disorders prevalence (%) of the sample.

BED: Binge Eating Disorder; NES: Night Eating Syndrome; GAD: Generalized Anxiety Disorder; MDD: Major Depressive Disorder; IND: Insomnia Disorder; PSYD: Psychotic Disorder; BD: Bipolar Disorder; BLPD: Borderline Personality Disorder; SUD: Substance Use Disorder; OTHERS: Obsessive-compulsive disorder, Epilepsy, Post-traumatic stress disorder, Dementia, Personality disorder

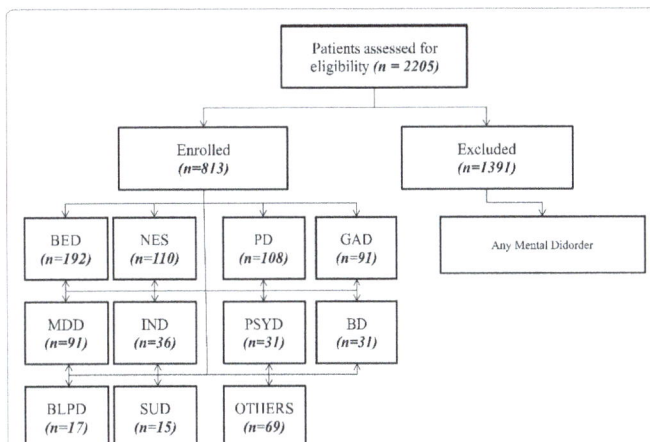

Figure 1: Recruitment flow chart.
BED: Binge Eating Disorder; NES: Night Eating Syndrome; GAD: Generalized Anxiety Disorder; MDD: Major Depressive Disorder; IND: Insomnia Disorder; PSYD: Psychotic Disorder; BD: Bipolar Disorder; BLPD: Borderline Personality Disorder; SUD: Substance Use Disorder; OTHERS: Obsessive-compulsive disorder, Epilepsy, Post-traumatic stress disorder, Dementia, Personality disorder

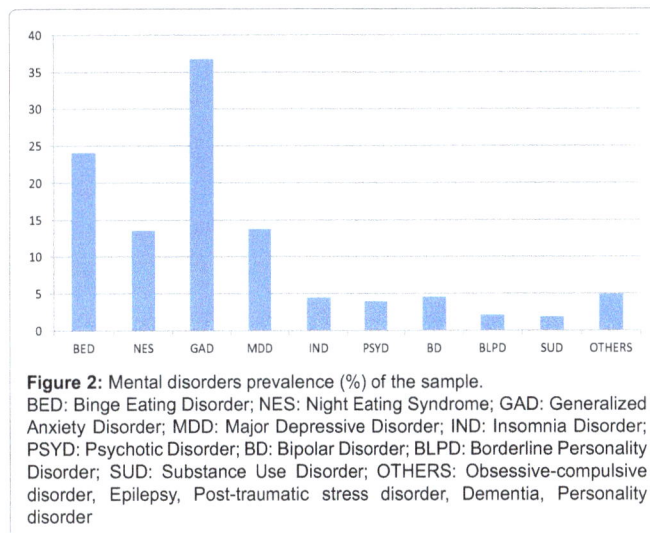

Figure 2: Mental disorders prevalence (%) of the sample.
BED: Binge Eating Disorder; NES: Night Eating Syndrome; GAD: Generalized Anxiety Disorder; MDD: Major Depressive Disorder; IND: Insomnia Disorder; PSYD: Psychotic Disorder; BD: Bipolar Disorder; BLPD: Borderline Personality Disorder; SUD: Substance Use Disorder; OTHERS: Obsessive-compulsive disorder, Epilepsy, Post-traumatic stress disorder, Dementia, Personality disorder

of obesity with mental disorders recognised by using the Diagnostic and Statistical Manual of Mental Disorders DSM 5 [18]. 1391 patients without psychiatric comorbidities were excluded from this study. All participants signed a written consent form before entering the study (Tables 1 and 2, Figures 1 and 2).

Demographic characteristics are shown in Table 1. Mean Body mass Index (BMI) was calculated on the whole sample, not considering each type of mental disorder because BMI is not yet considered a factor that can interfere with the severity of mental disorders. Type and prevalence of mental disorders are described in Table 2.

Every patient underwent psychiatric evaluation, which consisted of

1. Psychiatric examination to include or exclude mental disorders according to the DSM-5. It was performed to consider: patient's mood, level of anxiety, thought content and process, perception and cognition; investigation of the patient's trauma history; past psychiatric treatments (type, duration, and, where applicable,

doses); adherence to past and current pharmacological psychiatric treatments; response to possible past psychiatric treatments according to American Psychiatric Association (APA) guidelines statement for psychiatric evaluation of the mental state [19].

2. Structured eating interview based on the cognitive-behavioral model of Garner and Dalle Grave to identify the eating behaviours in gorging, snacking, sweeteating, grazing and binge created by Dalle Grave in Italian language [20].

3. Psychometric tools performed by rating scales validated in Italian language after the psychiatric examination for reinforcing the diagnosis. These were:

Beck Depression Inventory-II is one of the most widely psychometric tools to assess depression and its severity [21,22]. It was used for Major Depressive Disorders (MDD)

State Trait Anxiety Inventory (Form Y) for General Anxiety Disorders. It measures one's conscious awareness at two extremes of anxiety affect. Higher STAI scores suggest higher levels of anxiety [23].

Barratt Impulsiveness Scale (BIS-11) assesses the personality/behavioral construct of impulsiveness. It is the most widely cited instrument for the assessment of impulsiveness and has been used to advance our understanding of this construct [24-26].

Binge Eating Scale (BES) assesses the presence of binge eating behavior [27,28]. These latter scales were used to assess Binge Eating Disorder (BED) and binge behavior of the other mental disorders described herein.

Association of mental disorders with the prevalent eating behavior is established for each of them to investigate the type of relationship between mental disorder and eating behavior based on psychopathological traits. The study is a prevalence study.

Results

Mental disorders prevalence in our sample is described in Table 2. General Anxiety Disorder (GAD) and Binge Eating Disorder (BED) have the major prevalence. Data analysis shows that if we consider the prevalence of Night Eating Syndrome (NES), Eating Disorders are the most prevalent mental disorders among our sample of patients. Major Depressive Disorder (MDD) is also represented in a high percentage.

	Binge	Gorging	Snacking	Sweeteating	Grazing	Nocturnal eating
BED	100,00%	0,00%	0,00%	0,00%	0,00%	0,00%
NES	0,00%	0,00%	0,00%	0,00%	0,00%	100,00%
GAD	27,09%	39,46%	6,69%	9,36%	13,38%	4,01%
MDD	24,11%	33,04%	4,46%	7,14%	25,00%	6,25%
IND	19,44%	13,88%	8,33%	22,22%	13,88%	22,22%
PSYD	46,88%	28,13%	3,13%	6,25%	6,25%	9,38%
BD	43,24%	8,11%	8,11%	21,62%	13,51%	5,41%
BLPD	76,47%	17,64%	0,00%	0,00%	0,00%	5,88%
SUD	66,66%	0,00%	0,00%	0,00%	13,33%	20,00%
OTHERS	25,00%	12,50%	12,50%	30,00%	12,50%	7,50%

Table 3: Prevalence of eating behaviors of each mental disorder.

BED: Binge Eating Disorder; NES: Night Eating Syndrome; GAD: Generalized Anxiety Disorder; MDD: Major Depressive Disorder; IND: Insomnia Disorder; PSYD: Psychotic Disorder; BD: Bipolar Disorder; BLPD: Borderline Personality Disorder; SUD: Substance Use Disorder; OTHERS: Obsessive-compulsive disorder, Epilepsy, Post-traumatic stress disorder, Dementia, Personality disorder

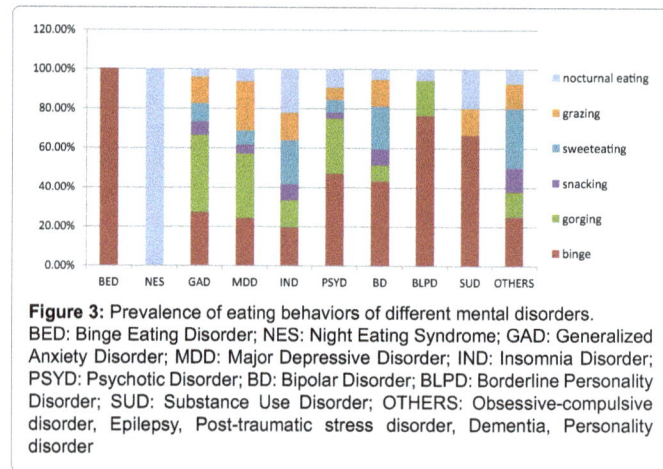

Figure 3: Prevalence of eating behaviors of different mental disorders. BED: Binge Eating Disorder; NES: Night Eating Syndrome; GAD: Generalized Anxiety Disorder; MDD: Major Depressive Disorder; IND: Insomnia Disorder; PSYD: Psychotic Disorder; BD: Bipolar Disorder; BLPD: Borderline Personality Disorder; SUD: Substance Use Disorder; OTHERS: Obsessive-compulsive disorder, Epilepsy, Post-traumatic stress disorder, Dementia, Personality disorder

Educational level, in our sample, does not have any significant influence on the mental disorders (Table 3 and Figure 3). Age does not change the psychopathological frame also because the elderly sample is not significant (Mean age 37,63 SD ± 12,07). The prevalence of eating behaviors associated to each mental disorder are described in Table 3. Data analysis shows that binge behavior is typical according to DSM 5 of Binge eating disorder but is also the most frequent behavior in patients suffering from Psychotic Disorder (PsyD), Bipolar Disorder (BPD), Borderline Personality Disorder (BlPD) and Substance Use Disorder (SUD). Gorging behavior is associated to General Anxiety Disorder (GAD) and Major Depressive Disorder (MDD) and it is totally absent in Substance Use Disorder. Grazing behavior is associated to MDD, Insomnia Disorder and Bipolar Disorder. Sweeteating is related to Insomnia Disorder and Bipolar Disorder. Nocturnal Eating is prevalent in Night Eating syndrome, Insomnia Disorders and Substance Use Disorder.

Discussion

Factors determining obesity are widely discussed in the scientific community. They are related to culture, emotional, metabolic and neurobiological aspects. Analysis of the studies show many controversial and different positions in the evaluation of the importance of environmental factors. One of these is the relationship with educational level. Some studies underline the importance of it on obesity development [29,30]. In our sample, the educational level does not have statistical significance probably because the prevalent status is of low educational level. This data is consistent with obesity distribution rate among the Campania population which indicates a major prevalence in the low cultural inhabitants.

General features and the association with eating behaviors are discussed in the following sections for each mental disorder.

Binge eating disorder: BED

Many studies underline the major frequency of BED in bariatric surgery population [31-34]. Its rate is increasing among obese and overweight population even if it is not related to BMI determining physical effects that lead to high socio-economic impact. DSM 5 included BED among the eating disorders describe binge as the marker symptom [30,35]. BED has a disorder of all mental dimensions concerning obesity: impulsivity, body image, mood and anxiety [7,36,37]. Impulsivity disorder is the most studied and researchers debate on the relation between BED and Impulse Control Disorders or the addictive disorders even if binge behavior is similar but not equal to craving [38-40]. In our sample, BED has the high prevalence (23,6%). Binge behavior is the only eating behavior according to DSM 5. In our experience, often BED is not recognized and is hidden by obesity. The screening for bariatric surgery that we adopted which stress the psychopathological traits allow us to establish specific psychiatric treatment before bariatric surgery. BED patients do not undergo bariatric surgery and begin psychiatric treatments, generally psychotherapy and psychopharmacology according to bariatric surgery follow-up studies that emphasize frequent weight regain in the long term [41].

Night eating syndrome: NES

NES is defined as an Eating Disorder characterized by "a dysfunction of circadian rhythms with a disassociation between eating and sleeping. Core criteria include a daily pattern of eating with a significantly increased intake in the evening and/or night time" [42-45]. Currently, many studies underline the prevalence of food intake at night related to specific cultural habits of every country [46,47]. Data analysis of our sample shows that: 1)NES has a prevalence of 13,53% among the mental disorders and nocturnal eating is the diagnostic marker. However, daily anorexia is not present and other eating behaviors are associated during the day, especially daily binge [44,45,48].The meaning of these data should be investigated to better understand the psychopathological features of NES. Bariatric surgery follow-up studies stress failure in weight loss in the long term related to high levels of impulsivity [49-51].

Generalized anxiety disorder: GAD

In our sample General Anxiety Disorder (GAD) has the higher prevalence among the mental disorders. Our study shows a prevalence in the female group compared to the male group in accordance with the study data [51-53]. The specific factors producing this association are not well defined. Some studies emphasize the role of psychological distress related to a negative judgment of the environment, feelings of exclusion typical to obese patients that can increase anxiety leading to Panic Disorder [54,55]. In our sample, the relationship with eating behavior shows a prevalence of binge, grazing and nocturnal eating which are all considered maladaptive behaviors. Data analysis lead us to hypothesize that personality trait anxiety can be a risk for developing GAD and its subtypes in obese populations and that eating behavior can act as a mediator. The prevalence of gorging behavior in our sample can be related to GAD, which determines hyperphagia and consequent obesity. Further studies on the relationship between GAD and obesity could explain if there is, like MDD, a bi-directional relationship between anxiety-obesity and obesity-anxiety. Moreover GAD is considered a risk for bariatric surgery. Many studies stress that it can worsen after surgery determining an increase of the symptoms and failure of weight loss [56-58].

Major depressive disorders: MDD

In our sample, the association between obesity and major depressive disorders (MDD) has a high prevalence. The causes of this finding is not yet clear. According with literature studies our sample also shows a bi-directional relationship obesity-depression and depression-obesity [59-61]. The analysis of the specific sample highlight that many patients assumed antidepressant therapy at the time of psychiatric evaluation and the effects on weight gain of SSRI antidepressant drugs as side effects are well known. However many studies emphasize that depression symptoms can influence the development of obesity over time especially feelings of sadness, emptiness, hopelessness, reduction of activities for most of the day or every day [59]. In our sample, the mean BDI-II score is 25,4 which points out the presence of depression. On the other hand, metabolic syndrome and the increase of adiposity which is typical in obese patients, determines the development of inflammatory processes and the consequent alteration of brain function [61-63]. Obesity also occurs as a consequence of the high caloric intake determined by maladaptive eating behaviors, such as in our sample binge and grazing [48,64,65].The association with grazing could be explained by the disorder of mood and anxiety that characterizes this behavior [7]. Further studies on psychopathological features must be done to clarify the meaning and the effects of grazing. Gorging and snacking eating behaviors seem to be a consequence of depression, reinforcing the depression-obesity pathway more than obesity-depression. In our sample, almost half of patients had SSRI + Benzodiazepine treatment for more than a year at our psychiatric assessment contributing to overeating and obesity. The association of binge or grazing behavior with depression is predictive of weight gain in the long term after bariatric surgery. International and Italian guidelines stress the necessity of depression treatment before surgery to avoid the worsening of symptoms and to prevent weight regain [14,15,65].

Insomnia disorder: IND

In our sample, Insomnia Disorder is one of the most frequent. In our experience this is provoked by physical impairment such as Sleep Apnea and mental factors related to neuroendocrine facets and anxiety structure. Moreover, insomnia contributes to obesity provoking psychosocial impairment and a reduction of physical activity [66-69]. In our sample, IND is predominantly associated with maladaptive eating behaviors particularly grazing and sweet-eating. We hypothesize that anxiety that is a facet of grazing behavior can interfere with the quality and quantity of sleep. Sweeteating, according to studies improves insulin resistance and determines short sleep through the alteration of Gut axis and neuroendocrine connections. We consider the association with Binge behavior as a symptom of other mental disorders that by themselves can produce IND. Sleep features must be investigated within the psychiatric assessment before bariatric surgery and treatment must be placed before the patient undergoes the operation.

Bipolar disorder and psychotic disorder: BD and PsyD

BD an PsyD are jointly discussed because the overall mechanism determining obesity and the influence of these diseases on obesity seems to be the same according to the overall analysis of the studies. Bipolar and psychotic patients have a high rate of obesity. This association has many related factors such as genetic, metabolic and treatment dependent factors [70-74].

In our sample, BD patients have binge as prevalent eating behaviors, but all maladaptive behaviors such as grazing and sweeteating are also significant. This finding leads us to think that obesity can be also the consequence of high caloric food-intake. The association with binge behavior is also explained by the high levels of impulsivity of BD particularly of maniac phase. BD is characterized by the disinhibition of impulse control and also by the dysregulation of the hunger/satiety system [75]. Similarly, the association with grazing and sweeteating which are considered maladaptive behaviors is related to the dysregulation of impulse control and belongs to Loss of Control (LOC) spectrum. Thus, eating behaviors can be considered symptoms of BD psychopathology. The same mechanisms can be described for Psychotic Disorders. Binge as a symptom of BD must be recognized above all in bariatric surgery candidates. Surgery is not able to determine weight loss. Follow-up studies show that BD patients do not achieve weight loss because they can't cope with post-operation program and because drug treatments on their own have an obesogenic side effect. Particularly patients suffering from psychotic disorders have a major cognitive impairment and are not able to follow the bariatric surgery post-operation program. This condition affects the choice of malabsorptive type of operation which can determine physical effects related to malnutrition and reduces the absorption of the specific drugs determining less control of BD and PsyD positive symptoms after surgery [76,77].

Borderline personality disorder: BPD

Borderline personality disorder (BPD) is a serious mental disorder marked by a pattern of ongoing instability in moods, behavior, self-image, and functioning. These experiences often result in impulsive actions and unstable relationships. The definition of Borderline underlines the link with addiction traits and this explains the prevalent association with binge behavior which we found in our sample. Binge is related to Impulse Control Disorder and addiction by neurobiological and emotional links as many studies underline [32,38,78]. Impulsive disorder is frequent in borderline patients and also in this case binge leads to obesity and the worsening of mental health. In our sample, the eating behaviors related to Borderline are binge and gorging. These data underline that binge is related to the incidence of impulse disorder. The presence of gorging, considered an eating behavior with low psychopathology, shows that a dysregulation of hunger/satiety system exists [7]. Further studies should investigate the relationship between obesity and BPD. Bariatric surgery must be chosen carefully above all for reduction of drug levels consequence of malabsorption and cannot be effective in patients with binge behavior.

Substance use disorder: SUD

Substance Use Disorder does not have a high prevalence in our study but the association with binge behavior or in general with all maladaptive eating behavior lead us to think about the relationship with craving and the disorder of the food-reward system. This result is according with the studies even if does not clarify the mechanism of this association [79-82]. Further studies could investigate the brain connection and the alteration of the regulation system. In our sample, SUD is related to binge, grazing and nocturnal eating. The association with binge and the others maladaptive eating behaviors characterized by medium impulsivity (grazing) and alteration of the food-reward system (nocturnal eating) could be considered as the expression of the same brain functioning related to addiction. The psychological analysis stresses the inability to stop using substances or food, low self-esteem, the necessity to escape from the social functions considered by patients as a continuous demonstration of their inability determining negative judgment and refusal by the environment. Bariatric surgery guidelines and follow-up studies show that patient suffering from SUD have a high risk of worsening after the operation and failure in weight loss.

Conclusion

This study emphasizes that the association between obesity and mental disorders is high among bariatric surgery candidates of our region. The relationship with eating behaviors is connected to the general features and to the alterations of brain functions of the mental disorders examined.

Limits

One limits of this study is that it does not present results that can

elucidate the quality of the relationship between mental disorders and eating behaviors on the basis of brain alteration. Further studies on the quality of mental dimensions concerning obesity and the relationship with brain function can be useful for a better understanding of the psychopathological mechanisms conducting to the association between mental disorders and obesity. Moreover this study does not show results based on retrospective analysis. It describes observational data.

References

1. OECD Reports obesity and the economics of prevention: Fit not Fat (2014) Obesity Update © OECD.

2. World Obesity Federation (2015) World map of obesity.

3. Gade H, Rosenvinge JH, Hjelmesæth J, Friborg O (2014) Psychological correlates to dysfunctional eating patterns among morbidly obese patients accepted for bariatric surgery. Obes Facts 7:111–119.

4. Gianini LM, White MA, Masheb RM (2013) Eating pathology, emotion regulation and emotional overeating in obese adults with binge eating disorder. Eat Behav 14: 309–313.

5. Noel C, Dando R (2015) The effect of emotional state on taste perception. Appetite 95: 89-95.

6. Ziauddeen H, Farooqi IS, Fletcher PC (2012) Obesity and the brain: How convincing is the addiction model? Nat Rev Neurosci 13: 279-286.

7. Micanti F, Iasevoli F, Cucciniello C, Costabile R, Loiarro G, et al (2016) The relationship between emotional regulation and eating behaviour: A multidimensional analysis of obesity psychopathology. Eat Weight Disord 2:1-11.

8. Van Strien T, Cebolla A, Etchemendy E, Gutiérrez-Maldonadod J, Ferrer-Garcíad M, et al (2013) Emotional eating and food intake after sadness and joy. Appetite 66: 20-25.

9. Lopresti AL, Drummond PD (2013) Obesity and psychiatric disorders: Commonalities in dysregulated biological pathways and their implications for treatment. Prog Neuropsychopharmacol Biol Psychiatry 45: 92-99.

10. Scott KM, Bruffaerts R, Simon GE, Alonso J, Angermeyer M, et al (2008) Obesity and mental disorders in the general population: Results from the world mental health surveys. I J Obes 32: 192–200.

11. Kivimaki M, Batty GD, Singh-Manoux A, Nabi H, Sabia S, et al (2009) Association between common mental disorder and obesity over the adult life course. Br J Psychiatry 195: 149–155.

12. Lin HY, Huang CK, Tai CM, Lin HY, Kao YH, et al (2013) Psychiatric disorders of patients seeking obesity treatment. BMC Psychiatry 13:1.

13. Livhits M, Mercado C, Yermilov I, Parikh JA, Dutson E, et al (2012) Preoperative predictors of weight loss following bariatric surgery: Systematic review. Obes Surg 22:70-89.

14. Mechanick JI, Youdim A, Jones DB, Garvey TW, Hurley DL, et al (2013) Clinical practice guidelines for the perioperative nutritional, metabolic and nonsurgical support of the bariatric surgery patient-2013 update: cosponsored by American Association of Clinical Endocrinologists, the Obesity Society and American Society for Metabolic and Bariatric Surgery. Surg Obes Relat Dis 19:337-372.

15. Fried M, Yumuk V, Oppert JM, Scopinaro N, Torres AJ, et al (2014) Interdisciplinary European guidelines on metabolic and bariatric surgery. Obes Surg 24: 42–55.

16. Yen YC, Huang CK, Tai CM (2014) Psychiatric aspects of bariatric surgery. Curr Opin Psychiatry 27: 374-379.

17. Müller A, Mitchell JE, Sondag C, de Zwaan M (2013) Psychiatric aspects of bariatric surgery. Curr Psychiatry Rep 15: 397.

18. American Psychiatric Association (2013) Diagnostic and statistical manual of mental disorders, DSM-5, 5th edn.

19. American Psychiatric Publishing, Arlington, VA; American Psychiatric Association (2016) The American psychiatric association practice guidelines for the psychiatric evaluation of adults. American Psychiatric Publishing, Arlington, VA.

20. Dalle Grave R (2001) Terapia cognitivo comportamentale dell'obesità. Verona Positive Press, Verona 249: 260.

21. Beck AT, Steer RA (1993) Manual for the beck depression inventory. Psychological Corporation San Antonio, TX.

22. Hayden MJ, Brown WA, Brennan L, O' Brien PE (2012) Validity of the Beck Depression Inventory as a screening tool for a clinical mood disorder in bariatric surgery candidates. Obes Surg 22:1666–1675.

23. Spielberger CD (1983) State: trait anxiety inventory form Y. Mind Garden Inc., Palo Alto, CA.

24. Patton JH, Stanford MS, Barratt ES (1995) Factor structure of the Barratt impulsiveness scale. J Clin Psychol 51: 768-774.

25. Vasconcelos AG, Malloy-Diniz L, Correa H (2012) Systematic review of psychometric properties of Barratt Impulsiveness Scale Version 11 (BIS-11). Clin Neuropsychiatry 9: 61-74.

26. Spinella M (2007) Normative data and a short form of the Barratt impulsiveness scale. Int J Neurosci 117:359-368.

27. Gormally J, Black S, Daston S, Rardin D (1982) The assessment of binge eating severity among obese persons. Addict Behav 7:981–989.

28. Grupski AE, Hood MM, Hall BJ, Azarbad L, Fitzpatrick SL, et al (2013) Examining the binge eating scale in screening for binge eating disorder in bariatric surgery candidates. Obes Surg 23:1–6.

29. Cohen AK, Rai M, Rehkopf DH, Abrams B (2013) Educational attainment and obesity: A systematic review. Obes Rev 14: 989–1005.

30. Devaux M (2011) Exploring the relationship between education and obesity. OECD Journal: Economic Studies vol.2011/1.

31. Amianto F, Ottone L, Abbate Daga G, Fassino S (2015) Binge eating disorder diagnosis and treatment: A recap in front of DSM5. BMC Psychiatry 15: 70.

32. Mitchell JE, King WC, Courcoulas A, Dakin G, Elder K, et al (2015) Eating behaviour and eating disorders in adults before bariatric surgery. Int J Eat Disord 48: 215-222.

33. Opolski M, Chur-Hansen A, Wittert G (2015) The eating related behaviours, disorders and expectations of candidates for bariatric surgery. Clin Obes 5:165–197.

34. Meany G, Conceição E, Mitchell JE (2014) Binge eating, binge eating disorder and loss of control eating: Effects on weight outcomes after bariatric surgery. Eur Eat Disord Rev 22: 87-91.

35. Kessler RM, Hutson PH, Herman BK, Potenza MN (2016) The neurobiological basis of binge-eating disorder. Neurosci Biobehav Rev 63: 223-238.

36. Grilo CM, White MA, Gueorguieva R, Wilson GT, Masheb RM (2013) Predictive significance of the overvaluation of shape/weight in obese patients with binge eating disorder: Findings from a randomized controlled trial with 12 month follow-up. Psychol Med 43: 1335-1344.

37. Elfhag K, Morey L (2008) Personality traits and eating behavior in the obese: Poor self-control in emotional and external eating but personality assets in restrained eating. Eat Behav 9: 285-293.

38. Micanti F, Pecoraro G, Costabile R, Loiarro G, Galletta D (2016) An explorative analysis of binge eating disorder impulsivity among obese candidates to bariatric surgery. J Addict Res Ther 7: 302.

39. Schulte EM, Grilo CM, Gearhardt AN (2016) Shared and unique mechanisms underlying binge eating disorder and addictive disorders. Clin Psychol Rev 44:125-139.

40. Schmidt F, Körber S, de Zwaan M, Müller A (2012) Impulse control disorders in obese patients. Eur Eat Disord Rev 20:144-1447.

41. Grilo CM, Masheb RM, Wilson GT, Gueorguieva R, White MA (2011) Cognitive-behavioral therapy, behavioral weight loss, and sequential treatment for obese patients with binge eating disorder: A randomized controlled trial. J Consult Clin Psychol 79: 675–685.

42. Cleator J, Abbott J, Judd P, Sutton C, Wilding JPH (2012) Night eating syndrome: Implications for severe obesity. Nutrition and Diabetes 2:44.

43. Gallant AR, Lundgren J, Drapeau V (2012) The night-eating syndrome and obesity. Obes Rev 13:528-536.

44. Meule A, Brahler E, Allison KC, de Zwann M (2014) The association between night eating syndrome and body mass depends on age. Eat Behav 15: 683-685.

45. Stunkard AJ, Grace WJ, Wolff HG (1955) The night-eating syndrome; a pattern of food intake among certain obese patients. Am J Med 19: 78-86.

46. Allison KC, Lundgren JD, O'Reardon JP, Geliebter A, Gluck ME, et al (2010) Proposed diagnostic criteria for night eating syndrome. Int J Eat Disord 43: 241-247.

47. Fischer S, Meyer AH, Hermann E, Tuch A, Munsch S (2012) Night eating syndrome in young adults: Delineation from other eating disorders and clinical significance. Psychiatry Res 200: 494-501.

48. Colles SL, Dixon JB, O'Brien PE (2007) Night eating syndrome and nocturnal snacking: Association with obesity, binge eating and psychological distress. Int J Obes 31:1722-1730.

49. Royal S, Wnuk S, Warwick K, Hawa R, Sockalingam S (2015) Night eating and loss of control over eating in bariatric surgery candidates. J Clin Psychol Med Settings 22:14-19.

50. Vinai P, Ferri R, Anelli M, Ferini-Strambi L, Zucconi M, et al (2014) New data on psychological traits and sleep profiles of patients affected by nocturnal eating. Sleep Med 16: 6.

51. de Zwaan M, Marschollek M, Allison KC (2015) The night eating syndrome (NES) in bariatric surgery patients. Eur Eat Disord Rev 23: 426-443.

52. Zhao G, Ford ES, Dhingra S, Li C, Strine TW, et al (2009) Depression and anxiety among US adults: Associations with body mass index. I J. Obes 33: 257–266.

53. Petry NM, Barry D, Pietrzak RH, Wagner JA (2008) Overweight and obesity are associated with psychiatric disorders: results from the National Epidemiologic Survey on Alcohol and Related Conditions. Psychosom Med 70: 288-297.

54. Gariepy G, Nitka D, Schmitz N (2010) The association between obesity and anxiety disorders in the population: A systematic review and meta-analysis. I J Obes 34: 407–419.

55. Lykouras L, Michopoulos J (2011) Anxiety disorders and obesity. Psychiatriki 22: 307-313.

56. de Zwaan M, Enderle J, Wagner S, Mühlhans B, Ditzen B, et al (2011) Anxiety and depression in bariatric surgery patients: A prospective, follow-up study using structured clinical interviews. J Affect Disord 133: 61-68.

57. Brunault P, Jacobi D, Miknius V, Bourbao-Tournois C, Huten N, et al (2012) High preoperative depression, phobic anxiety and binge eating scores and low medium-term. Psychosomatics 53: 363-370.

58. Legenbauer T, De Zwaan M, Benecke A, Muhlhans B, Petrak F, et al (2009) Depression and anxiety: Their predictive function for weight loss in obese individuals. Obes Facts 2: 227-234.

59. Luppino FS, de Wit LM, Bouvy PF, Stijnen T, Cuijpers P, et al (2010) Overweight, obesity and depression. Arch Gen Psychiatry 67: 220-229.

60. Faith MS, Matz PE, Jorge MA (2002) Obesity-depression associations in the population. J Psychosom Res 53: 935-942.

61. Atlantis E, Baker M (2008) Obesity effects on depression: Systematic review of epidemiological studies. Int J Obes (Lond) 32: 881-891.

62. Capuron L, Lasselin J, Castanon N (2017) Role of adiposity-driven inflammation in depressive morbidity. Neuropsychopharmacology Rev 42:115–128.

63. Dunbar JA, Reddy P, Davis-Lameloise N, Philpot B, Laatikainen T, et al (2008) Depression: An important comorbidity with metabolic syndrome in a general population. Diabetes Care 31: 2368–2373.

64. Pearl RL, White M A, Grilo CM (2014) Weight bias internalization, depression and self-reported health among overweight binge eating disorder patients. Obesity 22: E142–E148.

65. Fandiñoa J, Moreiraa RO, Preisslerb C, Gayab CW, Papelbauma M, et al (2010) Impact of binge eating disorder in the psychopathological profile of obese women. Comp Psychiatry 51:110-114.

66. Crönlein T (2016) Insomnia and obesity. Curr Opin Psychiatry 29: 409-412.

67. Hargens TA, Kaleth AS, Edwards ES, Butner KL (2013) Association between sleep disorders, obesity and exercise: A review. Nat Sci Sleep 5: 27-35.

68. Beccuti G, Pannain S (2011) Sleep and obesity. Curr Opin Clin Nutr Metab Care 14: 402–412.

69. Garaulet M, Ordovas JM (2013) Chronobiology and Obesity. Springer ed.

70. McElroy SL, Keck PEJr (2012) Obesity in bipolar disorder: An overview. Curr Psychiatry Rep 14: 650-658.

71. Goldstein BI, Liub SM, Zivkovic N, Schaffer A, Lung-Chang Chien LC, et al (2011) The burden of obesity among adults with bipolar disorder in the United States. Bipolar Disord 13: 387-395.

72. Bak M, Fransen AM, Janssen J, van Os J, Drukker M (2014) Almost all antipsychotics result in weight gain: A meta-analysis. PLoS ONE 9: 94112.

73. Correll CU, Detraux J, De Lepeleire J, De Hert M (2015) Effects of antipsychotics, antidepressants and mood stabilizers on risk for physical diseases in people with schizophrenia, depression and bipolar disorder. World Psychiatry 14:119-136.

74. Riordan HJ, Antonini P, Murphy MF (2011) Atypical antipsychotics and metabolic syndrome in patients with schizophrenia: Risk factors, monitoring and healthcare implications. Am Health Drug Benefits 4: 292-302.

75. Bernstein EE, Nierenberg AA, Deckersbach T, Sylvia LG (2015) Eating behavior and obesity in bipolar disorder. Aust N Z J Psychiatry 49: 566-572.

76. Brietzke E, Lafer B (2011) Long-acting injectable risperidone in a bipolar patient submitted to bariatric surgery and intolerant to conventional mood stabilizers. Psychiatry Clin Neurosci 65: 205.

77. Yogaratnam J, Biswas N, Vadivel R, Jacob R (2013) Metabolic complications of schizophrenia and antipsychotic medications-an updated review. East Asian Arch Psychiatry 23: 21-28.

78. Kessler RM, Hutson PH, Herman BK, Potenza MN (2016) The neurobiological basis of binge-eating disorder. Neurosci Biobehav R 63: 223-238.

79. Mitchell MR, Potenza MN (2014) Recent insights into the neurobiology of impulsivity. Curr Addict Rep 1: 309-319.

80. McIntyre RS, McElroy SL, Konarski JZ, Soczynska JK, Bottas A, et al (2007) Substance use disorders and overweight/obesity in bipolar I disorder: Preliminary evidence for competing addictions. J Clin Psychiatry 68:1352-1357.

81. Pelchat ML (2009) Food addiction in humans. J Nutr 139: 620-622.

82. Saules KK, Wiedemann A, Ivezaj V, Hopper JA, Foster-Hartsfield J, et al (2010) Bariatric surgery history among substance abuse treatment patients: Prevalence and associated features. Surg Obes Relat Dis 6: 615-621.

28

Organizational Commitment and its Predictors among Nurses Working in Jimma University Specialized Teaching Hospital, Southwest Ethiopia

Israel B[1]*, Kifle W[2], Tigist D[3] and Fantahun W[4]

[1]Department of Nursing, Faculty of Health Sciences, Jimma University, Ethiopia
[2]Department of Epidemiology, Faculty of Health Sciences, Jimma University, Ethiopia
[3]Department of Nursing, Faculty of Health Sciences, Jimma University, Ethiopia
[4]Specialized Teaching Hospital, Jimma University, Ethiopia

Abstract

Background: The idea of organizational commitment has intuitive appeal because of the relationship of commitment to turnover, absenteeism, and organizational performance. All of these are important to healthcare executives who are attempting to stabilize a nursing workforce in the presence of a growing nursing shortage.

Objective: The objective of the study was to determine the level of organizational commitment of nurses and its predictors among Jimma University specialized teaching hospital nurses, Southwest Ethiopia.

Methods: Institution based cross-sectional study design was conducted in Jimma University Specialized Teaching Hospital from March 2 to March 18, 2016 and systematic sampling technique was used to select a total of 242 study subjects. Data were collected using self-administered questionnaire and entered to Epi data version 3.1 and analyzed using SPSS version 16 software. One-way analysis of variance, independent sample T-tests and Multivariable linear regression analysis was conducted to identify predictors of organizational commitment and significance was checked at $p<0.05$.

Results: The respondents mean score of organizational commitment was 70.45 ± 8.22 and only 72 (32.9%) of the nurses score high level of organizational commitment. The independent t-test and One-way analysis of variance result revealed educational status and working ward were significantly associated with organizational commitment. The multivariable linear regression showed that perceived organizational support (ß=0.482, p<0.001), interpersonal relationship (ß=0.303, p=0.008), job satisfaction (ß=0.059, p=0.027), transformational leadership behavior (ß=0.165, p<0.001), educational qualification (ß=-1.860, p=0.02) and working ward (ß=-0.585, p=0.018) were significant predictors of organizational commitment among nurses.

Conclusion: The organizational commitment levels of nurses were low. Job satisfaction, perceived organizational support, transformational leadership behavior, interpersonal relationship, and working in ICU and OR are significant predictors of organizational commitment.

Recommendation: Human Resource Management, CEO and Nursing Leaders of JUSTH shall participate nurses in managerial decision making, using improved communication skills and give appreciation for their contributions to the organization.

Keywords: Institutional/facility; Commitment; Jimma; Nurse

Introduction

Background

Organizational commitment is defined as "the relative strength of an individual's identification with and involvement in a particular organization" [1]. Others described as employee's belief in the goals of the organization and determination to remain a part of the organization [2]. It is further conceptualized by the following three factors: "a) a strong belief in and acceptance of the organization's goals and values; b) a willingness to exert considerable effort on behalf of the organization; c) a definite desire to maintain organizational membership". It could also be referred to as the extent to which an employee develops an attachment and feels a sense of allegiance to his or her employer [3].

As cited by Mullins [4], committed employees in any organization must possess three major characteristics: sense of belonging to the organization, sense of excitement in the job and confidence in management leadership. One of the challenges facing modern organization involves maintaining employee commitment in the current working environment [5,6]. Studies have reported that nurses were more content with their work if they were committed to the believes, values and practices in the organization [7,8]. However, they are uncomfortable with job satisfaction, perceived organizational support, transformational leadership behavior and level of education [9].

Health service delivery is affected by human resources, service delivery system and infrastructures and cannot function effectively without sufficient, skilled, motivated and supported in health system performance [10,11].

Nowadays, in hospitals Nurses, are the largest group of professionals and that carry out the overall hospital activities, play an important role in determining the quality and cost of healthcare in their organizations' performance [12,13]. Nursing shortage is a major problem in the healthcare setting throughout the world and it is b/c of high turnover rate in the healthcare industry and this is significantly related with organizational commitment of nurses [14]. Researches on staff nurses suggested that organizational commitment indirectly influences turnover through its direct effect on antecedents of turnover, such as intent to leave [15,16]. Contemporary studies have continued

*Corresponding author: Israel B, Department of Nursing, Faculty of Health Sciences, Jimma University, Ethiopia, E-mail: israel.bekele90@gmail.com

to report a statistically significant relationship between organizational commitment and turnover behaviors in staff nurse populations [17].

In order to deal with nurses' turnover, most of the healthcare organizations increase the recruitment and retain nurses to maintain adequate staffing. Although increasing recruitment of nurses may help to offset the problem of nursing shortage in the short term, retaining them may be the best strategy in the long term because a healthcare objective is to maintain high quality of care at reduced costs. Among the factors that contributed to high retention, organizational commitment has been found as an antecedent [18-20].

Nurses enumerated different major factors that contribute to their commitment to the organization: perceived organizational support, transformational leadership behavior, relationships and interaction opportunities for learning, job satisfaction, a plan to retire from the organization, monetary benefits, patient care, co-workers, cultural factors, and job security, were related with level of organizational commitment [2,21,22].

There is a lack of research specifically related to level of organizational commitment and factors that predict nurses' commitment to the organization in Ethiopia. This study addresses this gap by identifying predictors of organizational commitment among staff nurses. It is also important for other researchers as a base who wants to investigate in different health institutions. This research might also offer managers insight into strategies for practices to improve nurse's organizational commitment, staff retention, job satisfaction, and performance.

The outcomes of this assessment would help to Jimma University, JUSTH administrators, and FMOH in drafting policies and guiding principles of nursing leadership in Ethiopia as well as for nursing leaders and staff nurses in providing information to confirm their organizational commitment and to examine factors associated with it. The objective of this study is to assess organizational commitment and its predictors among nurses working in Jimma University Specialized Teaching Hospital, southwest Ethiopia from March 2 to March 18 (Figure 1).

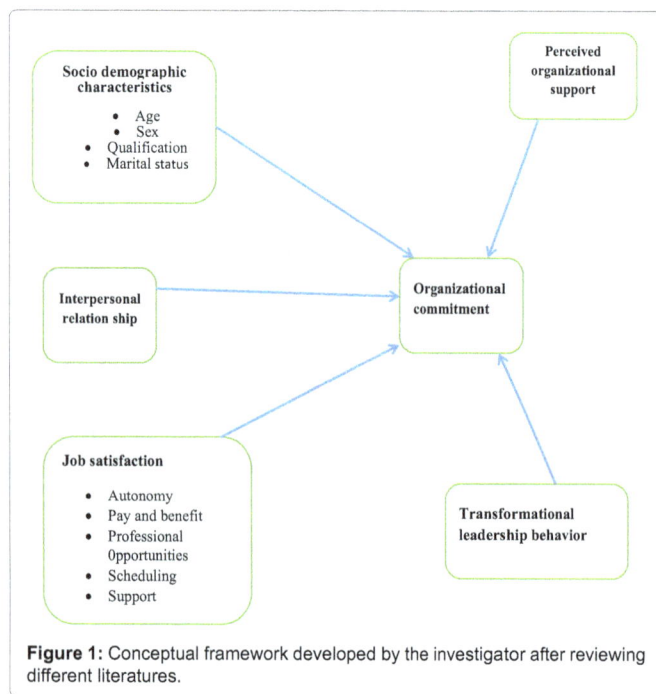

Figure 1: Conceptual framework developed by the investigator after reviewing different literatures.

Methods and Materials

The study was conducted in JUSTH, Jimma, Oromia Regional state from March 2-March 18, 2016. Jimma is the town of Jimma zone which is one of 18 zone of the Oromia Regional State found at 352 km from Addis Ababa, the capital city of Ethiopia, in the South western part of the country. There are two public hospitals found in the town which are called JUSTH and Shenen gibe hospital.

Jimma University specialized teaching hospital is one of the oldest public hospitals in the country. Geographically, it is located in Jimma city 352 km southwest of Addis Ababa. Currently it is the only teaching and referral hospital in the southwestern part of the country, providing services for approximately 15000 inpatient, 160000 outpatient attendants,11000 emergency cases, and 4500 deliveries in a year coming to the hospital from the catchment population of about15 million people.

Jimma university specialized teaching hospital is committed to reduce morbidity, mortality, disability and improve health status of the local people through providing a compressive package of high quality curative, preventive, promotive and rehabilitative health service to the public and providing clinical education to the next physicians, nurses, medical laboratory technologists, pharmacists and other clinical and public health students in collaboration with respective stakeholders [23].

It has a total of 1448 servants from which 861 are technical staffs and the remaining 587 are supportive staffs. From the technical staffs 242 physicians, 497 nurses, 45 midwives, 53 pharmacist, 48 laboratory technologist, 7 psychiatric nurses, 5 ophthalmic nurses, 2 dental nurses, 8 radiographer and the remaining 4 are M.Sc. Nurses professionals.

Facility based cross-sectional study design was employed. Sample size was determined using single population estimation formula with assumption of 95% confidence interval, 5% and considering the 50% proportion. Considering non-response rate of 10%, final total sample sizes was 242 and simple random sampling technique using lottery method was employed.

All Nurses who are served for six months or more in the hospitals at the time of the study and willing to participate was included and who were not available during data collection time due to Annual leave, maternal leave and sick leave were excluded.

Data collection procedures

To collect the data, self-administered structured questionnaire was used. Some of our tools were developed after review of different literatures [24].

Instrument

The organizational commitment scales was adopted from Stephen Jaros and originally it was developed by Meyer and Allen's [25] three-component model of organizational commitment, The job satisfaction and interpersonal relationship items was adapted from and these items will be answered on a five-point Likert scale with response options ranging from 1 (very dissatisfied) to 5 (very satisfied) and the perceived organizational support items was adopted from Format for the 8-itemSurvey of Perceived Organizational Support developed by Robert and Rubin [28] and this is also on a five point liker scale and the transformational leadership behaviors items was adopted [24-29].

Data analysis procedure

Data were checked for completeness, reversely coded items were backed, edited and entered into EpiData version 3.1 and exported to SPSS version 20.00 for analysis. The data were explored using descriptive statics such as frequencies to clean data. Scatter plots, skewness and kurtosis were examined to determine the shape of the data distribution. On the basis of this information, data were determined to be fairly normally distributed, so no transformations were required but 3 items were found to be an outlier for organizational commitment score and left out of respective analysis. One-way analysis of variance (ANOVA) and independent sample T-tests were used for comparing organizational commitment scores across the categories. For descriptive purpose data driven classification was done on perceived organizational support, job satisfaction, interpersonal relationship and transformational leadership behavior score in to two (two tiles), i.e., good/poor perceived organizational support, satisfied/unsatisfied job satisfaction, good/poor interpersonal relationship and good/poor transformational leadership behavior.

Simple linear regression was done to see the independent effect of predictors on the dependent variables and multiple linear regression analysis was conducted to identify final predictors of organizational commitment after controlling other independent variables. Variables $p \le 0.25$ in simple linear regression were entered in the final model. Participant's characteristics, perceived organizational support, job satisfaction, interpersonal relationship and transformational leadership behavior were entered independently.

Finally, variables with $P \le 0.05$ were assumed to be statistically significant. The assumptions in linear regressions (linearity, normality and multicollinearity) were checked.

Data quality assurance

Five percent of the questionnaires were pre-tested in Shenen gibe Hospital to assess the reliability, clarity, sequence, consistency and understandability and the total time it takes to finish the questionnaire before the actual data collection. To check the reliability and validity of questionnaires for each category the Crohnbach alpha was employed, for organizational commitment (0.83), perceived organizational support (0.819), for job satisfaction (0.87), relationship and interaction (0.88) and transformational leadership behavior was (0.85). Then after, the necessary comments and feedbacks were incorporated in the final tool. Training was given for the data facilitators on the objectives of the study and the way of collection.

Ethical consideration

Ethical clearance and approval to conduct the research was obtained from Jimma University College of health science, Ethical Review Board. Then a letter was secured from the university to respective hospital management to gain support for the study. Prior to administering the questionnaires, the aims and objectives of the study were explained to the participants and personal consent was obtained from study participant after explaining the objective of study. They were also told that participation is voluntarily and confidentiality and anonymity will be ensured throughout the execution of the study as participants were not required to disclose personal information on the questionnaire.

Results

Socio-demographic characteristics of the study participants

Out of the 242 distributed questionnaires 222 were collected from the respondents (9 questionnaires were unfilled, 3 questionnaires were not returned and 8 questionnaires were incomplete) giving the response rate of the study to be 91.7%. 3 outliers excluded from the analysis. From the study participants, 112 (51.1%) were male and 107 (48.9%) females. The participants' age ranged from 20 to 57 years with a mean age of 26.53 ± 5.057 years. One hundred thirty two (60.3%) were single and 87 (39.7%) married.

Regarding educational qualification, 114 (52.1%) of nurses were bachelor degree holders and only 2 (0.9%) were masters. They had work experience ranging from 1 year to 33 years with a mean of 4.33 ± 4.87years and 211 (96.3%) of them worked <10 years. Their monthly salary ranges from 1254 EBR to 8000 EBR with a mean of 2648.21 ± 1132.956 EBR.

Concerning the working area 57(26%) were in medical, 56 (25.6%) in surgical 0.30 (13.7%) in gynecology and obstetrics, 28 (12.8%) in pediatrics and neonatology, 19 (8.7%) in OPD and 29 (13.2%) were working in ICU and OR (Table 1).

Level of organizational commitment among nurses

The respondents mean score of organizational commitment was 70.45 ± 8.22, ranging from (44-99). From the given organizational commitment items (based on tertiale analysis); 71 (32.4%) of the respondents scored low level of organizational commitment; value ranging from (44-66), (34.7%) of them scored moderate level of organizational commitment; value ranges from (67-73) and only 72 (32.9%) of the nurses scored high level of organizational commitment; value ranges from (74-99) (Figure 2).

From the organizational commitment scale items" I think that people these days move from company to company too often "had maximum score frequency for agree (80 times) but this organization has a great deal of personal meaning for me had a minimum frequency of strongly agree (Figure 3).

Mean score were compared between marital status, educational status and sex category using independent sample t-test in relation to the "organizational commitment scale"-i.e. a higher score indicates a higher level of organizational commitment, and the result showed that

Participant characteristics		N	%
Sex	Male	112	51.1
	Female	107	48.9
Educational qualification	Diploma	103	47
	B.Sc. degree	114	52.1
	M.Sc. degree	2	0.9
Marital status	Married	87	39.7
	Single	132	60.3
Age category	20-29	195	89
	30-39	17	7.8
	>=40	7	3.2
Working unit category	Medical	57	26.0
	Gynecology and obstetrics	30	13.7
	Surgical	56	25.6
	Pediatrics and neonatology	28	12.8
	OPD	19	8.7
	ICU and OR	29	13.2

Table 1: Distribution of participant nurses by their characteristics working in Jimma University Teaching Hospital, South West Ethiopia, March 2016 (n=219).

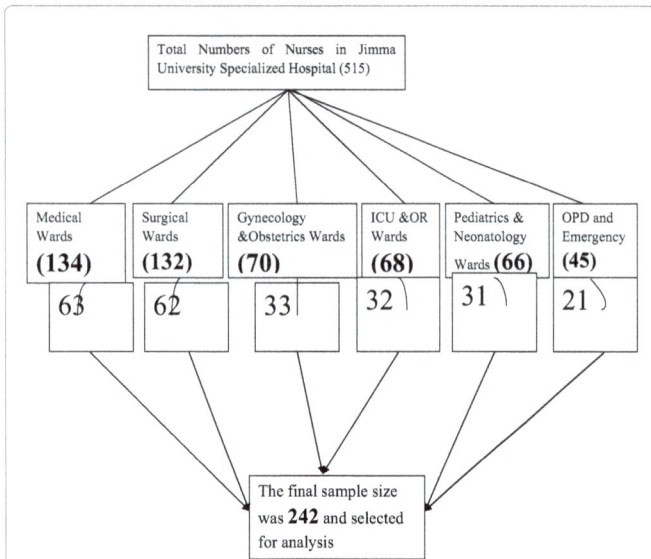

Figure 2: Flow chart of sample size.

Proportional allocation of nurses who were working in Jimma University Specialized Hospital in each wards indicated as follows in the following chart in order to gate the final sample size

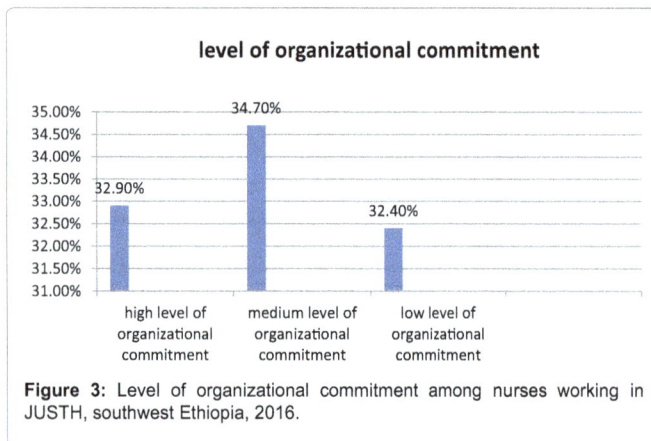

Figure 3: Level of organizational commitment among nurses working in JUSTH, southwest Ethiopia, 2016.

diploma holder mean score 72.0194 (SD=6.8599) was significantly higher than the mean of BSC degree and above holders mean score 69.0603 (SD=9.07101 at t=2.696 and p=0.008).

But, there were no significant mean difference seen between sex and marital status (Table 2).

Also mean scores were compared using one way ANOVA among different working ward groups of nurses. Organizational commitment mean score differed significantly among the six ward groups =7.726, p<0.001 (Table 3).

Associations of organizational commitment and independent factors

In the perceived organizational support assessment items 116 (53%) of the respondents fail to have good perception of organizational support. The top two factors with which the respondents strongly disagree from the perceived organizational support were "The organization really cares about my well-being "and "The organization cares about my general satisfaction at work". The top two strongly agree were" The organization fails to appreciate any extra effort from me" and "The organization takes pride in my accomplishments at work".

In job satisfaction assessment items (50.7%) of the respondents were not satisfied. The top two factors with which the respondents strongly disagree from the job satisfaction items were"

"I am satisfied with the amount of pay I receive in comparison with people in other occupations" and" I am satisfied with the degree to which I am fairly paid for what I contribute to this organization". The top very satisfied was" I am satisfied with the amount of time spent talking with my patients".

In interpersonal relationship assessment items (52.5%) of the respondents were satisfied. "I am satisfied with the relationship I have with other health-care workers" was the top to be described as very satisfied and very dissatisfied.

In transformational leadership behavior assessment items (51.6%) of the respondents were fail to have good perception of transformational leadership behavior. The top two factors with which the respondents strongly disagree from the transformational leadership behavior items were "Our immediate boss re-examines assumptions" and "rewards our

Variables category			Organizational commitment score			
Sex		N	Mean	SD	t	P
	Male	112	69.4732	9.3721	-1.825	0.69
Marital status	**Married**	87	70.2874	8.0664	-0.240	0.810
Educational status	**Diploma holders**	103	72.0194	6.8599	2.696	**0.008***

Table 2: Independent sample t-test showing the relationship between different categories of nurses and organizational commitment mean score among nurses working in Jimma University Hospital, 2016.

Variables		N	Mean	SD	F	p	95% Confidence Interval for Mean	
							Lower bound	Upper bound
Working wards	**Medical**	57	70.7895	7.2401	7.726	0.000	68.8684	72.7105
	Gynecology	30	69.9667	5.7684			67.8127	72.1206
	Surgical	56	73.4107	7.5070			71.4003	75.4211
	Pediatrics and neonatology	28	71.6786	9.56867			67.9682	75.3889
	OPD	19	71.3684	5.36667			68.7818	73.9551
	ICU and OR	29	62.7931	9.42405			59.2084	66.3778

Table 3: ANOVA table showing the relationship between working ward categories of nurses and organizational commitment mean score among nurses working in Jimma University Teaching Hospital, South West Ethiopia, 2016.

achievement". The top strongly agree was "our immediate boss has my respect" (Table 4).

Initial model of predictors of organizational commitment among nurses

Fifteen predictors (including five dummy variables) were entered independently to see their independent effect on level of organizational commitment and out of these perceived organizational support, level of job satisfaction, level of relationship and interaction, transformational leadership behavior and working in ICU and OR ward were found to have a significant association with level of organizational commitment among nurses (Table 5).

Predictors of organizational commitment among nurses

Variables with p-valve ≤ 0.25 in bivariate analysis were entered in the final model. In the model perceived organizational support, relationship and interaction, job satisfaction, transformational leadership behavior, educational status, working wards (ICU&OR and surgical ward) and salary were entered through enter method (Table 5).

	Satisfied	Unsatisfied
Jo satisfaction	49.30%	50.70%
Relationship and interaction	52.50%	47.50%
Transformational leadership behavior	48.40%	51.60%
Perceived organizational support	47%	53%

Table 4: Levels of different independent variables among nurses working in Jimma University Specialized Teaching Hospital using data driven classification, Southwest Ethiopia, 2016.

Perceived organizational support was found to have a positive association with organizational commitment and it explains slightly over 22.6% of the variance in bivariate analysis. For a unit increase in mean perceived organizational support organizational commitment score increases by .482 times at p<0.001; those nurses who have positive perceived organizational support have increased level of organizational commitment than those nurses with negative perceived organizational support.

Relationship and interaction was also shows a positive association with organizational commitment and it explains slightly over 20.7% of the variance in bivariate analysis. For a unit increase in relationship and interaction organizational commitment score increases by 0.303 times at p=0.008.Those nurses who have a good relationship and interaction have increased level of Organizational commitment than those who have not a good relationship and interaction.

Job satisfaction was also having a positive association with organizational commitment and it explains about 33% of the variance in bivariate analysis. For a unit increase in job satisfaction organizational commitment score increases by 0.059 times at p=0.027. Satisfied nurses have increased level of organizational commitment than those who were not satisfied.

Perceived Transformational leadership behaviors of managers have a positive association with organizational commitment and it explains 31.2% of the variance in bivariate analysis. For a unit increase in perceived transformational leadership behavior of managers organizational commitment score increases by 0.165 times

Model		Unstandardized Coefficients		p	95.0% Confidence Interval for B	
		B	Standard error		Lower bound	Upper bound
Perceived organizational support		0.844	0.105	0.000	0.637	1.050
Relationship and interaction		0.883	0.116	0.000	0.654	1.112
Job satisfaction		0.205	0.020	0.000	0.167	0.244
Transformational leadership behavior of managers		0.331	0.033	0.000	0.266	0.396
Age in years		0.007	0.110	0.948	-0.210	0.225
Sex	Male (ref)	1.647	1.108	0.139	-0.537	3.832
Educational status	Diploma(ref)	-2.959	1.098	0.008	-5.122	-0.796
Marital status	Married (ref)	0.273	1.138	0.810	-1.970	2.516
	Single					
Working ward/dummy variables	Medical (Ref)					
	Gynecology and obstetrics	-0.562	1.619	0.729	-3.754	2.629
	Surgical	3.975	1.248	0.002	1.516	6.434
	Pediatrics and neonatology	1.406	1.665	0.399	-1.875	4.688
	OPD	1.003	1.977	0.612	-2.894	4.901
	ICU and OR	-8.828	1.530	0.000	-11.843	-5.813
Work experience in years		0.042	0.115	0.711	-0.183	0.268
Income		0.000	0.000	0.128	-0.002	0.000

Table 5: Factors associated with organizational commitment in simple linear regression analysis among nurses working in Jimma University Teaching Hospital, South West Ethiopia, 2016.

at p<0.001.Those nurses who have positive perceived transformational leadership behavior of managers have increased level of organizational commitment than those who have negative perceptions.

Working in ICU and OR was found to have a negative association with organizational commitment; working in ICU and OR have shown to decrease mean organizational commitment by 3.62 times than working in other wards at p=0.004 (Tables 6 and 7).

Discussion

This study was carried out with the aim of determining the level of organizational commitment and its predictors among nurses. The study findings point to low level of organizational commitment among the studied nurses which is not similar as compared with findings in other studies [2,20]. Only about 72 (32.9%) of the nurses had a high level of organizational commitment. A number of factors might explain this

			Unstandardized Coefficients		Standardized Coefficients	t	Sig.	95% Confidence Interval for B	
Model			B	Std. Error	Beta			Lower Bound	Upper Bound
1	(Constant)		45.067	2.523		17.860	0.000	40.093	50.041
	Working wards	ICU and OR	-3.620	1.246	-0.150	-2.906	**0.004****	-6.076	-1.164
		Medical (ref)							
	Qualification	B.Sc. and above	-1.441	0.802	-0.088	-1.796	0.074	-3.022	0.141
		Diploma (ref)							
	Transformational leadership behavior		0.161	0.041	0.272	3.936	**0.000****	0.080	0.241
	Job satisfaction		0.058	0.026	0.162	2.200	**0.029****	0.006	0.110
	Relationship and interaction		0.291	0.112	0.151	2.602	**0.010****	0.070	0.511
	Perceived organizational support		0.462	0.096	0.263	4.798	**0.000****	0.272	0.652

Table 6: Factors associated with organizational commitment in multivariable analysis among nurses working in Jimma University Teaching Hospital, Southwest Ethiopia, 2016.
a. Dependent Variable: organizational commitment mean maximum VIF=2.368 minimum VIF=1.035
Adjusted R square=0 .498 **: significant for multivariable linear regression

Multiple Comparison							
LSD	Medical	Gynecology	0.82281	1.72636	0.634	-2.5801	4.2257
		surgical	-2.62124	1.44005	0.070	-5.4598	0.2173
		pediatrics	-0.88910	1.76629	0.615	-4.3708	2.5926
		OPD	-0.57895	2.02751	0.776	-4.5755	3.4176
		ICU and OR	7.99637*	1.74575	0.000	4.5552	11.4375
	Gynecology	Medical	-0.82281	1.72636	0.634	-4.2257	2.5801
		surgical	-3.44405*	1.73167	0.048	-6.8575	-.0306
		pediatrics	-1.71190	2.01115	0.396	-5.6762	2.2524
		OPD	-1.40175	2.24404	0.533	-5.8251	3.0216
		ICU and OR	7.17356*	1.99313	0.000	3.2448	11.1024
	Surgical	Medical	2.62124	1.44005	0.070	-.2173	5.4598
		gynecology	3.44405*	1.73167	0.058	0.0306	6.8575
		pediatrics	1.73214	1.77148	0.329	-1.7597	5.2240
		OPD	2.04229	2.03203	0.316	-1.9632	6.0478
		ICU and OR	10.61761*	1.75100	0.000	7.1661	14.0691
	Pediatrics	Medical	0.88910	1.76629	0.615	-2.5926	4.3708
		gynecology	1.71190	2.01115	0.396	-2.2524	5.6762
		surgical	-1.73214	1.77148	0.329	-5.2240	1.7597
		OPD	0.31015	2.27491	0.892	-4.1741	4.7944
		ICU and OR	8.88547*	2.02782	0.000	4.8883	12.8826
	OPD	Medical	0.57895	2.02751	0.776	-3.4176	4.5755
		gynecology	1.40175	2.24404	0.533	-3.0216	5.8251
		surgical	-2.04229	2.03203	0.316	-6.0478	1.9632
		pediatrics	-0.31015	2.27491	0.892	-4.7944	4.1741
		ICU and OR	8.57532*	2.25899	0.000	4.1225	13.0282
	ICU and OR	medical	-7.99637*	1.74575	0.000	-11.4375	-4.5552
		gynecology	-7.17356*	1.99313	0.000	-11.1024	-3.2448
		surgical	-10.61761*	1.75100	0.000	-14.0691	-7.1661
		pediatrics	-8.88547*	2.02782	0.000	-12.8826	-4.8883
		OPD	-8.57532*	2.25899	0.000	-13.0282	-4.1225

Table 7: The LSD Post Hoc test showing categories of working wards in Jimma University Specialized Teaching Hospital, 2016*.
The mean difference is significant at the 0.05 level

low level of organizational commitment. These are related to perceived organizational support, relationship and interaction, job satisfaction, perceived transformational leadership behavior and other work related factors and they are discussed in the following sections.

The result of the current study revealed low level of organizational commitment among nurses which was inconsistent with studies done in Malaysia using Meyer and Allen organizational commitment scale [25]. This discrepancy might be due to poor working environment and the attention given to nurses is low by the hospital management.

It's known that low level of organizational commitment leads to negative outcomes including increased staff turnover and decreased productivity of the organization [14,15]. It also affects retention of experienced nurses which serve the organization well and this may in turn affect the organization's objective of maintaining high quality of care at reduced costs [17-19]. In our countries 5 year health related GTP where health care organizations are required to strive to deliver quality of care and improve patient satisfaction and as a whole achieve the health related goals of the plan the importance of committed and devoted health personnel is very important. But, we cannot achieve all these goals by having nurses with low level of organizational commitment which takes the majority of health team in any health care settings.

With the increment of committed nurses to their organization, their roles will expand and as a result work environment will also change; the quality of nursing application in the hospital will increase and patient care will be enhanced. So, Jimma University Specialized Teaching Hospital may implement different strategies to increase organizational commitment among nurses.

Qualification of nurses was not a significant predictor of organizational commitment. Even if qualification is not a predictor of organizational commitment there is a significant mean difference between the two groups (BSc and above holders have lower organizational commitment score than diploma holders with p=0.008). This finding was inconsistent with that of a previous study conducted in USA and Tanzania and both stated that the nurses with higher educational levels showed a higher level of organizational commitment and the discrepancy might be no role difference between the two categories (the same job description) and this leads to BSC holders have lower scorer than diploma holders [9,13].

Working ward was a significant predictor of organizational commitment. Organizational commitment score decreases for those working in Intensive Care Unit (ICU) and Operation Theatre Room (OR) than other wards, their scores being 0.3620 times lower than those nurses working in other wards (p=0.004). This finding is consistent with that of a study conducted in Jordan that stated nurses working in ICU showed lower level of organizational commitment [30]. In our situation the benefit gained from working in ICU and OR is much less when compared to the burden they face and it might be this reason that contributes to this phenomenon.

So it is important to develop strategies that foster organizational commitment of nurses working in these highly burdened wards (units).

Perceived organizational support is another significant predictor of organizational commitment (p<0.001). The overall R square of 0.226 indicated that over 22% of the variance in organizational commitment could be explained by perceived organizational support. This result is consistent with a study conducted in Slovenia and USA showed that perceived organizational support was significant and substantial

predictor of organizational commitment explaining much of the variance in organizational commitment [2,9].The possible explanation is that, , if employees didn't feel empowered by their managers, they will likely have more negative working relationships with managers, which would be expected to negatively influence trust, increase conflict and lead to lower employee commitment toward the organization.

In the present study, there was no significant difference in organizational commitment score with nurse's age and experience which was inconsistent with the finding in Tanzania revealing both age and experience statistically significantly associated with organizational commitment. The findings of their research shows that the young (20-30 years) group nurses are more committed than the elder ones and in addition, less experienced nurses (1-10 years) showed to be more commitment [13]. The reason behind this discrepancy might be in our context the less experienced and younger nurses are always striving to get better job and they repeatedly move from one organization to the other compared to the older most of them have a family and not want to leave the organization.

The other findings from this study were transformational leadership behavior which was found to be significant predictor of organizational commitment at (p<0.001). The overall R square of 0.315 indicated that slightly over 31% of the variance in organizational commitment could be explained by transformational leadership behavior in bivariate analysis. The result of this study was consistent with researches done in Slovenia and USA which showed Significant positive correlation between organizational commitment and transformational leadership behaviors [2,9].This might be if nurses are believed that they are not treated well by their immediate leader they believe they are not part of the organization and not devote their time for the organization.

Job satisfaction was also found to be significant predictor of organizational commitment at (p=0.027).When mean job satisfaction increases by 1 unit mean organizational commitment is increased by 0.058 times. The result of this study is consistent with research done in Malaysia showing components of job satisfaction could explain 33% of variability in the organizational commitment among nurses in state hospitals of Malaysia [20]. The major reasons might be longer shift work, lack of motivation, insufficient resources and supplies, poor infrastructure, and inadequate human power.

The other finding from this study was relationship and interaction which was found to be significant predictor of organizational commitment (p<0.001). The overall R square of 0.333 indicated that over 33% of the variance in organizational commitment means score could be explained by relationship and interaction. Those nurses who have satisfied with their relationship and interaction scores 0.291 times more on organizational commitment score than from the unsatisfied ones (p=0.01) and this is consistent with the findings in Slovenia (r=0.730, p<0.001) [2].The possible explanation might be collaborative and trusting relationships with supervisors and co-workers have consistently been linked to organizational commitment specifically among nurses.

This study also showed that marital status and sex is not a predictor of organizational commitment in JUSTH, Which was consistent with the study conducted in kingdom of Saudi Arabia, showed that there was no significant relationship between organizational commitment and these two variables [12].

Limitations of the study

The finding of this study is limited to teaching hospital. Therefore the finding may not be generalized to nurses working at health centers, district hospitals and referral hospitals. There is also limitation of literature on this topic in our country because of this reason comparison of the results was done with other countries where the health institutions setup, health policy and other factors are quite different. Since it is organizational research there is also social or cultural desirable bias.

Conclusion

The results of this study indicate that the organizational commitment levels of nurses are at a low level and factors associated with this were; working wards, perceived organizational support, interpersonal relationship, job satisfaction and transformational leadership behavior. The finding of this study adds a small but essential piece to the puzzle of how to increase organizational commitment of nurses in Ethiopia.

Recommendations

Nursing director, Human Resource Personnel and CEO's of the hospital should develop various strategies to increase organizational commitment of nurses. It will be important if Human Resource Management, CEO and Nursing Leaders of JUSTH shall involve(participate) nurses in, decision-making processes and establish appropriate reward systems as such measures can result in the increment of level of commitment of nurses to the organization. The hospital management must give necessary support to nurses how they are important to this organization through close supervision, meetings and give appreciation for their contributions to the organization.

Hospital management must reform and continuously improve hospital organization through the effective use of leadership within teams and using improved communication skills. So, the hospital management should take necessary measures for the optimal provision of intrinsic and extrinsic job rewards to make their core workforce highly satisfied and committed. Further research is needed to examine the predictive ability of other variables such as empowerment on organizational commitment.

As a general recommendation; these findings indicate that leaders in Jimma University, Jimma University Specialized teaching hospital and Ministry of Health should initiate policies and encourage programs for the development of organizational commitment of nurses.

Acknowledgement

We would like to thank the followings for their contribution: Jimma University, College Health Sciences, for providing us ethical clearance; Jimma University specialized hospital , our data collectors, Study participants and others who participated directly or indirectly in this study.

References

1. Mowday RT (1998) Reflections on the study and relevance of organizational commitment. Human Resource Management Review 8: 387.

2. Mateja L, Brigita Skela-S (2014) Factors affecting nurses' organizational commitment. Obzornik Zdravstvene Nege 48: 294–301.

3. Porter LW, Steers RM, Mowday RT, Boulian PV (1974) Organizational commitment, job satisfaction, and turnover among psychiatric technicians. Int J Appl Psychol 59: 603-609.

4. Mullins LT (1999) Management and organizational behavior 5th Edn. London: Financial Times Management.

5. Harry ON, Joe-Akunne CO, Oguegbe T (2013) Job characteristics as predictors of organizational commitment among private sector workers in Anambra state Nigeria. Int J Asian Soci sci 3: 482-491.

6. Coetzee M (2005) The fairness of affirmative action: An organizational justice perspective. Faculty of Economic and Management Science in University of Pretoria etd. Chapter 5; Employee commitment 5:1-5.

7. Lichi H, Lily C, Hui C (2006) Development of an instrument for assessing factors related to nurses ' organizational commitment. Med Taiwan J Med 11: 9-19.

8. Christian U (2000) Working condition and employees commitment in indigenous private manufacturing firms in Nigeria. J Mod Afr Stud 38: 295-324.

9. Mahmoud Al-H (2009) Predictors of nurses' commitment to health care organizations. Aust J Adv Nurs.

10. Mowday R (2006) Strategies for adapting to high rate of employee turnover. Human resource management. Int J Nurs studies 39: 867-868.

11. Gilson L (2009) Developing a tool to measure health worker motivation in district hospitals in Kenya. Human Resources for Health.

12. Al-Aameri AS (2000) Job satisfaction and organizational commitment for nurses. Saudi Med J 21: 531-535.

13. Abdul Sattar K, Farooq (2015) The study of organization commitment and job satisfaction among hospital nurses: A survey of district hospitals of Dera Ismail Khan. Global Journal of Management and Business Research. Administration and Management.

14. Girma Alem G, Erdaw Tachbele B, Habtamu Abera H (2015) Assessment of factors affecting Turnover intention among nurses working at governmental health care institutions in East Gojjam, Amhara Region, Ethiopia. Am J Nurs 4: 107-112.

15. Wagner CM (2007) Organizational commitment as a predictor variable in nursing turnover research: Literature review. J adv Nurs 60: 235-247.

16. Holtom BC, O'Neill BS (2004) Job embeddedness: A theoretical foundation for developing a comprehensive nurse retention plan. J Nurs Adm 34: 216-227.

17. Laschinger HK, Purdy N, Cho J, Almost J (2006) Antecedents and consequences of nurse managers' perceptions of organizational support. Nurs Econ 24: 20-29.

18. Rhoades L, Eisenberger R (2002) Perceived organizational support: A review of the literature. J Appl Psychol 87: 698-714.

19. Zangaro GA (2001) Organizational commitment: A concept analysis. Nursing Forum 36: 14-22.

20. Siew PL, Chitpakdee B, Chontawan R (2011) Factors predicting organizational commitment among nurses in State Hospitals, Malaysia. Int med J Malaysia.

21. Ngozi IM, Ogwo Jay U (2014) How organizational commitment of critical care nurses influence their overall job satisfaction. J Nurs Educ Pract.

22. McNeese S, Donna K (2001) A nursing shortage: Building organizational commitment among nurses. J Healthc Manag.

23. www.ju.edu.et/jimma-university-specialized-hospital/wikipedia

24. Reza O (2013) Leadership style, organizational commitment and job satisfaction: A case study on high school principal in Tehran, Iran. Am J Humanity Soc Sci 1: 263-267.

25. Meyer JP, Allen NJ (1997) Commitment in the workplace: Theory, research and application. Thousand Oaks, CA; Sage Publications.

26. Agezegn A, Tefera B, Ebrahim Y (2014) Factors influencing job satisfaction and anticipated turnover among nurses in Sidama Zone Public Health Facilities, South Ethiopia. Nursing Research and Practice, Article ID 909768.

27. Murrells T, Clinton M, Robinson S (2005) Job satisfaction in nursing: Validation of a new instrument for the UK. J Nurs Manag 13: 296-311.

28. Robert E, Rubin H (1986) Perceived organizational support. J appl psychol 71: 500-507.

29. Dong I, Jung (1999) Re-examining the components of transformational and transactional leadership using the multifactor leadership questionnaire. J Occup and Org Psychol 72: 441-462.

30. Ali M, Saleh, Muhammad W, Darawad, Mahmoud Al-H (2014) Organizational commitment and work satisfaction among Jordanian nurses: A comparative study. Life Sci J 11: 31-36.

29

A Quantitative Survey on the Knowledge, Attitudes and Practices on Emergency Contraceptive Pills among Adult Female Students of a Tertiary Institution in Kaduna, Nigeria

Mohammed-Durosinlorun Amina[1]* and Krishna Regmi[2]

[1]Kaduna Polytechnic Clinic, Tudun Wada, Kaduna, Nigeria
[2]Department of Clinical Education and Leadership, University of Bedfordshire, UK

Abstract

Emergency contraception is of public health importance for preventing unintended pregnancies.

Objectives: To assess knowledge, attitude and practice of female students towards emergency contraceptive pills.

Methods: Quantitative cross-sectional survey of 220 fulltime female students of the Kaduna polytechnic, over the age of 18 years, by administering adapted questionnaires randomly.

Results: 14.6% of students had ever heard of ECP, most commonly postin or brand (54.8%) and 4.4% were aware of the correct timing of use. Majority (97.7%) had poor knowledge, poor attitude (80%) and low use (15.2%) of ECP. Bivariate analysis showed religion, "ever had sex" and use of regular contraception were associated with awareness of ECP ($p<0.05$) but not knowledge scores ($p>0.05$). Age, class level, religion, marital status, ever had sex, ever had an unintended pregnancy and ever had an abortion were associated with attitude to ECP ($p<0.05$). While marital status, ever had sex, current number of children, desired number of children, regular use of contraception, and ever had an abortion were associated with practice/use of ECP ($p<0.05$). Logistic regression showed religion to be predictor of knowledge of ECP ($p<0.05$); "ever had sex" in the past as a predictor of attitude of ECP ($p<0.05$).

Conclusion: Students had poor knowledge of ECP, poor attitude towards ECP and use of ECP was low. Increased uptake of ECP may be achieved using appropriate reproductive health messages emphasizing its benefits through healthcare professionals, teachers and peer educators.

Keywords: Contraceptive; Annual pregnancies; Progesterone

Introduction

Annually, 210 million women get pregnant, 80 million are unplanned and 46 million get aborted [1,2]. In developing countries, 76 million out of 182 million annual pregnancies are unintended [3], 66% of these among non-users of contraception. Nigeria has a youthful population [4] vulnerable to unintended pregnancies because of an early age of puberty and first intercourse, sexual activity and experimentation, multiple partners, alcohol, socio-economic problems, coercion, easier access to media that glamorizes sex, peer influence with less parental control, and they are less likely to use any form of contraception [5-7].

Unintended pregnancies pose significant public health problems, associated with higher rates of abortion and abortion related complications [1]. Especially in Nigeria where induced abortions are illegal unless medically indicated to save a mother's life, so are usually covert [1,2,8].

In Nigeria, 50% of women aged 15-49 reported unplanned pregnancies resulting in unsafe abortion in 10% [9]. An estimated 760,000 induced abortions occur annually [10] accounting for 20%-40% of maternal deaths [1,10]. Unintended pregnancies are also associated with smoking, drinking, physical abuse [6], depression [11], school dropout or disruption [12], poor antenatal attendance and obstetric outcomes, low birth weight and developmental deficits [6]. Resentment of the baby may lead to neglect [11,13-17]. Economic costs from disrupted schooling can worsen poverty due to unemployment from low level of skills, and government spends on welfare and skill acquisition programs [12]. Poverty may become a vicious cycle as offspring themselves may have unintended pregnancies, and become victims of physical abuse [13,18].

Levels of unintended pregnancies may reflect a country's state of women's reproductive rights [19,20] and worsens global population concerns on strained resources, threatening more environmental degradation and social tensions [6].

According to the WHO [21], emergency contraceptive methods offers women safe means of preventing unwanted pregnancies in event of unprotected sexual intercourse or contraceptive failure, and is a more accurate term than other synonyms. Hormonal methods of EC are mainly pills; estrogen only, combined estrogen-progesterone, progesterone only, Selective Progesterone Receptor Modulators (SPRM) such as Mifepristone (RU486) and Ulipristal Acetate (UPA). Non hormonal methods of EC include intrauterine contraceptive devices [22]. Other research drugs like anordrin, tamoxifen, danazol and misoprostol may offer no real advantage [23].

Materials and Methods

A quantitative cross-sectional survey was done of the knowledge,

*Corresponding author: Mohammed-Durosinlorun Amina, Kaduna Polytechnic Clinic, Tudun Wada, Kaduna, Nigeria, E-mail: ababdaze@yahoo.com

Attitude and Practice (KAP) of Emergency Contraceptive Pills (ECP) among selected female students of the Kaduna polytechnic, Nigeria. The Kaduna polytechnic, the largest polytechnic in Africa, South of the Sahara caters for an estimated staff and student population of 50,000. It is situated in North West zone of the country which has the lowest contraceptive rates; 3% as against the national rate of 15% and 32% in the southwest zone [24], and high mortality: estimated as 545 maternal deaths per 100,000 live births [25]. Using a national contraceptive prevalence rate of 15% from the 2008 Nigeria Demographic and Health Survey (NDHS) [24], and 10% attrition rate, the minimum required sample size was determined to be 216 using relevant statistical formulae [26].

Two- hundred and twenty full-time female students, over 18 years of age willingly participated after informed written consent.Male students, female students under 18 years, part time students or those that did not consent were excluded. The sampling frame was the most current list of students obtained from the statistics department of the polytechnic showing colleges (5), departments (40) and total number of students (13,953) segregated by level of study and sex. Levels of study for regular full-time students available at the polytechnic are national diploma one (NDI), national diploma two (ND2), higher national diploma one (HND1), higher national diploma two (HND2). There were 8,748 male students and 5,205 female students, and 220 adult female students were sampled in a multi-staged process; stratified by college, then departments' then level (class/year) of study. Simple random sampling was done in each stratum by balloting. The instrument of data collection was a piloted questionnaire adapted from previously validated studies [27-29], eliciting demographic information, and on the need for Emergency Contraception (EC), and KAP of EC.

The study anticipated minimal risks to participants; questionnaires were filled anonymously with no personal identifiers disclosed. Formal ethical approval for the study was obtained from the University of Liverpool and the Kaduna polytechnic. Data was analyzed using SPSS (version 17) computer software. Relevant descriptive and bivariate analysis was done. Levels of p<0.05 was considered statistically significant.

Results

Two- hundred and twenty questionnaires were administered and 200 retrieved, giving a response rate of 90.9%.

General and demographic characteristics of respondents (Table 1)

The mean age of respondents was 23.2 years (SD ± 3.4), with a minimum age of 18 years and maximum, 33 years. Most respondents were within the ages of 21 to 25 years and majority of students were single (151, 77.8%).

Reproductive health characteristics of respondents and need for ECP (Table 2)

Most (84.9%) of the students do not use regular contraception and 12.4% previously had an unintended pregnancy. Commonest reasons for unintended pregnancies were nonuse of contraception (34.9%) and contraceptive failure (34.9%). Similarly, 12.3% previously induced an abortion, with 35.7% of these experiencing various complications, most commonly pain and bleeding.

Characteristic	Frequency	Percent
Age (N= 197)		
<20	55	27.9
21-25	97	49.2
26-30	41	20.8
>30	4	2.0
Class level (N=200)		
National diploma (ND) 1	45	22.5
National diploma (ND) 2	88	44.0
Higher national diploma (HND) 1	32	16.0
Higher national diploma (HND) 2	35	17.5
Religion (N=194)		
Islam	112	57.7
Christianity	82	52.3
Marital status (N=194)		
Single	151	77.8
Married	43	22.2
Total	194	100

N= number or respondents

Table 1: Demographic characteristics of respondents.

Characteristic	Frequency	Percent
Ever had sex? (N=193)		
Yes	118	59.9
No	79	40.1
Current number of children (N=196)		
0	158	80.6
1-4	37	18.8
>4	1	0.5
Desired number of children (N=200)		
0	18	9.0
1-4	136	68.0
>4	46	23.0
Using regular contraception? (N=179)		
Yes	27	15.1
No	152	84.9
Ever had an unintended pregnancy (N=185)		
Yes	23	12.4
No	162	87.6
Reason for unintended pregnancy (N=43)		
Nonuse of contraception	15	34.9
Contraceptive failure	15	34.9
forced/coerced sex	1	2.3
others	12	27.9
Had an abortion? (N=187)		
Yes	23	12.3
No	164	87.7
Had complications of abortion? (N=42)		
Yes	15	35.7
No	27	63.4
Complications of abortion experienced (N=33)		
None	0	0
Pain	10	30.3
Bleeding	12	36.4
Infection	1	3.0
menstrual problems	6	18.2
infertility	0	0
others	4	12.1

N= number or respondents

Table 2: Reproductive health characteristics of respondents and need for ECP.

Knowledge, attitude and practice of emergency contraceptive pills

Only 27 students (14.6%) ever heard of ECP, mainly from friends/peers (54.2%), health personnel (41.7%), while none received information from teachers. More (75.0%) felt ECP were safe, while 25.0% felt otherwise. Students were most aware of the progesterone only (postinor) brands (63.3%), followed by combined estrogen and progesterone brands (13.6%).They were unaware of modern drugs like mifepristone and ulipristal. Most students were unaware if ECP can be gotten without prescription (78.1%). Only 6 students were aware of the correct timing of use of ECP as "within 72 hours" (4.4%). Few students had wrong beliefs about ECP causing abortion (27.9%) or future infertility (37%).

Seventy respondents (54.7%) felt that their partners would disapprove of ECP use and 45.3% felt their partners would approve. Potential barriers by 160 respondents ECP use were intolerable side effects (30%), moral/religious reasons (28.8%), ignorance (19.4%), inadequate fund (6.2%) and others (15.6%). Forty respondents (20%) had good attitude to ECP and 160 (80%) had poor attitude.

Only 27(15.2%) respondents previously used ECP and 2 (8.2%) used it within "within 72 hours". Others felt it was effective immediately only (37.5%), within 24hours (50%) and others (4.2%). All 21 respondents that used ECP found it to be effective but 14 (60.9%) experienced side effects such as menstrual abnormalities (50.3%), nausea and vomiting (29.2%), abdominal pain (8.3%) and others (12.5%).

Cross-tabulation

Bivariate analysis showed that religion , students that have "ever had sex"and use of regular contraception were significantly associated with increased awareness of ECP which can be used as a marker for knowledge (P value<0.05), while other factors were not. Muslim students (81.5%) were generally more aware than Christian students (18.5%); students that had sex before (85.2%) were more aware than students who had not (14.8%); and students that did not routinely use contraception (70.4%) were more aware than those using regular contraception (Table 3).

Several factors significantly affected attitude to ECP; age, class level, religion, marital status, ever had sex, ever had an unintended pregnancy and ever had an abortion (P value<0.05). While other factors such as current and desired number of children, and regular use of contraception did not significantly affect attitude to ECP (P value>0.05) (Table 4).

Several factors were significantly associated with the practice use of ECP; marital status, ever had sex, current number of children, desired number of children, regular use of contraception and ever had an abortion (P value<0.05). Other factors such as age, class level, religion, and ever had an unintended pregnancy were not significantly associated with the practice/use of ECP (P value>0.05) (Table 5).

Logistic regression

Logistic regression was used to analyze factors found to be significant on bivariate analysis (cross-tabulation) as predictors of KAP of ECP and these are attached in the appendices. Religion was found to be a predictor of knowledge of ECP using awareness as a marker for knowledge (p=0.010, CI=1.406-11.860). If respondents had ever

Characteristic	Ever heard of ECP		Test Statistic	df	p-value (significance)
	Yes N (%)	No N (%)			
Age (N=182)			Fishers exact test 1.172		0.769
<20	7 (25.9)	44 (28.4)			
21-25	15 (55.6)	78 (50.3)			
26-30	4 (14.8)	30 (19.4)			
>30	1 (3.7)	3 (1.9)			
Class level (N=185)			Pearson chi square 0.896	3	0.826
ND1	6 (22.2)	36 (22.8)			
ND2	13 (48.1)	71 (44.9)			
HND1	5 (18.5)	23 (14.6)			
HND2	3 (11.1)	28 (17.7)			
Religion(N=179)			Pearson chi square 7.785	1	**0.005**
Islam	22 (81.5)	80 (52.6)			
Christianity	5 (18.5)	72 (47.4)			
Marital status (N=179)			Pearson chi square 1.147	1	0.284
Single	19 (70.4)	121 (79.6)			
Married	8 (29.6)	31 (20.4)			
Ever had sex? (N=182)			Pearson chi square 8.119	1	**0.004**
Yes	23 (85.2)	87 (56.1)			
No	4 (14.8)	68 (43.9)			
Current number of children (N=181)			Fishers exact test 4.677		0.112
0	18 (66.7)	128 (83.1)			
1-4	9 (33.3)	25 (16.2)			
>4	0 (0)	1 (0.6)			
Desired number of children (N=185)			Pearson chi square 0.418	2	0.811
0	3 (11.1)	15(9.5)			
1-4	19 (70.4)	105 (66.5)			
>4	5 (18.5)	38 (24.1)			
Using regular contraception? (N=168)			Pearson chi square 4.384	1	**0.036**
Yes	8 (29.6)	19 (13.5)			
No	19 (70.4)	122 (86.5)			
Ever had an unintended pregnancy(N=173)			Pearson chi square 1.761	1	0.185
Yes	5 (19.2)	15 (10.2)			
No	21 (80.8)	132 (89.8)			
Had an abortion? (N=175)			Pearson chi square 3.674	1	0.055
Yes	6 (22.2)	14 (9.5)			
No	21 (77.8)	134(90.5)			

Table 3: Cross tabulation between awareness (as a marker for knowledge) and demographic and reproductive health characteristics of respondents and need for ECP.

Characteristic	Attitude to ECP		Test Statistic	df	p-value (significance)
	Good N (%)	Poor N (%)			
Age (N=197)					
<20	7 (17.5)	23 (14.6)	Pearson chi square 9.623	3	**0.022**
21-25	29 (72.5)	92 (58.5)			
26-30	2 (5.0)	40 (25.5)			
>30	2 (5.0)	2 (1.3)			
Class level (N= 200)					
ND1	9 (22.5)	36 (22.5)	Pearson chi square 8.304	3	**0.040**
ND2	22 (55.0)	66 (41.3)			
HND1	8 (20.0)	24 (15.0)			
HND2	1 (2.5)	34 (21.3)			
Religion (N=194)					
Islam	16 (40.0)	96 (62.3)	Fishers exact		**0.012**
Christianity	24 (60)	58 (37.7)			
Marital status (N=194)					
Single	37 (92.5)	114 (74.0)	Fishers exact		**0.010**
Married	3 (7.5)	40 (26.0)			
Ever had sex? (N=197)					
Yes	8 (20.0)	110 (70.1)	Fishers exact		**0.000**
No	32 (80.0)	47 (29.9)			
Current number of children (N=196)					
0			Pearson chi square 6.352	2	0.42
1-4	37 (94.9)	121 (77.1)			
>4	2 (5.1)	35 (22.3)			
	0 (0)	1 (0.6)			
Desired number of children (N=200)					
0			Pearson chi square 2.210	2	0.331
1-4	2 (5.0)	16 (10)			
>4	31 (77.5)	105(65.6)			
	7 (17.5)	39 (24.4)			
Using regular contraception? (N=179)					
Yes			Fishers exact		0.085
No	1 (3.4)	28 (17.3)			
	28 (96.6)	124 (82.7)			
Ever had an unintended pregnancy (N=185)					
Yes			Fishers exact		**0.016**
No	0 (0)	23 (15.1)			
	33 (100)	129 (84.9)			
Had an abortion? (N=187)					
Yes	0 (0)	23 (15.2)	Fishers exact		**0.009**
No	36 (100)	128 (84.8)			

Table 4: Cross tabulation between attitude and demographic and reproductive health characteristics of respondents and need for ECP.

had sex in the past was found to be a predictor of attitude to ECP (p value=0.004, CI=0.081-0.611). There were no predictors of use/practice of ECP (P value=>0.05).

Discussion

Not surprisingly, respondents were mainly single, sexually active and had sex without regular contraception. Premarital sex is not uncommon in Nigeria, 17.7 years is the median age at sexual debut [24]. Yet only a small number in this study (12.4%) reported unintended pregnancies.Quite unlike in Ilorin, among 600 mainly single sexually active students, 67.8% had unwanted pregnancies [10]. The reasons are unclear, but 12.3% reported previous abortions and [8] suggests Nigerian adolescents prefer induced abortion dealing immediately with their unwanted pregnancy, rather than contraception which they view as having unwanted long term complications. This is despite the fact that abortion is illegal and may in fact have more dangerous complications than EC. This is however only one opinion that needs to be verified. The awareness of ECP (14.6%) is much lower than other studies done in both northern [29], and southern [25,30,31]. Nigeria, lower than found in Cameroon [32], Nepal [28], America [33] and Austria [34]. The conservative nature of Nigeria may be responsible, especially in the north, where sensitive topics like contraception are hardly discussed at home or in schools [35-38].

As with other studies [29,31,39-43], knowledge was commonly from friends and peers. Information on source of contraceptive supplies assists logistic planning, and the 2008 NDHS reported private chemists as the chief provider of contraceptive methods in Nigeria [24]. Unfortunately no student heard about ECP from official school sources, indicating inadequate reproductive health education. Similarly, Postinor/progesterone only ECP was the commonest brand students knew [31,40], unaware of modern brands which have longer windows for use and fewer side effects; perhaps because service providers are themselves unaware [44].

Few knew the correct timing for effective use of ECP, similar to other studies [30,31]. Some studies present slightly higher levels of knowledge regarding correct timing of use [29,39,41-43]. Not knowing that ECP can be effective for up to 72hours or longer represents missed opportunities for higher impact in terms of efficacy. Advance prescription of ECP may perhaps be useful in situations like this. Most respondents had poor attitude to ECP due to their wrong beliefs that ECP can cause abortion and future infertility. Oladapo et al. [45] also noted respondents concerns about future fertility and sexual misbehavior. Ikeme et al. [40] however found that up to 40% of respondents would still recommend EC use to others.

The poor use of ECP is similar to findings of Oladapo et al. [45];

Characteristic	Practice(use) of ECP		Test Statistic	Df	p-value (significance)
	Yes N (%)	No N (%)			
Age (N= 175)					
<20	4 (14.8)	25 (16.9)	Pearson chi square 0.770	3	0.857
21-25	18 (66.7)	88 (59.5)			
26-30	5 (18.5)	33 (22.3)			
>30	0(0)	2(1.4)			
Class level (N= 178)					
ND1	8 (29.6)	34 922.5)	Pearson chi square 2.619	3	0.454
ND2	10 (37.0)	70 (46.4)			
HND1	2 (7.4)	21 (13.9)			
HND2	7 (25.9)	26 (17.2)			
Religion (N=172)					0.136
Islam	12 (44.4)	89 (61.4)	Fishers exact		
Christianity	15 (55.6)	56 (38.6)			
Marital status (N=172)					
Single	14 (51.9)	118 (81.4)	Fishers exact		**0.002**
Married	13 (48.1)	27 (18.6)			
Ever had sex? (N= 175)					
Yes	27 (100)	82 (55.4)	Fishers exact		
No	0 (0)	66 (44.6)			**0.000**
Current number of children (N=175)					
0			Pearson chi square 8.684	2	**0.013**
1-4	16 (59.3)	123 (83.1)			
>4	11(40.7)	24 (16.2)			
	0 (0)	1 (0.7)			
Desired number of children (N =178)					
0	6 (22.2)	10 (6.6)	Pearson chi square 9.089	2	**0.011**
1-4	13 (48.2)	110 (73.9)			
>4	8 (29.6)	31 (20.5)			
Using regular contraception? (N=162)					
Yes	9 (33.3)	16 (11.9)			
No	18 (66.7)	119 (88.1)	Fishers exact		**0.009**
Ever had an unintended pregnancy (N=164)					
Yes	7 (25.9)	17 (11.7)	Fishers exact		0.068
No	20 (74.1)	121(88.3)			
Had an abortion? (N=166)					
Yes	7 (29.2)	16 (11.3)	Fishers exact		**0.048**
No	17 (70.8)	126 (88.7)			

Table 5: Association between practice and demographic and reproductive health characteristics of respondents and need for ECP.

higher than Ibekwe and Obuna [25] and Obiechina and Mbamara [31]; and lower than others [29,39- 41]. Perhaps due to low levels of awareness, as one study in Nigeria revealed that respondents that terminated pregnancies would have used EC if they had known about it [42]. Also students may use less proven methods for EC not explored in this study, butdemonstrated in other studies [29,31,42,46], which are obtained easily, less stigmatized butin effective .

Logistic regression showed Muslims to be more aware of ECP than Christians. Yet, Muslims and Catholics are known to have conservative views on contraception, though this study did not fully explore religious views regarding contraception. Arowojolu and Adekunle [42] however found that Pentecostal Nigerian Christians were more likely to favor the use of ECP. In another study, religion was a significant factor determining where respondents source their contraceptive products; Catholics, and Muslims, showed a greater preference for chemist/patent medicine shops for their sources of contraceptives [47]. One Ethiopian study found emergency contraceptive use to be higher among the Protestant Christians than when compared to Orthodox Christians and Muslims [48].

As with other studies, previous sexual activity and contraception affected knowledge of ECP [39,49]. Those involved in sexual acts more prone to unintended pregnancies, so make more effort to find out how to prevent them. Marital status did not significantly affect knowledge of ECP, unlike findings from the 2008 NDHS [24], showing higher knowledge of EC among unmarried sexually active people than among

the married. Could this be because that was a household survey while this study specifically targeted students, and that most students are single? Ebuehi et al. [39] found marital status to affect practice of ECP.

Limitations

There is still a potential for responder bias and respondents may have filled in responses they perceive to be desirable rather than their actual perceptions. The study is limited by geography. Other parts of the country have different socio-cultural and religious characteristics which may affect findings. Findings may also not apply to student's females outside the school setting. Further studies can triangulate quantitative and qualitative methods.

Conclusion

Respondents have poor knowledge, attitude and practice of emergency contraceptive pills, and are at risk for unintended pregnancies, unsafe abortion which may worsen already bad maternal mortality statistics. Religion and previous use of contraception among those that have initiated sex are significant factors. Emergency Contraception (EC) has a potential to curb the menace of unintended pregnancies and offers female students a chance to complete their studies smoothly. So the school setting can be better utilized for positive health education messages regarding contraception and its benefits, while the country debates restrictions to abortion laws.

Lessons Learnt

- Emergency contraception has a role to play in reducing unintended pregnancies in this school setting if there is proper sensitization and awareness.

- Health providers, teachers, peers and religious leaders would serve as a good medium to disseminate correct information on emergency contraception and dispel myths.

- Sadly, newer, safer and more effective EC methods are unavailable in this setting.

Acknowledgment

This article is based on research undertaken for a public health project at the University of Liverpool. We thank to Dr Nigel Fuller (University of Liverpool), Dr Yinka Raji (UDUTH, Nigeria) and Dr Abdulkareem Durosinlorun (Federal ministry of agriculture, Kaduna) for their useful contributions.

References

1. Monjok E, Smesny A, Ekabua JE, Essien JE (2010) Contraceptive practices in Nigeria: literature review and recommendation for future policy decisions. Open Access J Contracept 1: 9-22

2. Guttmacher Institute (1999) Sharing responsibility: women, society and abortion worldwide. New York, NY: The Alan Guttmacher Institute.

3. Singh S, Darroch J, Vlassoff M, Nadeau J (2003) Adding it up: the benefits of investing in sexual and reproductive health. New York, New York: The Alan Guttmacher Institute.

4. National Population Commission Abuja (2006) Population and housing census of the federal republic of Nigeria priority tables (Volume 1). Abuja, Nigeria: Federal Republic of Nigeria.

5. World Health Organization (2011) WHO guidelines on preventing early pregnancy and poor reproductive health outcomes. WHO Geneva, Switzerland.

6. Blumenthal PD, Voedisch A, Gemzell-Danielsson K (2011) Strategies to prevent unintended pregnancy: increasing use of long-acting reversible contraception. Hum Reprod Update 17: 121-137.

7. Cadmus EO, Owoaje ET (2010) Patterns of contraceptive use among female undergraduates in the University of Ibadan, Nigeria. Int J Health 10: 2.

8. Otoide VO, Oronsaye F, Okonofua FE (2001) Why Nigerian adolescents seek abortion rather than contraception: Evidence from focus-group discussions. Int Fam Plan Perspect. 27: 77-81.

9. Bankole A, Oye-Adeniran B, Singh S, Adewole IF, Wulf D, et al. (2006) Unwanted Pregnancy and Unsafe Abortion in Nigeria: Causes and Consequences. New York: Guttmacher Institute.

10. Abiodun OM, Balogun OR (2009) Sexual activity and contraceptive use among young female students of tertiary educational institutions in Ilorin, Nigeria. Contraception 79: 146-149.

11. Tsui AO, McDonald-Mosley R, Burke AE (2010) Family planning and the burden of unintended pregnancies. Epidemiol Rev 32: 152-174.

12. Rich-Edwards J (2002) Teen pregnancy is not a public health crisis in the United States. It is time we made it one. Int J Epidemiol 31: 555-556.

13. Oringanje C, Meremikwu MM, Eko H, Esu E, Meremikwu A, et al. (2009) Interventions for preventing unintended pregnancies among adolescents. Cochrane Database Syst Rev: CD005215.

14. Koniak-Griffin D, Turner-Pluta C (2001) Health risks and psychosocial outcomes of early childbearing: a review of the literature. J Perinat Neonatal Nurs 15: 1-17.

15. Kosunen EA, Vikat A, Gissler M, Rimpelä MK (2002) Teenage pregnancies and abortions in Finland in the 1990s. Scand J Public Health 30: 300-305.

16. Phipps MG, Blume JD, DeMonner SM (2002) Young maternal age associated with increased risk of postneonatal death. Obstet Gynecol 100: 481-486.

17. Henshaw SK, Feivelson DJ (2000) Teenage abortion and pregnancy statistics by state, 1996. Fam Plann Perspect 32: 272-280.

18. Elfenbein DS, Felice ME (2003) Adolescent pregnancy. Pediatr Clin North Am 50: 781-800.

19. Mazharuarul MI, Rashid M (2004) Determinants of unintended pregnancy among ever married women in Bangladesh. J Fam Welf 50: 40-47.

20. United Nations (1994) Programme of Action. Adopted at the International Conference on Population and Development, Cairo, 5-13 September 1994. New York.

21. World Health Organization (2000) Emergency contraception. WHO/RHR/ Fact Sheet 244 . WHO, Geneva, Switzerland.

22. Bastianelli C, Farris M (2011) Emergency contraception: presently available formulations and controversies surrounding their use. Expert Rev Obstet Gynecol 6: 569-576.

23. Mittal S (2008) Interventions for emergency contraception: RHL commentary (last revised: 1 November). The WHO Reproductive Health Library; Geneva: World Health Organization.

24. National Population Commission Nigeria, ICF Macro (2009) Nigeria demographic and health survey 2008. Abuja, Nigeria: National Population Commission and ICF Macro.

25. Ibekwe PC, Obuna JA (2010) Awareness and practice of emergency contraception among university students in Abakaliki, southeast Nigeria. Niger J Clin Pract 13: 1.

26. Bruce N, Pope D, Stanistreet D (2008) Quantitative research methods for health research: a practical interactive guide to epidemiology and statistics. Chichester, UK: Wiley & Sons.

27. Wilder KJ, Guise JM, Perrin NA, Hanson GC, Hernandez R, et al. (2009) Knowledge, Awareness, Perceptions, and Use of Emergency Contraceptives among Survivors of Intimate Partner Violence. Obstet Gynecol Int 2009: 625465.

28. Adhikari R (2009) Factors affecting awareness of emergency contraception among college students in Kathmandu, Nepal. BMC Womens Health 9: 27.

29. Bako AU (1998) Knowledge and use of emergency contraception amongst Nigerian undergraduates. J Obstet Gynaecol 18: 151-153.

30. Abasiattai AM, Umoiyoho AJ, Bassey EA, Etuk SJ, Udoma EJ (2007) Misconception of emergency contraception among tertiary school students in Akwa Ibom State, South-south, Nigeria. Niger J Clin Pract 10: 30-34.

31. Obiechina J, Mbamara U (2010) Knowledge, attitude and practice of emergency contraception among students in tertiary schools in Anambra State Southeast Nigeria. Int. J Med Sci 2: 1-4.

32. Kongnyuy EJ, Ngassa P, Fomulu N, Wiysonge CS, Kouam L, et al. (2007) A survey of knowledge, attitudes and practice of emergency contraception among university students in Cameroon. BMC Emerg Med 7: 7.

33. Corbett PO, Mitchell CP, Taylor JS, Kemppainen J (2006) Emergency contraception: knowledge and perceptions in a university population. J Am Acad Nurse Pract 18: 161-168.

34. Mayerhofer C, Kirchengast S (2009) Contraception failure--what remains to be done? Knowledge and attitudes regarding the use of emergency contraception among Austrian women and men during reproductive phase. Int J Health Sci (Qassim) 2: 2.

35. Odoemelam A (1996) Incidence and management of male and female sexually maladjusted youngsters: gender and counseling implications. J Counc Assoc Niger 14: 160-171.

36. Okonkwo R, Eze I. (2000) Attitude of Nigerian Adolescents to premarital sexual behaviour. Implications for sex education. J Counc 1: 21-26.

37. Akerele JO, Egbochuku EO (2001) Sexual Risks and Practices in Nigeria. An update on the use of the condom. J Pharm Sci 7: 128-132.

38. Durojaiye M (1972) Guidance through sex education. In: Psychological guidance of the school-child. Evans Brothers Ltd.

39. Ebuehi OM, Ekanem EE, Ebuehi OA (2006) Knowledge and practice of emergency contraception among female undergraduates in the University of Lagos, Nigeria. East Afr Med J 83: 90-95.

40. Ikeme AC, Ezegwui HU, Uzodimma AC (2005) Knowledge, attitude and use of emergency contraception among female undergraduates in Eastern Nigeria. J Obstet Gynaecol 25: 491-493.

41. Akani C, Enyindah C, Babatunde S (2008) Emergency contraception: knowledge and perception of female undergraduates in the niger delta of Nigeria. Ghana Med J 42: 68-70.

42. Arowojolu AO, Adekunle AO (2000) Perception and practice of emergency contraception by post-secondary school students in southwest Nigeria. Afr J Reprod Health 4: 56-65.

43. Aziken ME, Okonta PI, Ando AB (2003) Knowledge and perception of emergency contraception among female Nigerian undergraduates. Int Fam Plan Perspect 29: 84-87.

44. Geidam AD, Kullima AA, Sadiq GU (2009) Knowledge, attitude and provision of emergency contraception among health professionals in Borno State Northern Nigeria. Int J Health Res 2: 339-346.

45. Oladapo OT, Adefuye PO, Odusoga OL, Okewole I, Daniel O J. (2005) Emergency contraception among female undergraduates in Ogun state, Nigeria. Sex health matters 6: 1.

46. Attahir A, Sufiyan MB, Abdulkadir A, Haruna MK (2010) Knowledge, perception and practice of emergency contraception among female adolescent hawkers in Rigasa suburban community of Kaduna State Nigeria. J Fam Reprod Health 4: 15-20.

47. Oye-Adeniran BA, Adewole IF, Umoh AV, Oladokun A, Gbadegesin A, et al. (2005) Sources of contraceptive commodities for users in Nigeria. PLoS Med 2: e306.

48. Tilahun FD, Assefa T, Belachew T (2010) Predictors of emergency contraceptive use among regular female students at Adama University, Central Ethiopia. Pan Afr Med J 7: 16.

49. Obi SN, Ozumba BC (2008) Emergency contraceptive knowledge and practice among unmarried women in Enugu, southeast Nigeria. Niger J Clin Pract 11: 296-299.

30

Plasmodium Malaria and ABO Blood Group among Blood Donors in Yenegoa, Bayelsa State, Nigeria

Abah AE[1]*, Grey A[2] and Onoja H[2]

[1]Department of Animal and Environmental Biology, University of Port Harcourt, Nigeria
[2]School of Science Laboratory Technology, University of Port Harcourt, Nigeria

Abstract

Background: Transmission of Malaria by blood transfusion remains a significant public health problem in the malaria endemic regions like Nigeria. This study therefore was to investigate *Plasmodium* malaria and ABO blood group among blood donors in Yenegoa, Bayelsa State, Nigeria.

Materials and methods: Prevalence of malaria infection was determined on 250 randomly selected blood donors (201 males and 49 females) using standard parasitological method and ABO blood group was done using the monoclonal antisera A, B, and D (murex Diagnostic, inc, Dartford, UK) on a slide and observing for agglutination.

Results: The overall prevalence was 91(36.4%) out of which 84(41.8%) were males and 7(14.3%) were females. Prevalence of infection in relation to age showed that subjects within age's 24-29 years were more infected with 48.6%. Followed by those within ages 30-35 years with 42.9%, and those within 42-47 years with 30.4% while the least infected age group were those within the ages 18-24 years with 23.7% rate of infections. ABO blood group of the population sampled showed that Blood group O+ was the most prevalent with 119(47.6%) followed by blood group B+ with 62(24.8%) and A+ with 31(12.4%) while the least prevalent was AB- with 0 prevalence. The prevalence of infection in relation to ABO blood group showed that blood group O+ had the highest prevalence with 42.9% followed by blood group A+ with 41.9% and groups AB+ and A- both tied with 33.3% while the least prevalence was recorded in blood group AB- with zero prevalence. The difference was not statistically significant (P>0.05).

Conclusion: The prevalence of malaria infection among blood donors is high and blood group O harbours more parasite than any other blood group in Bayelsa State.

Keywords: Malaria infection; ABO blood group; Donors; Bayelsa state; Nigeria

Introduction

Blood transfusion is a lifesaving procedure and has greatly increased over the years. According to the World Health Organization (WHO), every second, someone in the world needs blood and in every country. Surgery, trauma, severe anaemia and complications of pregnancy are among clinical conditions that demand blood transfusion [1]. Transmission of Malaria by blood transfusion is a significant public health problem especially in the malaria endemic regions of the world [2]. Malaria is endemic in Nigeria where it accounts for more cases and death than any other country in the world, and where high prevalence has been reported by many researchers [3-6].

Some studies have suggested that ABO blood groups have an impact on the infection status of an individual [7-10]. Pizzorno and Murray stated that malaria infected RBCs sometimes bind to uninfected RBCs to form clumps called rosettes [11]. The rosettes can obstruct flow in small blood vessel and lead to tissue damage and severe malaria disease. The virulence of *Plasmodium falciparum* has been associated with the capacity of the infected RBCs to adhere to uninfected RBCs, leading to rosetting of cells [12,13]. The ABO blood group types have been implicated in rosetting [14]. In Ethopia, Tekeste and Petros reported 25(35.7%), 15(21.4%), 14(20%) and 16(22.9%) to belong to blood group A, B, AB and O patients, respectively in a study using only severe malaria cases. Prevalence of malaria parasitemia and its possible association with ABO blood groups was investigated among inhabitants of Odakpu of Anambra State, Nigeria by Ilozumba and Uzozie [15,16]. They reported ABO blood group prevalence of 2.63%, 12.05%, 21.05% and 63.83% for groups AB, B, A and O respectively. Otajevwo reported a total prevalence of 138 (79.3%) in a study associating malaria parasitaemia with ABO blood groups among residents of Warri, Nigeria [17]. He observed that 6.9%, 19.0%, 20.7% and 53.3% of 174 blood samples analyzed belonged to blood groups AB, B, A and O respectively.

Few studies have been undertaken in to ascertain the prevalence of Malaria among blood donors in Nigeria. Falade et al. [18] reported 20.2% by microscopic method. Erhabor et al. [19] reported 10.2% among donors in the Niger Delta of Nigeria also Pondei et al. [20] reported 12.5% in screened blood in a tertiary health Centre in Niger Delta. Abah and Joe-Cliff [21] reported 28% among blood donors in Port Harcourt. Chikwem et al. [22] reported 4.1% in Maiduguri, Northern Nigeria. Akinboye and Ogunrinade [23] reported 7.8% at Ibadan, Nigeria. Uneke et al. [24] reported 40.9% in south-Eastern Nigeria. Epidi et al. [25] reported 51.5% in Abakaliki. Oladeinde et al. [26] reported 27.5% and 13.8% among commercial and volunteer donors respectively.

It is difficult to completely avoid the risk of transfusion-transmitted malaria without the exclusion of blood donation, hence asymptomatic carriers of *Plasmodium* species are still qualified to donate blood for transfusion purposes. The aim of this study therefore was to investigate *Plasmodium* malaria and ABO blood group among blood donors in Yenegoa, Bayelsa State, Nigeria.

*Corresponding author: Abah AE, Department of Animal and Environmental Biology, University of Port Harcourt, Nigeria, E-mail: austin.abah@uniport.edu.ng

Materials and Methods

Study area

Bayelsa State is located in the Niger Delta region, Southern Nigeria. Its capital is Yenagoa and it is bordered on the west by Rivers State, on the East and South by the Atlantic Ocean and on the North by Delta State. Rainfall in Bayelsa State varies in quantity from one area to another, the state experiences equatorial type of climate in the southern part and tropical rain towards the northern parts. Rain occurs generally every month of the year with heavy downpour. The mean monthly temperature is in the range of 25°C to 31°C. Mean maximum monthly temperatures range from 26°C to 31°C. The mean annual temperature is uniform for the entire Bayelsa State. The hottest months are December to April. The difference between the wet season and dry season temperatures is about 2°C at the most. Relative humidity is high in the state throughout the year and decreases slightly in the dry season. The Vegetation of the state is composed of four ecological zones. These include: Coastal barrier island forests, mangrove forests, freshwater swamp e.g. forests and lowland rain forests. These vegetation types are associated with the various soil units in the area. Bayelsa State has a population of about 1.5 million inhabitants and because of the favourable environment for vector breeding, malaria is the main cause of illness and death [27].

Ethical clearance

Permission was sought and obtained from Bayelsa State Ministry of Health. Verbal consent was obtained from the participants.

Sample collection

Venous blood was collected from 250 randomly selected blood donors (201 males and 49 females) at the Diete Koki Memorial Hospital Yenagoa, Bayelsa State, Nigeria. The donors were within the age of 18-60 years. Five milliliters of blood was collected from each participant and was dispensed into Ethylene Diamine Tetra-acetic Acid (EDTA) bottle, gently and properly mixed and transported to the parasitology laboratory of the Department of Animal and Environmental Biology.

Laboratory analyses

Both thick and thin blood films were prepared, stained and examined following the method described by Cheesbrough [28]. Thick and thin blood films were made and labeled on a clean glass slide as recommended by World Health Organization (WHO). The thin films were fixed with methanol and all films were stained with 3% Giemsa stain at pH 7.0 for 30 minutes. The blood films were examined under the microscope using the oil immersion (100x) objectives as described by Cheesbrough [28]. The thick films were used to determine the parasite density while the thin film was used to differentiate the species of the parasites.

Determination of blood group

The ABO blood grouping test was done using the slide method as described by Dacie et al. [29]. A drop of the monoclonal antisera A, B, AB and D (murex Diagnostic, Inc, Dartford, UK), was placed on a clean white tile respectively. A drop of the blood sample was added to each and with the help of a glass rod it was mixed properly, swirled for 2 minutes and observed for agglutination. Agglutination reaction signified the presence of the natural antigens A, B, AB or D and confirms ABO/Rhesus phenotypes.

Results

Out of the 250 blood samples analyzed, 91(36.4%) were positive for malaria parasites. Among them were 201 males out of which 84(41.8%) were positive and 49 females out of which 7(14.3%) were positive (Table 1). Prevalence of infection in relation to age showed that subjects within age's 24-29 years were more infected with 48.6%. Followed by those within age's 30-35 years with 42.9%, and those within 42-47 years with 30.4% while the least infected age group were those within the ages 18-24 years with 23.7% rate of infections (Table 2). ABO blood group of the population sampled showed that Blood group O+ was the most prevalent with 119(47.6) followed by blood group B+ with 62(24.8%) and A+ with 31(12.4%) while the least prevalent was AB- with 0 prevalence. The prevalence of infection in relation to ABO blood group showed that blood group O+ had the highest prevalence with 42.9% followed by blood group A+ with 41.9% and groups AB+ and A- both tied with 33.3% while the least prevalence was recorded in blood group AB- with zero prevalence (Table 3).Though the difference in prevalence of infection in relation to ABO blood group was not statistically significant (P>0.05).

Discussion

The prevalence of 36.4% recorded among blood donors in this study is relatively high. The high prevalence buttresses the fact that malaria is endemic in Nigeria where it accounts for more cases and death than any other country in the world [2]. Though high malaria prevalence has been reported by many researchers in Nigeria and blood donors are not isolated from other Nigerians, the high prevalence in the present study is worrisome due to the fact that the recipients of these blood are those that are vulnerable; mostly pregnant women, children under 5 years, accident victims and other immuno-suppressive patients

Sex	Number Examined	Number Infected	% infected
Male	201(80.4%)	84	41.80%
Female	49(19.6%)	7	14.30%
Total	250(100%)	91	36.40%

Table 1: Prevalence of malaria parasite among blood donors and in relation to sex in yenegoa.

Age-Group	Number Examined	Number Infected	% Infected
18-23	38	9	23.70%
24-29	72	35	48.60%
30-35	56	24	42.90%
36-41	47	13	27.70%
42-47	23	7	30.40%
48-53	14	3	28.60%
Total	250	91	36.40%

Table 2: Prevalence of parasite in relation to age group in yenegoa.

ABO Blood Group	Number Examiner	Number Infected	% Infected
O positive	119(47.6%)	51	42.90%
O Negative	11(4.4%)	3	27.30%
AB positive	12(4.8%)	4	33.30%
AB Negative	0(0%)	0	0.00%
A positive	31(12.4%)	13	41.90%
A Negative	6(2.4%)	2	33.30%
B positive	62(24.8%)	16	25.80%
B Negative	9(3.6%)	1	11.10%
Total	250	91	36.40%

Table 3: Prevalence of parasite in relations with blood group abo in yenegoa.

as reported elsewhere [4-6,21]. The prevalence of 36.4% is actually high when compared with results of Falade et al. [18] that reported 20.2% by microscopic method, Erhabor et al. [19] who reported 10.2% among donors in the Niger Delta of Nigeria, Pondei et al. [20] who also reported 12.5% in screened blood in a tertiary health Centre in Niger Delta. The 36.4% prevalence is still higher than results of Abah and Joe-Cliff, who reported 28% among blood donors in Port Harcourt, Chikwem et al. who reported 4.1% in Maiduguri, Northern Nigeria [21,22]. Akinboye and Ogunrinade that reported 7.8% at Ibadan and Oladeinde et al. that reported 13.8% among volunteer donors [23,26]. It is suggestive of the fact that rather than decrease, malaria prevalence among blood donors is on the increase and this trend was also established by the WHO report in which there were 214 million cases of malaria in 2015 as against an estimated 198 million cases of malaria worldwide in 2013 [30,31]. However, the prevalence recorded in this study is lower than reports of Uneke et al., who reported 40.9% in south-Eastern Nigeria and Epidi et al. who reported 51.5% among blood donors in Abakaliki [24,25]. The reason for the high prevalence of malaria infection in the area may be due to the prevailing environmental conditions such as high rainfall, high relative humidity and good vegetation which collectively enhance malaria vector breeding and consequently high transmission of infections.

Sex related prevalence showed that more males (41.8%) were infected than females (14.3%). This finding agrees with Muntaka and Opoku-Okrah but at variance with Otajevwo who reported that more females were infected than males among students of Igbinedion University Okada, Nigeria [32,33]. The fact that more male subjects 80.4% presented as donors than females (19.6%) and the reason for this discrepancy which had been explained by Bani and Giussani's who stated that gender plays key role in the motivation to give blood may explain the reason for the variation in the prevalence of infection among this population [34].

Prevalence of infection in relation to age showed that subjects within age's 24-29 years were more infected with 48.6%. This finding seems to agree with Muntaka and Opoku-Okrah who observed that individuals with age between 21-25 years had the highest infection among blood donors in a Ghanaian hospital [32]. The reason for this difference observed in terms of age was not actually clear and needs further investigation. It was, however, clear that the majority of the infected individuals were the young adults and the adolescence. Since these groups of people are the principal blood donors [35].

The prevailing blood group among the studied population showed that blood group O+ had the highest prevalence with 53.3%.This finding agrees with Enosolease and Bazuaye who reported 53.2% in Benin area of Niger-Delta, Abah and Joe-Cliff who reported that people in Blood group O were more than those of the other blood groups among blood donors in Port Harcourt and Odokuma et al. who also reported blood group O as the most common among students of the Abraka campus of Delta State University in Nigeria [21,36,37]. This supports the universal knowledge that blood group O is the commonest of all the blood groups.

The prevalence of infection in relation to ABO blood group showed that blood group O+ had the highest prevalence with 42.9% followed by blood group A+ with 41.9% and groups AB+ and A- both tied with 33.3% while the least prevalence was recorded in blood group AB- with zero prevalence. Similar findings were reported by Ilozumba and Uzozie and Otajevwo [16,17]. It has long been known that people with blood type O are protected from dying of severe malaria and that blood group O provides protection against severe malaria and that may explains why blood type O seems to be the commonest blood type in malaria

endemic countries and in the present study [38]. Goel et al. reported that because of endemicity of malaria in Nigeria, more than half of the population belongs to blood group O which protects against malaria [39]. That again may buttress the finding in this study where Blood group O has the highest prevalence of infection. Though Gupta and Rai chowdhuri had observed that people in blood group types A and other blood group types were more susceptible to malaria infections such observations may be for people who presented with symptoms as the present study was undertaken on subjects that were apparently healthy and could donate blood [38].

Conclusion

The prevalence of malaria infection among blood donors is high and blood group O harbours more parasite than any other blood group in Bayelsa State. However, severe blood shortages are widespread and would be exacerbated by rejecting blood that contained malaria parasites. This study confirms a high prevalence of transfusion-transmissible malaria among blood donors. Therefore, one would only align with earlier researchers that suggested that it would be of benefit to include screening for malaria parasitaemia in the routine investigation of potential blood donors in Nigeria.

References

1. WHO (World Health Organization) (2011) Department of essential health Technologies:Blood Transfusion Safety, Geneva.

2. WHO (World Health Organization) (1996) Blood Transfusion Safety, Geneva.

3. CDC (Centre for Disease Control): US Department and Health 2012. Atlanta co 800-CDC-info.

4. Kalu MK, Obasi NA, Nduka FO, Otuchristian G (2012) A comparative study of the prevalence of malaria in Aba and Umuahia urban areas of Abia State, Nigeria. Res J Parasitol 7: 17-24.

5. Olasehinde GI, Ajayi AA, Taiwo SO, Adekeye BT, Adeyeba OA (2010) Prevalence and management of Faciparium Malaria among infants and children in Ota, Ogun State, South western Nigeria. African Journal of Clinical and Experimental Microbiology 11: 159-163.

6. Abah AE, Temple B (2015) Prevalence of malaria parasite among asymptomatic primary school children in angiama community, Bayelsa State, Nigeria. Tropical Medicine & Surgery 4: 203-207.

7. Opera KN (2007) Onchocerciasis and ABO blood group status; a field based study. Inter J Trop Med 2:123-125.

8. Abdulazeez AA, Alo EB, Rebecca SN (2008) Carriage rate of human immunodeficiency virus (HIV) infection among different ABO and rhesus blood groups in Adamawa State, Nigeria. Biomed Res 19: 41-44.

9. Ndambaa Y, Gonoa E, Nyazemab N, Makazaa N, Kaonarea KC (1997) Schistosomiasis infection in relation to the ABO blood groups among school children in Zimbabwe. Acta Trop 65:181-190.

10. Blackwell CC, Dundan S, James VS, Mackenzie AC, Braun JM, et al. (2002) Blood group and susceptibility to disease caused by E.coli O157. J Inf Dis 185: 393-396.

11. Pizzorno E, Murray MT (2013) A textbook of Natural Medicine, (4thedn), Churchill livingstone, an imprint of Elservier inc 355.

12. Carlson J, Helmby H, Hill AVS, Brewster D, Greenwood BM, et al. (1990) Human cerebral malaria: association with erythrocyte rosetting and lack of anti-rosetting antibodies. Lancet 336: 1457-1460.

13. Ringwald P, Peyron F, Lepers JP, Rabarison P, Rakotomalala C, et al. (1993) Parasite virulence factors during falciparum malaria: rosetting, cytoadherence, and modulation of cytoadherence by cytokines. Infect Immun 61: 5198-5204.

14. Thakur A, Verma IC (1992) Malaria and ABO blood groups. Indian J Malariol 29: 241-244.

15. Tekeste Z, Petros B (2010) The ABO blood group and Plasmodium falciparum malaria in awash, Metehara and Ziway areas, Ethiopia. Malaria Jour 9: 280.

16. Ilozumba PC, Uzozie CR (2009) Prevalence of malaria parasitaemia and its association with ABO blood group in Odoakpu Area of Onitsha South Local Government Area, Anambra State Nigeria. Nig An Nat Sci 8:1-8.

17. Otajevwo FD (1997) ABO Blood groups Association with malaria parasitaemia among residents in Warri, Delta State. Warri J Sci Tech 4: 32-35.

18. Falade CO, Nash O, Akingbola TS, Michael OS, Olojede F et al. (2009) Blood banking in malaria endemic area: evaluating the problem posed by malarial Parasitaemias. Ann Trop Med Parsitol 103: 383-392.

19. Erhabor O, Ok O, Awah I, Uko KE, Charles AT (2007) The prevalence of Plasmodia parasitaemia among donors in the Niger delta of Nigeria. Trop Doc 37: 32-34.

20. Pondei K, Lawani E, Ndiok E (2012) Prevalence of the malaria Parasite In screened blood in a tertiary health centre in the malaria-endemic Niger Delta region of Nigeria. Global Adv Res J Microbiol 1:188-193.

21. Abah AE, Joe-Cliff O (2016) Current status of malaria parasite among blood donors in Port Harcourt, Rivers State, Nigeria. JASEM 20: 187 – 191.

22. Chikwem JO, Mohammed I, Okara GC, Ukwandu NCD, Ola TO (1997) Prevalence of transmissible blood infections among blood donors at the University of Maiduguri Teaching Hospital, Maiduguri, Nigeria. East Afr Med Jour 74: 213-216

23. Akinboye DO, Ogunrinade AF (1987) Malaria and Loaisis among blood donors at Ibadan, Nigeria. Trans R Soc Trop Med Hygi 81:398-399.

24. Uneke CJ, Ogbu O, Nwojiji V (2006) Potential risk of induced Malaria by blood transfusion in South-eastern Nigeria. Mcgill J Med 9: 8-13.

25. Epidi TT, Nwani CD, Ugorji NP (2008) Prevalence of malaria in blood donors in Abakaliki. Sc Res Es 3: 162-164.

26. Oladeinde BH, Omoregie R, Osakue EO, Onaiwu TO (2014) Asymptomatic malaria among blood donors in Benin city Nigeria. Iran J Parasitol 9: 415-422.

27. MSF (Medecins sans Frontiers): Fighting malaria in Niger Delta. International website of medecins Sans frontiers (msf). MSF USA 333 7th Avenue, New York, 2000. NY 10001-5004.

28. Cheesbrough M (2005) District Laboratory Manual for tropical countries. (2ndedn) update Vol. 1. Bulterworth –heinemann Ltd. Oxford ox28DP 249.

29. Dacie JV, Lewis SM (2002) Practical Haematology ix edition. Edinburgh Churchhill Livingstone 55.

30. WHO: World malaria report 2016. World Health Organization, 20 Avenue Appia, 1211 Geneva 27, Switzerland.

31. WHO: World malaria report 2014. World Health Organization, 20 Avenue Appia, 1211 Geneva 27, Switzerland.

32. Muntaka S, Opoku-Okrah C (2013) The Prevalence of malaria parasitaemia and predisposition of ABO blood groups to plasmodium falciparum malaria among blood donors at a Ghanaian Hospital. AU JTech 16: 255-260.

33. Otajevwo FD (2013) Prevalence of malaria parasitaemia and its association with ABO blood grouping among students of Igbinedion University Okada, Nigeria. British J Med Res 3:164-177.

34. Bani M, Giussani B (2010) Gender differences in giving blood: a review of the literature. Blood Trans 8: 278-287.

35. WHO (2003) Global defense against the infectious disease threat. Department of communicable diseases. WHO press.

36. Enosolease ME, Bazuaye GN (2008) Distribution of ABO and Rhesus D blood group in Benin area of Niger-Delta: Implication for regional blood transfusion. Asian J Trans Sci 2: 3-5.

37. Odokuma EI, Okolo AC, Aloamaka PC (2007) Distribution of ABO and rhesus blood groups in Abraka, Delta State, Nigeria. Nig J Physiol Sci 22: 89-91.

38. Gupta M, Rai chowdhuri AN (1980) Relationship between ABO blood groups and malariaBull. world Health Oragnization 58: 913–915.

39. Goel S, Palmkvist M, Moll K, Joanin N, Lara P, et al (2015) RIFINs are adhesins implicated in severe plasmodium falciparum malaria Nat. Med 21: 314–317.

31

Pragmatic Model for Integrating Complementary and Alternative Medicine in Primary Care Management of Chronic Musculoskeletal Pain

Miek C Jong[1-3]*, Martine Busch[3,4], Lucy PL van de Vijver[1], Mats Jong[2], Jolanda Fritsma[5] and Ruth Seldenrijk[6]

[1]*Department Nutrition & Health, Louis Bolk Institute, Driebergen, Netherlands*
[2]*Department of Nursing Science, Mid Sweden University, Sundsvall, Sweden*
[3]*National Information and Knowledge Centre for Integrative Medicine (NIKIM), Netherlands*
[4]*Van Praag Institute, Utrecht, Netherlands*
[5]*Zorgbelang Groningen, Groningen, Netherlands*
[6]*Patiënten Platform Complementaire Gezondheidszorg, Netherlands*

Abstract

Background: Integration of complementary and alternative medicine (CAM) into conventional care is driven by patients' needs for holistic care. This study aimed to develop a model for integration of CAM into primary healthcare in close collaboration with patients suffering from chronic musculoskeletal pain (CMP).

Methods: The study had a qualitative inductive approach following the principles of Grounded Theory, where data were collected and generated via several data sources and steps; individual and focus group interviews and meetings with patients, general practitioners (GPs), CAM practitioners, health insurers and other key informants.

Results: Consensus was reached on a model in which shared decision making was introduced to facilitate discussions on CAM between patients and GPs. Guided by evidence and best-practices, GPs refer patients to one of five selected and reimbursed CAM therapies (acupuncture, homeopathy, naturopathy, osteopathy or Tai Chi) and respective practitioner within their integrative network. CAM practitioners report treatment outcome back to the GP who follows-up on the patient for further evaluation.

Conclusions: In conclusion, it was feasible to develop a model for integration of CAM into primary healthcare management of CMP that was driven by patients' needs and obtained consensus of all stakeholders. The model is the first in the Netherlands to provide for integrative health services in primary care. It needs to be tested in a study setting before further implementation is recommended.

Keywords: Primary care; Complementary and alternative medicine; Integrative medicine; Chronic musculoskeletal pain

Abbreviations: CAM: Complementary and Alternative Medicine; CMP: Chronic Musculoskeletal Pain; GPs: General Practitioners; PPCG: Dutch Platform for Patients on Complementary Health Care; RET: Regional Expert Team

Introduction

Chronic musculoskeletal pain (CMP) is the most frequently occurring pain complaint managed in primary healthcare [1]. It can range from local pain, as in the common CMP types such as low back pain and knee pain, to more general bodily pain in fibromyalgia [2]. Musculoskeletal pain is considered chronic if the pain is still present after three months [3]. The prevalence of CMP is reported to range from approximately 20% to 48% in the general population [1,4-7]. As CMP is a major burden for patients and often causes long-term absence from work, adequate management and treatment of CMP poses a major health challenge for general practitioners (GPs) [8-10]. Pharmacological therapies have been reported to provide inadequate long-term pain relief for CMP [11-13]. Therefore, guidelines generally recommend lifestyle interventions such as exercise. Although shown to be effective, life-style changes are very difficult to maintain [14,15].

The use of complementary and alternative medicine (CAM) among people with CMP has become increasingly popular. CAM is defined as a group of diverse medical and health care systems, practices, and products that are not generally considered part of conventional medicine, such as acupuncture and homeopathy [16]. Estimates of CAM use in CMP patients differed between studies from on average 42 to 90% [17-23]. A previous Dutch study reported that 71% of patients with CMP had visited a CAM practitioner in either manual therapies, acupuncture, homeopathy, mind-body therapy or naturopathy [24].

Only a minority (30%) of those had actively communicated this CAM use with their GP. The majority of people with CMP surveyed in the study expressed their needs for a GP who inquires about CAM use and refers to CAM practitioners. As CAM is most commonly offered by practitioners in own private practices, rather than in conventional healthcare settings, no strategies, approaches nor models for integration of CAM into primary care exist in the Netherlands.

Several models for integration of CAM have been described [25]. In these models, the provision of conventional and CAM therapies varies from parallel practices, to consultative, collaborative, coordinated, multidisciplinary, interdisciplinary and totally integrated practices. Models for integrative primary care management of CMP, such as low back and neck pain, have been developed [26-29]. These models were designed according to the different health care delivery systems in the respective countries (UK, USA, Canada and Sweden) and are therefore not easily implemented in countries with other health care systems. More importantly, up till now, strategies on integration of CAM therapies largely rely on opinions and experiences of clinicians and researchers, rather than on criteria from the patient's perspective [26-

*Corresponding author: Miek C. Jong, Department Healthcare & Nutrition, Louis Bolk Institute, Hoofdstraat 24, 3972 LA Driebergen, Netherlands, Email: m.jong@louisbolk.nl

29]. Evaluation of such a model in practice has therefore demonstrated a mismatch between what patients wanted and what was estimated by the ones designing the model [26]. Nowadays, health care is evolving more and more toward a 'patient-centered model', in which patients become active participants and where care is designed to their individual needs and preferences [30]. It is therefore of great importance to actively involve patients and patients organizations into the development of models for integrative care.

The present study was initiated by the Dutch Platform for Patients on Complementary Health Care (PPCG). It aimed to develop a model for integration of CAM into primary care, in close collaboration with patients suffering from musculoskeletal pain. In order to enhance acceptability of the integrative model, key informants in primary care and CAM such as GPs, CAM practitioners, health insurance agencies and other health care associations were invited to participate in the study.

Methods and Materials

Study design and setting

This study was executed as phase 2 of a larger project, aimed to develop, implement and evaluate an integrative model for CMP in primary care and took place in the period May 2011- July 2012. Phase 1 of this project explored patient's perspectives towards integration of CAM [24]. The implementation and evaluation of the integrative model for CMP (Phase 3) was approved by the ethics committee (METOPP no: NL41527.028.12) and is expected to be finished by the end of 2015. The current study had a qualitative inductive approach, identical to the one previously used by others to successfully develop an integrative model for primary care [29,31]. In essence, this approach followed the principles of Grounded Theory in which experiences from participants provided the framework of explaining practice to further theory- and model development [32]. The study was conducted in primary care centers in the region of Amsterdam and in the region of Groningen. The project team performing the study consisted of one representative of a patient interest organization, one expert on CAM implementation and two senior researchers. The project team was supported by a Regional Expert Team (RET) as developed by Zorgbelang Groningen (regional patient interest organization). The RET consisted of six individual patients (one men, five women) who were experts by experience and able to communicate about their experiences. They all suffered from CMP for more than 5 years due to osteoarthritis, arthrosis, rheumatoid arthritis, fibromyalgia or a combination thereof. The project team was also supported by two GPs of primary care centers in Amsterdam.

Study procedures and participants

In an inductive study approach, following the principles of Grounded Theory, data can be generated from a multitude of sources, such as for example interviews, observations, documents and more [32]. Investigative procedures therefore involved focus group and key informant interviews with the following participants: 1. Patients, 2. Patient organizations, 3. GPs, 4. CAM practitioners, 5. Other key informants such as health insurance companies and health service research institutes, and 6. Regional Expert Team.

Four focus group interviews were conducted with the aim to collect "high quality data in a social context where people could consider their own views in the context of the views of others" [33]. All focus groups lasted approximately 2 hours. Sessions were recorded and field-notes were taken. The first focus group (May 2011) was with ten patients suffering from CMP. The opening question asked for patients'

experiences with CAM use. Subsequently, four questions followed on which health effects patients had experienced from CAM, how they communicated CAM use with their GP, how they envisioned the role of their GP with respect to CAM and which hurdles they encountered upon CAM use. At the end of the focus group interview, patients were asked; if they had one minute, what would they communicate about their CAM use with their GP? The second focus group (December 2011) was with six GPs working in primary care centers in the region of Amsterdam. It addressed four open questions exploring the needs, knowledge, general requirements and existing network of GPs towards integration of CAM in primary care. The third focus group (March 2012) was composed of ten members of the PPCG. An open discussion was initiated on the question how to envision, from a patients' perspective, the collaboration and communication between patients, GPs and CAM practitioners. The fourth focus group (April 2012) was with nine CAM practitioners. They were all physician, and presented a selection of members of the Dutch physician association for Integrative Medicine (AVIG). The central question for the open discussion was similar to that in the third focus group, but now from the perspective of the CAM practitioner.

Eight face-to-face interviews with key informants were conducted between May 2011 and February 2012. The first interview was with the Netherlands Organization for Health Research and Development (ZonMw) with whom further key informants were identified. Other key informants included two major health insurance companies in the Netherlands (Menzis and Agis), the foundation of health insurance companies on healthcare innovation (Innovatiefonds Zorgverzekeraars), two institutes for applied health services research (NIVEL, TNO), the national organization for primary care (LVG) and the Federation of Patient and Consumer Organizations in the Netherlands (NPCF). An open-ended interview guide was developed on the basis of patient's perspectives of integrative primary care as previously published [24]. Key informants were invited to also bring own themes and comments into the interview. The interviews lasted for one hour. The regional expert team of patients (RET) were invited to share their experiences with CAM use and their perspectives on integrative primary care by email via written questions. Written answers from all RET members were returned to the project team via email.

Data collection and analysis

Data collection and analysis was divided into two clearly distinct phases. In the first phase, field notes from individual and focus group interviews with key informants on their meaning and needs to enable a successful collaboration between providers were examined by two members of the project team by constant comparisons. Using these notes, a list of key themes and illustrative quotes was generated, categorized by key informant, providing the basis for a conceptual integrative model that was "grounded" in the perceptions and experiences of key informants. In the second phase, the generated themes and evolving conceptual integrative model were presented in confirmatory meetings to the RET, GPs, CAM practitioners and members of patient organizations (PPCG) for critique and refinement of the integrative model. Finalization of the integrative model was achieved in July 2012 by means of a consensus meeting in which the most important key informants were present: patients, GPs, CAM practitioners and Health Insurance Agencies.

Results

Development of the integrative model

After the first phase of data collection and analysis a set of themes appeared from focus groups and key informant interviews on how to integrate CAM into primary care. In table 1, generated themes and illustrative quotes of patients are shown. The patient is very well aware of the fact that GPs and CAM practitioners work in *two distinct worlds*, clearly separated from each other by philosophy. Patients value the expertise of both of them, and do not expect GPs to learn how to practice CAM themselves or vice versa. Integration of CAM into primary care is envisaged by referrals of GPs to CAM practitioners and by facilitating *communication on CAM* between them. Patients do not *disclose CAM use* to their GPs because they think the GPs are not knowledgeable on this topic and/or they are afraid of the GPs disapproval. Furthermore, patients want to have access to *reliable information* on CAM therapies and CAM practitioners. Enough *time* to properly discuss health problems and CAM with the GP came up, as well as the importance of *reimbursement* of CAM therapies (Table 1).

A theme derived from GPs was the *evidence-base of CAM* therapies for CMP (Table 2). Possible referrals to CAM should be done on the basis of available evidence and safety for a certain condition. Furthermore, *experiential exposure to CAM* therapies was a theme as to better understand the thoughts and ideas behind CAM. Another theme was *information and guidance* on which patients (related to health problems or diagnosis) can be referred to CAM practitioners. An additional theme generated through GP data was the *reliability and professional standard of CAM practitioners*. They should preferably be medical doctors as to not withhold patients from an active conventional treatment and refer patients back to the GP when needed.

A general theme brought up by CAM practitioners was that of *informing and guiding GPs* with respect to which patients could be referred to a CAM therapy (Table 3). Furthermore, *best CAM -practices* should be leading in the selection of CAM therapies in an integrative model. *CAM practitioner qualifications* was identified as a third theme as whether to select only medical doctors practicing CAM or also non-medic practitioners. Themes derived from other key informants were *cost-effectiveness of CAM* (health insurers) (Table 3). As CAM therapies are not covered by basic insurance, the question was raised whether cost-effectiveness of CAM integration could be expected. The theme of *gatekeeper* was brought up as to who has the general responsibility in the integrative model, the patient, the GP or the CAM practitioner. The theme of *shared decision making* was identified with respect to the importance of facilitating communication and referral to CAM between GPs and patients.

Themes	Quotes
Patients	
Two distinct worlds	"My GP does not have to practice a CAM therapy himself, he can better leave that to the CAM practitioner, he is already busy enough"
Communication on CAM	"If GPs dare to be open for other treatment options and talk about it with CAM practitioner, something essential can change in health care"
Disclosure of CAM use	"It is my experience that I am not been taken seriously if I tell my GP that I use CAM. I would like to get more understanding, now I only tell people in my direct environment from which I know that they are open to it"
Reliable information on CAM	"It is essential for my health problems that I have easy access to good and reliable information on CAM, for example a list of trustworthy CAM practitioners"
Time with GP	"I would like to have time with my GP to discuss which CAM treatment best fits me and what feels good for me to do, so that I can comply to it and can reach the results that we aim for"
Reimbursement of CAM	"I have used very expensive biologics that were reimbursed, while they did not work or gave side effects, but cheaper herbal medicines that are effective are not reimbursed"

Table 1: Themes and subsequent illustrative quotes derived from patients, patients organizations and RET interviews on how to integrate CAM into primary care.

Themes	Quotes
General Practitioners	
Evidence-base of CAM	"I very much would like to know which evidence there is for a CAM therapy, is it effective or inconclusive and how about safety?"
Experiential exposure to CAM	"How much information do you need on CAM in order to be able to refer? You have to know at least what it is about, to recognize it somehow, and to feel or experience for yourself as a GP what it is"
Information and guidance	'I would like to have information, simple facts sheets, as to which CAM therapy can be referred to, for which symptom and which result may be expected"
Reliability/professional standards CAM practitioners	"If I refer to a CAM practitioner that I know, that is OK, but if I do not know them, I have a preference that it is a medical doctor and member of a professional CAM organization"

Table 2: Themes and subsequent illustrative quotes from GPs on how to integrate CAM into primary care.

Themes	Quotes
CAM practitioner	
Informing and guiding GPs	"The GP should really know something about all CAM therapies in order to decide, on an individual basis, to which CAM therapy the patient should be referred to"
Best CAM practices	"I can treat arthritis of the knee and low back pain successfully with acupuncture, that is simple and straight forward"
CAM practitioner qualifications	"I wonder whether it is allowed by law for a general practitioner to share medical information in a referral letter to a CAM practitioner who is not a medical doctor"
Other key informants	
Cost-effectiveness CAM	"Referring patients to CAM might decrease the existing fear for enormous raises in costs, as giving people the choice what they really want, may be less expensive in the end"
Gatekeeper integrative model	"It remains the responsibility of the GP when he refers the patients to a CAM practitioner and those should to be trusted in which cases it is necessary to refer the patient back to the GP"
Shared decision making	"The relation between the professional and the patient should be central, different options should be discussed, taking into account the values and preferences of both"

Table 3: Themes and subsequent illustrative quotes from CAM practitioners other key informants on how to integrate CAM into primary care.

In the second phase of data collection more pragmatic questions and issues arose on how to refine and implement the integrative model: which CAM therapies should be selected as part of the integrative model? Should this be decided on best-practice experience, evidence, prevalence, patient's choice or therapies being recognized by health insurers? How many referrals to CAM therapies should be included and how many CAM treatment sessions per referral? Should the GP only refer to CAM practitioner or is self-use of CAM in the form of supplements and herbal supplements also advocated? How should the CAM practitioner provide feedback of his treatment to the GP? Is there enough time for shared decision making on CAM during a normal ten minute GP consultation? Furthermore, GPs wanted to make personal acquaintance with CAM practitioners as to build up an integrative collaborative network and GPs should initiate the discussion with the patient on CAM. This was felt to support the patients' feeling that the GP is taking their needs seriously. The questions and issues were discussed with all stakeholders as to prepare the documentation on which a decision for a model could be made. Consensus on the model was achieved in a final meeting with at least two or more representatives of the most important stakeholders: RET, GPs, CAM practitioners, PPCG and Health Insurers.

Integrative model in practice

The model for integration of CAM in primary care management of CMP that was agreed upon is schematically depicted in Figure 1. It starts with group or individual meetings between GPs and selected CAM practitioners aimed to get acquainted with each other and to exchange views, expertise and experiences in the management of CMP. Those CMP patients that contact their GP, are invited for a first consultation of 20 minutes in which the GP inquires about previous CAM use and informs patients on possible referral to one of the five selected CAM therapies: acupuncture, homeopathy, naturopathy, osteopathy, Tai Chi. These CAM therapies represented the top 5 most used CAM therapies for CMP in the Netherlands [24]. The GP provides the patient with an information leaflet on the CAM therapies and a second consultation between the patient and the GP is scheduled for one week later. During the second consultation of 20 minutes, the GP and patient mutually decide via the process of shared decision making whether or not to refer to one of the CAM therapies. This shared decision process includes discussion of the patients' health problems and history, CAM options, patients' preferences, values and expectations and pros/cons of CAM. The selection of a CAM therapy and individual CAM practitioner is guided by specifically developed tools for implementation (as described below). The GP writes a referral letter containing the necessary information to the CAM practitioner, which the patient hands over to the CAM practitioner upon the first consultation. The patient receives CAM treatment, of which full costs for maximum five CAM consultations are covered by the health insurance (and twelve classes for Tai Chi). The CAM practitioner sends a letter back to the GP on the treatment outcome of the patient and advice for follow up. The patient plans a third consult visit with his GP (2 x 10 min) to share the experiences and treatment outcome with CAM and discuss possible continuation and follow-up.

Practical tools for implementation

From the second phase of data collection and analysis, it became apparent that there was also a need to develop practical tools for implementation of the model. To support optimal shared decision making, an information leaflet was developed for patients, describing in general what CAM is and more specifically each of the selected CAM therapies. For GPs, a schematic table was developed depicting the available evidence for each selected CAM therapy and respective CMP related health problem. Since for half of the CMP conditions no studies with the selected CAM therapies could be found in literature, it was decided after consensus with stakeholders to also investigate personal practice experience of CAM practitioners in treating CMP. Through the Dutch professional CAM associations, five CAM practitioners per CAM therapy were selected to rate their clinical experience with CMP conditions. Results on clinical experience were depicted in a print-out table for GPs. Furthermore, a social map of selected CAM practitioners was created with the aim to facilitate the GPs in referring their patients to specific CAM therapies. CAM practitioners were selected by the project team on the following criteria: 1. Member of a recognized professional CAM association, 2. More than five years of

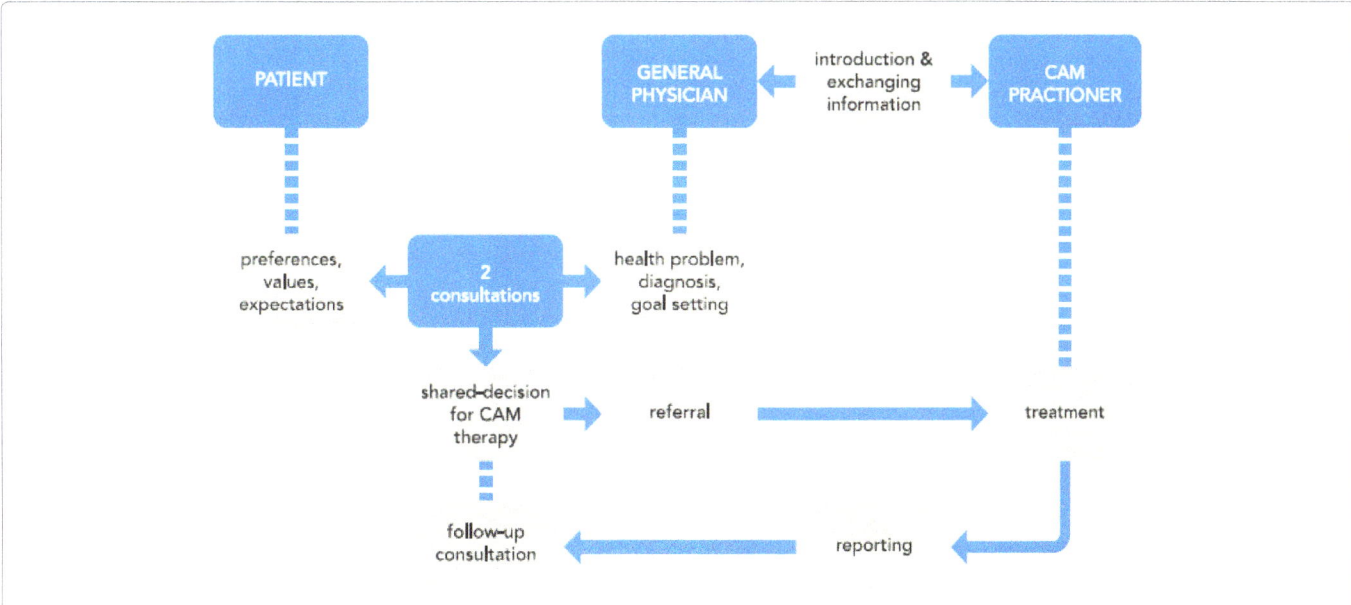

Figure 1: Schematic visualization of the integration of CAM into primary care management.

experience in practicing the specific CAM therapy, 3. At least more than two positive references from GPs in the area, 4. Private practice < 30 km from a GPs primary care center. At least two CAM practitioners for each CAM therapy per region (Amsterdam and Groningen) were selected. Selected CAM practitioners included both physicians and non-medic practitioners. The social map included photographs of each selected CAM practitioner, name and address of the practice and information on the specific expertise of the CAM practitioner. Last, two standardized concept letters were developed for GPs and CAM practitioners to use. A standardized referral letter that GPs could use to refer patients to CAM practitioners included patient information on the name, birth date, diagnosis, current (medical) treatment, reasons for referral and expected treatment outcomes. Another standardized letter for CAM practitioners was developed in order to report patients' therapy results back to the GP. It included information on name, birth date, diagnosis, description of treatment followed (how many times, no or yes medication), treatment outcome and advise for follow-up.

Discussion

It is very promising that in the present study consensus was reached among patients, GPs, CAM practitioners and health insurers on how to integrate CAM into primary care. In the range of different integrative models as described by Boon et al. [25], the integrative model on which consensus was reached was somewhere between a consultative model (expert advice is given from one professional to another) and a collaborative model (professionals who normally practice independently from each other, share information concerning a particular patient). The added value of the presented integrative model to those previously published in literature, is that the current model was developed together with patients [26-29]. Their perspectives were in many cases leading as to decide on the final model. It was for example quite clear that patients saw no need for full integration of CAM, but wanted best of "both worlds": being taken seriously by GPs in their search for CAM and get the GPs referral to a reliable CAM practitioner. Guiding them to select a CAM therapy was expected to be a thorough process. Therefore, the concept of shared decision making was built into the integrative model. The structural elements of shared decision making were expected to facilitate discussing patients' health problems, expectations and preferences as well as the available evidence and pro/cons of CAM. Dutch GPs were already familiar with this concept since implementation of shared decision making in clinical practice is strongly promoted in the Netherlands [34,35]. Patients also wanted time to discuss CAM use and referral with their GP. It was quite obvious to all stakeholders that the standard ten minute consultation time of GPs was not sufficient. Although GPs preferred to implement the integrative model within the existing schedule of consultation times, consensus was reached with all parties to use 20 minutes (double consultation time) for CAM use discussions in a first consultation and another 20 minutes for CAM referral in a second consultation.

Reimbursement of CAM was another big issue for patients. In contrast to some other EU countries, costs for CAM therapies are not covered by standard health insurance in the Netherlands [36]. Dutch citizens have the possibility to pay for additional insurance that (partly) covers some CAM therapies, however, health insurers are not obliged to accept people that apply for additional insurance. At the time of developing the integrative model, a Dutch study was published that demonstrated cost-effectiveness of CAM therapies in primary care [37]. These findings supported the process to reach consensus on reimbursement of CAM therapies by the participating health insurer (Menzis). It was decided by all stakeholders to maximal reimburse five CAM treatments (amounting to approximately €250 to €500). Questioned homeopaths, osteopaths and naturopaths shared the opinion that three to four treatments would suffice, whereas acupuncturists whished for more treatments (six to seven). A recent study in the Netherlands showed that chronic patients suffering from mitochondrial diseases spend up to €489 on CAM therapies per year out of the pocket [38]. Further studies are warranted to investigate what patients would be willing to pay themselves on CAM therapies and what should be reimbursed.

In the presented integrative model it was mutually decided that GPs could make referrals to CAM practitioners of both medical and non-medical background, a topic heavily debated. Many stakeholders are of the opinion that CAM practitioners with substantial medical knowledge, thus physicians practicing CAM, would fit better into integration initiatives as to facilitate communication with GPs [39]. Although more traditional forms of CAM, such as homeopathy and acupuncture are practiced by physicians in the Netherlands, most CAM therapies are practiced by non-medical or paramedical practitioners [40]. For patients in the present study it did not matter whether the practitioner was a physician or not, as long as the practitioner had good qualifications. GPs found it more important that the CAM practitioner worked within an ethical framework of a professional organization, with formal procedures for complaints, malpractice as to not withhold patients from effective conventional treatment. They also wanted to get personally acquainted with the CAM practitioner to build up a working relationship. It was decided that within the current integrative model, each physician should develop a list of trusted CAM practitioners in the area around his practice. This should be supported by facilitating meetings between them, as well as by a 'social map' of referral to CAM practitioners.

The integrative primary care model presented in this study also has its limitations. First of all, a qualitative inductive design was chosen, in line with the methods as published by others [29,31]. Although in essence, the methodological principles of Grounded Theory were followed, the integrative model might have been more "grounded" if the Grounded Theory research method would have been applied to the full extent. Another limitation of the present study is that with longer consultations times and reimbursement of CAM therapies, the integrative model operates to some extent outside the current context of conventional primary care. Primary care in the Netherlands is currently facing many changes, such as the introduction of multidisciplinary care groups for chronic patients [41,42]. Evaluation of the integrative model is therefore needed to adapt the model to better align with current changes in standard primary care. Since CAM practitioners work outside the realm of conventional medicine and therefore do not have access to the formal electronic patient registration system, it was not possible to directly document the prescription of CAM remedies into the registration system of the GP. Although feedback from the CAM practitioner to the GP is foreseen in the model through a written report, it would have been better for safety monitoring of possible interactions between conventional medication and CAM remedies to have this information during the process of treatment. Furthermore, all involved stakeholders unanimously decided that the GP should be the gatekeeper of the proposed integrative model as it seemed most appropriate with respect to promoting health and safety of the patient. Since nowadays the GP is overloaded with various tasks, it remains to be seen whether the GP is able to carry on another task as to monitor referrals and outcome of CAM therapy. Another limitation is that the CAM evidence tables and the social map of CAM practitioners, as developed for implementation of the model and being highly favored by GP's and patients, need structural updating. It is advised that these tools are embedded in a national center for integrative care to guarantee high quality and updated information.

In conclusion, it was feasible to develop a model for integration of CAM into primary care management of CMP that was driven by patients' needs and obtained consensus of all other participating stakeholders. The model will support patients in disclosing CAM use to GPs and aid in building up an integrative collaborative network of GPs and CAM practitioners. As a next step, the effects of the proposed integrative model on improving CMP management need to be investigated.

Acknowledgements

This study was financed by the PGO fund of the Dutch Ministry of Health, Welfare and Sports. All authors declare that they have no conflict of interest. We would like to thank the members of the RET and the PPCG for their valuable input. Jan Mehrtens and Ilonka Brugemann are acknowledged for giving their expert advice and assistance in developing the integrative model.

References

1. Cimmino MA, Ferrone C, Cutolo M (2011) Epidemiology of chronic musculoskeletal pain. Best Pract Res Clin Rheumatol 25: 173-183.

2. Croft PG, van-der-Windt D (2010) Primary care research and musculoskeletal medicine. Prim Health Care Res Dev 11:4-16.

3. Elliott AM, Smith BH, Penny KI, Smith WC, Chambers WA (1999) The epidemiology of chronic pain in the community. Lancet 354: 1248-1252.

4. Centers for Disease Control and Prevention Public health and aging: projected prevalence of self-reported arthritis or chronic joint symptoms among persons aged >65 years--United States, 2005-2030. MMWR Morbity Mortality Weekly Report. 52:489-91.

5. Hagen K, Linde M, Heuch I, Stovner LJ, Zwart JA (2011) Increasing prevalence of chronic musculoskeletal complaints. A large 11-year follow-up in the general population (HUNT 2 and 3). Pain Med 12: 1657-1666.

6. Parsons S, Breen A, Foster NE, Letley L, Pincus T, et al. (2007) Prevalence and comparative troublesomeness by age of musculoskeletal pain in different body locations. Fam Pract 24: 308-316.

7. Svebak S HK, Zwart J-A. One-Year Prevalence of Chronic Musculoskeletal Pain in a Large Adult Norwegian County Population: Relations with Age and Gender-The HUNT Study. Journal of Musculoskelatal Pain 14: 21-28.

8. Kroenke K, Outcalt S, Krebs E, Bair MJ, Wu J, et al. (2013) Association between anxiety, health-related quality of life and functional impairment in primary care patients with chronic pain. Gen Hosp Psychiatry 35: 359-365.

9. Rijksinstituut voor Volksgezondheid en Milieu. Klachten van het bewegingsapparaat (2000) Report no: 266807 002.

10. Stewart WF, Ricci JA, Chee E, Morganstein D, Lipton R (2003) Lost productive time and cost due to common pain conditions in the US workforce. JAMA 290: 2443-2454.

11. Curatolo M, Bogduk N (2001) Pharmacologic pain treatment of musculoskeletal disorders: current perspectives and future prospects. Clin J Pain 17: 25-32.

12. Häuser W, Walitt B, Fitzcharles MA, Sommer C (2014) Review of pharmacological therapies in fibromyalgia syndrome. Arthritis Res Ther 16: 201.

13. Turk DC (2002) Clinical effectiveness and cost-effectiveness of treatments for patients with chronic pain. Clin J Pain 18: 355-365.

14. Hayden JA, Cartwright JL, Riley RD, Vantulder MW; Chronic Low Back Pain IPD Meta-Analysis Group (2012) Exercise therapy for chronic low back pain: protocol for an individual participant data meta-analysis. Syst Rev 1: 64.

15. Van Gool CH, Penninx BW, Kempen GI, Rejeski WJ, Miller GD, et al (2005) Effects of exercise adherence on physical function among overweight older adults with knee osteoarthritis. Arthritis Rheum 53: 24-32.

16. National Center for Complementary and Integrative Health (2015) Definition of CAM.

17. Breuer GS, Orbach H, Elkayam O, Berkun Y, Paran D, et al. (2006) Use

18. Callahan LF, Wiley-Exley EK, Mielenz TJ, Brady TJ, Xiao C, et al. (2009) Use of complementary and alternative medicine among patients with arthritis. Prev Chronic Dis 6: A44.

of complementary and alternative medicine among patients attending rheumatology clinics in Israel. The Israel Medical Association Journal 8:184-187.

19. Ernst E (2008) Complementary treatments in rheumatic diseases. Rheum Dis Clin North Am 34: 455-467.

20. Herman CJ, Allen P, Hunt WC, Prasad A, Brady TJ (2004) Use of complementary therapies among primary care clinic patients with arthritis. Prev Chronic Dis 1: A12.

21. Katz P, Lee F (2007) Racial/ethnic differences in the use of complementary and alternative medicine in patients with arthritis. J Clin Rheumatol 13: 3-11.

22. Lapane KL, Sands MR, Yang S, McAlindon TE, Eaton CB (2012) Use of complementary and alternative medicine among patients with radiographic-confirmed knee osteoarthritis. Osteoarthritis Cartilage 20: 22-28.

23. Rossy LA, Buckelew SP, Dorr N, Hagglund KJ, Thayer JF, et al. (1999) A meta-analysis of fibromyalgia treatment interventions. Ann Behav Med 21: 180-191.

24. Jong MC, van de Vijver L, Busch M, Fritsma J, Seldenrijk R (2012) Integration of complementary and alternative medicine in primary care: what do patients want? Patient Educ Couns 89: 417-422.

25. Boon H, Verhoef M, O'Hara D, Findlay B (2004) From parallel practice to integrative health care: a conceptual framework. BMC Health Serv Res 4: 15.

26. Cheshire A, Polley M, Peters D, Ridge D (2011) Is it feasible and effective to provide osteopathy and acupuncture for patients with musculoskeletal problems in a GP setting? A service evaluation. BMC Fam Pract 12: 49.

27. Maiers MJ, Westrom KK, Legendre CG, Bronfort G (2010) Integrative care for the management of low back pain: use of a clinical care pathway. BMC Health Serv Res 10: 298.

28. Mior S, Barnsley J, Boon H, Ashbury FD, Haig R (2010) Designing a framework for the delivery of collaborative musculoskeletal care involving chiropractors and physicians in community-based primary care. J Interprof Care 24: 678-689.

29. Sundberg T, Halpin J, Warenmark A, Falkenberg T (2007) Towards a model for integrative medicine in Swedish primary care. BMC Health Serv Res 7: 107.

30. Agency for Healthcare Research and Quality (2002) Expanding patient-centered care to empower patients and assist providers.

31. Frenkel MA, Borkan JM (2003) An approach for integrating complementary-alternative medicine into primary care. Fam Pract 20: 324-332.

32. Corbin J, Strauss A (2008) Basics of qualitative research : techniques and procedures for developing grounded theory. 3rd ed. Thousand Oaks: SAGE.

33. Patton M (2002) Qualitative research and evaluation methods. 3rd ed. London: SAGE.

34. Makoul G, Clayman ML (2006) An integrative model of shared decision making in medical encounters. Patient Educ Couns 60: 301-312.

35. Van der Weijden T, van Veenendaal H, Drenthen T, Versluijs M, Stalmeier P, et al (2011) Shared decision making in the Netherlands, is the time ripe for nationwide, structural implementation? Zeitschrift fur Evidenz, Fortbildung und Qualitat im Gesundheitswese 105:283-288.

36. Wiesener S, Falkenberg T, Hegyi G, Hök J, Roberti di Sarsina P, et al. (2012) Legal status and regulation of complementary and alternative medicine in Europe. Forsch Komplementmed 19 Suppl 2: 29-36.

37. Kooreman P, Baars EW (2012) Patients whose GP knows complementary medicine tend to have lower costs and live longer. Eur J Health Econ 13: 769-776.

38. Franik S, Huidekoper HH, Visser G, de Vries M, de Boer L, et al. (2015) High prevalence of complementary and alternative medicine use in patients with genetically proven mitochondrial disorders. J Inherit Metab Dis 38: 477-482.

39. Chung VC, Ma PH, Hong LC, Griffiths SM (2012) Organizational determinants of interprofessional collaboration in integrative health care: systematic review of qualitative studies. PLoS One 7: e50022.

40. Van Dijk P (2004) Geneeswijzen in Nederland: compendium van alternatieve geneeswijz. Deventer: Ankh-Hermes bv.

32

Prevalence of High-Risk Underlying Conditions for Pneumococcal Disease among People over 50 Years in Catalonia, Spain

Angel Vila-Corcoles[1,2*], Imma Hospital[1], Olga Ochoa-Gondar[1,2], Cinta de Diego[1], Eva Satue[1], Maria Aragon[3]

[1]Primary Health Care Service "Camp de Tarragona", Institut Catala de la Salut, Tarragona, Spain
[2]Primary Care Research Institute (IDIAP Jordi Gol), Barcelona, Spain
[3]Information System for the Improvement of Research in Primary Care (SIDIAP), Primary Care Research Institute Jordi Gol, Universitat Autonoma de Barcelona, Barcelona, Spain

Abstract

Background: Published data on the frequency and distribution of high-risk factors for pneumococcal disease are limited. This study investigated the prevalence of high-risk underlying conditions for pneumococcal disease among people over 50 years in Catalonia, Spain.

Methods: Cross-sectional population-based study including 2,033,465 individuals aged 50 years or older registered at 01/01/2015 in the Catalonian Health Institute. A previously validated institutional research clinical Database was used to identify high-risk conditions to suffer pneumococcal disease (functional or anatomic asplenia, cochlear implants, cerebrospinal fluid [CSF] leaks and/or immunocompromising conditions). Prevalence of risk conditions was compared according to gender and age strata.

Results: Of the total 2,033,465 study population, an amount of 176,600 persons (8.7%) had any high-risk condition. Prevalence of high-risk subjects did not substantially differ by gender (9.2% in men *vs.* 8.2% in women; p<0.001), but considerably increased with increasing age (5.1% in 50-64 years *vs.* 10.6% in 65-79 years *vs.* 16.1% in people 80 years or older; p<0.001).

Overall, 294 individuals (<0.1%) had anatomical or functional asplenia, 76 (<0.1%) cochlear implants, 41 (<0.1%) CSF leaks, 3,854 (0.2%) had immunodeficiency/AIDS, 16,815 (0.8%) had severe renal disease (nephrotic syndrome or renal failure), 5,034 (0.2%) had received bone marrow transplantation, 103,948 (5.1%) had recent cancer (diagnosed within 5 prior years) and 72,040 (3.5%) received immunosuppressive medication/radiotherapy.

Conclusion: In our setting, almost ten percent of people over 50 years have any high-risk factor for pneumococcal vaccination, basically immunocompromising conditions.

Keywords: *Streptococcus pneumonia*; Risk factors; Underlying conditions; Pneumococcal disease; Pneumococcal vaccines

Introduction

Infections due to *Streptococcus pneumoniae* are a major cause of morbidity and mortality worldwide. According to the World Health Organization, pneumococcal disease causes an estimated 1.6 million deaths annually among all-age populations throughout the world [1]. To date, after the introduction of routine childhood immunization, high-risk individuals and older adults suffer the greatest burden of pneumococcal disease in developed countries. At present, two antipneumococcal vaccines are available for using in adults: the "classical" 23-valent pneumococcal polysaccharide vaccine (PPV23) and the "new" 13-valent protein-polysaccharide conjugate vaccine (PCV13).

Among adult populations, apart from the presence of low socioeconomic status or high-risk behaviours (e.g. smoking and/or alcohol abuse), it is known that the risk of developing invasive pneumococcal disease (IPD) is greatest in persons with certain high-risk underlying medical conditions, such as anatomic or functional asplenia, cochlear implants, cerebrospinal fluids (CSF) leaks, immunodeficiency's and immunocompromising conditions [2-4].

Although some studies have reported major comorbidities and underlying conditions among hospitalised patients with IPD, population-based data on the prevalence of these high-risk conditions is limited. Indeed, despite these patients are considered a major target group for pneumococcal vaccination, data about its true prevalence in most settings is unknown [4-10].

The accurate knowledge of prevalence for distinct risk conditions is important to estimate the true magnitude of at-risk groups and

estimate the size of distinct target populations to implement different antipneumococcal vaccination strategies. In the present study, we investigated the prevalence of distinct high-risk medical conditions for pneumococcal disease among middle-aged and older adults in Catalonia, Spain.

Methods

This is a cross-sectional study involving 2,033,465 individuals aged 50 years or older, who were registered in any of the Primary Health Care Centres (PHCCs) of the Catalonian Health Institute on January 1, 2015 (date of survey). The study was approved by the ethical committee of the institution (file P14/134) and was conducted in accordance with the general principles for observational studies.

In Catalonia, there are 358 PHCCs (comprised by family physicians, nurses, social workers and support staff) which are distributed by geographical area and are responsible for the health care of the population in their areas. The *Catalonian Health Institute* manages 274

---

*Corresponding author: Angel Vila Corcoles, Primary Health Care Service "Camp de Tarragona", Institut Catala de la Salut, Tarragona, Spain, E-mail: avila.tarte.ics@gencat.cat

PHCCs (76.5%), serving a population of approximately five millions people; the remaining 84 PHCCs are managed by other providers. Doctors and nurses systematically use electronic medical records to record medical diagnoses, underlying conditions, prescriptions, and other clinical, patient management activities coded according to the International Classification of Diseases, 10the Revision (ICD-10).

The *Catalonian Health Institute Information System for the Development of Research in Primary Care* ("SIDIAP" database) compiles coded clinical information from the Electronic PHCC's records, and it has been used as main data source for this report. Quality criteria for clinical data and research utility of the SIDIAP database have been reported [11,12]. The SIDIAP sample is representative of the general Catalan population in terms of geography, age and gender distributions, according to the official census [11].

The "SIDIAP" research database was used to identify the following high-risk conditions in each study subject: functional or anatomic asplenia (ICD10 codes D57, D73 and Q89), cochlear implants (Z96.2 and Z45.3), CSF leaks (Z98.2), immunodeficiency/AIDS (D80-D84 and B20-B24), severe renal disease (including nephrotic syndrome [N04 and N39.1] and/or chronic renal failure with glomerular filtration ≤ 30 ml/min), bone marrow transplantation (Z94), solid organ or haematological neoplasia diagnosed within previous 5 years (C00-C97) and/or immunosuppressive medication/radiotherapy in prior 12 months (specific SIDIAP codes). We assumed that information in electronic clinical records was complete, so a condition was considered absent if it was not recorded.

The statistical differences between prevalence for distinct risk conditions according distinct population subgroups were evaluated using the Chi-squared tests or Fisher's test as appropriate, considering statistical significance at p<0.05 (two-tailed). Data were analyzed using the SPSS 18 statistical package.

Results

Of the total 2,033,465 study population, mean age was 66.1 years old (SD: 11.5), being 935,705 (46%) men and 1,097,760 (54%) women. By age strata, 1,021,648 (50.2%) were 50-64 years old, 691,283 (34.0%) were 65-79 years old and 320,534 (15.8%) were aged 80 years or more.

Overall, 294 persons (<0.1%) had anatomical or functional asplenia, 76 (<0.1%) cochlear implants, 41 (<0.1%) CSF leaks, 3,854 (0.2%) immunodeficiency/AIDS, 16,815 (0.8%) had severe renal disease, 5,034 (0.2%) had received bone marrow transplantation, 103,948 (5.1%) had recent cancer and 72,040 (3.5%) received immunosuppressive medication/radiotherapy.

A total of 176,600 persons (8.7%) had any of the above mentioned risk condition and may be considered high-risk subjects for pneumococcal vaccination. Of them, 152,221 presented one high-risk condition, 23,301 presented two conditions and 1,078 presented three or more conditions.

Prevalence of high-risk subjects did not substantially differ by gender (9.2% in men *vs.* 8.2% in women; p<0.001), but considerably increased with increasing age (5.1% in 50-64 years *vs.* 10.6% in 65-79 years *vs.* 16.1% in 80 years or older; p<0.001). Prevalence for each one of the distinct high-risk conditions, according to gender and age strata, is shown in Tables 1 and 2, respectively.

Discussion

Published data about population-based prevalence of risk factors/underlying conditions to suffer pneumococcal diseases is limited [7,13,14]. The present study, which included more than 2 millions people 50 years or older in Catalonia (Spain), estimates the prevalence for most high-risk factors/conditions related to severe pneumococcal infections described in the literature [4,7,15].

Gender Risk condition	MEN N=935,705 n (%)	WOMEN N=1,097,760 n (%)	p	Total N=2,033,465 n (%)
Asplenia	141 (<0.1)	153 (<0.1)	0.504	294 (<0.1)
Cochlear Implant	27 (<0.1)	49 (<0.1)	0.067	76 (<0.1)
CSF Leaks[1]	17 (<0.1)	24 (<0.1)	0.559	41 (<0.1)
Immunodeficiency/AIDS	2,762 (0.3)	1,092 (0.1)	<0.001	3,854 (0.2)
Severe Renal Disease[2]	6,931 (0.7)	9,884 (0.9)	<0.001	16,815 (0.8)
Bone Marrow Transplantation	3,096 (0.3)	1,938 (0.2)	<0.001	5,034 (0.2)
Recent Neoplasia[3]	55,475 (5.9)	48,473 (4.4)	<0.001	103,948 (5.1)
Immunosuppressive Medication/Radiotherapy[4]	29,408 (3.1)	42,632 (3.9)	<0.001	72,040 (3.5)

Table 1: Prevalence of distinct high risk conditions for pneumococcal disease, by gender among Catalonian people 50 years or older.
[1]CFS: Cerebrospinal Fluid
[2]Severe renal disease includes nephrotic syndrome and/or chronic renal failure with glomerular filtration ≤ 30 ml/min
[3]Recent neoplasia includes solid organ or haematological neoplasia diagnosed within previous 5 years
[4]Immunosuppressive medication/radiotherapy administered in prior 12 months

Age group Risk condition	50-64 years N=1,021,648 n (%)	65-79 years N=691,283 n (%)	≥ 80 years N=320,534 n (%)	p
Asplenia	186 (<0.1)	83 (<0.1)	25 (<0.1)	<0.001
Cochlear Implant	23 (<0.1)	31 (<0.1)	22(<0.1)	<0.001
CSF Leaks[1]	11 (<0.1)	16 (<0.1)	14 (<0.1)	<0.001
Immunodeficiency/AIDS	3,111 (0.3)	618 (0.1)	125 (0.0)	<0.001
Severe Renal Disease[2]	1,605 (0.2)	4,783 (0.7)	10,427 (3.3)	<0.001
Bone Marrow Transplantation	2,415 (0.2)	2,251 (0.3)	368 (0.1)	<0.001
Recent Neoplasia[3]	30,339 (3.0)	47,047 (6.8)	26,562 (8.3)	<0.001
Immunosuppressive Medication/Radiotherapy[4]	22,319 (2.2)	28,902 (4.2)	20,819 (6.5)	<0.001

Table 2: Prevalence of distinct high risk conditions for pneumococcal disease, according to age strata in study population.
[1]CFS: Cerebrospinal Fluid
[2]Severe renal disease includes nephrotic syndrome and/or chronic renal failure with glomerular filtration ≤ 30 ml/min
[3]Recent neoplasia includes solid organ or haematological neoplasia diagnosed within previous 5 years
[4]Immunosuppressive medication/radiotherapy administered in prior 12 months

According our results, almost ten percent (8.7%) of the general population over 50 years in our setting have any high-risk condition to suffer pneumococcal disease. This proportion is too similar in men (9.2%) and women (8.2), but it is considerably higher in older than in younger subjects (5.1% in 50-64 years *vs.* 16.1% in 80 years or older).

Our results may have implications for policy makers, having special interest to known the true magnitude of certain target population subgroups and evaluate possible cost-effectiveness of different prevention strategies. To date, there are not universal consensus for pneumococcal vaccination schedules in adults [1,9,10,16,17].

At present, experts are evaluating different alternative vaccination strategies for adults (basically, maintaining "classical" PPV23 recommendations for adults, changing PPV23 for "new" PCV13 recommendation in some risk groups, or adding PCV13 recommendation for all or some target adult population subgroups). Nevertheless, a direct comparison between clinical effectiveness of PPV23 *vs.* PCV13 in adults, together a better knowledge of the magnitude of possible indirect effects from PCV13 childhood vaccination in adults, is necessary before a well informed decision can be made [18]. Apart from its possible better efficacy than PPV23, the lower serotype coverage of the PCV13 is a shortcoming for routine use of PCV13 alone in adult populations. A sequential strategy using both PCV13 and PPV23 vaccines could be a way to achieve greater effectiveness among high-risk subjects. In this way, according to current recommendations of the Advisory Committee on Immunization Practices (ACIP) of the Center for Diseases Control and Prevention, a sequential dual pneumococcal vaccination (PCV13 plus PPV23) is recommended for persons aged 65 years or older (with or without underlying conditions) and persons 19-64 years with CSF leaks, cochlear implants, functional or anatomic asplenia, sickle cell disease or other hemaglobinopathy, congenital or acquired asplenia, immunocompromised persons (congenital or acquired immunodeficiency, human immunodeficiency virus infection, chronic renal failure, nephrotic syndrome, leukemia, lymphoma, Hodgkin disease, generalized malignancy, iatrogenic immunosuppression [treatment with immunosuppressive drugs, including long-term systemic corticosteroids and radiation therapy], solid organ transplant and multiple myeloma) [10,16]. At present, ACIP recommends pneumococcal vaccination using exclusively PPV23 for immunocompetent persons 19-64 years with other comorbidities or risk conditions such as pulmonary or cardiac disease, diabetes mellitus, alcoholism and smoking) [9].

Our study has several strengths. Study design was population-based and large enough to assess accuracy prevalence of main high-risk conditions related to invasive pneumococcal infections. As limitation, although the validity of clinical data source was previously checked, information bias may have occurred if some comorbidity/underlying condition was not recorded, but such misclassification would likely be small considering that the prevalence observed for most risk conditions fit with data previously reported in the literature [7,12,15]. In North Europe, a population-based study including 5.2 million Finnish all-age people, approximately four percent of the population had any high-risk condition for pneumococcal disease (organ or bone marrow transplantation, chronic renal failure, cancer diagnosed within previous 5 years, immunodeficiency or HIV infection) [19]. The impact of possible information bias may be higher in relation to diseases such as AIDS (stigma and legal problems if the patient does not authorize registration) or diseases that are managed in the hospital setting (especially if survival after diagnosis was short).

We have not available data about the prevalence of some high-risk conditions (e.g. solid organ transplantations); so, the global burden of high-risk group for pneumococcal infections may have been slightly underestimated. In addition, the global magnitude of certain high-risk conditions may also have been underestimated in some cases considering that the study population did not include persons less than 50 years of age.

Conclusion

Our data shows that a considerable proportion (almost ten percent) of overall people 50 years or older in our setting have any high-risk condition (especially immunocompromising conditions) to suffer invasive pneumococcal disease and, consequently, they should be considered serious candidates for pneumococcal vaccination. We emphasize that it is important to estimate accurately the prevalence of high-risk individuals because these persons are at the center of the current debate on whether or not to extend the possible vaccination programs (PPV23, PCV13 or PPV23+PCV13) for all or only certain high-risk individuals.

Acknowledgement

This work is supported by a grant from the "Fondo de Investigación Sanitaria" (FIS) of the "Instituto de Salud Carlos III" (call 2015) for the "Acción Estratégica en Salud 2013-2016 del Programa Estatal de Investigación Orientado a los Retos de la Sociedad", framing in the "Plan Estatal de Investigación Científica y Técnica y de Innovación 2013-2016"; code file PI15/01230, cofinanced by the European Union through the "Fondo Europeo de Desarrollo Regional" (FEDER). This work is also funded by a grant from the IDIAP Jordi Gol, Barcelona (grant SIDIAP 13/049). The authors thank Angel Vila-Rovira for his help in the production of this paper.

Contributors

A. Vila-Corcoles and O. Ochoa-Gondar designed the study, assessed outcomes, wrote and edited the paper; M. Aragon obtained the data; O. Ochoa-Gondar did statistical analyses.

˙ The following persons are members of the EPIVAC study group: A. Vila-Corcoles, O. Ochoa-Gondar, I. Hospital, C. de Diego, E. Satue, E. Salsench, J. Blade, X. Ansa, JA. Guzman, F. Gomez, X. Raga, MO. Perez, F. Ballester, R. Magarolas, L. Esteban, E. Figuerola and F. Ramos.

A. Vila-Corcoles, I. Hospital, O. Ochoa-Gondar, C. de Diego and E. Satue designed the study, assessed outcomes wrote and edited the paper; M. Aragon obtained the data; I. Hospital did statistical analyses; the two first listed authors contributed similarly to this work.

References

1. World Health Organization (2012) Weekly epidemiological record. Pneumococcal vaccines. WHO position paper.

2. Ortqvist A, Hedlund J, Kalin M (2005) *Streptococcus pneumoniae*: Epidemiology, risk factors and clinical features. Semin Respir Crit Care Med 26: 563-574.

3. Lynch JP 3rd, Zhanel GG (2010) *Streptococcus pneumoniae*: Epidemiology and risk factors, evolution of antimicrobial resistance and impact of vaccines. Curr Opin Pulm Med 16: 217-225.

4. Centers for Disease Control and Prevention (1997) Prevention of pneumococcal disease: Recommendations of the Advisory Committee on Immunization Practices (ACIP). MMWR Morb Mortal Wkly Rep 46:1–24.

5. Pastor P, Medley F, Murphy TV (1998) Invasive pneumococcal disease in Dallas County, Texas: Results from population-based surveillance in 1995. Clin Infect Dis 26: 590–595.

6. Harrison LH, Dwyer DM, Billmann L, Kolczak MS, Schuchat A (2000) Invasive pneumococcal infection in Baltimore, Md: Implications for immunization policy. Arch Intern Med 160: 89-94.

7. Kyaw MH, Rose CE Jr, Fry AM, Singleton JA, Moore Z, et al. (2005) The influence of chronic illnesses on the incidence of invasive pneumococcal disease in adults. J Infect Dis 192: 377-386.

8. Nuorti JP, Butler JC, Farley MM, Harrison LH, McGeer A, et al. (2000)

Cigarette smoking and invasive pneumococcal disease. Active Bacterial Core Surveillance Team. N Engl J Med 342: 681-689.

9. Centers for Disease Control and Prevention (CDC) Advisory committee on immunization practices (2010) Updated recommendations for prevention of invasive pneumococcal disease among adults using the 23-valent pneumococcal polysaccharide vaccine (PPSV23). MMWR Morb Mortal Wkly Rep 59: 1102-1106.

10. Centers for Disease Control and Prevention (CDC) (2012) Use of 13-valent pneumococcal conjugate vaccine and 23-valent pneumococcal polysaccharide vaccine for adults with immunocompromising conditions: Recommendations of the Advisory Committee on Immunization Practices (ACIP). MMWR Morb Mortal Wkly Rep 61: 816-819.

11. Information system for the development of research in primary care (SIDIAP data base).

12. García-Gil M del M, Hermosilla E, Prieto-Alhambra D, Fina F, Rosell M, et al. (2011) Construction and validation of a scoring system for the selection of high-quality data in a Spanish population primary care database (SIDIAP). Inform Prim Care 19:135-145.

13. Klemets P, Lyytikäinen O, Ruutu P, Ollgren J, Nuorti J (2008) Invasive pneumococcal infections among persons with and without underlying medical conditions: Implications for prevention strategies. BMC Infect Dis 8: 96.

14. Vila-Corcoles A, Aguirre-Chavarria C, Ochoa-Gondar O, de Diego C, Rodriguez-Blanco T, et al. (2015) Influence of chronic illnesses and underlying risk conditions on the incidence of pneumococcal pneumonia in older adults. Infection 43: 699-706.

15. Schoenmakers MCJ, Hament JM, Fleer A, Aerts PC, van Dijk H, et al. (2002) Risk factors for invasive pneumococcal disease. Reviews in Medical Microbiology 13: 29-36.

16. Tomczyk S, Bennett NM, Stoecker C, Gierke R, Moore MR, et al. (2014) Use of 13-valent pneumococcal conjugate vaccine and 23-valent pneumococcal polysaccharide vaccine among adults aged >65 years: Recommendations of the Advisory Committee on Immunization Practices (ACIP). MMWR Morb Mortal Wkly Rep 63: 822-825.

17. European Centre for Disease Prevention and Control. Vaccine Schedule. Recommended immunisations for pneumococcal disease.

18. Vila-Corcoles A, Ochoa-Gondar O (2013) Preventing pneumococcal disease in the elderly: Recent advances in vaccines and implications for clinical practice. Drugs Aging 30: 263-276.

19. Klemets P, Lyytikäinen O, Ruutu P, Ollgren J, Nuorti J (2008) Invasive pneumococcal infections among persons with and without underlying medical conditions: implications for prevention strategies. BMC Infect Dis 8: 96.

33

Quality of Life Predictors and Glycemic Control among Type 2 Diabetic Patients Attending Primary Health Care Centers in Qatar

Mohamed Salem Nasralla Saleh[1]*, Zeliakha Alwahedi[2], Muna Taher[2], Ahmed Mostafa[2], Mohamed Hashim[2] and Hisham Almahdi[2]

[1]*Department of Family Medicine, Faculty of medicine - Suez canal University – Egypt*
[2]*Primary Health Care Corporation - Qatar*

Abstract

Introduction: Diabetes is one of the most worldwide prevalent chronic diseases that impact the quality of life. The aim of treatment in diabetes must go beyond glycemic control to include quality of life. The aim of this study is to assess quality of life and glycemic control among diabetic patients attending Primary Health Care Centers in Qatar.

Methods: Descriptive cross sectional study was conducted to assess quality of life in 281 adult patients with type 2 diabetes attending non-communicable disease clinics in Primary Health Care Centers in Qatar. patients completed SF-36 checklist and information about socio demographic data and disease characters which include some measurements from patient files (BMI,HBA1C,LDL). Data analysis was applied to identify the significant predictors of quality of life with significant limit of $P < 0.05$.

Results: Total sample include 281 patients adult diabetics of whom mean age 53 ± 10.4, 62.1% were males while 37.9% were females, 28.6% were Qatari patients, diabetics with duration more than 10 years represent 37.2%, the average quality of life score is 64.4 ± 24.6, increasing age is significantly associated with less quality of life scores, males were having significantly higher scores than females. Single patients, higher education, type of medications (tablets), controlled LDL and employed were having significant high scores in different quality of life domains. Prolonged duration of diabetes and complications is significantly associated with less quality of life scores, while obesity and HBA1c were not significantly associated with quality of life domains.

Conclusion: Complications, insulin users and women appear to be the most incremental correlate for poor quality of life so special consideration before shifting to insulin and future research on gender specific attributes to improve quality of care to this vulnerable group.

Keywords: Quality of life; Predictors; Glycemic control; Type 2 diabetic patients; Primary health care; Qatar

Introduction

Diabetes mellitus is one of the most daunting challenges posed today by chronic diseases. Recent data show that approximately 130 million people suffer from diabetes mellitus worldwide and that this number will rise to almost 300 million by the year 2025. This more than two fold rise is projected to occur because of population aging, unhealthy diets, obesity and sedentary lifestyle [1]. In Qatar, the overall prevalence of type 2 DM among the adult population has been estimated to be as high as 17%, and a high proportion of pre-diabetes in Qatari adults predicts an increase the prevalence of DM in the next few years [2]. Diabetes substantially increases the risk of blindness, renal diseases, coronary arterial disease, cerebrovascular disease, and peripheral vascular disease [3]. Diabetes mellitus is becoming a major health problem in Qatar, changes in the lifestyle of the population are accused as an important factor in the increase of its prevalence, and Quality of life (QOL) is an important outcome in clinical trials and health care interventions [4]. Sometimes QOL, health and satisfaction with life are used synonymously [5]. The World Health Organization (WHO) defines QOL as an "individual's perception of their position in life in the context of the culture and value systems in which they live and in relation to their goals, expectations, standards and concerns, it is a broad-ranging concept, affected in a complex way by the person's physical health, psychological state, personal belief and social relationships to salient features of their environment" [6]. Diabetes mellitus is a common and demanding health problem that has a great effect on the everyday life of patients [7]. Diabetes complications have important effects on patient quality of life as well as socioeconomic implications [8]. The two major approaches to measuring health related quality of life are generic and disease specific instruments and the two have been compared in diabetes patients and shown to

demonstrate complementary, with generic ones perhaps providing more information than their specific counterparts [9-11]. Therefore the aim of this study was to assess quality of life and glycemic control among diabetic patients attending Primary Health Care Centers in Qatar and to determine the significant predictors of quality of life and glycemic control.

Materials and Methods

Study design

Descriptive cross sectional study to assess quality of life among diabetic patients attending primary health care centers in Qatar.

Study setting

This study was conducted at Primary Health Care Corporation in Qatar, where diabetic patients seen in primary health care centers by specialists or consultants in family medicine through non communicable disease clinics, these clinics are scheduled to be one to two clinics in each health center arranged in morning or evening duty according to each health center situation, the capacity of each clinic reaches average of 25 patients per clinic time.

*Corresponding author: Mohamed Salem Nasralla Saleh, Faculty of medicine - Suez canal University – Egypt, E-mail: msalem@phcc.gov.qa

Study subject

It includes all diabetic patients who fulfill the inclusion criteria: Male and female type 2 diabetic patients who are registered in the non-communicable disease clinic in the selected health centers and agreed to participate in the research during the study period.

Exclusion criteria includes

Type 1 DM, Gestational DM, previously diagnosed depressed patients, patients with communication problems, severe disabling complication.

Sampling

The sample size was calculated according to expected prevalence of good QOL in a previous study done in Saudi Arabia 2013 of 29.8% and another study in Nigeria estimate 20.7% [12,13]. we used 25.25% as average from both studies Assuming a margin of error of 5%, and 95% confidence level, the calculated sample size is 291, according to Daniel equation it includes all patients attending central health centers chosen for their high registration number of diabetic patients who fulfilled the inclusion criteria, selection is based on systematic random sampling technique every 2nd patient until reaching the required number, this was done in 3 months period from 1st June to the end of August 2015 [14]. However due to incomplete information in 10 checklists, so the total sample size reached 281.

Data collection

During the clinic visit, patients completed the Rand 36-item short form health survey (SF-36), and gave the completed form to the interviewers who also explained to them the used form. This process done after approval from institutional review board and signing consent form by patients. The SF-36 data were scored according to the methods suggested in the SF-36 Health Survey: Manual and Interpretation Guide [15]. The eight domains used to assess patient health status in this analysis were: Physical Functioning, Role-Physical, Bodily Pain, General Health, Vitality, Role- Emotional, Social Functioning, and Mental Health. Raw scale scores were transformed to 0–100 scales, in which higher scores consistently represent better health status in all the dimensions measured.

Another questionnaire for the patients was developed by the research team, which includes questions about their personal characteristics, duration of type 2 diabetes, and other potential determinants of quality of life, for example, smoking status, blood pressure measurement, body mass index metabolic control including HbA1c and LDL and complications (micro albuminuria, fundus changes, foot problems and coronary heart disease), type of treatment and compliance. The definition of outcome variables was as following: control of blood pressure if it is less than 140/90 - control of diabetes if HbA1c less than 7% - LDL less than 100 mg/dl are controlled - BMI more than 25 (overweight) if more than 30 (obesity).

Mean (SD) Age (years)			53.8 (±10.4)	Duration of Diabetes	Less than 5 years	96	34.10%
					5 – 10 Years	81	28.70%
Gender	Male	175	62.10%		More than 10 Years	105	37.20%
	Female	106	37.90%	Presence of DM complications	Present	234	83.30%
					Not present	47	16.70%
Ethnicity	Qatari	80	28.60%	Co-morbidities	None	115	40.90%
	Arab	91	32.40%		Cardiovascular	119	42.40%
	Others	110	39.00%		Others	47	16.70%
Social status	Single	12	4.30%	Type of DM medications	Tablets	151	53.70%
	Married	246	87.60%		Insulin and tablets	107	38.10%
	Divorced/Widowed	23	8.10%		Others	23	8.20%
Educational Level	Primary	88	31.40%	Compliance on DM medications	Compliant	218	77.60%
	Intermediate	25	8.80%		Non-compliant	63	22.40%
	Secondary	69	24.70%	LDL Level	Controlled	135	48.00%
	Graduate or higher	99	35.10%		Uncontrolled	146	52.00%
				Target Hemoglobin A1c	Achieved	88	31.30%
					Not achieved	193	68.70%
Job status	Housewife	72	25.60%	BMI	Normal	86	30.60%
	Manual worker	44	15.80%		Overweight or Obese	195	69.40%
	Admin/Business	101	35.80%	Target Blood pressure	Achieved	205	72.90%
	Others	37	13.00%		Not achieved	76	27.10%
	Not working	28	9.80%	Mean (SD) SF- 36 scores	Physical functioning		67.2 (±25.6)
Income	Enough	253	90.10%		Role functioning/physical		70.3 (±39.9)
	Not enough	26	9.20%		Role functioning/emotional		72.1 (±38.9)
					Energy/fatigue		56.1 (±17.8)
Smoking status	Smoker	46	16.20%		Emotional well being		68.3 (±16.8)
	Ex- or non-smoker	235	83.80%		Social Functioning		72.7 (±21.0)
					Pain		55.3 (±16.0)
					General Health		53.4 (±20.5)
					Average		64.4 (±24.6)

Table 1: Socio-Demographic & Disease Characteristics of Patients and distribution of SF-36 scales, BMI: Body Mass Index, SF-36: Rand 36-item Short Form Health Survey, DM: Diabetes Mellitus, LDL: Low density Lipoprotein.

Ethical considerations

Participation in the study was completely voluntary, the investigators explained purpose of research and every patient was able to withdraw at any time, confidentiality was maintained. Approval by Institutional Review Board from research section – Primary Health Care Corporation in Qatar was obtained before conducting the study PHCC/RC/14/07/2014 – RS/RC/FL6/15/05 – Date: 30th April 2015.

Data analysis

Data collected will be analyzed using Epi Info and statistical significant tests suitable for different variables will be used. Categorical data will be tested by X2. Student t test will be used for continuous data. Multivariate analysis will be done to verify the independent factors that could affect the quality of life response.

Results

Table 1 shows the respondent characters: total sample include 281 patients adult diabetics of whom mean age 53 ± 10.4, 62.1% were males while 37.9% were females, 28.6% were Qatari patients, married in 87.6%, less than secondary educated in 40.2% not currently employed in 35.4% and smokers in 16.2% while disease characters of respondent : diabetics with duration more than 10 years represent 37.2%, diabetic complications in 83.3%, diabetics comorbidity in 49.1%, compliance to treatment represent 77.6%, controlled LDL in 48%, achieved HBA1C in 31.3%, obesity in 69.4%, and achieved blood pressure goal in 72.9%. The average quality of life score is moderate 64.4 ± 24.6 in all scale items except (Energy/Fatigue – Pain – General health).

Table 2 shows respondents sociodemographic characters and quality of life domains :increasing age is significantly associated with less quality of life domains (physical functioning, role physical, emotional wellbeing, social functioning and pain), males were having significantly higher scores than females in all quality of life domains except in (emotional wellbeing and social functioning), Qatari patients have higher significant score regarding social wellbeing while Arab patients have higher significant score in two domains (physical function and role functioning physical) but other nationalities have significant higher scores in four domains (role functioning emotional, energy/ fatigue, social functioning and pain). With regard to other parameters such as (single patients, higher education and employed) were having significant high scores in different quality of life domains.

Table 3 shows respondents disease characters and quality of life domains: prolonged duration of diabetes is significantly associated with less quality of life scores specially in (physical functioning, role functioning physical, social functioning, pain and general health). Presence of complications were significantly associated with less quality of life scores (role functioning physical, role functional emotional, energy/fatigue and pain) while no comorbidities were significantly higher scores in quality of life domains (pain and general health). Type of medications (tablets) are significantly associated with high scores in quality of life domains specially (physical functioning, role functioning physical, energy/fatigue, and pain) it was from 60% to 80% range of moderate quality of life. Compliance is significantly associated with higher scores in (role functioning emotional and emotional wellbeing). Controlled LDL is significantly associated with higher scores in quality of life domains (physical function, social functioning and pain) while obesity and HBA1c were not significantly associated with quality of life domains.

Patient characteristics / SF-36 subscales		Physical function	Role functioning/ Physical	Role functioning/ Emotional	Energy / Fatigue	Emotional well being	Social functioning	Pain	General Health	
Duration of Diabetes	Less than 5 years	74.1 (26.3)**	80.3 (35.6) **	77.5(37.9)	61.4(18.0)	67.1(16.5)	77.2 (20.6) **	78.6 (21.3) **	59.3(14.4) **	
	5 – 10 Years	65.6 (25.0)	67.3(41.3)	68.4(38.7)	52.9(16.0)	67.1(16.2)	69(20.1)	71(21.6)	51.6(16.5)	
	More than 10 Years	62.0 (26.0)	63.1(43.3)	71.8(40.4)	54.8(19.1)	71.4(17.3)	71.9 (22.8)	67(27.5)	54.4(16.4)	
Presence of DM complications	Present	68.1 (24.9)	54.3 (46.7)**	61.7 (45.6) **	51.2 (20.4) **	68.5 (16.3)	72.9 (20.5)	61 (31.7) **	56 (16.1)	
	Not present	62.2 (28.6)	73.5 (37.7)	74.2 (37.1)	57.1 (17.1)	67.1 (18.8)	71.9 (23.8)	74.5 (21.1)	51.6(15.6)	
Co-morbidities	None	68.6 (24.7)	76.1(35.3)	72.8(36.3)**	57.0(17.6)	71.4(16.9)**	73.4(19.0)	77.6(18.9)	58.6(14.8)**	
	Cardiovascular	66.4 (26.9)	67.4(42.8)	71.4(42.1)	57.2(17.1)	66.6(16.9)	71.6(22.1)	70.5(25.2)	55.1(16.3)	
	Others	65.5 (24.8)	63.3(42.3)	72.3(37.0)	50.9(19.5)	64.8(15.0)	73.9(23.4)	63.4(27.3)	47.6(16.0)	
Type of DM medications	Tablets	72.1 (23.9)**	73.1(38.5) **	73.3(38.9)	59.1(16.7)**	67.0(15.8)	73.9(20.0)	76.3(21.7)**	56.9(15.8)	
	Insulin and tablets	60.0 (27.6)	63.6(44.0)	72.9(39.4)	52.9(18.7)	71.1(17.9)	70.8(23.6)	65.1(26.3)	53.2(16.4)	
	Others	67.8 (18.3)	82.6(20.6)	60.9(35.8)	51.5(17.3)	63.8(15.9)	73.9(14.1)	78.2(13.4)	54.6(15.6)	
Compliance on DM medications	Compliant	68.0 (25.9)	71.2(40.6)	75.4(38.0)**	57.1(18.1)**	69.7(16.6) 71.8(21.0)	72.1(24.0) 55.2(16.3)			
	Non-compliant	64.4 (24.7)	67.1(37.8)	60.1(40.0)	52.6(16.4)	63.4(16.4)	76.0(21.1)	72.7(22.7)	55.6(15.3)	
LDL Level	Controlled	72.0 (24.8)**	74.6(38.9)	71.6(39.8)	56.5(17.4)	67.4(15.3)	77.4(22.2)**	76.3(23.4) **	56.5(16.0)	
	Uncontrolled	62.7 (25.6)	66.3(40.6)	72.6(38.1)	55.7(18.2)	96.2(18.0)	68.4(19.0)	68.5(23.4)	54.1(16.1)	
Target Hemoglobin A1c	Achieved	69.5 (24.9)	73.6(38.7)	75.0(37.6)	55.6(16.3)	66.5(16.6)	75.3(19.6)	74.0(23.3)	54.6(14.6)	
	Not achieved	66.1 (25.9)	68.8(40.5)	70.8(39.5)	56.3(18.5)	69.1(16.8)	71.6(21.6)	71.4(23.9)	55.6(16.7)	
BMI	Normal	70.9 (25.6)	71.2(39.4)	74.4(38.5)	56.7(17.8)	67.7(16.2)	74.7(20.9)	(75.0)23.7	54.6(17.2)	
	Overweight or Obese	65.5 (25.5)	70.0(40.4)	71.1(39.1)	55.8(17.8)	68.6(17.0)	71.9(21.1)	71.0(23.6)	55.6(15.6)	
Target Blood pressure	Achieved	69.1 (25.5)**	69.1(25.5)**	72.7(39.4)	73.5(38.4)	57.0(17.7)	67.8(16.6)	73.1(21.2)	72.5(23.6)	56.1(15.3)
	Not achieved	61.8 (25.2)	61.8(25.2)	63.8(40.9)	68.4(40.0)	53.7(17.9)	69.6(17.2)	71.7(20.7)	71.5(24.1)	53.0(17.8)

Table 2: Socio-Demographic characteristics and SF-36 subscales (Mean scores of the sub-scales and SD), Notes: ** P values < 0.05 - Abbreviations: BMI: Body Mass Index, SF-36: Rand 36-item Short Form Health Survey, DM: Diabetes Mellitus, LDL: Low density Lipoprotein.

Patient characteristics / SF-36 subscales		Physical function	Role functioning/ Physical	Role functioning/ Emotional	Energy / Fatigue	Emotional well being	Social functioning	Pain	General Health
Age groups	< 55 years	74.8 (23.7)**	80.5 (34.6) **	71.7 (38.8)	57.4 (16.5)	65.0 (15.5)**	77.2 (19.5) **	76.1 (21.7) **	56.4 (14.7)
	55 – 69 years	61.6 (24.5)	62.5 (42.5)	71.6 (40.0)	55.2 (19.0)	70.8 (17.5)	69.5 (21.5)	68.1 (24.0)	53.1 (16.4)
	> 69 years	48.8 (33.0)	51.5 (48.0)	82.4 (35.6)	52.6 (22.0)	74.8 (18.3)	60.3 (24.3)	61.4 (34.2)	55.0 (22.4)
Gender	Male	70.8 (24.8)**	74.4 (37.0) **	75.8 (35.9) **	58.1 (18.9)**	67.4 (17.0)	73.7 (21.5)	74.8 (22.5) **	56.2 (16.4)**
	Female	61.5 (26.6)	64.0 (44.7)	65.3 (43.4)	53.2 (15.3)	69.0 (16.2)	71.0 (20.6)	65.9 (25.1)	52.2 (14.9)
Ethnicity	Qatari	55.3 (27.9)**	52.0 (45.3) **	69.8 (39.5)	51.5 (16.9)**	71.8 (17.6)**	66.0 (22.3) **	63.3 (25.4) **	52.0 (15.2)
	Arab	74.7 (21.1)	78.9 (34.8)	69.0 (40.3)	54.5 (16.1)	63.5 (17.4)	73.8 (20.6)	74.6 (21.6)	54.8 (15.9)
	Others	70.6 (25.9)	77.2 (37.6)	78.6 (37.3)	61.5 (19.3)	70.6 (14.6))	77.4 (20.4)	76.1 (24.2)	57.8 (16.1)
Social status	Single	85.9 (16.3)**	95.5 (10.1) **	75.8 (36.8)	65.0 (12.0)**	71.3 (9.1)	76.1 (18.1) **	75.9 (17.9) **	61.4 (10.7)**
	Married	68.9 (25.2)	72.7 (39.2)	74.3 (38.3)	57.1 (17.8)	67.8 (16.8)	74.4 (20.6)	73.3 (23.9)	55.7 (15.8)
	Divorced/ Widowed	46.0 (28.1)	34.5 (47.7)	58.7 (47.0)	46.9 (18.3)	76.6 (17.3)	54.8 (24.2)	56.9 (26.9)	45.2 (15.8)
Educational Level	Primary	61.5 (28.9)**	52.0 (47.5) **	62.2 (44.0) **	52.5 (18.4)**	72.3 (18.0)	72.0 (23.7)	66.2 (27.0) **	51.2 (14.6)**
	Intermediate	71.7 (22.7)	92.9 (22.6)	93.7 (22.7)	63.1 (17.1)	73.1 (15.4)	75.0 (20.1)	72.9 (23.5)	56.0 (13.4)
	Secondary	67.2 (27.2)	69.1 (39.2)	71.8 (38.6)	55.1 (17.9)	65.8 (15.3)	70.1 (23.0)	69.4 (23.4)	52.2 (17.0)
	Graduate or higher	75.7 (22.4)	81.0 (33.7)	77.8 (36.7)	59.6 (17.4)	67.6 (16.2)	76.5 (19.3)	77.6 (22.5)	59.0 (16.1)
Job status	Housewife	55.2 (27.5)**	46.4 (47.3) **	58.2 (46.3) **	48.7 (14.7)**	69.7 (18.0)	67.4 (22.5) **	57.6 (25.3) **	49.6 (15.0)**
	Manual worker	82.6 (21.4)	84.0 (33.2)	75.2 (38.8)	64.9 (17.7)	72.9 (16.9)	84.0 (19.5)	84.0 (20.5)	54.2 (13.8)
	Admin/Business	72.0 (21.7)	76.7 (34.1)	76.9 (36.6)	57.6 (17.8)	66.5 (15.9)	74.7 (20.1)	73.8 (20.4)	56.9 (15.7)
	Others	76.6 (25.4)	89.8 (25.3)	81.3 (32.7)	65.9 (18.1)	71.1 (17.9)	72.7 (20.4)	82.3 (21.1)	62.5 (17.0)
	Not working	55.8 (25.3)	61.5 (44.2)	80.6 (29.4)	49.2 (15.7)	67.0 (15.3)	66.1 (22.3)	63.4 (28.5)	50.8 (18.0)
Income	Enough	67.6 (26.2)	70.5 (40.9)	73.9 (38.7)	56.5 (18.0)	68.8 (16.4)	73.6 (21.5)	71.7 (24.4)	55.0 (15.4)
	Not enough	68.0 (27.5)	71.0 (41.3)	65.3 (43.5)	58.8 (17.8)	65.0 (20.1)	70.5 (22.5)	72.2 (23.8)	55.8 (20.4)
Smoker		76.4 (21.0)**	76.7 (33.4)	73.6 (38.2)	57.3 (17.1)	64.3 (15.6)**	75.9 (20.1)	74.7 (21.0)	54.8 (14.3)
Ex- or non-smoker		65.5 (26.6)	69.1 (41.4)	72.9 (39.1)	56.3 (18.3)	69.8 (16.6)	72.4 (21.7)	71.8 (24.8)	55.6 (16.4)

Table 3: Disease-related characteristics and SF-36 subscales (Mean scores of the sub-scales and SD), ** P values < 0.05 Abbreviations: BMI: Body Mass Index, SF-36: Rand 36-item Short Form Health Survey, DM: Diabetes Mellitus, LDL: Low density Lipoprotein.

Discussion

In this study of the quality of life and its determinants in diabetic patients in Qatar, we found that regarding sociodemographic factors and its relation to quality of life that increasing age, prolonged diabetes duration, female patients, less educated patients, and no employment have significant less scores in different quality of life domains. These findings are in agreement with who reported that some demographic factors are associated with quality of life in general population as well as diabetic patients such as: men seem to report better quality of life than women, increasing age seems to be associated with decrements in some domains of quality of life also more education is associated with better quality of life [16].

This study found that smoking is significantly associated with higher score in physical function domain of quality of life while it is significantly with lower scores in emotional wellbeing domain; this in agreement of a study found that current smoking is associated with decrease mental health [17]. Giving higher score in physical function domain is self-reported and may not reflect the truth and this finding may be due to high prevalence of smoking in the studied population which is 16.2%. With regard to disease character and its relation to quality of life domains it is found that duration of diabetes, presence of complications or comorbidities and insulin use are significantly associated with less scores in different quality of life domains which is matched with which stated that the strongest correlates of health related quality of life are diabetic complications and its comorbidities, the prolonged duration of diabetes is usually associated with complications which may explain its relation to poor quality of life, also same finding in review of health related quality of life by who found that macro vascular disease reported to be the strongest predictor of poor quality

of life, in our study the cardiovascular comorbidity represent 42.4% which could explain previous results also controlled LDL in our study is associated with higher score in quality of life, at the same time another important finding in our study which is use of treatments other than drugs is significantly associated with less quality scores which is in concordance with study done by which reported that less quality of life satisfaction with insulin use. In regard to BMI, HBA1C, and targeted blood pressure all these factors show no significant relation with quality of life, this is in contradictory to which reported less quality of life among diabetic obese patients [18-21].

Limitations

This study is based on self-reported measure specially may affect complication and comorbidity reporting, it is cross sectional study which may not establish temporal relationship between exposure and outcome measures, there are other factors that may affect quality of life not well assessed in this study such as lifestyle, psychosocial aspects, and health education.

Conclusions

Complications appears to be the most incremental correlate for poor quality of life, so interventions to prevent it may improve quality of life, poor quality of life among insulin users makes special consideration before shifting patients to insulin, and finally women with diabetes appeared to have less score in quality of life domains which mandates future research on gender specific attributes to improve quality of care to this vulnerable group

Acknowledgement

The data referred in current report have been gathered with budget support from research section in primary health care corporation (PHCC) in Qatar. Authors acknowledge participation in data collection of the following residents affiliated to Hamad medical Corporation in Qatar (Dr: Reem Kamal, Dr: Noura Alnachawi, Dr: Ehab Fadel, Dr: Ahmed Abdelrazek, Dr: Adel Abbass, Dr: Aza Ziyada). Acknowledgement is extended to Dr: Mansoura Fawaz, consultant family medicine, PHCC and Dr.Nagah Selim Consultant Community Medicine PHCC.

References

1. WHO (1997) The world health report: conquering suffering humanity world health organization Geneva.

2. Bener A, Zirie M, Janahi IM, Al-Hamaq AO, Musallam M, et al. (2009) Prevalence of diagnosed and undiagnosed diabetes mellitus and its risk factors in a population-based study of Qatar. Diabetes Res. Clin Pract 84: 99-106.

3. Thommasen HV, Berkowitz J, Thommasen AT, Michalos AC (2005) Understanding relationships between diabetes mellitus and health-related quality of life in a rural community. Rural Remote Health 5: 441.

4. Fayers PM, Machin D (2000) Quality of life: assessment, analysis, and interpretation. New York, John Wiley.

5. Snoek FJ (2000) Quality of life: a closer look at measuring patients' well-being. Diabetes spectrum

6. 13: 24-29.

7. Study protocol for the World Health Organisation project to develop a Quality of Life assessment instument (WHOQOL) (1993) Quality of life research 2: 153-159.

8. Faro B (1999) The effect of diabetes on adolescent quality of life. Pediatr Nurs 25: 247-254.

9. Massi-Benedetti M (2002) The cost of diabetes type 2 in Europe. The code 2 study. Diabetologia 45: S1-S4.

10. Anderson RM, Fitzgerald JT, Wisdom K, Davis WK, Hiss RJ (1997) A comparison of global versus disease specific quality of life measures in patients with NIDDM. Diabetes Care 20: 299-305.

11. Woodcock AJ, Julious SA, Kinmonth AL, Campbell MJ (2001) Problems with the performance of SF- 36 among people with type 2 diabetes in general practice. Qual Life Res 10: 661-670.

12. Parkerson GR, Connis RT, Broadhead WE, Patrick DL, Taylor TR, et al. (1993) Disease specific versus generic measurement of health related quality of life in insulin dependent diabetic patients. Med Care 31: 629-639.

13. Abolfotouh M, Salam M, Sukiman w, Alturiaf D, Al-Issa N, et al. (2013) Predictors of Quality of Life and Glycemic Control among Saudi Adults with Diabetes. International Journal of Medicine and Medical Sciences 46: 1360.

14. Issa BA, Baiyewu O (2006) Quality of life of patients with diabetes in a nigerian teaching hospital. HongKong. J Psychiatry 16: 27-33.

15. Daniel WW (1999) Biostatistics: A Foundation for Analysis in the Health Sciences (7th edtn) John Wiley & Sons, New York.

16. Ware JE, Snow KK, Kosinski M, et al. (1993) SF-36 Health Survey Manual and Interpretation Guide. The Health Institute, New England Medical Center, Boston, Massachusetts.

17. Ashraf Eljedi, Rafael T Mikolajczyk, Alexander Kraemer, Ulrich Laaser (2006) Health Related quality of Life in diabetic Patients and Cntrols without Diabetes in refugee camps in the Gaza strip:a cross sectional study .BMC Public health 6: 268.

18. Camacho F, Anderson RT, Bell RA, Goff DC Jr, Duren-Winfield V, et al. (2012) Investigating correlates of health related quality of life in low income sample of patients with diabetes. Qual Life Res 11: 783-796.

19. Li C, Ford ES (2010) Healthy Lifestyle Habits and Health Related Quality Of Life in diabetes. Centre of Disease Control and Prevention. Springer Science and Business media 2096- 2114.

20. Wandell PE (2005) Quality of life of patients with diabetes mellitus. An overview of research in primary health care in the Nordic countries. Scand J Prim Health Care 23: 68-74.

21. Wexler DJ, Grant RW, Wittenberg E, Bosch JL, Cagliero E, et al. (2006) Correlates of health related quality of life in type 2 diabetes. Diabetologia 49: 1489-1497.

22. Huang IC, Frangakis C, Wu AW (2006) The relationship of excessive body weight and health related quality of life:evidence from a population study in Taiwan. Int j Obes (Lond) 30: 1250-1259.

34

Risk Factors Associated with Diabetes Mellitus in a Saudi Community

Khlid Al A[1], Abbas Al M[2*] and Nisha S

[1]Department of Respiratory therapy, Inaya Medical College, Riyadh, Saudi Arabia
[2]Department of Nursing, Inaya Medical College, Riyadh, Saudi Arabia.

Abstract

Background: According to World Health Organization (WHO) statistics almost seven million of the Saudi population are diabetic and three million are pre-diabetic. The risk of developing diabetes increases with some risk factors including family history, age, obesity and lack of physical activity. It is highly significant to allocate resources to quantify the prevalence of diabetes through preforming an assessment of the blood glucose level of the target population. Therefore, we designed this study to determine the association between certain demographic and clinical variables and random blood sugar among Saudi population.

Methods: Cross-sectional design using survey was used to recruit subjects from business location in the capital city of Riyadh. A total of 144 subjects were recruited using Simple random sampling technique. Information gathered included age, gender, family history, history of gestational diabetes, hypertension, level of physical activity, body mass index (BMI) and results of random blood sugar (RBS).

Results: The study provided information about the association between certain demographic and clinical variables and Random Blood Sugar among Saudi population. The age and physical activity were significantly associated with high blood sugar level. Also, females who were diagnosed with Gestational Diabetes Mellitus (GDM) demonstrated a high score of RBS and therefore are at high risk for type 2 Diabetes Mellitus (DM).

Conclusion: In conclusion, this study revealed that there is a significant association between certain demographic and clinical variables and Random Blood Sugar among Saudi population. A prevention program at the level of the community should be initiated targeting those risk factor groups to prevent diabetes mellitus. Also, further studies to modify the risk factors are highly recommended to control and reduce the DM prevalence in Saudi Arabian population.

Keywords: Diabetes mellitus; Gestational diabetes; Risk factors; Prevalence Saudi Arabia

Introduction

Diabetes mellitus is one of the largest global health emergencies of the 21st century and a major public health problem in Saudi Arabia in parallel with the worldwide diabetes pandemic. The adoption of a modern lifestyle is a predisposing factor to this emerging pandemic. The indigenous Saudi population seems to have a special genetic predisposition to develop type 2 DM, which is further amplified by a rise in obesity rates, and the presence of other variables of the insulin resistance syndrome. [1].

As per the statistics of World Health Organization (WHO) Saudi Arabia ranks seventh in the world for the diabetes rates. Approximately seven million of the population in Saudi Arabia is diabetic and around 3 million are pre-diabetic. Indeed, diabetes has approximately shown a ten-fold increase among Saudi population in the past three eras. [2]. DM is irreversible once established. Diabetes develops slowly but progresses from pre-diabetes to diabetes without proper treatment. [3]. As time progresses more and more people live with diabetes, which leads to serious life-changing complications. In addition to the 415 million adults who are estimated to currently have diabetes, there are 318 million adults with impaired glucose tolerance, which puts them at high risk of developing the disease in the future. It has been estimated that two out of five adults with diabetes are undiagnosed in the Middle East [4]. The risk of developing type 2 diabetes increases with family history, age, obesity and lack of physical activity. Besides members of certain racial/ethnic groups, women with prior GDM and individuals with impaired glucose tolerance (IGT) or impaired fasting glucose (IFG) are prone to develop diabetes as well.

Diabetes mellitus is known to affect quite a few body systems and thereby affect the individual's health in different ways such as having coronary artery disease (CAD), renal failure, diabetic retinopathy, etc.

Therefore, many countries attempted to study the consequences of diabetes on the population. However, it is interesting to note that the prevalence of DM is extremely variable among different populations though it increases with aging. The urban areas of Saudi Arabia have high prevalence of DM, owing to changes in the lifestyles of people particularly over the past few decades. [5]. A study conducted in rural areas of Saudi Arabia showed that there was an escalation of prevalence with age and higher-income groups with an overall prevalence in women as twice as that for men. The blood glucose was significantly affected by the factors such as age, income and BMI [6]. An investigation on the prevalence and associated factors for glucose intolerance among Saudi populations in urban and rural communities revealed that the measurement of mean random plasma glucose (RPG) from the urban population was considerably higher than that of the rural population. The world's highest age adjusted prevalence of DM was found in the urban population of Saudi Arabia [7].

In nutshell, the modernization and resultant shift in lifestyle to more sedentary activity with higher-fat diets and obesity are the causes of the increased prevalence of diabetes mellitus in the Saudi community. Rational planning and allocation of resources would be effective with the quantification of prevalence of DM among the Saudi population

*Corresponding author: Dr. Abbas Al M ,Department of Nursing, Inaya Medical College, Riyadh, Saudi Arabia. E-mail: aalmutair@inaya.edu.sa

[8]. Type 2 DM is diagnosed by analyzing an elevated blood glucose concentration. Therefore, it is essential to perform an assessment with blood glucose determination in the target population in order to determine the prevalence of type 2 DM. Considering this, the main objective of our study was to determine the prevalence of type 2 DM in a representative sample among the visitors of a business location in Riyadh. Furthermore, we also intended to identify the risk factors associated with the development of diabetes mellitus.

Materials and Methods

Subjects were recruited from the visitors of a business location in Riyadh. A total of 144 subjects were selected using simple random sampling technique. Information gathered include demographic factors such as age, gender, family history, history of gestational diabetes, hypertension, level of physical activity, Body Mass Index (BMI) and results of Random Blood Sugar (Tables 1 and 2). The exclusion criteria included subjects with other chronic diseases such as hypertension, renal and liver diseases and infectious diseases. Visitors with chronic and infectious diseases were directed to visit a medical center to do further medical investigations. Incompletely filled questionnaires also were removed resulting in a total sample size to n=144.

SPSS software, version 23 (SPSS Inc., Chicago, Illinois, USA) was used for data entry and analysis. The data were presented as scores using a predefined scoring system for each variable. The main outcome was resting blood sugar level, which was calculated on a continuous scale. The Pearson correlation test was used to infer any significant correlation between demographic, clinical variables and main outcome. On the other hand, for analysis of the association between the studied variables and the outcome, generalized linear model (GLM) was used. All analyses were carried out at a significance level of 0.05.

Results

Two variables, specifically age of the participants and physical activity, were significantly associated with the outcome (P=0.027,

P=0.03, respectively) (Table 3). Significant associations in the analysis were used in a generalized linear model to determine the independent factors associated with high RBS levels. The final model showed that being 50 years or older and with no physical activity will increase the risk of having a higher score of RBS, hence will be at high risk of type 2 diabetes. On the other hand, after adjusting for gender, female who were diagnosed with gestational diabetes increase the risk of higher score of RBS and therefore a higher risk of type 2 DM.

After Combining the variable scores for each participant, a linear regression model was used to interpret any association between the total score and final resting blood sugar level (Table 4). Our model revealed a significant association between the total score and RBS (P=0.007). Moreover, using this model, we can conclude that that for each added one unit score unit and increase of 8.437 in resting blood sugar level was recorded (P=0.007). Therefore, increase in the total score of the submitted survey is associated with a higher risk of type 2 DM (Figures 1-3).

Discussion

This cross-sectional survey provides information about the association between certain demographic and clinical variables and Random Blood Sugar among Saudi population. In the results, age of the participants and physical activity were significantly associated with the Random Blood Sugar level RBS (p=0.027, p=0.03, respectively). This confirms a study conducted in rural Saudi Arabia to assess the prevalence of diabetes mellitus. It is also in congruent with a study examining the longitudinal relation among physical activity, BMI and development of type 2 DM in a high risk population [9].

In fact, there were several studies which showed that a physically active lifestyle results in lower incidence of diabetes mellitus. A study conducted among 5990 male alumni of University of Pennsylvania revealed that the leisure time physical activity such as walking, stair climbing, sports etc. are inversely related to the development of type 2 DM. It is not only effective in preventing the type 2 DM but also provides a pronounced protective effect among persons who are at high risk for

Parameter Estimates							
Parameter	B	Std. Error	95% Wald Confidence Interval		Hypothesis Test		
			Lower	Upper	Wald Chi-Square	df	Sig
(Intercept)	243.682	115.8177	16.683	470.680	4.427	1	0.035
[Age=0]	0.705	106.6664	-208.358	209.767	0.000	1	0.995
[Age=1]	26.750	114.7790	-198.213	251.713	0.054	1	0.816
[Age=2]	265.773	119.8827	30.807	500.739	4.915	1	0.027
[Age=3]	0[a]						
[Physically Active=0]	-158.682	53.6132	-263.762	-53.602	8.760	1	0.003
[Physically Active=1]	0[a]						
(Scale)	10539.366[b]	3042.4530	5985.408	18558.173			
Dependent Variable: RBS Model: (Intercept), Age, Physically Active							
a. Set to zero because this parameter is redundant							
b. Maximum likelihood estimate							

Table 1: Model 1.

Coefficients[a]							
Model		Unstandardized Coefficients		Standardized Coefficients	t	Sig.
		B	Std. Error	Beta		
1	(Constant)	75.311	17.742		4.245	0.000
	T_score	8.437	3.070	0.230	2.749	0.007
a. Dependent Variable: RBS						

Table 2: Model 2.

Variable	Score	Frequency (%)
Age (groups)	Less than 40 years	95 (65.5)
	40-49 years	27 (18.6)
	50-59 years	18 (12.4)
	60 years older	4 (2.8)
Gender	Male	31 (21.4)
	Female	113 (77.9)
Gestational Diabetes	Yes	20 (13.8)
	No	11 (7.6)
Family History	Yes	52 (35.9)
	No	92 (62.1)
Hypertension Diagnosis	Yes	117 (80.7)
	No	19 (13.1)
Physically Active	Yes	67 (46.2)
	No	70 (48.3)
BMI	BMI less than 18.50	10 (6.9)
	BMI 18.50-24.99	33 (22.8)
	BMI 25:00-29.99	57 (39.3)
	BMI 30 or more	43 (29.7)

Table 3: Sociodemographic data.

Mean	121.56
Std. Deviation	67.42

Table 4: RBS descriptive statistics.

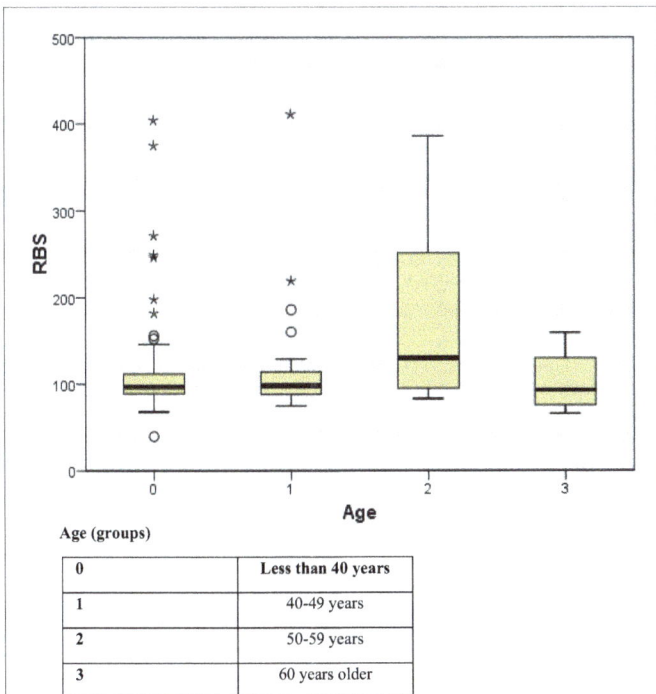

Age (groups)

0	Less than 40 years
1	40-49 years
2	50-59 years
3	60 years older

Figure 1: From the histogram above, we can observe that the data is skewed to the left. As the RBS scores are not normally distributed as shown, we can explain this by the fact of our small sample size.

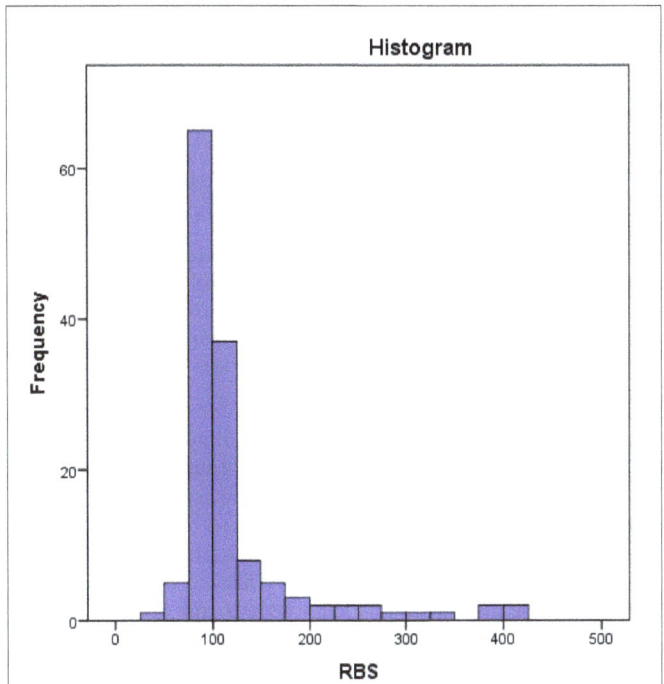

Figure 2: A boxplot representing the age and physically active variables in relation with RBS scores. It can be clearly noticed that older participants with no physical activity are at higher risk of increase in their RBS score, hence higher risk of type 2 DM (RBS 0-500 mg/dL).

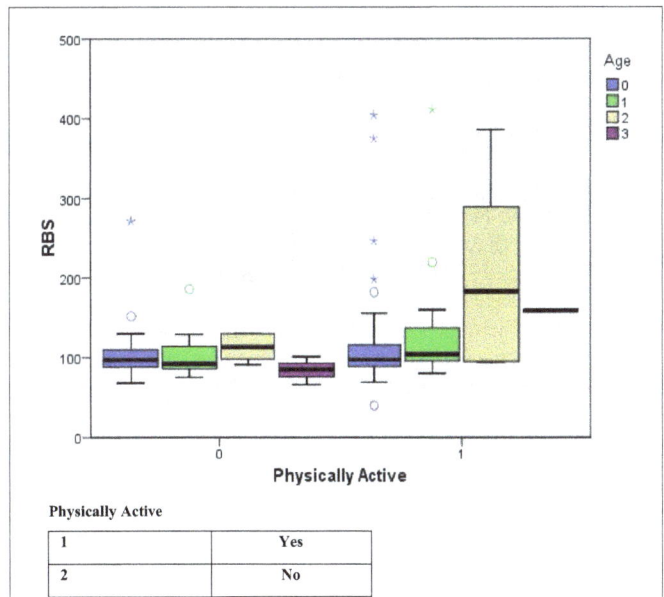

Physically Active

1	Yes
2	No

Figure 3: A line graph representing the increase in mean RBS score as the total score of the survey participants' increase. A steep increase is noticed beyond the total score of 8, which is explained by our previous regression analysis. As most probably, participants who recorded more than 8 in their total scores are from older age groups.

the disease [10]. A prospective cohort study including 5 years follow-up among US male physicians yielded similar results. Apparently, even after adjusting for BMI, the development of type 2 DM was reduced by exercise. It also identified the increased physical activity as a primary prevention strategy for type 2 DM [11]. Comparable findings were observed between regular vigorous exercise and incidence of type 2

DM in a prospective cohort study including 87253 US women aged between 34-59 years, even after doing multivariate adjustments for age, BMI, etc., the reduced risk for type 2 DM found with exercise was not altered [12]. A review of literature about physical inactivity among the population of Saudi Arabia exposed a high prevalence (43.3%-99.5%) of physical inactivity among Saudi children and adults. Additionally, the Saudi population is at high risk for coronary heart disease due to physical inactivity owing to major life style changes in recent years [13].

The results of the present study are very much consistent with the abovementioned prospective studies. However, diabetes was diagnosed by measuring Random Blood Glucose level in the present study, whereas subjective reporting was used in some of the previous studies. Precisely, the incidence of diabetes increases with decreased physical activity in higher age group.

1-3% of all pregnant women develop Gestational Diabetes Mellitus (GDM). Pregnancy induced insulin resistance coupled with decreased production of insulin are considered as the primary causes of GDM. A systematic review on patients with type 2 DM with a history of GDM, reported that once diagnosed with GDM, the progression to type 2 DM was at more similar rates, there was a marked rise of cumulative incidence in the first 5 years and followed by a slow rise after 10 years [14]. The prevalence of postpartum diabetes is found in women with the diagnosis of GDM at less than 24 weeks of gestation [15]. Even non obese glucose tolerant women with a history of GDM were showing a metabolic profile of type 2 DM [16].

The results of the current study are in congruent with the above findings. The females who were diagnosed with GDM, demonstrated a high score of RBS and therefore are at high risk for type 2 DM

A cross-sectional study conducted among adults in Bangladesh revealed that older age, higher socioeconomic status, hypertension and obesity are significantly correlated to the development of type 2 DM [17]. Likewise, a cross-sectional epidemiological study conducted in Greece showed that the prevalence of type 2 DM increased significantly with older age (p<0.001) [18]. Similarly, the prevalence of diabetes in the adult population of US between 40-74 years of age is increasing [19]. A household survey conducted in Saudi Arabia showed a significant increase in the prevalence of type 1 DM, type 2 DM and Impaired Glucose Tolerance in the age group >30 years and a slight decrease in the incidence of type 1 DM among those over the age of 60 years .It also shed light to the fact that Saudi Arabia is one among the countries that have a high prevalence for DM and a moderate risk for Impaired Glucose Tolerance [20].

The prevalence of diabetes mellitus was found to increase with age in the Al Kharj area of Saudi Arabia as 23% of the diabetic patients belonged to the age group more than 65 years whereas, only 0.3% remained in the age group below 24 years. [21].

Conclusion

The findings of the present study also showed that being 50 years or older with less physical activity will increase the risk of having high score of RBS, hence will be at high risk for type 2 DM.

In summary, the current study reemphasize the need for devising a nationwide awareness program about a lifestyle modification including increased physical activity (30-45 min/day), weight reduction, improved eating habits as well as early detection of diabetes. Being health care providers in Saudi Arabia, we have the responsibility for an immediate action to save the country from this alarming condition before it exceeds the capacity of adjustment. A large prospective study is recommended to assess the effectiveness of a lifestyle modification program on the reduction of prevalence of type 2 DM among Saudi population.

References

1. Elhadd TA, Al-Amoudi AA, Alzahrani AS (2007) Epidemiology, clinical and complications profile of diabetes in Saudi Arabia: A review. Ann Saudi Med 27: 241-250.

2. Abdulaziz Al, Dawish M, Alwin Robert A, Braham R, Abdallah Al Hayek A, et al. (2016) Diabetes mellitus in Saudi Arabia: a review of the recent literature. Curr Diabetes Rev 12: 359-368.

3. Guariguata L, Nolan T, Beagley J (2014) International Diabetes Federation. IDF Diabetes Atlas.

4. Lindström J, Peltonen M, Eriksson JG, Ilanne-Parikka P, Aunola S, et al. (2013) Improved lifestyle and decreased diabetes risk over 13 years: long-term follow-up of the randomised Finnish Diabetes Prevention Study (DPS). Diabetologia 56: 284-293.

5. Al-Nozha MM, Al-Maatouq MA, Al-Mazrou YY, Al-Harthi SS (2004) Diabetes mellitus in Saudi Arabia. Saudi Med J 25: 1603-1610.

6. Fatani HH, Mira SA, El-Zubier AG (1987) Prevalence of diabetes mellitus in rural Saudi Arabia. Diabetes Care 10: 180-183.

7. Al Nuaim AR (1997) Prevalence of glucose intolerance in urban and rural communities in Saudi Arabia. Diabet Med 14: 595-602.

8. Alqurashi K, Aljabri K, Bokhari S (2011) Prevalence of diabetes mellitus in a Saudi community. Ann Saudi Med 31: 19-23.

9. Kriska AM, Saremi A, Hanson RL, Bennett PH, Kobes S, et al. (2003) Physical activity, obesity and the incidence of type 2 diabetes in a high-risk population. Am J Epidemiol 158: 669-675.

10. Helmrich SP, Ragland DR, Leung RW, Paffenbarger Jr RS (1991) Physical activity and reduced occurrence of non-insulin-dependent diabetes mellitus. N Engl J Med 325: 147-152.

11. Manson JE, Nathan DM, Krolewski AS, Stampfer MJ, Willett WC, et al. (1992) A prospective study of exercise and incidence of diabetes among US male physicians. JAMA 268: 63-67.

12. Manson JE, Stampfer MJ, Colditz GA, Willett WC, Rosner B, et al. (1991) Physical activity and incidence of non-insulin-dependent diabetes mellitus in women. The Lancet 338: 774-778.

13. Al-Hazzaa H (2004) Prevalence of physical inactivity in Saudi Arabia: A brief review. East Mediterr Health J 10: 663-670.

14. Kim C, Newton KM, Knopp RH (2002) Gestational diabetes and the incidence of type 2 diabetes. Diabetes Care 25: 1862-1868.

15. Kjos SL, Buchanan TA, Greenspoon JS, Montoro M, Bernstein GS, et al. (1990) Gestational diabetes mellitus: The prevalence of glucose intolerance and diabetes mellitus in the first two months post-partum. Am J Obstet Gynecol 163: 93-98.

16. Damm P (1998) Gestational diabetes mellitus and subsequent development of overt diabetes mellitus. Dan Med Bull 45: 495-509.

17. Chowdhury MAB, Uddin MJ, Khan HM, Haque MR (2015) Type 2 diabetes and its correlates among adults in Bangladesh: A population based study. BMC public health 15: 1070.

18. Tentolouris N, Andrianakos A, Karanikolas G, Karamitsos D, Trontzas P, et al. (2012) Type 2 diabetes mellitus is associated with obesity, smoking and low socioeconomic status in large and representative samples of rural, urban and suburban adult Greek populations. Hormones (Athens) 11: 458-467.

19. Harris MI, Flegal KM, Cowie CC, Eberhardt MS, Goldstein DE, et al. (1998) Prevalence of diabetes, impaired fasting glucose and impaired glucose tolerance in US adults: The Third National Health and Nutrition Examination Survey, 1988-1994. Diabetes care 21: 518-524.

20. Bacchus RA, Bell JL, Madkour M, Kilshaw B (1982) The prevalence of diabetes mellitus in male Saudi Arabs. Diabetologia 23: 330-332.

21. El-Hazmi M, Warsy A, Al-Swailem A, Al-Swailem A, Sulaimani R, et al. (1996) Diabetes mellitus and impaired glucose tolerance in Saudi Arabia. Ann Saudi Med 16: 381-385.

35

Self-Management Support (SMS) from a Chronic Disease Worker in a Rural Primary Health Service

Ervin K[1]*, Koschel A[1] and Campi S[2]

[1]*Department of Rural Health, University of Melbourne, Graham St, Shepparton, 3630, Australia*
[2]*Violet Town Bush Nursing Centre, Cowslip St, Violet Town, 3669, Australia*

Abstract

The benefits of self-management in chronic disease have been proven and are a recommendation by the peak body for primary care in Australia. In a region of rural Victoria Self-Management Support (SMS) programs have had limited success due to a lack of implementation by trained staff? In this study a small rural health service trained and supported staff to provide SMS care and evaluated the effect compared to usual general medical practitioner (GP) care.

All clients (over the age of 18) allocated a GP care plan at local consenting medical clinics and those receiving SMS care at the rural health service were invited to participate in a survey using the Patient Assessment of Care for Chronic Conditions survey (PACIC). The PACIC is a brief, validated patient self-report instrument to assess the extent to which clients with chronic illness report care that is patient-centred, proactive, planned and includes collaborative goal setting; problem-solving and follow-up support. Responses were compared using non-parametric testing to determine differences between the SMS group and the patients from the GP group (usual care).

Overall the SMS group reported higher frequencies of always or often receiving care that supported a patient centred, planned approach to chronic disease management. In particular for client involvement in making the plan, choosing their own goals, having a written list, understanding how their own self-care influences their condition and post visit contact. Client feedback supported the provision of the SMS program.

Keywords: Chronic disease; Self-management support

Introduction

The prevalence of chronic conditions is increasing in Australia with more than half of the population aged 65-84 years having five or more long term conditions, which now contributes to 80% of disease burden in Australia [1-3]. It is imperative that successful models of care are implemented to manage the growing burden. There is a growing consensus that clients have a more active role to play in defining and reforming healthcare, particularly in chronic disease management, where clients monitor and manage the majority of their own care, related to their illness, day-to-day [4-6]. Benefits of self-management support programs have been provided and are recommended by the Australian Institute for Primary Care [1,7-9].

In Australia, people with chronic or terminal conditions present for six months or longer are eligible for a General Practitioner (GP) management plan. The management plan provide financial rebates for GPs to manage chronic or terminal medical conditions by preparing, coordinating, reviewing or contributing to plans for ongoing care. The rebates for GPs recognise the increased time required to structure and co-ordinate the often complex care required for these clients [10].

Clients with chronic conditions often require multiple service providers in addition to their GP care. Self-management support (SMS) programs are delivered by health care staff trained in delivering SMS. There are many models of self-management strategies currently in use in Australia including Stanford, Flinders, motivational interviewing, and health coaching [11]. Key principles of SMS includes; shared decision making, which encompasses formulating health goals, using planned evidence based care, improving support and access to resources to assist in self- management and systematic monitoring of the patients health status at agreed intervals [12].

Previous research in SMS in the area under study had been limited to staff implementation of SMS training [13,14]. The findings from these studies highlighted difficulty in implementation of SMS related to staff's perception that current service delivery models did not accommodate SMS and the difficulty in changing clinician practice from traditional information provision models to shared decision making with clients [13-16].

A new model of primary health care in rural Victoria, Australia, undertook provision of a chronic disease worker (CDW) with a component of the role to accept referrals from GP's for clients with chronic conditions. The CDW utilised the GP care plan to implement the required care and coordinate referral to various providers, while at the same time build self-management skills with each client. The CDW had previously undertaken training in SMS for chronic disease. This pilot project aimed to explore the difference between clients receiving care under the usual General Practice care plan model versus that receiving self-management support from a CDW.

Methodology

The area of the study was three small townships with a total combined population of 9,486 people, located in one shire and serviced by one community health and wellbeing program as a consortium. The shire has a known ageing population with high rates of chronic disease [17-19].

*Corresponding author: Kaye Ervin, Department of Rural Health, University of Melbourne, Graham St, Shepparton 3630, Australia, E-mail: ervink@humehealth.org.au

Recruitment

The chronic disease worker identified all clients from the local community health service receiving SMS. The researcher provided a plain language statement describing the study, a survey and a reply paid envelope to all clients receiving SMS, which was mailed out by the administrative staff, two months post visit. The CDW was blinded to the survey to prevent change in practice which may have biased results.

Practice nurses at the medical clinics in the three townships agreed to identify and mail out a plain language statement describing the study, a survey and a reply paid envelope to clients with a GP care plan for chronic conditions. The practice nurses were not blinded to the survey in order to gain compliance with recruiting for the research study. The surveys took approximately 10 minutes to complete and were voluntary. All surveys were returned by reply paid post to the researcher.

Sample Size

All clients (over the age of 18) allocated a GP care plan at consenting medical clinics were invited to participate in this study. This was estimated to be approximately 27 clients. This was the usual care group (GP). In the SMS group an estimate of approximately 36 people were expected to be eligible to participate.

Evaluation Tool

Clients were surveyed using the Patient Assessment of Care for Chronic Conditions (PACIC) survey. The PACIC is a 20 item survey which asks clients opinions about their contribution to their care and treatment, the provision of information, collaborative goal setting, person-centred care planning and referral networks. The PACIC is a brief, validated patient self-report instrument to assess the extent to which clients with chronic illness receive care that aligns with the chronic care model-measuring care that is patient-centred, proactive, planned and includes collaborative goal setting; problem-solving and follow-up support [17].

The PACIC tool consists of five scales and an overall summary score, each having good internal consistency. The PACIC is only slightly correlated with age and gender, and unrelated to education. It is only slightly correlated (r=0.13) with the number of chronic conditions. The PACIC demonstrates moderate test-retest reliability (r=0.58 during the course of 3 months) and is correlated moderately, (r=0.32-0.60, median=0.50, P<0.001) to measures of primary care and patient activation [17].

The PACIC is a practical, client-level assessment of the chronic care model implementation. It is suggested as the preferred tool for evaluating the chronic care model, and demonstrates significant positive correlation with improved client outcomes such as medication adherence, improved rates of exercise, quality of life, reduced hospital admission and self-rating of overall health [18,19].

SMS Intervention

The proposed SMS intervention supports and enhances the goals set by clients as part of their GP care plan. The aim of the SMS intervention is to provide a healthcare environment that delivers information in a way that supports; patient- centred care, health literacy, evidence based practice, timely referrals and healthcare recommendations that are appropriate to the clients health conditions. Clients receive an initial assessment including six areas for current best practice management. The assessment is focused on relevancy of needs, in terms of capacity, including financial, physical and cognitive needs. Clients self-rate how they are managing in each of these areas. The six areas addressed are;

1. Manage medications effectively

2. Engage in specific treatment activities

3. Monitor and act on symptoms

4. Attend services and appointments

5. Manage triggers and risk factors

6. Manage healthy lifestyle factors

Current health behaviours are assessed using the stages of change model and goals are set by the client and documented in a personal self-management plan. Goals are reviewed at subsequent visits with the CDW. When the client feels that they are managing in these areas and can continue working on their health care goals themselves they are discharged from the self-management program.

Analysis

The study utilised a survey with both quantitative questions and the ability to record open ended comments. The qualitative comments are reported as recorded with no thematic analysis undertaken, given the brevity of responses.

Quantitative data analysis was limited to descriptive statistics and describing trends. Data was analysed using Stata, fishers exact testing for categorical variables and Mann Whitney U tests for continuous responses. Power to detect a difference was calculated using results of participants for the GP and SMS groups, resulting in a power of 50% to detect a difference. Given this power and the small sample size non parametric testing, Monte Carlo, was undertaken to detect potential differences. Qualitative comments are presented as client feedback.

Results

Survey responses were collected from 15 clients (55.5%) in the GP group and 23 (95.8%) in the SMS group. In the SMS group seven clients were referred to other services for care, one client was deceased and three clients refused to participate in the SMS program.

The majority of SMS clients were referred to the CDW by their GP. During the course of six months the CDW completed 98 telephone calls with clients, 14 telephones consults with other service providers, 40 home visits and 13 other visits. Fourteen clients had logistical support as part of care co-ordination needs identified through the SMS process in addition to their SMS management plan and 14 clients were discharged from the SMS management program.

Reasons for referral were for varied health conditions but specifically for opinion, support and management of a chronic condition. Goals were closely aligned with referral reasons with independence and staying at home and increased understanding and knowledge being the most commonly reported goals.

The range of self-reported chronic conditions in the GP group included; cardiovascular, arthritis, spinal injuries, obesity and diabetes. In the SMS group conditions included; cardiovascular, arthritis, spinal injuries, mental health issues and diabetes. The majority in the SMS group were listed as multiple conditions. Table 1 reports on the demographic characteristics of the two groups.

Table 2 presents the results of the PACIC survey for the GP and SMS groups. Client feedback was recorded by the CDW. Responses were

		GP group	SMS group	P value
Age	Median	66.3 years	66.5 years	*0.47
	Range	61-73	55 - 80	
Gender	Male	8 (53%)	8 (35%)	#0.3
	Female	7 (47%	15 (65%)	
Length of time associated with service	1 month or less	1 (6.7%)	5 (21.7%)	^0.002
	1–6 months	2 (13.3%)	14 (60.9%)	
	6–12 months	2 (13.3%)	1 (4.3%)	
	Over 12 months	10 (66.7%)	3 (13.0%)	
Know why they have a care plan	Yes	14 (93.3%)	22 (95.6%)	#0.6
	No	1 (6.7%)	1 (4.3%)	

* Mann Whitney U test
\# Fishers Exact test
^ Monte Carlo test

Table 1: Comparison of demographic characteristics.

		GP group	SMS group	P value
Asked for my ideas when we made a treatment plan	None of the time	0	0	0.14
	A Little/Some of the Time	2 (14.3%)	2 (8.6%)	
	Most of the Time/Always	12 (85.7%)	21 (91.3%)	
Helped to make a treatment plan that I could carry out in my daily life	None of the time	0	0	0.03
	A Little/Some of the Time	3 (20%)	1 (4.3%)	
	Most of the Time/Always	12 (80%)	22 (95.6%)	
Given a copy of my treatment plan	None of the time	0	0	0.001
	A Little/Some of the Time	4 (28.5%)	2 (8.7%)	
	Most of the Time/Always	10 (71.4%)	21 (91.2%)	
Asked to talk about my goals	None of the time	1 (7.1%)	0	0.01
	A Little/Some of the Time	3 (21.4%)	2 (8.7%)	
	Most of the Time/Always	10 (71.4%)	21 (91.3%)	
Helped to set specific goals	None of the time	1 (7.1%)		0.06
	A Little/Some of the Time	3 (21.4%)	3 (13%)	
	Most of the Time/Always	10 (71.4%)	20 (86.9%)	
Asked questions about my health habits	None of the time	1 (7.1%)	0	0.09
	A Little/Some of the Time	3 (21.4%)	3 (13%)	
	Most of the Time/Always	10 (71.5%)	20 (86.9%)	
Asked how my chronic condition affects my life	None of the time	0	0	1.0
	A Little/Some of the Time	2 (13.3%)	1 (4.6%)	
	Most of the Time/Always	13 (86.7%)	21 (95.4%)	
Given choices about treatment to think about	None of the time	0	0	0.13
	A Little/Some of the Time	2 (14.2%)	1 (4.3%)	
	Most of the Time/Always	12 (85.7%)	22 (95.7%)	
Asked to talk about any problems with my medicines or their effects	None of the time	1 (7.1%)	1 (4.3%)	0.25
	A Little/Some of the Time	2 (14.2%)	1 (4.3%)	
	Most of the Time/Always	11 (78.6%)	21 (91.3%)	
Given a written list of things I should do to improve my health	None of the time	2 (14.3%)	1 (4.3%)	0.001
	A Little/Some of the Time	4 (28.5%)	0	
	Most of the Time/Always	8 (57.2%)	22 (95.6%)	
Satisfied that my care was well organized	None of the time	0	0	0.11
	A Little/Some of the Time	1 (7.1%)	1 (4.3%)	
	Most of the Time/Always	13 (92.8%)	22 (95.7%)	
Shown how what I did to take care of myself influenced my condition	None of the time	0	0	0.01
	A Little/Some of the Time	3 (21.4%)	1 (4.3%)	
	Most of the Time/Always	11 (78.6%)	22 (95.6%)	
Helped to plan ahead so I could take care of my condition even in hard times	None of the time	0	0	0.07
	A Little/Some of the Time	5 (33.4%)	2 (8.6%)	
	Most of the Time/Always	10 (66.7%)	21 (91.3%)	

Encouraged to go to a specific group or class to help me cope with my chronic condition	None of the time	2 (14.3%)	7 (30.4%)	0.18
	A Little/Some of the Time	6 (42.8%)	3 (13%)	
	Most of the Time/Always	6 (42.9%)	13 (56.5%)	
Referred to a dietician, health educator, or counsellor	None of the time	3 (20%)	8 (36.4%)	0.70
	A Little/Some of the Time	2 (13.3%)	2 (9.2%)	
	Most of the Time/Always	10 (66.7%)	12 (54.5%)	
Contacted after a visit to see how things were going	None of the time	4 (28.6%)	1 (4.3%)	0.04
	A Little/Some of the Time	1 (7.1%)	1 (4.3%)	
	Most of the Time/Always	9 (64.3%)	21 (91.3%)	

Table 2: Comparison of PACIC.

recorded at multiple time points during the SMS program. Responses from clients after the first initial visit included;

- Very helpful and informative, now feeling motivated and wanting to make changes to diet and exercise regime. Information given in a way that you feel like you can actually start to achieve something.

- When asked what the client understands about his diabetes and his management plan. He stated that he has little understanding at present and that the entire doctor said to him was go for a walk 20 minutes 3 times a week to manage his diabetes.

- It has been great to be able to sit and have a talk to someone who can answer all your questions and give you information in a way that is understood. I wish that I had had those years ago. It has been very helpful.

During the program responses recorded included;

- After visiting I have become so much of confidence in processing in my life. It has made me want to continue looking after myself to the fullest and enjoy a future retirement.

- Client states that after setting goals and working on them she now feels more independent, more in control of her life and more settled in the family home. She also stated that she followed up our referral to review her medications and her asthma is being controlled better, she feels a lot better and is less breathless.

- It was very helpful to have someone help me to get on track. The self-management support helped me by explaining what diabetes was and how to manage it. It was helpful to talk through what the dietician and the doctor had said. It made it clearer for me. It was very confusing before that. Lots of appointments and information, etc.

Responses were also recorded from family during the program with the following examples;

- Mum seems more relaxed and less edgy since our service has been in place. The shopping lists are a great idea. This has helped mum manage. Mum is very comfortable talking to you about things. This is a great improvement on her refusing all services and not letting anyone into the home. (all services were reinstated to allow the couple to remain living in their home)

- Wife stated I don't know what you said to my husband but he has now got me buying cottage cheese. He received the information in the mail, that you sent, and he has read over it all very carefully. Since you spoke with him he has had a complete change in his thinking, he realises that he needs to change his lifestyle to improve his health so that he can live longer.

Responses recorded at the point of discharge included:

- Client stated that prior to seeing me she had thought there was no point in living. She now says that she feels like a new woman and her whole outlook has changed. She feels stronger both physically and mentally. She has completely changed her life around in that she is now exercising daily, attending appointments with navigating life, setting boundaries around family relationships, managing pain and making better food choices.

- Got motivated to get back on track and manage my type 2 diabetes. I have lost weight, more motivated, diabetes under better control, feeling better, lot more energy, feeling like I can manage a full day's work and enjoying life more. I feel that I can manage my health now.

- Very helpful, I was able to discuss my concerns and then I was given helpful advice

Discussion

There was a significant difference in response rate between the GP and the SMS group. The GP group relied on practice nurses identifying patients and mailing out the survey. Clients in the SMS group had recent contact with the CDW within 2 months of the survey; however in the GP group contact with the GP may have occurred longer ago than two months. Recent contact may influence a person to respond in comparison to a patient who has not had recent contact; this may explain the difference in responses.

There was no difference between age and gender or knowledge of having a care plan between the two groups. The SMS group reported being associated with providing service for less time than those in the GP group, not surprising given it was a new program.

The value of having a CDW is demonstrated in the statistically significant differences in SMS group in relation to the following:

- Involvement of the client when making a treatment plan to carry out in their daily life,

- Being given a copy of their treatment plan,

- Being asked to talk about their own goals,

- Receiving a written list,

- Understanding how self-care influences condition, and

- Being contacted after the visit for follow up.

Broader literature shows that involving the client in their treatment plan and talking about goals results in improved outcomes, both for compliance to the plan and resulting improvements in their condition [20]. Education for clients regarding their conditions and ensuring that information is understood has been shown in other studies to improve clinical outcomes for clients [21]. In contrast, many other studies show that compliance is poor when clients do not have an understanding of the reasons or the impact that treatment has on their condition [22]. It has long been recognised that time constraints for GP's prevent them undertaking the level of client education required [23]. Given the demands of GP's and the associated costs of extended visits, it makes good economic sense to utilise other health workers to undertake this role.

Although there was no significant difference overall for the remainder of elements assessed however there were some differences in frequency worthy of discussion. Compared to the GP group, clients in the SMS group reported higher frequencies of the following often occurring:

- Assisted in goal setting to achieve improved eating and exercise,

- Being asked about their health habits,

- Asked how their condition affected their life,

- Being given choices about their treatment,

- Being asked to talk about problems with their medications,

- Helped to make plans so they could take care of themselves even in hard times, and

- Recommended specific groups of class activities for those with chronic conditions.

Choices and preferences for clients regarding treatment is a fundamental tenet of client autonomy and self-determination [24]. Involving clients in their care and treatment by elucidating their values and what matters most to them more likely results in better compliance and resultant improved health outcomes [24]. Models of care, where the GP advises the client what to do, without consideration of the clients preferences but based on the GP's expertise, have not been acceptable models of care for some time [25]. The best recommendations in the world are wasted, if the client does not follow them [26]. There is also compelling evidence that patients who are active participants in managing their health and health care have better outcomes than patients who are passive recipients of care [27].

There was no difference between groups for being satisfied that care was well organised or being encouraged to attend community programs. The GP group reported higher frequencies of being referred to an allied health professional compared to the SMS group. This is potentially because the CDW was able to meet the needs of client without referral.

Qualitative responses provided and reported above suggest that the support of the CDW has been invaluable immediately after initial assessment, during the program and prior to discharge. Clients report better understanding of their conditions and support to initiate and maintain changes to poor health behaviours contributing to their conditions. This suggests that CDW's have time to elucidate root-cause behaviour issues which impact on the chronic condition as well as a viable process that addresses the underpinning issues. These positive results demonstrate the usefulness of initiating and maintaining the motivation of clients with chronic conditions.

It should be acknowledged that the sample size was small and power to detect a difference therefore compromised by this; however the qualitative results are consistent with the survey results suggesting that the positive outcomes achieved are valid.

Conclusion and Recommendations

There were several significant differences in the SMS group in relation to CDW support that advocate for the continued use of such health professionals. Where specific items assessed were not statistically different between the GP group and the SMS group the SMS group fared better for consistency in always receiving care compared to mostly in the GP group. Comments provided by clients further support the benefits in relation to initiating change and maintaining change in clients to improve health outcomes.

Previous evaluations of SMS in the Hume region have demonstrated that staff trained in SMS failed to implement the training and therefore achieve improved service delivery and support for clients with chronic conditions [14-18]. Anecdotally, previous poor uptake of SMS is also reportedly a result of the need to make government targets for care delivery and the onerous reporting involved. The framework of support in this project enabled the CDW to work collaboratively with clients at a suitable pace, reflecting a person-centred culture, with resultant better uptake and outcomes. This evaluation demonstrated that staff commitment to service delivery change to support clients with chronic conditions resulted in much improved support for clients. It is the first evidence in the region to demonstrate the benefits of SMS training and achievable implementation.

Acknowledgement

We acknowledge the Australian Government Department of Health University Department of Rural Health Program for funding.

References

1. Australian Institute for Primary Care (2008) Early intervention in chronic disease in community health services initiative. Statewide Evaluation, Technical and Data Report.

2. Australian Institute of Health and Welfare (2014) Australia's health Canberra: AIHW.

3. Stone GR, Packer TL (2010) Evaluation of a rural chronic disease self-management program. Rural Remote Health 10: 1203.

4. Wagner EH, Austin BT, Davis C, Hindmarsh M, Schaefer J, et al. (2001) Improving chronic illness care: translating evidence into action. Health Aff (Millwood) 20: 64-78.

5. The MacColl Center for Health Care Innovation (2004) Group Health Cooperative. Improving Chronic Illness Care. Group Health's MacColl Center for Health Care Innovation.

6. Wagner EH (1998) Chronic disease management: What will it take to improve care for chronic illness? Eff Clin Pract 1: 2-4.

7. Bodenheimer T, Lorig K, Holman H, Grumbach K (2002) Patient self-management of chronic disease in primary care. JAMA 288: 2469-2475.

8. Bundy C (2004) Changing behaviour: using motivational interviewing techniques. J R Soc Med 97 Suppl 44: 43-47.

9. Coleman MT, Newton KS (2005) Supporting self-management in patients with chronic illness. Am Fam Physician 72: 1503-1510.

10. Department of Health, A. Primary care fact sheet - Chronic disease 2014.

11. Department Health Victoria. Common models of chronic disease self-management support. A fact sheet for Primary Care Partnerships.

12. Gale J (2010)Health coaching guide for health practitioners: Using the HCA model of health coaching.

13. Jeffery V, Ervin K (2014) Early intervention in chronic disease--four years on: barriers to implementing self-management strategies. J Allied Health 43: e1-3.

14. Ervin K, Jeffery V (2013) Staff perceptions of implementing health coaching as a tool for self management in chronic disease: A qualitative study. Journal of Nursing Education and Practice 9.

15. Ervin K, Jeffery V, Koschel A (2012) Evaluating the implementation of health coaching in a rural setting. Journal of Hospital Administration.

16. Ervin K, Jeffrey V (2015) Does peer leader support improve implementation of SMS training? Asia Pacific Journal of Health Management.

17. Glasgow RE, Wagner EH, Schaefer J, Mahoney LD, Reid RJ, et al. (2005) Development and validation of the Patient Assessment of Chronic Illness Care (PACIC). Med Care 43: 436-444.

18. Robert Wood Johnson Foundation (2015) Improving Chronic Illness Care: The Chronic Care Model.

19. Robert K, Lyon R, Slawson J (2011) Delivering better chronic disease care is a team sport that requires a clear game plan. Family Practice Management 18: 27-31.

20. Strickland PA, Hudson SV, Piasecki A, Hahn K, Cohen D, et al. (2010) Features of the Chronic Care Model (CCM) associated with behavioral counseling and diabetes care in community primary care. J Am Board Fam Med 23: 295-305.

21. Bowen JL, Provost L, Stevens DP, Johnson JK, Woods DM, et al. (2010) Assessing Chronic Illness Care Education (ACIC-E): a tool for tracking educational re-design for improving chronic care education. J Gen Intern Med 25 Suppl 4: S593-609.

22. Burke B L, Dunn C W, Atkins D C, Phelps J S (2004) The Emerging Evidence Base for Motivational Interviewing: A Meta-Analytic and Qualitative Inquiry. Journal of Cognitive Psychotherapy18: 309-322.

23. Yarnall KS, Pollak KI, Østbye T, Krause KM, Michener JL (2003) Primary care: is there enough time for prevention? Am J Public Health 93: 635-641.

24. Elwyn G, Frosch D, Thomson R, Joseph-Williams N, Lloyd A, et al. (2012) Shared decision making: a model for clinical practice. J Gen Intern Med 27: 1361-1367.

25. Charles C, Gafnia A, Whelan T (1999) Decision-making in the physician patient encounter: revisiting the shared treatment decision-making model. Soc Sci Med 651-661.

26. Novella S (2013) Patient Participation in Decision-Making. Science-Based Medicine.

27. Coulter A, Collins A (2011) Making shared decision-making a reality. No decision about me, without me. The Kings Fund.

36

Stability and Sterility Data in Pre-Filled Syringes for Zuclopenthixol Acetate and Haloperidol used in Emergency Tranquilisation

Hana Morrissey[1]* and Patrick Ball[2]

[1]Grad Cert Wound Care, Dip Hosp Pharm Admin, Senior Lectuer in Pharmacy, MHFA Instructor, School of Psychological and Clinical Sciences, Charles Darwin University, Ellengowan Drive, Darwin NT 0909, Australia
[2]Patrick Ball, Charles Darwin University, Ellengowan Drive, Darwin NT 0909, Australia

Abstract

Background: Needle stick injuries are a known risk in the acute hospital setting especially where the patient is agitated. The emotional burden on the staff experiencing this occupational injury is well reported, however there is insufficient data to support storing pre-filled syringes, out of the manufacturer's pack for longer than for immediate administration.

Aim: The aim was to investigate the stability and sterility of zuclopenthixol acetate and haloperidol in pre-filled syringes to allow their use as an alternative to drawing the dose from an ampoule or vial prior to administration.

Method: Two of the commonly used products in rapid tranquilisation were aseptically drawn in suitable syringes and tested for stability and sterility to establish shelf-life. Ten invited medical and nursing staff involved in rapid tranquilisation were invited to a focus group for feedback on the product practicality of use, cost and logistics of stock management.

Results: The stability and sterility tests show that zuclopenthixol acetate and haloperidol retained stability and sterility when stored under 25°C in a 3 mL disposable plastic syringes, for a period of 60 days with cost of AU$67 and AU$30 per syringe respectively.

Conclusion: The prefilled syringes provide ease and speed of administration, potential reduction in needle-stick-injuries and proved to maintain sterility. This study demonstrated that zuclopenthixol acetate 150 mg/3mL and haloperidol 15mg/3mL retained stability and remained sterile when stored under 2-8°C in plastic syringes for a period of 60 days. However the proposal was not adopted as dose flexibility was considered a greater priority than the safety gains.

Keywords: Tranquilisation; Needle-stick injuries; Stability; Sterilisation; Zuclopenthixol acetate; Haloperidol

Introduction

Needle stick injury (NSI) is a known risk in the acute hospital setting. While the prevalence is low in Australia [1] the emotional burden on health professionalsfollowingan incident is high and may require absence from duty and interruption to the person's life-style until their safety is ensured [1]. It is also known that needlestick injuries are under-reported, especially from practitioners outside the public hospital setting [2-4], with administration and re-capping needles found to be the most common causes [3].

In mental health facilities, patients who require the administration of rapid tranquilisation medications are likely to be agitated, increasing the risk of needlestick injuries for the staff administering the medication, and the supporting staff involved in the de-escalation intervention or restraining the patient. The time from the decision to administer medication to the deliverycan be critical to patient safety. The nature of this procedure does not lend itself to the use of cannulation and needle-less injection systems. The ECRI Institute [5,6] reported that 59% of health staff injuries from sharps are caused by needles.

The most common infections found with needlestick injuries in Australia were Hepatitis B, Hepatitis C and HIV [5,6]. When compared, the prevalence of positively diagnosed conditions was similar to the data from the United Kingdom and United States of America (Table 1).

The same report presented data on the direct and indirect cost of needle stick injuries. This included the investigation, treatment and lost productivity due to time off for investigations, anxiety and distress [5,6].

To gain understanding of the rapid tranquilisation (RT) process (calming without full sedation) and the dynamics of the situation, an

Virus type	Australia	United Kingdom	United States of America
Hepatitis C	1.6-40%	30%	6-30%
Hepatitis B	1.8-10%	3%	1.8%
HIV	0.1-0.3%	0.3%	0.3%

*Value of Technology: Needle stick and Sharps Injuries and Safety-Engineered Medical Devices[5]&[6], at: http://www.mtaa.org.au/docs/vot/vot-needlestick-and-sharpscopytosend.pdf?sfvrsn=0. Revised on: 22/12/13

Table 1: Needlestick Injuries and transmission risks of Hepatitis C, Hepatitis B and Human Immunodeficiency Virus*.

RT administration in the hospital was attended. It was observed that the patient distress and the staff stress surrounding the whole process could easily lead to needle stick injury during the process of preparing the required dose. The nursing and medical staff feedback remains a crucial part in establishing the practicality and safety of the product.

Method

No ethical approval was required as the project involved only laboratory testing.

*Corresponding author: Hana Morrissey, Grad Cert Wound Care, Dip Hosp Pharm Admin, MHFA Instructor, FACP, AACPA, RP. School of Psychological and Clinical Sciences, Charles Darwin University, Ellengowan Drive, Australia, E-mail: Hana.morrissey@cdu.edu.au

Identifying the medications will be tested

The most commonly used medications in rapid tranquilisations in this facility were midazolam, haloperidol and zuclopenthixol acetate. Olanzapine was sometimes used but at the time was "special access scheme medicine," not approved or funded for general use in Australia. In addition, its form as a lyophilised powder and poor stability after reconstitution limited its potential in this context, accordingly it was not considered to be feasible. Benztropine was also used, but it was not used often and is used only after initial sedation to control side effects, when the situation has calmed. Midazolam was excluded as the Therapeutics Good Administration (TGA) of Australia had a previously established profile and identified a 60 days shelf-life, from production date, if the syringes were prepared in an approved Pharmaceutical Inspection Convention and Pharmaceutical Inspection Cooperation Scheme (PIC/S) clean room environment and aseptic manufacturing process. Accordingly haloperidol and zuclopenthixol acetate were chosen to be tested.

The products tested for stability were: zuclopenthixol acetate, clear glass single use ampule (Clopixol Accuphase™, Lundbeck Australia Pty. Ltd) 30 mg/3 mL and haloperidol glass single use ampule (Serenace™, Sigma Pharmaceuticals Pty. Ltd) 5 mg/mL, the syringes used were Becton, Dickinson and company™ manufactured 5 mL plastic disposable syringes containing a final volume of 3 mL. Storage condition of the original products was nominated to be 25°C. Acquisition of all items required and all processes and process documentation involved in aseptic compounding of these products were conducted in accordance with PIC/S. The supplier provided the testing laboratory with one batch of each of the test products. Each syringe contained the exact content of one ampule and was directly filled from that ampule. The aseptic filling process was completed in an accredited clean room utilising a laminar flow cabinet by a validated clean room technician under supervision of a registered pharmacist.

Testing after the aseptic manufacturing

Two aspects were tested, stability and sterility. Stability was tested in the TGA'sapproved laboratories and the microbiology, sterility and endotoxin content were conducted in the AMS™ Laboratories (Silverwater Australia) (AMS).

Stability testing TGA Laboratories

The method was designed (Table 2) by the TGA, based upon the methods of the British Pharmacopeia. Additional information was requested by the TGA to guide the development of the testing method; such as the desirable storage condition at the point of use in health facilities and frequency of use of the two products. The time stability trial required that:

- The pre-filled syringes must be filled by the selected manufacturer with the same commercial products as would be used in future production in accordance to the manufacturer's validated aseptic compounding process.

- The syringes used in the testing process must be the same to that will be used in future production.

- If any of the batch production conditions or material changed the stability data would no longer be valid and new stability trial would be required.

Three packs of 10 syringes of each of the two products were delivered to the TGA laboratories and the master code, batch number and expiry date for the syringes were recorded on receipt. A sample identification code was then assigned to each product by the TGA scientists and stored in a temperature controlled store room under 22 ± 1°C.

- In lots of five syringes of each medicine per time-point for plus one lot of five used as control. The pilot batch of syringes was produced and transported from the manufacturer to the TGA laboratories under the same transport conditions as to be used to deliver to the health facilities, and at the same temperature (25°C) the product will be stored during transportation of the manufacturer product requirement.

- Haloperidol syringes were tested at weeks 1, 3, 6 and 9 after receipt date, and zuclopenthixol acetate syringes were tested at weeks 2, 4, 7 and 10 after receipt date.

- The products were tested to using the methods specified in the British Pharmacopoeia 2008 (Table 2).

Sterility testing AMS laboratories

- Ten syringes of each of the two products were delivered to the AMS laboratories under the same transport conditions as to be used to deliver to the health facilities, and at the same temperature (25°C) the product will be stored during transportation of the manufacturer product requirement.

- A sample identification code was then assigned to each product by the AMS scientist and stored in a temperature controlled store room under 22 ± 1°C.

- Appearance was noted on both samples, using a 3 mL syringe of each of the two products.

- The laboratory used the Limulus Amoebocyte Lysate (LAL) kinetic chromogenic method TM125 for sample validation.

Clopixol Accuphase™ zuclopenthixol acetate 150 mg/3mL samples were initially diluted in pyrogen-free water (PFW) with 0.5%

Product / presentation	Test / procedure	Test method
Serenace™ Haloperidol 15 mg/3mL syringes for injection	Appearance	Visual inspection
	Content and ID of haloperidol	HPLC
	Related substances	TLC
	pH	British pharmacopeia
	Particulate matter (at week 9 only)	British pharmacopeia
Clopixol Accuphase™ zuclopenthixol acetate 150mg/3mL	Appearance	Visual inspection
	Content and ID of zuclopenthixol acetate	HPLC
	Related substances	HPLC
	Colour saturation at 440 nm	UV
	Particulate matter (at week 10 only)	British pharmacopeia

Table 2: Products tested to Pharmacopoeial specifications.

pyrosperse (supplied by Cambrex / Lonza) and vigorously vortexed as a pre-treatment step. Further dilution was then made in PFW to investigate the inhibition and enhancement effect by spiking a known amount of endotoxinand testing for recovery. A dilution of 1/100 in PFW was shown to have a satisfactory recovery, indicating an adequate prevention of inhibition and enhancement by the product.

Serenace™ Haloperidol 15 mg/3 mL sample did not require a pre-treatment; dilutions were made in PFW to also to investigate the inhibition and enhancement effect by spiking a known amount of endotoxin and testing for recovery. Dilution of 1/100 in PFW was shown to have a satisfactory recovery, indicating an adequate prevention of inhibition and enhancement by theproduct.

After validation tests were performed the TM125 (kinetic chromogenic) LAL test was performed on the samples.

Results

Stability tests results

The samples met the specified physical characteristics of the two products as specified in the 2008 British Pharmacopeia with no changes or trends identified in their visual appearance. There were no changes in the parent products or their related substances. The particulate matter

remained within the 2008 British Pharmacopeia range. The parent product remained within the British Pharmacological requirement (2008) ranges (95-105% for Clopixol Accuphase™ and 90-110% for Serenace™) with insignificant changes recorded as 2.4% and 4.2% for Clopixol Accuphase™ and 90-110% for Serenace™ respectively. The results are shown in Tables 3 and 4. Only Haloperidol required pH testing as indicated by the British Pharmacopeia 2008.

Sterility tests results

The results for the Kinetic Chromogenic LAL assay which performed to detect endotoxin units (EU)/mL was <0.5 EU/mL (Limit is 0.5 EU/mL) for Clopixol Accuphase™ zuclopenthixol acetate and Serenace™ Haloperidol 15 mg/3mL samples (Table 5).

Clopixol Accuphase™ zuclopenthixol acetate 150 mg/3mL sample validations for sterility was conducted and growth was recovered within 72hours at respective incubation temperatures (Table 6) indicating that the sample testing procedures and specification were conducted in accordance with the test for sterility specified in the TM115 section 5, British 2008 and European Pharmacopeia 2008.

The sterility test results for Clopixol Accuphase™ zuclopenthixol acetate and Serenace™ Haloperidol 15 mg/3mL samples indicated no

Time Point	Test Results / Specifications				
	Visual appearance	Assay of zuclopenthixol acetate HPLC	Related substances (including transisomer) HPLC	Colour of the solution at 440 nm HPLC	Particulate matter BP method
	Clear yellowish oil	95-105%	Complies with BP	NMT 0.2	Complies
Week 2	Satisfactory	101.2	Complies	0.054	Complies
Week 4	Satisfactory	100.4	Complies	0.047	Complies
Week 7	Satisfactory	98.9	Complies	0.054	Complies
Week 10	Satisfactory	98.8	Complies	0.056	Complies

Table 3: Clopixol Accuphase™ zuclopenthixol acetate 150mg/3mL samples specification for stability test.

Time Point	Test Results / Specifications				
	Visual appearance	Assay of haloperidol HPLC	Related substances By TLC	pH	Particulate matter BP method
	Clear colourless solution	90-110%	Complies with BP	2.8-3.6	Complies
Week 2	Satisfactory	102.1	Complies	3.3	Complies
Week 4	Satisfactory	98.7	Complies	3.3	Complies
Week 7	Satisfactory	98.5	Complies	3.4	Complies
Week 10	Satisfactory	97.9	Complies	3.4	Complies

Table 4: Serenace™ Haloperidol 15 mg/3mL syringes for injection samples specification for stability test.

Sample Reference	LAL Assay Detection Limit Endotoxin units (EU)/mL	LAL Result EU/mL
Serenace™ Haloperidol 15 mg/3mL syringes for injection Diluted 1/100 in PFW	0.5	<0.5
Clopixol Accuphase™ zuclopenthixol acetate 150 mg/3mL Initial dilution of 1/10 in PFW with 0.5% pyrosperse made and vortexed. Further dilution then made to 1/100 in PFW	0.5	<0.5

Table 5: Kinetic Chromogenic LAL test results.

Test organism	Strain number	Media used	Incubation temperature in ºC	Inoculum A (cfu/mL)	Inoculum B (cfu/mL)	Mean (cfu/mL)	Evaluation (growth/no growth)
Staphylococcus aureus	ATCC 6538	THO	30-35ºC	35	39	37	Growth
Pseudomonas aeruginosa	ATCC 9027	THO	30-35ºC	14	17	16	Growth
Clostridium sporogenes	ATCC 11437	THO	30-35ºC	43	49	46	Growth
Bacillus subtillis	ATCC 6633	TO5	20-25ºC	70	85	78	Growth
Candida albicans	ATCC 10231	TO5	20-25ºC	19	22	21	Growth
Aspergillus niger	ATCC 16404	TO5	20-25ºC	27	34	31	Growth

Table 6: ClopixolAccuphase™ zuclopenthixol acetate 150mg/3mL and Serenace™ Haloperidol 15 mg/3mL samples validation.

Media / Incubation Clopixol Accuphase™ zuclopenthixol acetate 150mg/3mL	Observation Growth / No growth
Fluid Thioglycollate USP+ 0.5% Tween 80 at 30-35ºC / 14 days	No growth
Tryptone Soya Broth + 0.5% Tween 80 at 20-25ºC / 14 days	No growth

Table 7: ClopixolAccuphase™ zuclopenthixol acetate 150 mg/3mL sterility tests results after 60 days.

Media / Incubation Serenace™ Haloperidol 15 mg/3mL syringes for injection	Observation Growth / no growth
Fluid Thioglycollate USP+ 0.5% Tween 80 at 30-35ºC / 14 days	No growth
Tryptone Soya Broth + 0.5% Tween 80 at 20-25ºC / 14 days	No growth

Table 8: Serenace™ Haloperidol 15 mg/3mL syringes for injection sterility tests results after 60 days.

growth when treated with fluid thioglycollate USP + 0.5% tween 80 at 30-35ºC / 14 days and tryptone Soya Broth + 0.5% Tween 80 at 20-25ºC / 14 days (Table 7 and 8), which complies with British 2008 and European Pharmacopeia 2008.

Discussion

Due to financial constraints and limitation in suitable facilities and equipment for aseptic dispensing and testing, the two processes were contracted out to accredited compounding provider and laboratories. The compounder the TGA good manufacturing practice guidelines which based on the PIC/S principles, the ISO Standards 14644.1-4 and 13408-7:2012, the Australian standards AS 1386 – Cleanrooms and clean workstations for aseptic preparations.The laboratories conducting the testing were accredited by the National Association of Testing Authorities, Australia and applied the established testing methods for pharmaceutical products by those products manufacturers and the methods specified in the British Pharmacopeia 2008. This arrangement imposed some limitations on the possibility of repeating any testing to.

The sample tested (Serenace™ Haloperidol 15 mg/3mL syringes, Clopixol Accuphase™ zuclopenthixol acetate 150 mg/3mL) for stability and sterility met the Pharmacopoeial requirements (British Pharmacopeia and European pharmacopeia 2008 edition) for parameters tested, during the testing period when stored below 25°C and protected from light. No significant changes or trends were observed in the stability trial for any parameters in either product. Particulate matter was tested and was acceptable for both products.

- The tested doses (Haloperidol 15 mg/3 mL, zuclopenthixol acetate 150 mg/3mL and Midazolam 5mg/1mL) are not the only doses used. 100 mg zuclopenthixol acetate, 10-20 mg haloperidol, and benztropine 2 mg are also used.

- Prefilled syringes may be of significant use in facilities with large number of acute cases.

- There may be need to use of multiple syringes or part syringe content, which may lead to medication administration errors. Nursing staff preferred to mitigate the needle stick injury risk themselves over taking the risk of causing medication dose or administration error (measuring and drawing the dose from the original manufacturer ampule rather than discarding the excess from the pre-filled syringes).

- The short shelf life of 60 days would lead to increased turnover and wastage compared to the shelf-life of the manufacturer's ampoules and empty syringes, and was considered unlikely to be cost-effective.

Conclusion

This study demonstrated the possibility of providing a safer pre-filled syringes product when compared to current practice in many mental health facilities. Filling syringes and label them with short-drug name or description using a wound dressing-tap rather than what we achieved with this study to produce appropriately labelled pre-filled syringes which carry shelf-life, storage details, drug name/strength/dose and rout of administration, based on scientific finding rather than guessing.

This study demonstrated that Clopixol Accuphase™ (zuclopenthixol acetate) 150 mg/3 mL and haloperidol 15 mg/3 mL retained stability and remained sterile over 10 and 9 weeks respectively when stored under 25°C in disposable plastic syringes for a period of 60 days, when tested using the British Pharmacopeia and the European Pharmacopeia methods and criteria (Tables 7 and 8).

Acknowledgement

The authors express their thanks to the TGA and AMS for their analytical input.

References

1. Bowden FJ (2001) Needle-stick injuries in primary care. Aust Prescr 24: 98-100.

2. http://anmf.org.au/media-releases/entry/media_100504

3. Fourie WJ, Keogh JJ (2011) The need for continuous education in the prevention of needle stick injuries. Contemporary Nurse 39:194-205.

4. Bi P (2008) Sharps injury and body fluid exposure among health care workers in an Australian tertiary hospital. Asia-Pacific J Pub Hlth 20: 139-147.

5. Anon (2013) Value of Technology: Needle stick and Sharps Injuries and Safety-Engineered Medical Devices. (Archived by WebCite® at http://www.webcitation.org/6McEAIPQ2)

6. Anon (2014) Guidance for Industry Pyrogen and Endotoxins Testing: Questions and Answers. Office of Communications, Division of Drug Information.. Accessed: 2014-01-14. (Archived by WebCite® at http://www.webcitation.org/6McEL6aPI)

37

Survey of Australian Father's Attitudes towards Infant Vaccination: Findings from the Australian Father's Study

Natasha Prosser[1], Rodney Petersen[2] and Julie Quinlivan[1,3]*

[1]Department of Obstetrics and Gynaecology, Joondalup Health Campus, Joondalup, WA 6027, Australia
[2]Women's and Babies Service, Women's and Children's Hospital, North Adelaide, SA 5006, Australia
[3]Institute for Health Research, University of Notre Dame Australia, Fremantle, 6160, WA, Australia

Abstract

Objective: To investigate the attitudes of expectant Australian fathers towards vaccination, and to identify factors which may influence these attitudes.

Methods: A cross-sectional survey study of 407 Australian men with expectant partners, mean age 30.4 (SD 6.7). Self reported attitude, level of knowledge and information resources accessed regarding pregnancy related issues. Participant demographics collected included: Age, number of children, relationship status, level of education, employment information and smoking status.

Results: Majority (89%) of participants had a positive attitude towards infant vaccination, 9% felt neutral and 2% had negative attitudes. Positive attitudes towards vaccination were associated with lower self-reported knowledge of pregnancy issues but a higher likelihood of discussing pregnancy issues with health care providers rather than sourcing information from the internet (both $p<0.001$).

Conclusion: A majority of Australian expectant fathers have a positive attitude towards infant vaccination. Fathers with negative attitudes to vaccination self-reported higher levels of knowledge. They were more likely to obtain information from the Internet instead of healthcare staff.

Implication for public health: Including fathers in health discussion with knowledgeable health care providers may result in increased vaccine uptake.

Keywords: Fathers pregnancy; Attitudes, Mixed methods study; Prospective study; Cohort study; Infant vaccination; Conscientious objector

Background

Vaccine preventable diseases place a heavy burden on the community and the introduction of widespread immunization regimens have resulted in the reduction or eradication of many diseases, saving millions of lives. It is considered one of the most significant contributions to the improvement in global health outcomes [1-6]. Some protection for non-immunized people may be achieved via 'herd immunity', when the majority of the population are vaccinated thus restricting the spread of disease [7].

Despite the success of immunization programs, many children still contract vaccine preventable illnesses, some with tragic outcomes [6,8]. Many of these children were too young to be vaccinated, unable to receive them for medical reasons or contracted disease as a result of vaccine failure. However, some parents choose not to vaccinate their children, citing political, personal or philosophical motives for declining [9-12]. Other vaccine opponents question the safety, efficacy and necessity of recommended vaccines [9-12].

While there is literature on parental attitudes to vaccination, there is a paucity of information on father's attitudes. Most studies reported that the mother was the primary source of information [9-12]. Given fathers play an important role in child rearing and exert influence on decision making processes as co-parent, we have sought to explore the attitudes of expectant fathers towards newborn vaccination.

Methods

Study design

A self-reporting survey of expectant fathers.

Setting

This study was undertaken as part of The Australian Father's Study (AFS), a longitudinal study of Australian father's experiences of parenthood from the third trimester of their partner's pregnancy until 6 weeks post-partum [13,14]. Participants were identified through the antenatal clinic at Joondalup Health Campus (JHC). JHC incorporates both public and private hospitals and is located in the North Metropolitan region of Perth, Western Australia. This study was reviewed and granted ethics approval by the JHC Human Research Ethics Committee. Data were collected between 2013 and 2015.

Participants

Expectant fathers, who were the acknowledged father of the child, were recruited via the pregnant mother on her attendance at antenatal clinic after 20 weeks gestation. Recruiters were qualified medical practitioners or midwives affiliated with the AFS. The mother's consent for the father's participation was sought and participants were provided an information brochure outlining the requirements of involvement to enable informed consent to enter the trial to be given. Individual consent was obtained from each participant. Exclusion criteria were: pregnancy complicated by known foetal anomaly, fathers with limited

***Corresponding author:** Julie Quinlivan, Department of Obstetrics and Gynaecology, Joondalup Health Campus, Joondalup, WA 6027, Australia, E-mail: Julie.Quinlivan@nd.edu.au

English language abilities, not acknowledged as biological parent status.

Data sources

This mixed methods study was a predefined sub-study of the AFS collected between January and July 2014. The number of new antenatal bookings in this recruitment period was 981. This is a longitudinal study of Australian men who are the acknowledged father of the unborn child of their pregnant partner. Data were collected via a self-reported questionnaire consisting of demographic details including: age, country of birth, living arrangements with the mother, employment status, education level, other children, and smoking status [13,14]. A Likert scale was used to assess attitudes to infant vaccination and a self- reported level of knowledge about pregnancy issues. In addition, participants were asked to explain their attitude toward vaccination via an open-ended question. Qualitative information was extracted from written comments. Three questionnaires were administered in the antenatal period to be filled in six weeks prior to birth (Q1), immediately post partum (Q2) and six weeks post partum (Q3). Overall return rate of questionnaires following consent is 79% with individual return rates of 85%, 79% and 73% for Q1, Q2 and Q3 respectively. The data for the vaccination study comes from Q1.

Variables

Participant responses from the Likert scale regarding attitudes to vaccination were assigned as either 'Positive', 'Neutral' or 'Negative' for analysis.

Bias

Potential sources of bias in this self-reported study are information bias, selection bias, non-response bias, and response bias. Attempts to minimise these sources of bias included: Extended data collection period, standard response forms, de-identified and confidential respondent surveys.

Sample size

The primary hypothesis was that education would positively influence attitudes towards infant vaccination. Fathers with a positive attitude towards infant vaccination would have undertaken more formal years of education compared to those with a negative or neutral attitude. We estimated 80% of fathers with a positive attitude would have 12 or more years of education, whereas only 30% of fathers with a neutral or negative attitude would have this degree of education. Assuming two samples, with alpha error of 0.05, beta of 0.2 and power of 80%, then 22 expectant fathers with negative or neutral attitude towards vaccination were required to test the hypothesis.

Given the percentage of 12-15 month-olds fully vaccinated in Australia ranges from a high of 92.3% to a low of 86.2%, and rates of specific conscientious objection ranged from 0% to 7.1% across different Medicare Local catchment areas, we estimated 6% of expectant fathers might have a negative or neutral attitude towards vaccination [15,16]. We therefore recruited 407 expectant fathers into the vaccination study.

Statistical analysis

Statistical analysis was performed using Minitab® (version 16, University of Melbourne). Difference in attitudes to vaccinations was assessed using Chi Square test or Fisher Exact test if cell size was less than 5. Responses to the open-ended questions were assessed using inductive content analysis. Responses were independently read by the principal researchers and an abstraction process used to summarize and

conceptualize the overall meaning and implications of the comments. Open coding was performed to maximize the number of headings in order to describe all aspects of the content [17].

Results

Participants

407 expectant fathers were recruited into the vaccination study.

Descriptive data

The demographic characteristics of the study participants are summarised in Table 1. Of the 407 Fathers included in the study, the mean age was 30.4 years, (SD 6.7). Of these, 147 (41%) indicated Australia was not their country of birth, a figure higher than the average Australian overseas born general population (28.5%) [18]. Most men reported that they were living with the mother of the child (94.1%) and had achieved an education level of year 12 or higher (82.5%). Nearly 10% of the fathers reported they were unemployed or in retraining. Of those who were employed, 66.3% worked more than 40 h per week.

Outcome data

Table 2 summarises demographic details, vaccination knowledge, and information sources regarding pregnancy issues by attitude towards vaccination. The majority of participants had a positive attitude towards infant vaccination (N=357, 89%). However, 9% (N=35) of fathers had a neutral and 2% (N=8) a negative attitude. Seven participants did not indicate their attitude to vaccination and were treated as missing data (not included in table).

The key finding was that fathers with neutral and negative attitudes towards infant vaccination reported self-assessed higher levels of knowledge of vaccination issues (p=0.01 and <0.001 respectively). These same men also reported they were more likely to have gained their knowledge from the Internet than from a healthcare professional (both p<0.001).

Qualitative data

Of the 357 men with positive attitudes to vaccination, 66 commented on their beliefs, the main themes identified were: Vaccination as

Variable	Australian Fathers Study N=407
Age in years Mean (Std. Dev.)	30.4 (6.7)
Country of birth N (%) Australia Overseas	227 (56%) 180 (44%)
Relationship living arrangements N (%) Living with mother Not living with mother	383 (94.1%) 17 (4.2%)
Level of education N (%) Less than 12 years of school 12 years of school or more	65 (16%) 336 (82.5%)
Employment N (%) Not currently employed Yes and work locally Yes and fly in fly out worker	39 (9.6%) 296 (72.7%) 65 (16%)
Hours worked each week Less than one hour a week 1-15 h per week 16-40 h per week More than 40 h per week	16 (4%) 5 (1.2%) 108 (26.5%) 270 (66.3%)
First time father N (%) Yes No	210 (51.5%) 195 (48%)

Table 1: Demographics of study cohort.

	Positive attitude N=357 (87.7%)	Neutral attitude N=35 (8.6%)	Negative attitude N=8 (2%)
Age Mean (SD) p-value	30.43 (6.7)	30.14 (6.8) 0.55	29.85 (5.0) 0.21
Country of birth N (%) Australia Overseas p-value	210 (59%) 147 (41%)	14 (40%) 21 (60%) 0.03	3 (37.5%) 5 (62.5%) 0.28
Relationship with mother of baby N (%) Living with mother Not living with mother p-value	338 (94.7%) 17 (4.7%)	35 (100%) 0 (0%) 0.38	6 (75%) 2 (25%) 0.06
Level of education N (%) Less than 12 years of school 12 years of school or more p-value	60 (16.8%) 296 (82.9%)	4 (11.4%) 31 (88.6%) 0.63	1 (12.5%) 7 (87.5%) 1.00
ATSI Race N (%) Yes No p-value	55 (15.4%) 301 (84.3%)	8 (23%) 27 (77%) 0.24	1 (12.5%) 7 (87.5%) 1.00
Employment type N (%) Not currently employed Yes and work locally Yes and fly in fly out worker p-value	31 (8.7%) 264 (74%) 61 (17%)	8 (23%) 25 (71%) 2 (6%) 0.015	2 (25%) 5 (62.5%) 0 (0%) 0.13
Hours worked per week N (%) 0-1 h a week 1-40 h per week 40+ h per week p-value	13 (4%) 104 (28.5%) 239 (67%)	3 (9%) 6 (17%) 26 (74%) 0.45	2 (25%) 2 (25%) 3 (37.5%) 0.23
Smoker N (%) Yes No p-value	92 (25.8%) 262 (73.4%)	5 (14%) 30 (86%) 0.15	4 (50%) 3 (37.5%) 0.08
First time father N (%) Yes No p-value	188 (53%) 165 (46%)	18 (51%) 17 (49%) 0.86	2 (25%) 5 (62.5%) 0.26
Self-assessed knowledge of vaccination Likert scale 0-10 Mean (Std Dev) p-value	6.6 (1.7)	7.7 (0.9) 0.01	9.2 (0.2) <0.0001
Source of knowledge N (%) * Healthcare staff * Internet * Friends and family * Other p-value	254 (71.2%) 23 (6.4%) 65 (18.2%) 15 (4.2%)	15 (43%) 18 (51%) 2 (6%) 0 (0%) 0.001	0 (0%) 7 (87.5%) 1 (12.5%) 0 (0%) <0.0001

Table 2: Differences between fathers with positive versus neutral or negative attitudes toward infant vaccination.

medical advancement, health benefits, anger towards those who do not immunise and the importance of high rates of vaccination. No participants who reported neutral feelings towards vaccinations commented on their viewpoint. Of the 8 participants with a negative attitude towards vaccinations, all commented on their decisions, with the main themes identified being: risks of vaccination, persecution, and the redundancy of vaccinations.

Advancement of modern medicine

A number of respondents commented that they believed vaccinations were a demonstration of the progress of medicine and a sign of an advanced society. One participant wrote:

"I'm going to make sure my child is vaccinated. When you think back how entire families were wiped out, in the old cemeteries and such, I mean why you wouldn't vaccinate your child. They are progress."

Another participant wrote:

"Vaccines are one of the wonders of modern medicine."

Health benefits

Many expectant fathers felt that vaccinations were essential and saved lives and unvaccinated children were at risk.

"Everyone knows vaccines save lives. Those parents who don't vaccinate their children put all other children at risk."

Another father discussed the risk versus benefit of vaccinations

"The side effects listed are pretty mild – sore arm, irritable for a few hours. The benefits are huge. It can save your child's life or stop them getting deaf or brain damaged. I know the baby's not here yet but already I feel very strongly protective. I will do anything to reduce the risk of my child being hurt."

Anger towards those who did not vaccinate

A common theme expressed by some fathers was anger towards people who did not vaccinate their children because it placed their own child at increased risk.

"I read abut (sic) a baby that died cause a mother took her unvaccinated child to day care. That's crazy. If not vaccinated you (sic) kid can die. If that happened to me I'd want those parents to pay. Maybe they should go to prison or something because really, they've killed that child by their actions."

This theme was also reflected by expectant fathers with a positive attitude towards vaccination whose partners, the baby's mother, had a negative attitude. Two participants in this situation wrote detailed comments about their frustration that hospital staff ignored them because the mother's views carried greater weight. In one case where the mother had signed a "Refusal of vaccination" form the father wrote:

"Why should my child be put at risk because we disagree about this? Why does her opinion matter more than my own? I want Hepatitis B and Vitamin K injections at birth. She thinks they are dangerous. Father's opinions and values don't count. We are ignored – even when we are the one saying and doing the right thing and agreeing with the doctors. I was so angry that the midwife ignored me I had to leave the room"

Another father who separated from his partner after enrolling in the study wrote in his questionnaire:

"She's bitter about me leaving and taking it out on our baby. She knows I want him to have all the needles and tests. I asked the hospital to give them but they said only the mother can say so. Why is that the case? I mean, why is her word worth more than mine? It's my baby as much as it is hers. I just want what is best for my baby. She just wants to hurt me."

Importance of high vaccination rates

Another common theme addressed was the importance of high vaccination rates in protecting the community. One participant wrote:

"You need most people to have injections so everyone is safe. Babies are only safe if everyone is injections (sic)."

Risks of vaccination

In the sub-group of fathers with a negative attitude towards vaccination, one theme was that the risks of vaccination outweighed benefits. One participant wrote:

"The absolute risk of our child contracting a disease is very low. The risks of vaccination disease such as autism and ADD are high."

Another participant agreed

"There are 100s of studies that show a link between vaccines and poor outcomes for children. Papers about autism, nerve damage, immune damage, cancer and death (sic). I mean you risk killing your child just to supposedly keep it safe from disease, but you give it a disease instead. Even if you don't get a bad event, the needles hurt your child and cause them to suffer."

Persecution

Some participants felt that people who conscientiously objected to immunization where being unfairly punished for their choices.

"The government overstate this issue and try to make you feel guilty following your own free will."

"Now the government penalises parents like us. We have to fill in extra forms for childcare. Just because we have gone to the trouble to look into it ourselves and not be mindless numbers we get penalized."

Redundancy of vaccines

One participant reflected on the necessity of vaccinations.

"...vaccines are not needed anymore. The disease's they protect against have basically disappeared. One paper said no cases of diphtheria had been seen in the world for decades so why do you need a vaccine against it".

Discussion

This paper evaluates the attitudes of Australian fathers towards vaccinations and factors that may be associated with particular attitudes to vaccination.

We found that the majority of fathers in the survey were supportive of infant and childhood vaccinations, while a small proportion demonstrated a neutral (9%) or negative (2%) attitude.

Participants with a neutral or negative attitude towards vaccination felt they were better informed about vaccination compared to fathers with a positive attitude, self-reporting higher levels of knowledge (p=0.01 and p<0.001 respectively). However, while there was social, financial and educational parity across the groups, fathers with neutral and negative attitudes were more likely to use the Internet as a source of knowledge rather than a health care professional (both p<0.001).

Vaccinations have made a significant contribution to the global health picture yet despite their success; there has been a notable decline in voluntary uptake. Their very success may well have contributed to the reduction in uptake secondary to a newfound complacency toward vaccine-preventable diseases. Disease is no longer present as a reminder to vaccinate, thus the perceived risk of the severity of diseases is low [9,11,19].

Consumer confidence in vaccines can also challenge uptake, with concern for safety and side effects driving a reluctance to vaccinate. Adverse publicity in the media has previously raised questions about safety, efficacy and side effect profiles result in lack of trust by some parents [10,11,20,21]. Some studies have suggested that socioeconomic factors such as level of education and income were more important than parental perceptions in vaccination uptake by parents [11,12,22]. Our study did not reflect this, with no statistically significant difference in education and employment outcomes between fathers with positive, neutral or negative attitudes (p>0.05).

Conflict can arise where there are two opposing, yet strongly held opinions with regards to the health care decisions of the child. Fathers may feel disregarded by perinatal staff and thus excluded from a unified parental team when the wishes of the mother take preference over those of the father.

Overwhelmingly, fathers reported that benefits of protection against disease outweighed side effects and chose to endorse vaccination. These fathers were more likely to accept advice on vaccination from health care providers [10-12,20].

Limitations

This study has several limitations due to its self-reporting design, which may introduce response and non-response bias. However, this is limited by the adequate sample size to obtain information on fathers with neutral and negative attitudes. This study was undertaken in a single public hospital in Perth, Western Australia, which may reduce the generalizability of the results. This study does not link attitudes with actual vaccine uptake and may not differentiate between partial uptake or late vaccine adaptors.

Conclusion

This paper emphasises the importance for health professionals to be able to provide up to date information in the face of vast quantities of material available for public consumption on the Internet. Their role as a reliable source of information should not be underestimated. Where possible, involving fathers in discussions around the benefits of vaccinations may help to increase vaccination rates.

Acknowledgement

The AFS is registered at the Australian and New Zealand Clinical Trials Registry with the number ACTRN 12613001273774 and the trial website is located at http://australianfathersstudyresearchtrial.weebly.com

References

1. Maródi L (2006) Neonatal innate immunity to infectious agents. Infect Immun 74: 1999-2006.

2. Roush SW, Murphy TV (2007) Historical comparisons of morbidity and mortality for vaccine-preventable diseases in the United States. JAMA 298: 215-2163.

3. World Health Organization. Immunization coverage. Fact sheet 2015.

4. WHO, UNICEF, Bank W (2009) State of the world's vaccines and immunization. In: Organization WH 3rd ed.

5. Andre FE, Booy R, Bock HL (2008) Vaccination greatly reduces disease, disability, death and inequity worldwide. Bulletin of the World Health Organization.

6. Gilbert L (2012) Immunisation and vaccine preventable diseases. The Royal College of Pathologists of Australia.

7. Fine P, Eames K, Heymann DL (2011) "Herd Immunity": A Rough Guide. Clinical Infectious Diseases 52: 911-916.

8. Martin N, Foxwell AR (2009) Measles status in Australia, outbreaks in the first quarter of 2009. Commun Dis Intell Q Rep33: 225-231.

9. Brown KF, Kroll JS, Hudson MJ (2010) Factors underlying parental decisions about combination childhood vaccinations including MMR: A systematic review. Vaccine 28: 4235-4248.

10. Ramsay ME, Yarwood J, Lewis D (2002) Parental confidence in measles, mumps and rubella vaccine: Evidence from vaccine coverage and attitudinal surveys. Br J Gen Pract 52: 912-916.

11. Dannetun E, Tegnell A, Hermansson G (2005) Parents' reported reasons for avoiding MMR vaccination. A telephone survey. Scand J Prim Health Care 23:149-153.

12. Gust D, Brown C, Sheedy K (2005) Immunization attitudes and beliefs among parents: beyond a dichotomous perspective. Am J Health Behav 29: 81-92.

13. Jeffery T, Luo KY, Kueh B (2015) Australian fathers' study: What influences paternal engagement with antenatal care? J Perinat Educ 24:181-187.

14. Atkinson A, Petersen RW, Quinlivan JA (2013) Employment may protect fathers in the setting of maternal teenage pregnancy fromanxiety and depression: Findings from the Australian father's study. Reprod Syst Sex Disord 5:161.

15. National Health Performance Authority (2014) Healthy communities: Immunisation rates for children in 2012-13.

16. Department of Health. Immunise- ACIR - Annual Coverage Historical Data. Department of Health, 2015.

17. Elo S, Kyngäs H (2008) The qualitative content analysis process. J Adv Nursing. 62:107-115.

18. Australian Bureau of Statistics. 3412.0 - Migration, Australia, 2014-2015.

19. Bardenheier B, Yusuf H, Schwartz B (2004) Are parental vaccine safety concerns associated with receipt of measles-mumps-rubella, diphtheria and tetanus toxoids with acellular pertussis, or hepatitis B vaccines by children? Arch Pediatr Adolesc Med 158: 569-575.

20. Wu AC, Wisler-Sher DJ, Griswold K (2007) Postpartum mothers' attitudes, knowledge and trust regarding vaccination. Matern Child Health J 12:766-773.

21. Godlee F, Smith J, Marcovitch H (2011) Wakefield's article linking MMR vaccine and autism was fraudulent. BMJ 342: c7452.

22. Danis K, Georgakopoulou T, Stavrou T (2010) Socioeconomic factors play a more important role in childhood vaccination coverage than parental perceptions: A cross-sectional study in Greece. Vaccine 28:1861-1869.

38

The Role of Geographical Access in the Utilization of Institutional Delivery Service in Rural Jimma Horro District, Southwest Ethiopia

Kiflom Zegeye[1], Abebaw Gebeyehu[2]* and Tesfahun Melese[3]

[1]*Communicable disease control Team, Kellem Wollega Zonal Health Department, Oromia Regional State, Ethiopia*
[2]*Department of Reproductive Health, Institute of Public Health, University of Gondar, Ethiopia*
[3]*Department of Health Informatics, Institute of Public Health, University of Gondar, Ethiopia*

Abstract

Introduction: Access to skilled maternal care in a suitable setting at all births is momentous to reduce maternal mortality. The role of geographical access particularly in rural Ethiopia is not sufficiently investigated. Hence, the central intention of this study was to estimate the effect of geographic access of rural mothers on institutional delivery care use in Jimma Horro District, Southwest Ethiopia.

Methods: A community-based cross-sectional survey was conducted in April 2012 in six randomly selected *kebeles*. Data on socio-demographic, maternal history and maternity services use were collected from 528 eligible mothers using structured questionnaire. Geo-referenced data on respondents' houses and health institutions as well as walking tracks from each village center to the nearest health center were recorded using hand-held Global Positioning System (GPS) instrument and mapped using Arc GIS 9.3. Multivariate logistic regression analysis was performed to estimate the effect of distance on facility delivery use by controlling for range of confounders.

Results: Only 8% of the mothers gave birth to their last babies in health facilities. One third of the respondents live within 5-kilometer walking distance of the nearest health center. Each kilometer increase in walking distance to the nearest health center resulted in a reduction of institutional delivery service by 22% (AOR=0.78, 95% CI: 0.64 to 0.96). Use of institutional delivery service was also significantly higher among mothers who faced obstetric complications, and those who attended four and more ANC visits.

Conclusion: Geographic access to health centers plays a major role in institutional delivery care use among rural mothers. Tackling the geographical dimension of access is pivotal in elevating institutional delivery care utilization.

Keywords: Geographic access; Institutional delivery

Background

Access to skilled maternal care at all births is a central strategy for ensuring safe motherhood [1]. It is also well documented that, apart from the skill, an enabling environment, where there is access to the necessary equipments, drugs, and other supplies that improve management of pregnancy-related complications has substantial impact on the reduction of both maternal and neonatal deaths [2,3].

Despite such proven interventions, the issue of maternal mortality remains to be a major public health problem of many developing countries to this day [4,5]. Sub-Saharan Africa alone accounts for 56% of the global maternal deaths, where rural women bear the highest burden [5-7]. Maternal deaths occur mostly during labor, delivery, and the immediate postpartum period [4]. The Ethiopian Demographic and Health Survey (EDHS) 2011 reported 676 maternal deaths per 100,000 live births, which is almost the same with that of 2005 EDHS figure (673) [7].

Historical and contemporary evidences ascribed the fundamental grounds for such high mortalities and morbidities at least partly to lack of access and timely use of appropriate delivery care services [8,9]. Majority of these deaths could be averted by improving access to the interventions for addressing complications of pregnancy and childbirth and utilization of these services by all mothers [4]. This requires both the availability of such services as well as the will of pregnant women to seek apposite care at delivery.

Despite decades of ongoing efforts to strengthen delivery care services, institutional delivery service utilization by women during childbirth has been persistently very low in Ethiopia [10]. The situation is more serious in rural areas where only 4.1% of the deliveries occur in health facilities compared to 49.8% for urban areas [7].

While the likelihood of a woman giving birth in a health facility depends on multitude of factors, poor geographic access has been identified as one of the major barriers facing rural women in seeking and using life-saving maternity care services in many developing countries including Ethiopia [2,11].

Geographic access, the distance (or time) needed in order to reach a health facility, is not only a direct physical barrier that precludes women from reaching health institutions but it also affects even the decision to look for care. It could have more influence in rural areas of Ethiopia, where it is norm to see women in labor being carried on men's shoulder traveling many kilometers to reach a health facility [12].

Many of the studies, particularly in Ethiopia, assess geographic accessibility in terms of subjective data on distance or travel time to health facilities as study participants or "informants" reported [13,14]. This kind of assessment often raises the question of internal validity of the data. Hence, this study was conducted to shed light on the extent to which geographic access of rural women to health facilities can influence the use of institutional delivery care by adjusting for

*Corresponding author: Abebaw Gebeyehu, Department of Reproductive Health, Institute of Public Health, University of Gondar, Ethiopia,
E-mail: abebawgebeyehu@yahoo.com

the effects of some socio-demographic, maternal and other service utilization related factors. Objective distance measurements were also employed by integrating some features of Geographic Information System (GIS). Findings could be helpful to understand the pattern of geographic accessibility of rural women to health facilities and the role it plays in utilization of institutional delivery service.

Methods

A community-based cross-sectional survey was conducted in Jimma Horro District in April 2012. Jimma Horro lies in Kellem Wellega Zone of Oromia Regional State, Southwest of Ethiopia with 8° 57' 41.314" North 34° 49' 16.864" East geographic coordinates. Nunnu, the capital of the district, is found 663 km of Addis Ababa, the capital of Ethiopia. According to the 2007 census, total population of the district for the year 2011/2012 was 54,081. The district was organized into one urban and 19 rural *kebeles* - the smallest administrative unit in Ethiopia (Figure 1). The district's health care system is made up of two health centers and 20 health posts [15]. During the data collection period, there was neither ambulance nor public transport services within the district available.

The required sample size was computed using single population proportion formula under the assumptions of 95% confidence level, 4.1% rural mothers delivered in health facility [7] and 2.5% margin of error (d). After taking into account design effect of two and 10% possible non-response rate, the final sample size was calculated to be 530. The outcome of interest was institutional delivery service utilization, which was dichotomized as "Yes" and "No". In this study, childbirths took place in hospitals or health centers were considered as institutional deliveries whereas those occurred in health posts or at home were not.

Cluster sampling technique was employed to select the study units considering rural *kebeles* as logical clusters. From the 19 rural *kebeles,* six were selected by simple random sampling. Each household within the selected *kebeles* was visited. All women in the selected *kebeles* who had reported to have at least one birth (≥ 28 weeks of gestation) within the two years preceding the data collection period were included in the survey regardless of the birth outcome.

Geographic access to health facilities was determined in terms of walking distance from center of each village to the nearest health center. A village (locally known as '*Gere*') is a neighborhood or group of people, which comprises roughly 20 households. The distance was measured in kilometers; and implemented as continuous walking distance. Moreover, means of transportation used to reach health facilities, socio-demographic, and other factors like history of service utilization were included as independent variables.

The data were collected in April 2012. The *Garmin* H72 GPS handheld device was used to collect all the geo-referenced data. Data were collected using structured survey questionnaire, which was developed first in English and translated into local language, Oromo, by native speaker. The questionnaire included socio demographic information, obstetric history (age at first marriage, age at first pregnancy, ANC, birth complication, and birth attendant), and health facility delivery service utilization information (place of delivery, birth attendant, mode of transportation, time needed to reach health facility, distance).The field data collectors were divided into six teams - one team per *kebele*. Each team comprises two data collectors with handheld GPS device and two *kebele* informants. Two supervisors coordinated movements of teams.

Data collectors together with kebele and village informants determined center of 52 villages. Then, track data on routes from each village center to the nearest health center (following the path the study participants commonly use to reach health center close to the village) were registered. Besides, geo-referenced location data (x-y coordinates) on interviewee houses, health centers and health posts were recorded. All the GPS data were collected in Geographic Coordinate System (GCS), Adindan, and datum D_Adindan in decimal degrees with five places of precision (dd.ddddd). Finally, the GPS data were re-projected to Projected Coordinate System (PCS), Adindan _UTM_Zone_37N. *Kebele* and District boundaries and polygon maps for the entire study area and other geographic features within it were obtained from the Ethiopian Central Statistics Authority (CSA) (Figure 2). For each woman a face-to-face interview procedure was done by female data collectors.

The GPS (walking track, household and facility location) data were entered into Arc GIS version 9.3 and integrated into respective *kebeles'* polygon map, and were processed for interpretations. In addition, all the other collected data were entered into Epi Info version 3.5.1. Eventually, both the data in the Epi Info and Arc GIS were transferred to SPSS version 16.0 for further analysis. Logistic regression analysis was used to control possible confounders.

Training was given to data collectors and supervisors prior to the actual data collection time focusing on skills of conducting interview, field GPS and questionnaire data collection and recording. The questionnaire was pretested and checked for its cultural appropriateness and clarity. This study was reviewed and approved by the Institutional Review Board (IRB) of the University of Gondar. Formal permission

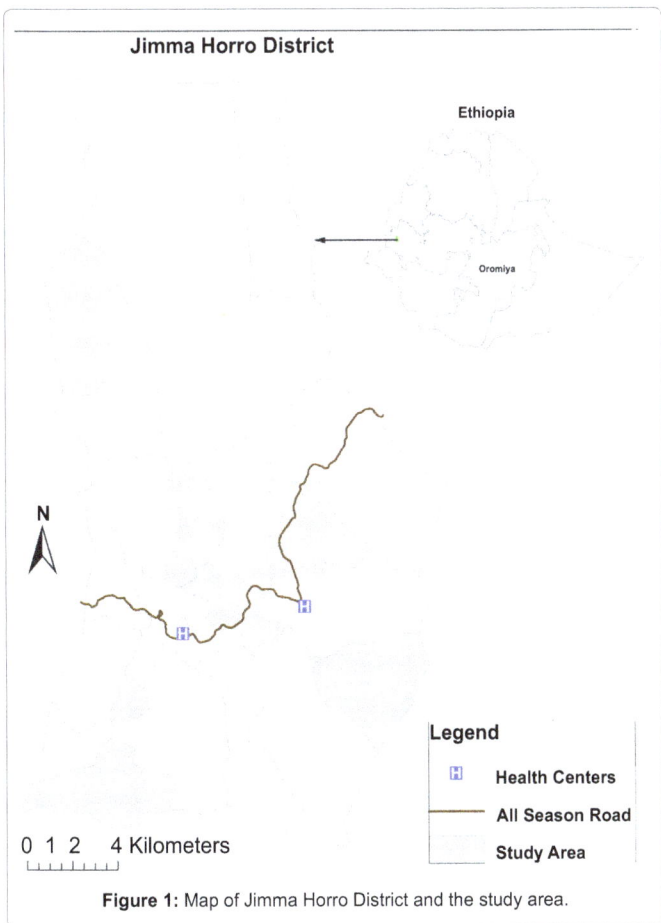

Figure 1: Map of Jimma Horro District and the study area.

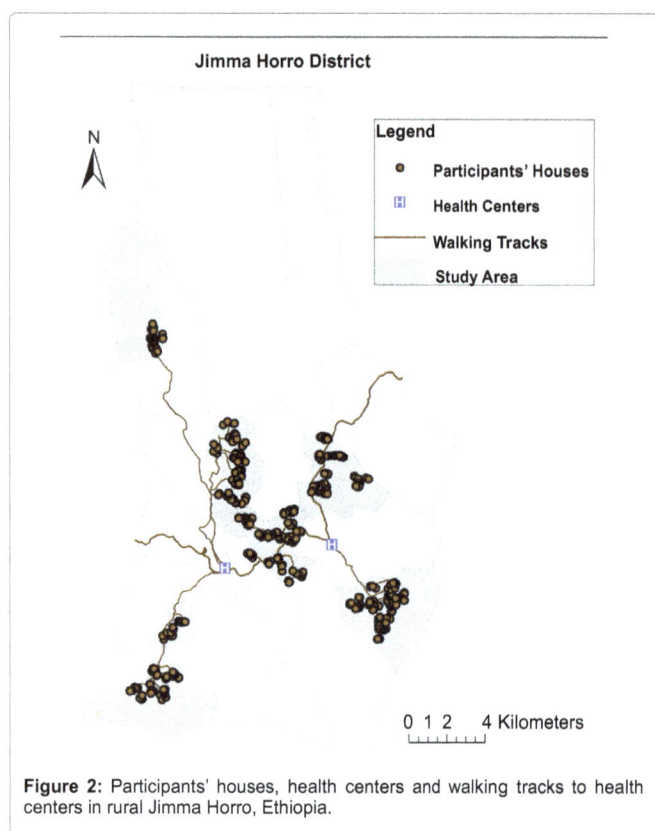

Figure 2: Participants' houses, health centers and walking tracks to health centers in rural Jimma Horro, Ethiopia.

to conduct the study was obtained Kellem Wellega Zone Health Department and Jimma Horro District Health Office. Verbal informed consent was also obtained from each study subject.

Results

Socio-demographic characteristics of the study participants

In the study, 528 eligible mothers were identified. The mean age was 28 ± 6.1 SD years. About three-fourth (73.3%) were between 20-34 years of age. Most, 97.7%, 94.1%, of them were married and were housewives respectively. About 80% of the women and 47% of their husbands did not attend any formal education. More than half (65.7%) reported to have more than four family members (Table 1).

Institutional delivery service utilization

Out of 528 mothers, 42 (8%) delivered in health institutions (37 mothers in health center and 5 in hospital)

During delivery, three-forth (74.2%) and 16.5% of the mothers were assisted by relatives and/or neighbors and Traditional Birth Attendants (TBAs), respectively. Skilled health workers and Health Extension Workers (HEWs) assisted only 8.1% and 0.8% mothers, respectively.

The role of geographic access in the utilization of institutional delivery service (before and after controlling of confounders)

In the study, 189 (35.8%) of the mothers were found to live within 5 kilometer, 495 (93.8%) of the mothers reside within 10 km walking distance of the nearest health center. Proportion of institutional delivery service utilization was 13.2% among those who live within 5 km of a

Characteristics		Institutional delivery		Total
		Yes n (%)	No n (%)	n (%)
Mother's age at interview	15-19	19(15.2)	106(84.8)	125(23.7)
	20-24	8(5.5)	138(94.5)	146(27.7)
	25-29	4(3.4)	112(96.6)	116(22)
	30-34	9(8.1)	102(91.9)	111(21)
	35+	2(6.7)	28(93.3)	30(5.7)
	Mean (Standard deviation)		28(6)	
Marital status	Married	42(8.1)	474(91.9)	516(97.7)
	Others (separated, divorced and widowed)	0(0)	12(100)	12(2.3)
Religion	Protestant	31(11.4)	240(88.6)	271(51.3)
	Muslim	4(3.1)	126(96.9)	130(24.6)
	Orthodox	7(5.5)	120(94.5)	127(24.1)
Mother's education	No formal education	28(6.7)	393(93.3)	421(79.7)
	Primary and above	14(13.1)	93(86.9)	107(20.3)
Mother's occupation	House wife	41(8.2)	456(91.8)	497(94.1)
	Others (farmer, employed [waged], student)	1(3.2)	30(96.8)	31(5.9)
Husband's Education (n=517)	No formal education	9(3.7)	233(96.3)	242(46.8)
	Primary and above	33(12)	242(88)	275(53.2)
Husband's occupation (n=517)	Farmer	40(8)	461(92)	501(96.9)
	Others (Merchant, employed[waged])	2(12.5)	14(87.5)	16(3.1)
Monthly family income	83-250 ETB	6(3.6)	159(94.6)	165(31.2)
	251-417 ETB	6(4.5)	128(95.5)	134(25.4)
	418-832 ETB	9(10.2)	79(89.8)	88(16.7)
	≥ 833 ETB	21(14.9)	120(85.1)	141(26.7)
	Mean (Standard deviation)		574.7(531.3)	
Family size	1-4	22(12.2)	159(87.8)	181(34.3)
	>= 5	20(5.8)	327(94.2)	347(65.7)
	Mean (Standard deviation)		5.6(1.9)	
Have radio	Yes	27(11.2)	215(88.8)	242(45.8)
	No	15(5.2)	271(94.8)	286(54.2)

Table 1: Socio-demographic characteristics of rural women in relation to delivery service use in Jimma Horro, Southwest Ethiopia.

Characteristics		Institutional delivery		Total
		Yes n (%)	No n (%)	n (%)
Age at 1st marriage	15-19	30(8.2)	338(91.8)	368(69.7)
	20-24	12(8.8)	125(91.2)	137(25.9)
	25-29	0(0)	23(100)	23(4.4)
	Mean (Standard deviation)		18.3(2.9)	
Age at 1st pregnancy	15-19	21(6.9)	284(93.1)	305(57.8)
	20-24	19(10.6)	160(89.4)	179(33.9)
	25-29	2(4.8)	42(95.2)	44(8.4)
	Mean (Standard deviation)		19.6(3.1)	
Pregnancy planned	Yes	40(8.5)	431(91.5)	471(89.2)
	No	2(3.5)	55(96.5)	57(10.8)
Gravidity	1	16(16.2)	83(83.8)	99(18.8)
	2-4	16(6.2)	242(93.8)	258(48.9)
	≥ 5	10(5.8)	161(94.2)	171(32.3)
	Mean (Standard deviation)		3.7(2.2)	
Birth order	1	17(16.3)	87(83.7)	104(19.7)
	2-4	15(5.9)	240(94.1)	255(48.3)
	≥ 5	10(5.9)	159(94.1)	169(32)
	Mean (Standard deviation)	3.6(2.2)		
Any abortion	Yes	2(7.7)	24(92.3)	26(4.9)
	No	40(8)	462(92)	502(91.9)
Obstetric complication	Yes	9(20.9)	34(7.1)	43(8.1)
	No	33(6.8)	452(93.2)	485(91.9)
ANC visit	Yes	38(10.9)	310(89.1)	348(66)
	No	4(2.2)	176(97.8)	180(34)
Number of ANC visit(s)	No visit	4(2.2)	176(97.8)	180(34)
	1-3 visit(s)	7(4.5)	148(95.5)	155(29.4)
	≥ 4 visits	31(16.1)	162(83.9)	193(36.6)
Distance (home to HC)	<5 km	25(13.2)	164(86.8)	189(35.8)
	>5 km	17(5)	322(95)	339(64.2)

Table 2: Maternal history and service use characteristics of rural women in relation to delivery service use in Jimma Horro, Southwest Ethiopia.

health center and 5% among those who were reside in more than 5 km of the nearby health center (Table 2). The longest and shortest one-trip distances to a nearby health center were 15.8 and 2.6 kilometers respectively.

The bivariate analysis indicated that there was statistically significant association between distance and use of institutional delivery service. One-kilometer increase in walking distance to the nearest health center resulted in a reduction of odds of institutional delivery service use by a factor of 0.78 (COR=0.78, 95%CI: 0.65 to 0.93) (Table 3).

The association between distance to a nearest health center and use of institutional delivery was significant even after the model was adjusted for the selected socio-demographic, obstetric and other factors. As walking distance to the nearest health center increased by a kilometer, institutional delivery declined by 22% that means by a factor of 0.78(AOR=0.78, 95%CI: 0.64to 0.96) (Table 3). Concerning mode of transportation to reach health facilities during childbirth, all mothers delivered in health facilities was taken to a health center or health post with locally made stretcher-like "bed" carried by relatives and or neighbors. Those who gave birth in hospital used trucks which are not made for such purpose (such as *NPR ISUZU*) to reach a hospital.

In addition to distance to the nearest health center, experience of complications, presence of ANC visits and number of ANC visits showed statistically significant association with institutional delivery service utilization (Table 3).

Discussion

The present study has emphasized the importance of geographical access in the use of institutional delivery services in such rural areas with extremely low facility delivery service.

Despite of the fact that institutional delivery care is an important factor for health of the mother and the newborn, utilization of institutional delivery service by rural mothers in the study area was very low, where fewer than 1 in 10 mothers gave birth in health institution. Comparable previous findings were reported from rural mothers in different parts of Ethiopia (Metekel, 6.8%, rural Jimma, 6.2%) [16,17]. This finding was higher than the recent EDHS estimate; merely 4.1% of rural births took place in health facilities [7]. The difference in facility delivery use in this study when compared to the national figure could be attributed partly to differences in methodological settings.

In this study, an attempt has been made to look at the pattern geographic access to health facilities in light of two access standards. The first one is the international standard for access to clinical/curative services, which defines good geographic access as being within five kilometers distance of service delivery point. The other one is the potential coverage or access standard of the Federal Ministry of Health of Ethiopia (FMHE), as having access to health facilities within distance of 10 km [18]. The later standard might not pose substantial difficulties in having access to many preventive services. Yet, considering the former benchmark is instrumental, particularly in rural Ethiopia where

Characteristics		Crude Odds Ratio (95% CI)	Adjusted Odds Ratio (95% CI)
Religion	Protestant	4.07(1.41-11.78)	3.48 (0.98,10.86)
	Muslim	1.84(0.53-6.44)	1.82(0.47, 7.00)
	Orthodox	1	1
Mother's education	No formal education	1	1
	Primary and above	2.11(1.07-4.17)	1.45(0.59, 3.58)
Husband`s Education	No formal education	1	1
	Primary and above	3.530(1.65-7.54)	2.09(0.87, 5.02)
Monthly family income	83-250 ETB	1	1
	251-417 ETB	1.23(0.39-3.89)	0.79(0.25, 2.55)
	418-832 ETB	2.82(0.97-8.19)	1.53(0.47, 4.97)
	≥ 833 ETB	4.81(1.88-12.29)	2.48(0.91, 6.77)
Family size	1-4	2.26(1.20-4.27)	1.64(0.63, 4.25)
	≥5	1	1
Have radio	Yes	2.27(1.18-4.37)	1.68(0.75, 3.77)
	No	1	1
Birth order	1	3.11(1.36-7.08)	3.05(0.86, 10.78)
	2-4	0.99(0.44-2.27)	0.94(0.35, 2.54)
	≥5	1	1
Obstetric complication	Yes	3.63(1.60-8.19)	4.08(1.49, 11.14)
	No	1	1
ANC visit	Yes	5.39(1.89-15.36)	3.79(1.21, 11.85)
	No	1	1
Number of ANC visit	No visit	1	1
	1-3 visit(s)	2.08(0.60-7.25)	1.39(0.38, 5.06)
	≥ 4 visits	8.42(2.91-24.37)	5.72(1.90, 17.19)
Distance to health center		0.78(0.65-0.93)	0.78(0.64, 0.96)

1 - Reference category

Table 3: Association of distance and other factors with institutional delivery service utilization among rural women in Jimma Horro, Southwest Ethiopia.

virtually the only means of reaching health facilities is traveling on foot or by stretcher, which might deteriorate the mothers' condition along the way and make treatment more complicated [4,12,18].

When the 5 km criterion was taken, around one third of the mothers have access to health centers. When the 10 km standard was considered, however, great majority of the mothers have access to health centers. Rural mothers in the study area travel an average of 7.3 kilometers to reach the nearest health center; a 10 km discrepancy was noticed between the shortest and the longest walking distances to reach the nearest health center.

Geographic access to health centers was materialized to be a strong predictor of facility delivery utilization. Use of institutional delivery service declined as distance from the nearest health center became longer and longer. Institutional delivery utilization among mothers living within 5 km distance of the nearest health center was virtually 3 fold higher than those who live more than 10 km of a health center near to them. Such role of distance was observed in many developing countries. In rural Uttar Pradesh, India, women who live within a radius of 3 km from health facility were more likely to seek institutional delivery service than those living 8 km or more from the facility [19]. A study from rural Haiti also indicated as distance to hospital increased from 5 km to 30 km the utilization of institutional delivery deceased by 12% [20]. Women within 5 km of health facility were almost 4 times more likely to deliver in health facility than those of 6+ km in southern Tanzania [21].

The odds of institutional delivery service use among these rural mothers declined by 22%, as distance to the nearest health center increased by a kilometer. In rural Zambia 29% decrease in odds of

facility delivery was observed for every doubling of distance [22]. Possible explanation for this might be pregnant women do not even attempt to reach a facility for delivery since walking many kilometers is difficult in labor and worse if labor starts at night and transport means are traditional and often unavailable particularly in such rural area [4,11,23]. Apart from this, women in higher monthly income families were more likely to opt for institutional delivery service than those in lower monthly income families. This finding was in line with previous studies in India [23,24]. The main reason for mothers with higher monthly income to deliver in health facilities is that delivery service requires extensive costs during transportation and care which is difficulty for the lower income families to afford.

Though not significant, the probability of giving birth in health facilities increased in lower birth orders. First births were more likely to take place in health facilities than fifth and more births. This finding was supported by previous studies [25]. There are a number of explanations for this. It could be because mothers often face more difficulty in their first pregnancy and are less experienced in childbirth that increases the probability of using health facilities during delivery. Contrarily, mothers with high birth orders could have previous experience in childbirth that might build their confidence, which in turn increase chance of home delivery [24-26].

Mothers who had experience of obstetric complications were more likely to use health institutions during their pregnancy and/or childbirth. Similar previous studies from rural Nepal supported this finding [27]. This might be due to the fact that experience of complications during pregnancy and/or delivery might make women seek skilled assistance from health professionals in health institutions [26].

The current study also showed mothers who had ANC visits, and who had four and more ANC visits during their most recent pregnancy were more likely to use health institutions during their childbirth than those who had never visited. Similar results were also found from previous studies in rural Cambodia, rural India and Bangladesh [2,24,28]. This might be because ANC visit especially when it is more than four ANC visits expose the women to more health education and counseling which are both likely to increase service utilization [26].

It is worth considering that due to its cross-sectional nature, recall and interviewer bias could be potential limitations of this study. Besides, while the use of such smaller geographic areas reduces unmeasured geographic access variations within area of aggregation in large studies, it does not consider the border crossing issue. It is important to note that, the nearest health facilities are not necessarily health facilities actually the mothers gave their birth.

Conclusion

The present study documented that institutional delivery service utilization among mothers in rural Jimma Horro district was very low (8%). The study identified that geographic access to health centers plays a major role in the utilization of institutional delivery care. Strong emphasis is commendable to consider the geographical dimension when planning expansion of maternity care services particularly delivery care service to reach the remote rural women. Increased attention should be given for distant mothers to boost up their access to health centers. However, this should be interpreted in cautious since distance alone is not always informative which depends on seasonal variation, mode of transportation and nature of roads. In this regard, efforts such as establishing affordable and sustainable emergency transport services should be given due weight, as it could minimize the effect of long distance.

Authors' Contributions

All authors contributed equally during the process of proposal development. KZ handled the data collection process. All authors involved during data analysis. KZ prepared the draft. Then AG and TM revised drafts of the paper. All authors read and approved the final manuscript.

Acknowledgements

We are very grateful to University of Gondar for the approval of the ethical clearance and its technical and financial support. We would like to extend our heartfelt thanks to the Kellem Wellega Zonal Health Department, Jimma Horro District Health Office, and the Ethiopian Central Statistics Authority Head Office for their kind collaboration. Special thanks go to Dereje Abdena and Yaddesa Hailu, for their valuable support during data collection. Authors are also highly indebted to data collectors and study participants.

References

1. UNFPA (2012) Skilled Attendance at Birth.

2. Yanagisawa S, Oum S, Wakai S (2006) Determinants of skilled birth attendance in rural Cambodia. Trop Med Int Health 11: 238-251.

3. Campbell OM, Graham WJ; Lancet Maternal Survival Series steering group (2006) Strategies for reducing maternal mortality: getting on with what works. Lancet 368: 1284-1299.

4. Ronsmans C, Graham WJ; Lancet Maternal Survival Series steering group (2006) Maternal mortality: who, when, where, and why. Lancet 368: 1189-1200.

5. Prata N, Graff M, Graves A, Potts M (2009) Avoidable maternal deaths: three ways to help now. Glob Public Health 4: 575-587.

6. Hailu S, Enqueselassie F, Berhane Y (2009) Health facility-based maternal death audit in Tigray, Ethiopia Ethiop J Health Dev 23: 115-119.

7. CSA, Ethiopia, ICF International (2012) Ethiopia Demographic and Health Survey 2011.

8. Prata N, Passano P, Sreenivas A, Gerdts CE (2010) Maternal mortality in developing countries: challenges in scaling-up priority interventions. Womens Health (Lond Engl) 6: 311-327.

9. Ronsmans C, Etard JF, Walraven G, Høj L, Dumont A, et al. (2003) Maternal mortality and access to obstetric services in West Africa. Trop Med Int Health 8: 940-948.

10. FDR, Ethiopia, MOH (2010) Health Sector Development Program IV: 2010/11 - 2014/15 2010. Ministry of Health: Addis Ababa.

11. Wagle RR, Sabroe S, Nielsen BB (2004) Socioeconomic and physical distance to the maternity hospital as predictors for place of delivery: an observation study from Nepal. BMC Pregnancy Childbirth 4: 8.

12. Ethiopian (2008) Maternal Health Care Seeking Behaviour in Ethiopia: Findings from EDHS 2005: In-depth Analysis of the Ethiopian Demographic and Health Survey 2005. UNFPA: Addis Ababa.

13. Abera M, Gebremariam A, Belachew T (2011) Predictors of Safe Delivery Service Utilization in Arsi Zone, South-East Ethiopia. Ethiop J Health Sci 21: 95-106.

14. Teferra AS, Alemu FM, Woldeyohannes SM (2012) Institutional delivery service utilization and associated factors among mothers who gave birth in the last 12 months in Sekela District, north west of Ethiopia: a community-based cross sectional study. BMC Pregnancy Childbirth 12: 74.

15. Jimma Horro, Woreda Health Office (2012) Annual Report of Jimma Horro Woreda Health Office for the year 2011/2012. Jimma Horro Woreda Health Office 1-86.

16. Tura G, Mariam AG (2008) Safe delivery service utilization in Metekel zone, North West Ethiopia. Ethiopian Journal of Health Sciences 17: 213-222.

17. Kruk ME, Paczkowski MM, Tegegn A, Tessema F, Hadley C, et al. (2010) Women's preferences for obstetric care in rural Ethiopia: a population-based discrete choice experiment in a region with low rates of facility delivery. Journal of epidemiology and community health 64: 984-988.

18. The World Bank and Ministry of Health Ethiopia (2005) A Country Status Report on Health and Poverty (In Two Volumes) Volume II: Main Report.

19. Varma DS, Khan ME, Hazra A (2010) Increasing institutional delivery and Access to emergency obstetric care Services in rural Uttar Pradesh. The Journal of Family Welfare 56: 23-30.

20. Gage AJ, Guirlène Calixte M (2006) Effects of the physical accessibility of maternal health services on their use in rural Haiti. Popul Stud (Camb) 60: 271-288.

21. Mpembeni RN, Killewo JZ, Leshabari MT, Massawe SN, Jahn A, et al. (2007) Use pattern of maternal health services and determinants of skilled care during delivery in Southern Tanzania: implications for achievement of MDG-5 targets. BMC Pregnancy Childbirth 7: 29.

22. Gabrysch S, Cousens S, Cox J, Campbell OM (2011) The influence of distance and level of care on delivery place in rural Zambia: a study of linked national data in a geographic information system. PLoS Med 8: e1000394.

23. Agha S, Carton TW (2011) Determinants of institutional delivery in rural Jhang, Pakistan. Int J Equity Health 10: 31.

24. Kesterton AJ, Cleland J, Sloggett A, Ronsmans C (2010) Institutional delivery in rural India: the relative importance of accessibility and economic status. BMC Pregnancy Childbirth 10: 30.

25. Nigussie M, Haile-Mariam D, Mitike G (2004) Assessment of safe delivery service utilization among women of childbearing age in north Gondar Zone, north west Ethiopia. Ethiop J Health De 18: 145-152.

26. Gabrysch S, Campbell OM (2009) Still too far to walk: literature review of the determinants of delivery service use. BMC Pregnancy Childbirth 9: 34.

27. Dhakal S, van Teijlingen E, Raja EA, Dhakal KB (2011) Skilled care at birth among rural women in Nepal: practice and challenges. J Health Popul Nutr 29: 371-378.

28. Pervin J, Moran A, Rahman M, Razzaque A, Sibley L, et al. (2012) Association of antenatal care with facility delivery and perinatal survival - a population-based study in Bangladesh. BMC Pregnancy Childbirth 12: 111.

39

Perinatal Death and Associated Factors in Wolaita Sodo Referral Hospital, Southern Ethiopia: A Facility Based Cross-Sectional Study

Mihiretu A[1]*, Negash T[2] and Elazar T[1]

[1]*School of Public Health, College of Health Sciences and Medicine, Wolaita Sodo University, Ethiopia*
[2]*Boloso Bombe Primary Hospital, Wolaita Zone, Ethiopia*

Abstract

Background: Birth is a critical time for the mother and fetus. In Ethiopia rates of new born morbidity and mortality are among the highest in the world. Even though many African mothers including Ethiopian mothers' pregnancies are ending up in perinatal mortality, little was investigated to identify the associated factors.

Methodology: A facility based retrospective cross-sectional study was conducted in July, 2015 in Wolaita Sodo University teaching and referral Hospital by collecting data through record review of all women who gave birth at the hospital within the past one year preceding the survey. Systematic sampling technique was used to select 300 subjects. Epi-data version 1.4.4.0 and SPSS version 20 were used to enter and analyze data respectively. Proportions and means were used to describe the study population by explanatory variables whereas; Bivariate and multivariable logistic regression were used to identify the candidate and predictor variables respectively. All statistical tests were considered significant at alpha <0.05.

Result: Among the 300 mothers who delivered their index child at Wolaita Sodo University teaching and referral hospital, 52(17.3%) of them had a dead perinatal outcome. Antenatal care visit, obstructed labor, referral from other health facility, cord prolapse, preeclampsia and birth weight were identified as predictors of perinatal outcome.

Conclusion: Perinatal death in Wolaita Sodo referral hospital is tremendously high, which seeks a due attention. Hence, to avert the situation, improvement in antenatal care service (supported with ultrasound examination); improving obstetrics care; and early diagnosis and appropriate management of severely asphyxiated fetus at the time of delivery could reduce the prevalence. Easily accessible health facilities (which provide comprehensive essential and emergency obstetric services) could reduce perinatal death attributable to referral related causes. Besides, to have a safe delivery, health facilities should give due attention to the use of partograph.

Keywords: Perinatal death; Wolaita Sodo; Birth outcome; Southern Ethiopia; Still birth

Introduction

Birth is a critical time for the mother and fetus. However, an estimated 1.02 million intra-partum stillbirth and 0.9 million intra-partum related neonatal deaths occur annually. Around 42% of the 535900 maternal deaths each year, most of the burden (90%) occurs in lowest and middle income countries. Neonatal mortality rates are 25 fold higher in low income counties and stillbirth rates are up to 50 fold higher as compared to their counterparts; with more than three-quarters occurring in south Asia and sub-Saharan Africa [1].

In Sub Saharan Africa approximately 30 million women become pregnant in a year. Of those, about 1 million deliveries are still birth; at least 1million babies die in their first month of life and 0.5 million die on the first day. About 4 million low birth weight babies and others with neonatal complications may live but not reach their full potential. Africa accounts for 11% of world's population but more than 25% of the worlds' new born deaths. Of the 20 countries with the highest risk of neonatal death, 15(75%) are in Africa [2].

In Ethiopia rates of new born morbidity and mortality are among the highest in the world. The overall perinatal mortalities reported from ten hospital based studies in Ethiopia were in the range of 66 to 124 per 1000 births. The reports of the large scale community based perinatal mortalities were in the range of 37 to 52 per 1000 births. The proportion of stillbirths and early neonatal deaths reported from the hospital based and community based studies was very high (60-110 and 20-34/1000 births) [3].

The etiological factors for perinatal outcomes are different in developed and developing world. The primary obstetric causes identified and modified for developing world include ante-partum hemorrhage, hypertensive disorders, preterm labor, infections, obstructed labor, cord accidents, fetal abnormalities and unexplained deaths [4]. Similarly, the major causes of perinatal mortality in Ethiopia as compiled from hospital data are obstructed labor, mal-presentation, hypertensive disorder, infection, hemorrhage and prematurity [3].

The aim of safe delivery service is to have healthy mother and baby with a little intervention as possible. Proper medical attention and hygienic condition during delivery can reduce the risk of complication and infections that may cause the death or serious illness of the mother and the baby or both. Hence, an important component in the effort to reduce the risks of mothers and children is to increase the proportion of babies delivered in a safe and clean environment and under the supervision of health professional [5].

There are significant differences in the fetal outcome by their presentation. Neonates delivered vaginally for breech presentations had lower APGAR scores, greater admission rates to neonate intensive care unit (NICU) and higher neonatal death rates. Similarly, infants born by operative vaginal delivery and Caesarean section had increased risk of admission to NICU compared to normal vaginal delivery [6].

*Corresponding author: Mihiretu A, School of Public Health, College of Health Sciences and Medicine, Wolaita Sodo University, Ethiopia,
E-mail: mihiretua@gmail.com

In developed countries, 10-25% of all stillbirths appear to be caused by a maternal/fetal infection. In developing countries, which often have far higher stillbirth rates, the relative contribution of infection is known to be greater. An infection in the uterus or elsewhere in the mother's body (such as a urinary tract infection) may precipitate pre-term labor, and there by contribute to a stillbirth. In developed countries, screening for many infectious organisms and subsequent rapid treatment has resulted in a significant reduction in this etiological component of still birth. However, in certain developing countries, the stillbirth rate remains quite high due to infection with modest hope as to achieving a substantial reduction in both [7].

Since this study reveals important determinants of perinatal mortality in Wolaita Sodo University teaching and referral hospital, the result can be utilized as a valuable evidence for determinants of perinatal mortality in similar settings of Ethiopia and other developing countries.

Methodology

A facility based retrospective cross-sectional study was conducted in Woliata Sodo University teaching and referral Hospital from, July 1-30/ 2015. The hospital is located in Sodo town, which is found 327 km south from Addis Ababa (the capital city of Ethiopia).

The hospital is expected to serve around two million people. The total number of beds in the hospital was 200, Out of which 60 beds were in obstetrics and gynecology department. The services delivered by these departments were pre-operative, post-operative, in patient, post abortion care, safe abortion services, labor, delivery, and others. Currently 257 health professionals serve permanently in the hospital including specialists, general practitioners, nurses, midwives, pharmacists and others [8]. This study covered a 12 month (July1/ 2014 to June, 30/ 2015) facility based retrospective cross-sectional study.

Data was collected by reviewing records of all women who gave birth at Wolaita Sodo university teaching and referral hospital within the time period between July1/ 2014 to June30/ 2015. The data was collected by preparing structured checklist and reviewing delivery registration books, operation theatre books and patients' charts.

Sample size was calculated using single population formula based on the following assumptions. Using 95% confidence interval, 5% precision, 26.3% estimation of perinatal death proportion [5], 10% probability of incomplete data and a population correction formula, the final sample size was calculated to be 300.

Systematic sampling technique was used to select representative study subjects by including every 11th mother from the whole 3320 mothers who gave birth at the hospital in the specified time period. A pretested structured checklist was used to collect data by four midwives.

One day training was given before data collection. Regular checkup was made on daily basis for its consistency and completeness.

Epi-data version 1.4.4.0 and SPSS version 20 were used to enter and analyze data respectively. Proportions and means were used to describe the study population by explanatory variables. Bivariate logistic regression was done to identify the differentials of perinatal outcome in the study population. The important predictor variables were determined using multivariable logistic regression model. Stepwise backward procedure was used for modeling by including variables with significant or marginally significant association in the bi-variate logistic regression. All statistical tests were considered significant at alpha <0.05.

As a secondary data analysis, ethical approval & clearance were obtained from Wolaita Sodo University College of medicine & health science ethical review committee. Permission was obtained from Wolaita Sodo university teaching and referral hospital. To keep the privacy of study subjects' information, their name was substituted by code number with respect to their chart.

Result

Socio-demography

All the 300 study subjects were addressed yielding 100% response rate. Majority of study subjects, i.e. 238(79.3%) were rural residents whereas 283(94.3%) were between age of 18-34 years. The lowest number 5(1.7%) of study subjects were under the age of 18 years.

Medical and health Care factors

Out of 300 mothers enrolled in the study 13(4.3%) were hypertensive and 13(4.3%) were diabetic. Nineteen (6.3%) mothers were diagnosed as having an infection of Chorioamnionitis. Nearly half (149) of study subjects didn't ever visit health facility for antenatal care service during their pregnancy period (Table 1).

Maternal and fetal factors

Maternal factors: About 123(41%) study participants were primi-para while their counterparts were multi-para. The onset of labor had begun before admission to hospital among 274(91.3%) mothers. Prolonged labor (the duration of labor beyond 12 hours) before admission was recorded in 74(27%) of mothers. The labor started spontaneously in 275(91.7%) of mothers whereas it started deliberately in hospital by induction on their counterparts. Thirty seven (12.3%) mothers had history of previous stillbirth and majority of deliveries 262(87.3%) were term while only 28(9.3%) and 10(3.3%) of mothers had a preterm and post term pregnancies respectively. Twenty four (8%) mothers were diagnosed with obstructed labor, whereas 18(6%) and 20(6.7%) had cord prolapsed and ante-partum hemorrhage, respectively (Table 2).

Fetal factors: Around 265(88.3) mothers gave birth to a normal birth weight, while 18(6%) and 10(3.3%) gave birth to underweight and overweight neonates. Majority of births 226(75.3%) were attended by integrated emergency surgeons. Forty one (13.7%) and 40 (13.3%) of infants had APGAR score of <4/10 in the 1st and 5th minutes respectively. Out of total deliveries, 6(2%) of them had congenital anomalies (Table 3).

Birth outcome of study participants: Among the 300 study participants who delivered their index child at Wolaita Sodo University teaching and referral hospital, 52(17.3%) of them had a dead perinatal outcome; whereas their counterparts gave birth to alive babies.

Predictors of perinatal outcome: Multivariable logistic regression

Variables		Frequency (percent)
Hypertension	Yes	13 (4.3)
	No	287 (95.7)
Diabetes Mellitus	Yes	13 (4.3)
	No	287 (95.7)
Chorio-amnionitis	Yes	19 (6.3)
	No	281 (93.7)
Antenatal Care	Booked	151 (50.3)
	Unbooked	149 (49.7)

Table 1: Distribution of medical and health related characteristics among mothers who gave birth at WSUTRH - Sodo, southern Ethiopia, 2015.

Variables		Frequency (percent)
Parity	Primi-para	123 (41)
	Multi para	177 (59)
Previous Still-birth	Yes	37 (12.3)
	No	263 (87.7)
Previous c/s scar	Yes	12 (4)
	No	288 (96)
GA at delivery	Term(37-42 weeks)	262 (87.3)
	Preterm (28–36 weeks)	28 (9.4)
	Post term (>42 weeks)	10 (3.3)
Obstructed Labor	Yes	24 (8)
	No	276 (92)
Cord Prolapsed	Yes	18 (6)
	No	282 (94)
Ante-partum hemorrhage	Yes	20 (6.7)
	No	280 (93.3)
Preeclampsia	Yes	21 (7)
	No	279 (93)
Eclampsia	Yes	5 (1.7)
	No	295 (98.3)
Come with referral	Yes	188 (62.7)
	No	112 (37.3)
Labor onset	Spontaneous	275 (91.7)
	Induced	25 (8.3)
Duration of labor	<20 h	200 (66.7)
	>20 h	74 (24.7)
Mode of Delivery	Vaginal	181 (60.3)
	Caesarean	87 (29)
	Instrumental	32 (10.7)
Episiotomy	Yes	106 (35.3)
	No	194 (64.7)

Table 2: Distribution of maternal factors among mothers who gave birth at WSUTRH, Southern Ethiopia, 2015.

Variables		Frequency (percent)
Fetal presentation	vertex	265 (88.3)
	Non-vertex	35 (11.7)
Birth weight	2.5-4.0 kg	272 (90.7)
	<2.5 kg	18 (6)
	> 4.0 kg	10 (3.3)
Fetal number	Single	289 (96.3)
	Twin	11 (3.7)
Sex of neonate	Male	188 (62.7)
	Female	112 (37.3)
APGAR score 1st min	<4/10	41 (13.7)
	4-6/10	84 (28)
	7-10/10	175 (58.3)
APGAR score 5th min	<4/10	40 (13.3)
	4-6/10	15 (5)
	7-10/10	245 (81.7)
Congenital anomaly	Yes	6 (2)
	No	294 (98)

Table 3: Distribution of fetal factors among mothers who gave birth at WSUTRH, Southern Ethiopia, 2015.

analysis revealed that antenatal care visit, obstructed labor, referral from other health facility, cord prolapse, preeclampsia and birth weight were significantly associated with perinatal death (Table 4).

Mothers with un-booked ANC were 4 times more likely to have perinatal death than those who booked [(AOR=3.950, 95% CI (1.546, 10.094)]. Similarly mothers with obstructed labor were 9 times more likely to have perinatal death as compared to their counterparts [(AOR=8.791, 95% CI (2.248, 34.381)]. Mothers presented with cord prolapse were 8 times more likely to have perinatal death than their counterparts [(AOR=8.041, 95% CI (1.951, 33.140)]. Similarly, mothers with preeclampsia were 8 times more likely to have perinatal death than those who had no history of preeclampsia [(AOR=7.600, 95% CI (1.739, 33.222)].

Mothers who gave birth to low birth weight were 9 times more likely to have perinatal death as compared to those who gave birth to a normal birth weight baby [(AOR= 8.8, 95% CI (2.1, 36.5)]. And mothers who came with referral to the hospital were 7 times more likely to end up in perinatal death as compared to mothers who came to hospital by themselves [(AOR =7.320, 95% CI (2.476, 21.637)] (Table 4).

Discussion

Overall, 17.3% of mothers gave birth to a dead fetus. This finding is significantly higher than the national prevalence of 4.6 as reported by Ethiopian Demographic and Health Survey [9]. This is also higher than a study conducted in Nigeria, in which the world's highest newborn mortality rate of 6.6% was reported [10]. This might be due to hospital related factors and institutional set up such as absence of well-equipped neonatal ward, suboptimal obstetric care during ante partum, intra-partum, postpartum and delay from client or service provider.

Backward stepwise multivariable logistic regression was done and revealed that mothers with unbooked ANC, referred mothers from other health facility, obstructed labor, mothers presented with cord prolapse, mothers with preeclampsia and those who gave birth to low birth weight baby were identified as significant predictors of perinatal death. Accordingly, mothers presented with unbooked ANC follow-up were 4 times more likely to experience perinatal death than the booked ones. This is consistent with a study done at Jos university teaching hospital 2006-2007, Niger, which suggests that unbooked study participants were more likely to end up in still birth as compared to their counterparts (X2 = 40.628; P<0.0003) [11].

Mothers who came with referral to the hospital were 7 times more likely to end up with perinatal death than those come with self-referred. And also those who had obstructed labor were 9 times more likely to end up in perinatal mortality than those with normal labor. This is in line with a cross sectional Study done in Jimma University Specialized Hospital which showed that most cases of perinatal death were referred from health centers, and delayed referral was the cause for 45.8% of dead fetal outcome [12].

Mothers presented with cord prolapse were 8 times more likely to have perinatal death than those who do not. This is similar with a cross sectional study done on maternal and fetal outcomes at Senegal and Mali, which showed umbilical cord accidents as an important cause of fetal death which accounts approximately 15% of all still births [7].

Mothers with preeclampsia were 8 times more likely to end up in perinatal death than those who did not have preeclampsia. This in

Variables	Dead	Alive	COR (95% CI)	AOR
Gestational age				
Term (37-42 weeks)	33	229	1	1
Preterm (28-36 weeks)	18	10	12.491 (5.313,29.366)*	18.623 (5.490,63.170)
Post term (>42 weeks)	1	9	0.771 (0.095,6.284)	0.370 (0.024,5.820)
Antenatal care visit				
Yes	10	142	1	1
No	42	107	5.535 (2.657, 11.531)**	3.950 (1.546, 10.094)**
Come with referral				
Yes	45	143	4.72 (2.048, 10.882)**	7.320 (2.476, 21.637)**
No	7	106	1	1
Obstructed labor				
Yes	15	9	10.766 (4.395, 26.374)**	8.791(2.248, 34.381)**
No	37	239	1	1
Cord prolapse				
Yes	11	7	9.237 (3.237, 25.204)**	8.041 (1.951, 33.140)**
No	41	242	1	1
Preeclampsia				
Yes	8	13	3.287 (1.287, 8.395)*	7.600 (1.739, 33.222)**
No	44	234	1	1
Fetal presentation				
vertex	39	226	1	1
Non vertex	13	22	3.424 (1.593, 7.361)*	0.350 (0.075, 1.627)
Episiotomy				
Yes	7	99	1	1
No	45	149	4.271 (1.852, 9.853)**	1.148 (0.373, 3.532)
APGAR score				
<4/10	39	2	833.625 (147.398, 4714.642)	
4-6/10	9	75	5.130 (1.532, 17.180)**	4.288 (0.934, 19.680)
7-10/10	4	170	1	1
Birth weight				
2.5-4.0 kg	36	237	1	1
<2.5 kg	13	5	17.044 (5.734, 50.664)**	8.767 (2.105, 36.522)**
>4.0 kg	3	7	2.810 (0.695, 11.362)	
Congenital anomaly				
Yes	4	2	10.250 (1.826,57.547)**	0.127 (0.010, 1.547)
No	48	246	1	1

*- p-value < 0.05, ** -p-value < 0.01

Table 4: Predictors of perinatal death among mothers who gave birth at WSUTRH -southern Ethiopia, 2015.

line with a study done on trend of mode of delivery in Australia over study period of 1998-2008, which revealed that women with maternal diabetes mellitus, gestational diabetes mellitus, maternal hypertension, and preeclampsia were significantly associated with perinatal death [14].

Mothers who gave birth to low birth weight baby were 9 times more likely to have dead fetal outcome as compared to those who gave birth to normal birth weight baby. This finding is similar with a cross sectional study done in Senegal and Mali from 2007-2008 which suggested that low birth weight was significantly associated with perinatal death [13].

Conclusion and recommendations

Perinatal death in Wolaita Sodo referral hospital is tremendously high, which seeks a due attention. Un-booked antenatal care visit, obstructed labor, preeclampsia, cord prolapse, referral from other health facility and low birth weight delivery were significant predictors of perinatal death. Hence, to avert the situation, improvement in antenatal care service (supported with ultrasound examination);

improving obstetrics care; and early diagnosis and appropriate management of severely asphyxiated fetus at the time of delivery could reduce the prevalence. Easily accessible health facilities (which provide comprehensive essential and emergency obstetric services) could reduce perinatal death attributable to referral related causes. Besides, to prevent adverse birth outcome and to have a safe delivery, health facilities should give due attention to the use of partograph.

References

1. Joy EL, Gary LD, Robert LG (2009) Evidence for intra-partum deaths: Evidence for action. Int J Gynaecol Obstet:107.

2. World Health Organization, 2003. Surgical care at district hospital.

3. Yifru B, Asres B (2014) Perinatal mortality trends in Ethiopia. Ethiop J Health Sci 24: 29-40.

4. Patterson R, Woods D, Greenfield D, Sithembiso V (2005) Improving survival rates of new-born infants in South Africa. Reproductive health 2: 1-8.

5. Prevalence of adverse neonatal outcome and association with HIV infection among postnatal women in Mtwara Regional Hospital-Tanzania: 2009.

6. Fatma YZ, Fatma AM, Ghazala MM, Essa MD (2009) Relation between

prenatal care and pregnancy outcome at Benghazi. Sudanese Journal of Public Health 4: 403-410.

7. Briand V, Dumont A, Abrahamowicz M, Sow A, Traore M, et al. (2012) Maternal and perinatal outcomes by mode of delivery in Senegal and Mali: A cross-sectional epidemiological survey. PLoS ONE 7: 1-8.

8. Woliata Sodo University Teaching and Referral Hospital (2014/2015) HMIS report.

9. Ethiopia Demographic and Health Survey (2011) Central statistical agency and ICF International.

10. World Health Organization (2006) Neonatal and perinatal mortality; country, regional and global estimates. Geneva, Switzerland.

11. Mutihir JT, Eka PO (2010) Incidence, risk and etiological factors of stillbirths at the Jos University Teaching Hospital. Niger J Clin Pract 14.

12. Shimelis F, Hailemariam S, Fessehaye A (2010) Incidence, causes and outcome of obstructed labor in Jimma University Specialized Hospital. Ethiop J Health Sci 20: 145-151.

13. Shah A, Fawole B, Jams M, Amokrane F, Nafion I, et al. (2009) Cesarean delivery outcomes from the WHO global survey on maternal and perinatal health in Africa. Int J Gynaecol Obstet.

14. Graham J, Zhang L (2010) Factors associated with negative birth outcome. Findings from birth cohort study.

40

Back Pain during Pregnancy and Quality of Life of Pregnant Women

Ibanez G[1,2]*, Khaled A[1], Renard JF[1], Rohani S[1], Nizard J[3], Baiz N[4], Robert S[1], Chastang J[1]

[1]Department of Education and Research in General Medicine, Pierre-and-Marie-Curie, Sorbonne University, France
[2]Pierre Louis Institute of Epidemiology and Public Health, Sorbonne University, France
[3]Department of Obstetrics and Gynecology, Pitié Salpêtrière Hospital, Sorbonne University, France
[4]Department of Epidemiology, Allergic and Respiratory Diseases, Pierre Louis Institute of Epidemiology and Public Health, Sorbonne University, France

Abstract

Background: This study aimed to compare the quality of life (QOL) of women with low back pain and women without low back pain during pregnancy.

Methods: We conducted a cross-sectional study on pregnant women recruited in a hospital maternity or in primary care settings. Data collection was carried out through a self-administered questionnaire including the QOL Short Form Health Survey SF12-V2 scale. Independent sample t-tests were calculated to compare differences in QOL between women with and without low back pain. Multivariate regression models then examined the effect of low back pain on QOL, adjusting for covariate factors.

Results: Among the 218 pregnant women included in the study, 137 were suffering from low back pain (LBP). The mean intensity of pain (numerical scale) in the LBP group was 5.04 ± 1.73 (range 0 to 10 for maximum pain). Among women with low back pain, 21% of them (n=29) reported having received the following treatments for their pain. There was a significant difference in the quality of life between the group of women with low back pain (LBP) and the one without low back pain (NLBP) in the areas of mental health, physical health as well as social relations. The mental health and social relationships dimensions seemed more affected than the physical scores.

Conclusion: Low back pain decreased physical and psychosocial health during pregnancy. A greater support should be promoted in the medical follow-up of pregnant women with low back pain.

Keywords: Back pain; Pregnancy; Pregnant women

Introduction

Low back pain is a frequently reported complaint during pregnancy [1-3]. According to a Cochrane literature review more than two-thirds of pregnant women suffered from back pain during their pregnancies [4]. These pains often remain underestimated and undertreated [1-3]. According to Skaggs et al. [5] 85% of patients suffering from back pain did not receive any treatment from their caregiver and among those who were treated, only 1% stated that they were relieved by the proposed therapy.

The known risk factors of low back pain during pregnancy are previous history of back pain, maternal age and multiparity and physical activity [1,2,6]. Increase in Body Mass Index during pregnancy is a much-debated risk factor in the occurrence of low back pain [7]. The consequences in terms of economic impact have been described in several publications. In a study by Skaggs et al., these pains were found to be at the origin of many sick leaves during pregnancy [5]. A recent Norwegian study reported an average duration of 6.5 weeks of sick leave as a result of moderate lumbar pain [8]. This subject would therefore be important from a public health perspective in Scandinavian countries with an estimated cost of $2.5 million in 1990 [9].

During pregnancy, the occurrence of low back disorders could have global consequences involving physical, psychological and social impacts among women and their unborn children [4,10]. Few studies have evaluated the impact of these pains on the quality of life and the progress of the pregnancy; the results of these studies are controversial. In France, no data are available on this subject [11-13]. The main objective of our study was to determine the relation between low back pain and quality of life of pregnant women. The secondary objective was to find a correlation between the intensity of pain related to low back disorders and Quality of Life (QOL) scores.

Materials and Methods

Design of the study and population

A cross-sectional study was conducted between May and December 2013. The research sample consisted of 361 pregnant women going for regular checkups at the Pitié Salpêtrière maternity hospital (Paris) or at primary care settings including general medicine and midwife practices (in three departments in Parisian suburbs: Val-de-Marne, Seine-et-Marne and Hauts-de-Seine). Inclusion criteria were all pregnant women speaking French with a singleton pregnancy. Exclusion criteria were women consulting the gynecologic obstetric emergencies as well as those hospitalized. Participants were excluded from the study when having an adverse obstetric history (stillbirth, neonatal death, preterm birth or low birth weight in a previous pregnancy) or a high-risk pregnancy (gestational diabetes, gestational hypertension, hemorrhage during the second or third trimester, abnormal fetal growth or hospitalization for threatened preterm labor).

Data collection

Data for this study were collected through self-administrated questionnaires. Eligible women were invited to participate in the study during their prenatal consultations. Low back disorders were defined

*Corresponding author: Ibanez G, Department of Education and Research in General Medicine, Pierre-and-Marie-Curie, Sorbonne University, France, E-mail: gladys.ibanez@upmc.fr

as pain beside the lumbo-sacral spine, located at the iliac crests level or lower, central or lateral. A body diagram helped differentiate low back disorders from sacro-iliac pain. The first part of the questionnaire was devoted to pregnant women's socio-demographic and medical information and to the localization of low back disorders. A second part was devoted to the measurement of the quality of life.

Studied variables

The quality of life was measured through the questionnaire SF-12v2 (Short Form with 12 items). This is a validated tool in the international literature to measure the QOL and it is commonly used worldwide [14]. This tool is easy to use in its short version, with only 7 questions, and explores the eight main areas of health of the SF-36: physical functioning, physical role, bodily pain, general health, vitality, social functioning, emotional role and mental health. Two general scores summarize the physical component (PCS) and the mental component (MCS). It is a self-administered survey requiring short filling time (estimated at approximately 2 min). An updated version was developed by researchers specialized in QOL assessment. It has good psychometric properties as demonstrated in numerous studies.

The socio-demographic and medical characteristics considered were: age, term of pregnancy, body mass index (BMI) before the pregnancy, couple's marital situation, number of children, socio-professional category and back pain background outside of pregnancy. The presence of low back pain was assessed through a single question and was completed by a drawing indicating the exact location of the pain. The intensity of pain was evaluated using a numerical scale rated from 0 to 10. The medical treatment (including analgesics) was clearly reported.

Number of subjects needed

The number of required subjects was assessed on the basis of a difference of 4 on the score of quality of life (52 for group 1 versus 48 for group 2), a standard deviation of 10, a power of 80% and an alpha risk of 5%. In order to observe a significant difference between the two groups, a total of 156 subjects were needed. The statistical analysis (standard deviation, confidence interval, risk p) was carried out using the SAS Software 2.1 based on an Excel database summarizing the results.

First, the analysis included a description of the population and the quality of life of pregnant women. The QOL between the two groups, with and without low back pain, was then compared. Comparisons used Chi-square or Student tests as appropriate. Then associations were studied taking into account the following socio-demographic characteristics: maternal age, term of pregnancy, couple situation, women's socio-professional category, back pain history and place of recruitment (hospital or primary care settings). Statistical significance was defined as p<0.05. The statistical analyses were performed using the SAS 9.2 software (SAS Institute Inc., Cary, NC, USA).

Ethics committee

The questionnaire was distributed in the waiting room by two investigators. The research protocol had been validated by the Advisory Committee on the Treatment of Information in Research (CCTIRS).

Results

Out of the 339 women invited to participate in the study, 77 (22.7%) refused to participate and 44 (13.0%) were ineligible (Figures 1-3). 262 (77.3%) questionnaires were collected and 218 (64.3%) pregnant

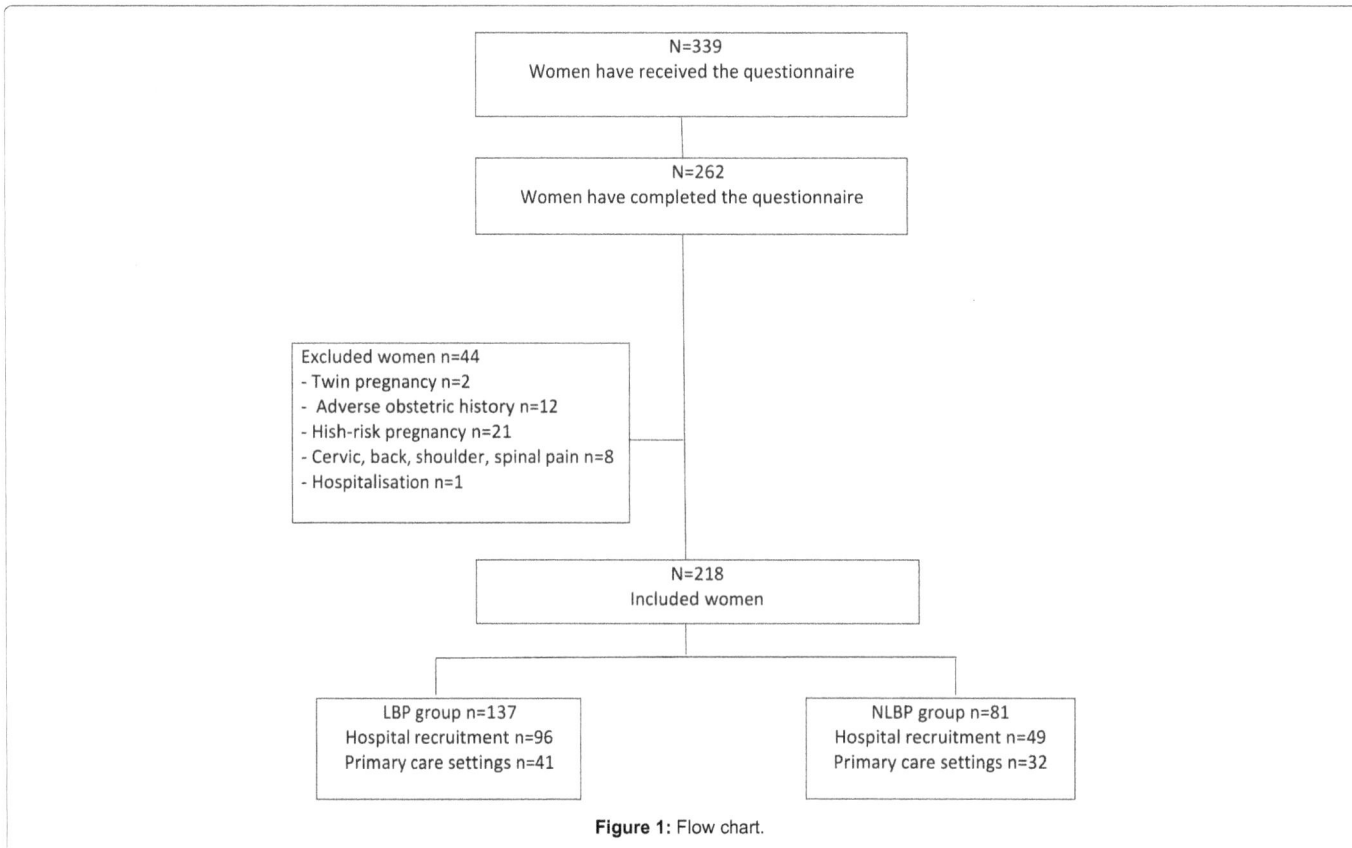

Figure 1: Flow chart.

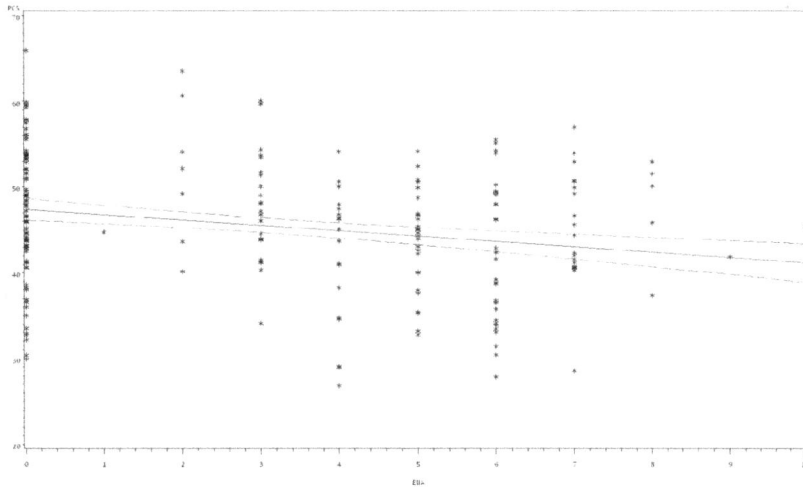

Figure 2: Correlation between the intensity of the pain and the PCS score.

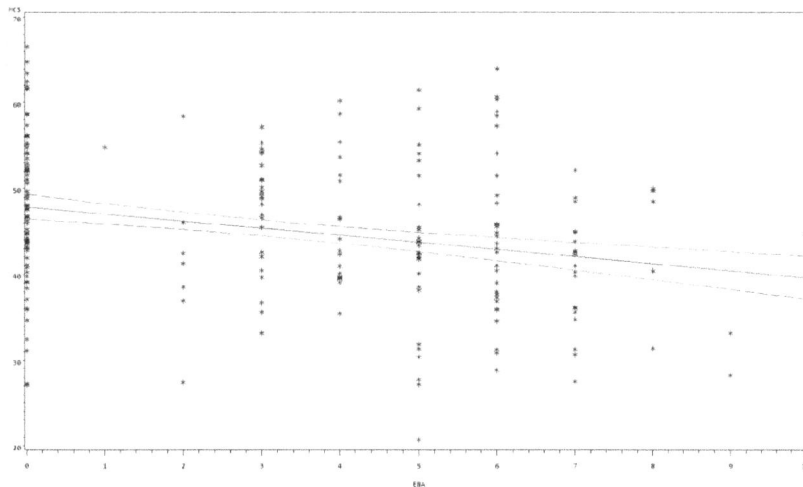

Figure 3: Correlation between the intensity of the pain and the MCS score.

women were included, divided into two groups: "Group with low back pain" (LBP, n=137) and "Group without low back pain" (NLBP, n=81).

Women's characteristics

Women in our sample were aged 18 to 44 years. They mainly lived with a partner and were more often primiparous women (Table 1). Women recruited at hospital or primary care settings had similar socio-demographic characteristics, except for women recruited at hospital who more often tended to live alone (respectively 11.8% and 4.11%, $p=0.06$) (data not shown).

The mean intensity of pain (numerical scale) in the LBP group was 5.04 ± 1.73 (range of 0 to 10 for maximum pain). At the first, second, and third trimester, it was respectively 1.44 ± 0.93, 2.84 ± 0.37 and 3.40 ± 0.23 ($p=0.07$). Among women with low back pain, 21% (n=29) reported having received the following treatments for such pain: osteopathy (7 women), paracetamol (6 women), acupuncture (4 women), physiotherapy (3 women), phloroglucinol (3 women), lumbar belt (1 women), magnesium (1 woman) or combination of these treatments (4 women).

Comparison of QOL scores

Prior to the adjustment of statistical analyses, women with low back disorders had lower physical scores with PCS scores respectively at 44.39 ± 2.47 (LBP group) and 47.34 ± 3.22 (NLBP group) ($p=0.006$) (Table 2). They also had lower mental scores with MCS scores respectively at 43.81 ± 2.18 (LBP) and 47.73 ± 2.65 (NLBP) ($p=0.001$). The "Physical role", "Bodily pain", "General health", "Social functioning", "Emotional role" and perceived "Mental health" were significantly poorer and lower. No differences were found in terms of "Physical functioning" and "Vitality".

After taking into account the potential confounding factors, women with low back disorders had lower physical scores with PCS scores respectively at 48.40 ± 2.37 (LBP group) and 50.75 ± 3.05 (NLBP group) ($p=0.03$) (Table 3). They also had lower mental scores with MCS scores respectively at 39.8 ± 2.98 (LBP group) and 43.5 ± 3.72 (NLBP group) ($p=0.004$). The "Physical role", "Bodily pain", "Social functioning", "Emotional role" and perceived "Mental health" were significantly poorer and lower. No differences were found in terms of "Physical functioning", "General health" and "Vitality".

	Total population % (n)	Low back pain group %(n)	No low back pain group %(n)	P value
Age:				
- Less than 20 years	1.8 (4)	2.2 (3)	1.2 (1)	
- 20 years to 30 years	36.9 (80)	40.2 (55)	31.3 (25)	
- 30 years to 40 years	56.7 (123)	54.0 (74)	61.2 (49)	0.47
- >40 years	4.6 (10)	3.6 (5)	6.3 (5)	
BMI (kg/m²) before pregnancy:				
- Less than to 19	10.1 (22)	7.3 (10)	14.8 (12)	
- 19 to 25	70.1 (152)	72.8 (99)	65.4 (53)	
- 25 to 30	15.2 (33)	16.2 (22)	13.6 (11)	0.25
- >30	4.6 (10)	3.7 (5)	6.2 (5)	
Term of pregnancy:				
- First Trimester (4 to 16)	4.2 (9)	2.9 (4)	6.2 (5)	
- 2nd Trimester (16 to 28)	25.8 (56)	24.8 (34)	27.5 (22)	0.42
- 3rd Trimester (>28)	70.0 (152)	72.3 (99)	66.3 (53)	
Couple:				
- Yes	90.8 (197)	88.2 (120)	95.1 (77)	0.09
- No	9.2 (20)	11.8 (16)	4.9 (4)	
Number of children:				
- No children	56.7 (123)	56.6 (77)	56.8 (46)	
- 1 children	29.0 (63)	30.9 (42)	25.9 (21)	
- 2/3 children	13.4 (29)	12.5 (17)	14.8 (12)	0.30
- >3 children	0.9 (2)	0 (0)	2.5 (2)	
Socio-professional category:				
- Managerial and professional occupations	27.5 (60)	25.6 (35)	30.9 (25)	
- Intermediary businesses, craftsmen, shopkeepers	47.7 (104)	47.5 (65)	48.2 (39)	
- Clerical support workers, service and sales workers, skilled workers	16.5 (36)	19.6 (27)	11.1 (9)	
- No job, student	8.3 (18)	7.3 (10)	9.9 (8)	0.36
Previous history of back pain outside of pregnancy:				
- Yes	32.6 (71)	45.3 (62)	11.1 (9)	
- No	67.4 (147)	54.7 (75)	88.9 (72)	<0.0001
Place of recruitment:				
- Hospital	66.5 (145)	70.1 (96)	60.5 (49)	
- Primary care settings	33.5 (73)	29.8 (41)	39.5 (32)	0.15

Table 1: Socio-demographic and medical characteristics of the population (n=218).

	Low back pain Group (n=137) Mean ± SD	No low back pain Group (n=81) Mean ± SD	P value
Physical Component Summary (PCS)	44.39 ± 0.65	47.34 ± 0.84	0.006
Physical Functioning (**PF**)	43.52 ± 0.87	45.21 ± 1.12	0.24
Physical Role (**RP**)	39.51 ± 0.71	44.14 ± 0.92	<0.0001
Bodily Pain (**BP**)	41.40 ± 0.79	47.37 ± 1.02	<0.0001
General Health (**GH**)	52.18 ± 0.54	54.33 ± 0.71	0.02
Mental Component Summary (MCS)	43.81 ± 0.72	47.73 ± 0.95	0.001
Vitality (**VT**)	45.19 ± 0.76	46.27 ± 0.99	0.39
Social Functioning (**SF**)	43.79 ± 0.74	48.11 ± 0.96	0.0004
Emotional Role (**RE**)	40.65 ± 0.83	43.99 ± 1.08	0.02
Mental Health (**MH**)	44.03 ± 0.74	49.41 ± 0.96	<0.0001

Table 2: Comparison of QOL between two groups (unadjusted analyses).

	Low back pain Group Mean ± SD	No low back pain Group Mean ± SD	P value
Physical Component Summary (PCS)	48.40 ± 1.50	50.75 ± 1.63	0.03
Physical Functioning (**PF**)	47.35 ± 2.11	48.39 ± 2.28	0.50
Physical Role (**RP**)	42.80 ± 1.69	46.80 ± 1.83	0.001
Bodily Pain (**BP**)	43.60 ± 1.91	48.41 ± 2.07	0.001
General Health (**GH**)	52.23 ± 1.35	54.06 ± 1.46	0.07
Mental Component Summary (MCS)	39.82 ± 1.75	43.54 ± 1.90	0.004
Vitality (**VT**)	41.96 ± 1.87	43.05 ± 2.03	0.43
Social Functioning (**SF**)	42.22 ± 1.84	47.00 ± 2.00	0.001
Emotional Role (**RE**)	40.19 ± 2.04	43.57 ± 2.21	0.03
Mental Health (**MH**)	41.75 ± 1.80	45.75 ± 1.95	0.003

* Analyses were adjusted for the following variables: Maternal age, term of pregnancy, family status, socio-professional category of women and low back pain history

Table 3: Comparison of QOL between two groups (adjusted analyses N=215/218).

A significant correlation between the intensity of pain and the QOL has been found for PCS and MCS (supplementary data). The more intense the pain was, the worse the perceived quality of life was, both physically and morally. The correlation coefficients for the PCS score and the MCS score were equal to ß1=-0.63 ± 0.18 and ß2=-0.83 ± 0.20, respectively. The correlation between the intensity of pain and the QOL was stronger for the mental component.

Discussion

Summary of results

In our study, the quality of life of women suffering from low back pain was poorer than that of women without low back pain. Women of the LBP group had significantly lower scores on the "Physical role", "Bodily pain", "Social Functioning", "Emotional role" and "Mental Health" sub-scales of the SF12-V2 questionnaire. Therefore, low back pain decreased physical and psychosocial health during pregnancy. In addition, few women with back pain received treatment for these low back disorders.

Strengths and limitations of the study

Few studies have assessed the impact of low back disorders during pregnancy. To the best of our knowledge, this is the first study on this topic conducted in France. In order to avoid bias related to co-morbidity, we decided to exclude women with a history of chronic diseases or hospitalized women, because their perception of the quality of life in this context of anxiety could be biased. The SF12-V2 is a commonly used tool for the assessment of the QOL of patients with low back pain.

Our study also presented limitations. This cross-sectional study does not establish a clear cause and effect relationship between QOL and low back pain, but rather an association between the presence of low back pain and an altered quality of life. Moreover, we carried out a brief exploration of the QOL. It would have been relevant to tackle other aspects of the QOL, such as the quality of sleep or sexuality, which are impaired among women suffering from back pain during pregnancy. The response rate of 69.2% in patients with and 57.9% in patients without low back pain is quite low, especially for those without back pain. Therefore, there was a risk of a certain selection bias. For example, subjects who are very interested in QOL research or those with bad QOL were more likely to participate. Furthermore, this study focused on low back pain during pregnancy and excluded patients with neck pain, shoulder pain or sacro-iliac pain. The reasons were that low back pain is a frequent reason for doctor consultation during pregnancy. Moreover, specific pathophysiological mechanisms were described for low back pain during pregnancy, including mechanical constraints, neuromuscular efficiency and fatigability of back extensor muscles, functional changes in back muscle activity, hormonal changes, psychosocial factors, etc. [7,15-17]. Moreover, we chose to recruit in hospital and primary care settings in Paris and Parisian suburb, and as such, this population is not representative of the French pregnant women population.

Comparison with others studies

In a study conducted in Sweden on pregnant women between the 34th and 37th weeks of pregnancy the QOL was significantly altered in the group suffering from back pain, with observed impact on sleep, energy, physical pain, and mobility, but also limitations in work, achievement of domestic tasks, social life and leisure [11]. In a case-control study conducted in 2009 by Coban et al. there was no clear evidence of impact of back pain on the QOL during pregnancy, though a strong correlation

was found between the intensity of the pain and the physical capacity of women to perform daily tasks [12]. Mogren et al. [11] found that the perception of health was declining during pregnancy among women suffering from lumbo-pelvic pain, with an increased risk of reporting poor health (OR 3.05 [95% CI 1.70 -5.46]).

Several studies have found that pregnancy in itself contributes to a decrease in the QOL with a gradual decline in physical capacity and to emotional disorders such as anxiety and depression [18-21]. Our study found that the mental health of women suffering from back pain was perceived as poorer; they often felt depressed and discouraged. According to several authors, mental disorders such as depression, anxiety, or prenatal stress could have a short-term and long-term negative impact on women's health as well as on the children's physical and mental health [22,23]. These findings are based on the concept of "Fetal Programming", which describes how fetal or perinatal events are act on the fetus and have influence on the outbreaks of diseases upon adulthood. After birth, these antenatal psychological disorders are associated with an increased risk for the child to develop emotional problems, attention deficit disorder with hyperactivity, and impaired cognitive development [24].

Conclusion

The World Health Organization (WHO) declared that health is "a state of complete physical, mental and social well-being and not merely the absence of disease or infirmity". Positive and negative dimensions of health vary from one person to another in a continuum. Common mental health disorders include depression and anxiety and are well known to health professionals. The positive dimension of mental health includes quality of life, well-being and has recently become the central focus of international policy, such as in Canada and the United Kingdom [25].

According to the WHO, quality of life is a broad ranging concept affected by the person's physical health, psychological state, level of independence, social relationships, personal beliefs, and relationship with salient features of their environment. The results of our study support the strong association between physical, social, and psychological health. Low back pain is a common reason for consultation during pregnancy and is strongly associated with an altered quality of life among pregnant women. Well-being and quality of life of pregnant women should be included within the scope of pregnancy monitoring and preventive health programs. All health professionals involved in pregnancy care (primary health care and hospital professionals) should thus be more sensitive to the different dimensions of health.

References

1. Wang SM, Dezinno P, Maranets I, Berman MR, Caldwell-Andrews AA, et al. (2004) Low back pain during pregnancy: prevalence, risk factors and outcomes. Obstet Gynecol 104: 65-70.

2. Vermani E, Mittal R, Weeks A (2010) Pelvic girdle pain and low back pain in pregnancy: A review. Pain Pract 10: 60-71.

3. Kovacs FM, Garcia E, Royuela A, Gonzalez L, Abraira V; Spanish Back Pain Research Network (2012) Prevalence and factors associated with low back pain and pelvic girdle pain during pregnancy: A multicentre study conducted in the Spanish National Health Service. Spine 37: 1516-1533.

4. Pennick VE, Young G (2007) Interventions for preventing and treating pelvic and back pain in pregnancy. Cochrane Database Syst Rev: CD001139.

5. Skaggs CD, Prather H, Gross G, George JW, Thompson PA, et al. (2007) Back and pelvic pain in an underserved United States pregnant population: A preliminary descriptive survey. J Manipulative Physiol Ther 30: 130-134.

6. Sabino J, Grauer JN (2008) Pregnancy and low back pain. Curr Rev Musculoskelet Med 1: 137-141.

7. Mogren IM, Pohjanen AI (2005) Low back pain and pelvic pain during pregnancy: Prevalence and risk factors. Spine (Phila Pa 1976) 30: 983-991.

8. Malmqvist S, Kjaermann I, Andersen K, Økland I, Brønnick K, et al. (2012) Prevalence of low back and pelvic pain during pregnancy in a Norwegian population. J Manipulative Physiol Ther 35: 272-278.

9. Norén L, Ostgaard S, Nielsen TF, Ostgaard HC (1997) Reduction of sick leave for lumbar back and posterior pelvic pain in pregnancy. Spine (Phila Pa 1976) 22: 2157-2160.

10. Olsson C, Nilsson-Wikmar L (2004) Health-related quality of life and physical ability among pregnant women with and without back pain in late pregnancy. Acta Obstet Gynecol Scand 83: 351-357.

11. Mogren I (2006) Perceived health, sick leave, psychosocial situation, and sexual life in women with low-back pain and pelvic pain during pregnancy. Acta Obstet Gynecol Scand 85: 647-656.

12. Coban A, Arslan GG, Colakfakioglu A, Sirlan A (2011) Impact on quality of life and physical ability of pregnancy-related back pain in the third trimester of pregnancy. J Pak Med Assoc 61: 1122-1124.

13. Gandek B, Ware JE, Aaronson NK, Apolone G, Bjorner JB, et al (1998) Cross-Validation of item selection and scoring for the SF-12 Health Survey in nine countries: Results from the IQOLA Project. J Clin Epidemiol 51: 1171 1178.

14. Dumas GA, Leger A, Plamondon A, Charpentier KM, Pinti A, et al. (2010) Fatigability of back extensor muscles and low back pain during pregnancy. Clin Biomech (Bristol, Avon) 25: 1-5.

15. Albert H, Godskesen M, Westergaard JG, Chard T, Gunn L (1997) Circulating levels of relaxin are normal in pregnant women with pelvic pain. Eur J Obstet Gynecol Reprod Biol 74: 19-22.

16. Ostgaard HC, Andersson GB, Schultz AB, Miller JA (1993) Influence of some biomechanical factors on low-back pain in pregnancy. Spine (Phila Pa 1976) 18: 61-65.

17. Wang P, Liou SR, Cheng CY (2013) Prediction of maternal quality of life on preterm birth and low birth weight: A longitudinal study. BMC Pregnancy Childbirth 13: 124.

18. Otchet F, Carey MS, Adam L (1999) General health and psychological symptom status in pregnancy and the puerperium: What is normal? Obstet Gynecol 94: 935-941.

19. Lee AM, Lam SK, Sze Mun Lau SM, Chong CS, Chui HW, et al. (2007) Prevalence, course and risk factors for antenatal anxiety and depression. Obstet Gynecol 110: 1102-1112.

20. Manber R, Blasey C, Allen JJ (2008) Depression symptoms during pregnancy. Arch Womens Ment Health 11: 43-48.

21. Da Costa D, Dritsa M, Larouche J, Brender W (2000) Psychosocial predictors of labor/delivery complications and infant birth weight: A prospective multivariate study. J Psychosom Obstet Gynecol 21: 137-148.

22. Glynn LM, Schetter CD, Hobel CJ, Sandman CA (2008) Pattern of perceived stress and anxiety in pregnancy predicts preterm birth. Health Psychol 27: 43-51.

23. Talge NM, Neal C, Glover V (2007) Early stress, translational research and prevention science network: Fetal and neonatal experience on child and adolescent mental health. Antenatal maternal stress and long-term effects on child neurodevelopment: How and why? J Child Psychol Psychiatry 48: 245 261.

24. Canadian Institute for Health Information (2009) Exploring positive mental health. Ottawa, Canadian Population Health Initiative.

25. The British Psychological Society (2009) Psychological health and well-being: A new ethos for mental health. A report of the working group on psychological health and well-being. Leicester, The British Psychological Society.

41

Assessment of Sexual Activity and Contraceptive use among Young Ages of Jimma Teachers Training College Students, Jimma Town, South West Ethiopia, Cross Sectional Study

Sena Belina Kitila[1]*, **Ashagre Molla Asaye**[1] and **Anuwar Yusuf Issa**[2]

[1,2]*Department of Nursing and Midwifery, College of Health Science, Jimma University, Ethiopia*

Abstract

Background: Young age in Ethiopia are estimated to be 19.3% of total population. Despite their number, they lack access to the reproductive health service information like sexuality and family planning methods. Most of them get their peers whose views are often inaccurate and based on remorse. The aim of this study was to assess sexual activity and contraceptives use among young ages of Jimma teachers training college students.

Methods: Cross sectional study design with quantitative methods of data collection was employed from February to March 2013 using pre tested self-administering questionnaire.

Results: Data was extracted from 257 respondents that makes response rate 100%. Out of the total of 257 study participants, 127(49.45%) of the students were from 20 -22 years age, 89 (34.63%) were males, 230(89.49%) were Oromo, 106(41.24%) of them were Muslim, 237(89.49%) of them were unmarried, 189 (77.04%) of them were from farmer families and 168(65.4%) were from illiterate family. Half 118(45.9%) were currently sexually active, 95(80.5%) those sexually active were using any types of contraceptive.

Conclusion and Recommendation: 45.9% of the study participants were sexually active, and among those sexually active 80.5% were using any types of contraceptive methods. Age of the respondents, sex, religion and educational level of the family found to be associated with sexual activity , and age of the respondents, marital status, age at first sexual intercourse, parent occupation and educational level of the family were found to be associated with contraceptive sue. Further prospective studies with both qualitative and quantitative method of data collection is recommended .

Keywords: Young age; Sexual activity; Contraceptive; Jimma teachers training college

Abbrevations: EDHS - Ethiopian Demographic and Health Survey; FP - Family Planning ; HIV/AIDS - Human Immune Virus/Acquired Immune Deficiency Syndrome; JTTC - Jimma Teacher Training College; MOH - Ministry Of Health; RH - Reproductive Health; STD - Sexually Transmitted Disease; UN - United Nation; USA - United State of America; WHO - World Health Organization.

Introduction

Young age is a period in human development characterized by significant physiological, psychological and social changes [1]. Majority of the world Young age peoples are living in the developing countries, moreover nine out of ten of them face profound challenges from obtaining education to simple staying alive [2] and they are lack access to basic Reproductive Health (RH) information like sexuality and family planning service, most of them get information about this from their peers whose views are often inaccurate and based on remorse [3]

Demographic and sociologic study shows as there is association between ages, sex, races, income, socio economic changes, self-esteem, biological factors, peers pressures, physiologic maturation urbanization, civilization, life style and family structure and sexual activities [4,5]

Initiation of sexual activity at an earlier age can leads to an increase life time number of sexual partners, lower probability of using modern contraceptive methods [6].Worldwide half of the contraception occurring per day are unplanned and about one fourth are unwanted [7]. Young sexual activity vary from culture to culture and those who experiencing first coitus at earlier ages are less likely to take the necessary precautions to prevent unwanted pregnancy or STDS [8].

The study conducted in South African high school students

indicates as morbidity and mortality among young ages become a focus of policy initiatives in developing countries, due to low contraceptive use; rising pregnancy rates and reliance on clandestine abortion [9,10]

The study done in 2003, in developed nation like United States, Canada, Great Britain, Netherland and France, showed as the average typical age sexual initiation is around 17.5 years and in US, it is 17.2, in Canada 17.3, in Great Britain 17.5, in Netherland 17.7 and in France 18.0 years [11].

Study conduct in southern Nigeria secondary school on sexual activity, contraceptive knowledge and use showed as only 36%(886/2460) knew the most likely time for contraception to occur , 40% of them were sexually active , of this sexually active 26% of them started at age of 19 years, 25% of them had involved with older business man [11].

The study conducted in Cameron on 670 young age's school student to evaluate their knowledge and practice of sexuality indicated as 53%were sexually active, 41% used any contraceptive method during their recent intercourse [12]. Also the study in Kenya on premarital

*Corresponding author: Sena Belina Kitila, Department of Nursing and Midwifery, College of Health Science, Jimma University, Ethiopia, E-mail: Senabalina26@gmail.com or sena.belina@ju.edu.et

sexual activities among school young ages on 300 enrolled in 46 educational college students 48-77% of male have had coitus compared with 17% to 67% of females, nearly half of sexually active males report multiple sexual partners [13].

The fertility survey conducted in Uganda on age 15-24years in both rural and urban on 4510 subjects revealed, 84% of the male and 81.5% of female were sexually active and the mean age at first coitus was 15.1 years for male and 15.5 for females, greater than 80% had awareness on contraceptive but only 25% used contraceptive [14].

The very low level of economic development, widespread poverty, very poor and inadequate health services make the consequences of adolescent sexuality much more serious in the Ethiopian context than those of the developed countries and this reflected by the highest HIV prevalence in the group 15-24 years 12.1% [15].

The study done in Ethiopia at Addis Ababa on college students indicated as 60% of them were sexually active, the mean age at first coitus was 15.3years for females and 16.4 for male. In Harar 50% of female and 25% male experienced sexual intercourse at mean age of 16.9 years and only one fourth of them used family planning methods. The study at Jimma University showed as 228 (39.9%) students sexually active, 195 (41.7%) males and 33 (31.7%) [16,17]. Also in Ethiopia 32% had sexual intercourse before age 15, 65 % before age 18 and the trends in age at sexual initiation have increased little between 2000 and 2005 EDHS [18].

Methods and Materials

A cross sectional the study was conducted from February to March 2013 at Jimma teacher training college (JTTC) which is located 352kms from Addis Ababa towards south west and 2.5Kms to the East of Jimma town. It is one of regional teachers training colleges in Ethiopia. It was established 1969 as teachers training institute (TTI) and upgrade in to TTC in 2002.

The source population for this study were all students of Jimma teacher training college regular graduating class of academic year 2013 and the study population were all sampled students selected using systematic random sampling technique using their attendance list as sampling frame and available during the study period.

Data was collected through self-administrated questionnaire using pre-tested structured questionnaire which has both close and open ended questions

The quality of the data was assured by using validated pre-tested questionnaires. Prior to the actual data collection, pre-testing was done on 5% of the total study subjects. Data collection facilitators were trained for one day intensively on the study instrument and data collection procedure that includes the relevance of the study, objective of the study, about confidentiality of the information and informed consent.

Data analysis was conducted using SPSS version 16.0. In addition to descriptive statistics, the chi-square test was employed to assess for associations between dependent and independent variables of the study to determine degree of association. P-value of <0.05 considered significant and the results presented using tables, graphs, and charts.

Ethical approval letter for the study was granted from Jimma University College of public Health and Medical sciences department of Nursing. Informed consent was received from all the participants after explaining the purpose of the study before distributing the questionnaire and it ensured during each activity of data collection. The

Variables		Frequency(n=257)	Percentage
Age	19	21	8.17
	20-22	127	49.45
	22-24	109	42.4
Sex	Male	89	34.63
	Female	168	65.37
Religion	Muslim	106	41.24
	Orthodox	98	38.13
	Protestant	43	16.73
	Others	10	3.89
Ethnicity	Oromo	230	89.49
	Amhara	21	8.17
	Others	6	2.33
Marital status	Unmarried	237	92.2
	Married	20	7.78
Parent occupation	Farmer	189	77.04
	Merchant	42	16.34
	Employed	13	5.06
	Others	4	1.56
Educational level of the family	Illiterate	168	65.4
	Literate	89	34.6

Table 1: Distribution of study participants by their socio-demographic characteristics, among Jimma teacher training college students, Jimma town, February to March, 2013.

respondents also were reassured on confidentiality of their responses during and after the study.

Results

The data were collected from a total of 257 study subjects from February to March 2013 (Table 1) that makes the response rate 100% and the results are presented under subheadings as follows.

Socio demographic characteristics of the respondents

127 (49.45%) of the students were from 20 -22 years age groups. 168 (65.37%) of the respondents were females. As to ethnicity majority 230 (89.49) were Oromo followed by Amhara 21 (8.17%). Majority 106 (41.24) of them were Muslim and 237 (89.49%) of the respondents were unmarried. Concerning their parent occupation and educational level 189 (77.04%) of them were farmers and 168 (65.4%) were from illiterate families respectively (Error! Reference source not found) (Table 2).

Sexual activity of the respondents

118 (45.9%) of respondents were currently sexually active. Among sexually active, 44 (37.3%), age at sexual debut was 16-19 years of age, 72 (61.02%) were reported that first sexual intercourse was unplanned, 75 (63.56%) of them had first sexual intercourse with their boy/girlfriend, 75 (65.5%) had two life time sexual partners, 80 (67.79%) were being with their regular partner. 104 (83.14%) of them have had sexual intercourse with other than their regular partner and 75 (72.11%) had one sexual partner other than their regular partner and 23 (19.49%) ever receive money, gift or that favor to sex (Error! Reference source not found) (Table 3).

Contraceptive use practice

Among sexually active 118 study participants 95 (80.5%) were using any types of contraceptive methods, Out of this 38 (40%) of them reported as they have used condom, 57 (60%) were reported as they use contraceptive sometimes and 25 (21.18%) of them responded as they used condom at first sexual intercourse. The respondents also asked

Variables		Frequency(n=257)	Percentage
Ever started sex	Yes	118	45.9
	No	139	54.1
Age at first sexual intercourse	≤15	35	29.7
	16-19	44	37.3
	20-24	28	23.73
	≥ 25	11	9.32
First sex is planned	Yes	46	38.08
	No	72	61.02
Partner at first sexual intercourse	Boy/girl friend	75	63.56
	Husband/Wife	16	13.56
	Commercial sex works	17	14.4
	Others	10	8.47
No. of partner	1	14	11.86
	2	75	65.5
	≥ 3	29	24.57
Now with regular partner	Yes	80	67.79
	No	38	32.21
Reason to remain with regular partner**	To protected from STDs	51	63.17
	To protected from HIV	63	78.75
	Increased the trust of partner	46	57.5
Have sex other than regular partner	Yes	104	83.14
	No	14	11.86
No. of partner other than regular partner	1	75	72.11
	2	19	18.26
	≥ 3	10	9.61
Ever receive money, gift or favor to sex	Yes	23	19.49
	No.	95	80.5

**More than one answer is possible

Table 2: Distribution of study participants by their sexual activity, among Jimma teacher training college students, Jimma town, February to March, 2013.

Variables		Frequency	(%)
Ever used contraceptive	Yes	95	80.5
	No	23	19.49
Type of contraceptive used	Pills	15	15.79
	Inject able	35	36.84
	Condoms	38	40
	Others	7	7.36
Frequency of using contraceptive	Some times	57	60
	Always	29	30.52
	Rarely	9	9.47
Use condom during at first sexual intercourse	Yes	25	21.18
	No	93	78.81
Reason not for using condom at first sexual intercourse*	Not available	57	61.29
	Not trust condom	15	16.13
	Due to partner pressure	27	29.03
	In hurry	9	9.67
	Increased the trust of partner	38	40.86
	Others	11	11.83
purpose of using condom*	To protected from STDs	49	51.58
	To protected from HIV	61	63.21
	To protected from unwanted pregnancy	38	40
	Others	7	7.37

*More than one answer is possible.

Table 3: Distribution of study participants by their contraceptive use practice, among Jimma teacher training college students, Jimma town, February to March, 2013.

for the reason why they did not use condom and why they use, and 57 (61.29%) of them were responded that as it was not available, while 61 (63.21%) of respondents were used it to prevent from HIV/AIDS. (Error! Reference source not found.)

Association between dependent and independent variables

Dependent and independent variables were cross tabulated with each socio demographic characteristics related factors, and Sexual activity and practice of contraceptive. There were statistically significant associations observed between age of the respondents ($\chi^2=0.09$, p=0.0187), sex ($\chi^2=0.01$, p=0.00), religion ($\chi^2=0.15$, p=0.0242), educational level of the family ($\chi^2=0.01$, p=0.000) with sexual activity and There were statistically significant associations between age ($\chi^2=18.00$, p=0.00), marital status ($\chi^2=21.5$, p=0.00), age at first sexual intercourse ($\chi^2=11.5$, p=0.009) parent occupation ($\chi^2=11.7$, p=0.00) and educational level of the family ($\chi^2=43.1$, p=0.00) with contraceptive use, however there is no associations between sex, religion and ethnicity with ever used contraceptive.

Discussion

Initiation of sexual activity at earlier age can leads to an increase life time number of sexual partners, lower probability of use of contraceptive and higher probability of having STIs [6].

This study revealed that, 45.9% students were sexually active, out of these sexually active 37.3%, started it at 16-19 years of age, and 29.7% them starts early at age of 15 and below years.

This finding was higher than what has been identified in the study conduct in southern Nigeria where 40% of them were sexually active and 26% of them started it at age of 19 years [11], the study at Jimma University in which 228(39.9%) students were sexually active and what reported on EDHS where 32% had sexual intercourse before age 15 years [18]. Conversely , lower than what has been observed in Cameron where 53% of the students were sexually active [12] , the study in Kenya where 48-77% of male have had coitus , 17% to 67% of females [13] , the study conducted in Uganda where 84% of the male and 81.5% of female were sexually active and the mean age at first coitus was 15.1 years for male and 15.5 for females [14] and the study done in Ethiopia at Addis Ababa where 60% of them were sexually active, the mean age at first coitus was 15.3years for females and 16.4 for male [18].

The likely expiations for this dissimilarity might be due to difference in study period, level of education of the study subjects involved, operationalisation variables, policy concern, geographical location and cultural background of the study population, the college students came from different corners with different experiences and separation from the family.

This study also identified that among sexually active students 80.5% were using any types of contraceptive methods.

This finding was by far higher than the study conducted in Cameron where 41% of those sexually active used any contraceptive method during their recent intercourse [12], the study conducted in Uganda where greater than 80% sexually active students had awareness on contraceptive but only 25% used contraceptive [14].

The likely expiations for this dissimilarity might be due to difference in study period, level of education of the study subjects involved, operationalisation variables, policy concern about contraceptive, geographical location and sociocultural difference, knowledge about contraceptive and variation of attitude toward contraceptive and custom of the study population in different country on the world.

This study further revealed the association between socio demographic characteristics such as age of the respondents, sex, religion and educational level of the family found to be associated with sexual activity , and age of the respondents, marital status, age at first sexual intercourse, parent occupation and educational level of the family were found to be associated with contraceptive sue

The finding of this study is comparable with what has been reported Demographic and sociologic study where is association between ages, sex, races, income, socio economic changes, self-esteem, biological factors, peers pressures, physiologic maturation urbanization, civilization, life style and family structure and sexual activities [4,5].

Conclusion and Recommendation

This cross sectional study revealed that, 45.9% respondents currently sexually active, and among sexually active students 80.5% were using any types of contraceptive methods. Socio demographic characteristics such as age of the respondents, sex, religion and educational level of the family found to be associated with sexual activity , and age of the respondents, marital status, age at first sexual intercourse, parent occupation and educational level of the family were found to be associated with contraceptive sue. Further prospective studies with both qualitative and quantitative method of data collection is recommended.

Competing Interests

There no financial and non-financial competing interests and the study was funded by the Jimma University. There have been no reimbursements, fees, funding, nor salary from any organization that depends on or influence the results of this study. The authors do not hold any stocks or shares in an organization that may in any way might be affected by this publication.

Acknowledgement

We would like to express our deepest gratitude to Jimma University College of Health Sciences for financially supporting us. Our appreciation also goes to our data collectors, supervisors and study participants for their valuable contribution in the realization of this study.

References

1. Rewnge M (2008) international family planning perspective

2. Kora A,Haile M (2005) sexual behavior and level of awareness of reproductive health. EMJ 13: 108-113.

3. Young age (2008) reproductive health family planning, standards of practice manual Eth. AA MOH 120-124.

4. Karen giffen M (2009) Young age, reproductive health behavior social science and medicine 15.

5. Contraceptive use in young age America family physical. File format; PDF / adobe acrobat view: HTML Org: UCSF edu. (Science) pesters 2005/deepeners. PDF.

6. Radheshan B (2006) international family planning perspective 27.

7. WHO (2007) unsafe abortion ;global and regional estimate of in dependence and morality due to unsafe abortion with lasting available country data, Geneva

8. WHO (2008) health of young people's: challenge and promise.

9. Federal office of statistics and institute (2005)for resource development/Macro Internanatiol, Nigeria Demographic and Health Survey, Columbia MJ, USA, 2005.

10. Couper ID, Alexander TJD (2005) Family planning: attitudes of rural high school students. SA FamPract 16: 602-609.

11. National campaign to prevent teen age pregnancy half way their prospection for continued progress in preventing teen age pregnancy. Washington Dc the

campaign 2009.

12. Kahn (2006) results from national school based 2008 youth risk behavior survey and progress toward achieving related health objectives for the nation. (public report) 108: 47-55

13. Saving William Arc (2008) Verbal physical abuse stressors in the lives of lesbians male and bisexual youth; association with school problems running away J consult psychology 261-269

14. JSTR (2006) International family planning perspective. 23: 28-33.

15. Taylor D, Chavez G, Habra A, Boggs J (2007) Risk factors for adult paternity in births to Adolescents. Obstetric Gynecology 89: 199-205.

16. Ache. Amazing (2009) a new version for young age sexual health transition.10.

17. Fikirte M (2009) Assesment of Parent Adolecant Communication on Sexual and Reproductive Health Matters in Awwasa Town. SNNPR, Ethiopia. Addis Ababa University: Faculty of Medicine Department of Community Health (MPH thesis). Addis Ababa Ethiopia.

18. Attawell K (2005) Going to Scale in Ethiopia: Mobilizing Youth Participation in a National HIV/AIDS Program. Social & Scientific Systems Inc. /the Synergy Project, Washington, D.C.

19. Shivered (2011) Assessment of Knowledge, Attitude and Risk Behavior towards HIV AIDS and Other STDs. Among Preparatory Students of Gonder Town, North West Ethiopia. BMC Research Notes 4: 505.

Permissions

The contributors of this book come from diverse backgrounds, making this book a truly international effort. This book will bring forth new frontiers with its revolutionizing research information and detailed analysis of the nascent developments around the world.

We would like to thank all the contributing authors for lending their expertise to make the book truly unique. They have played a crucial role in the development of this book. Without their invaluable contributions this book wouldn't have been possible. They have made vital efforts to compile up to date information on the varied aspects of this subject to make this book a valuable addition to the collection of many professionals and students.

This book was conceptualized with the vision of imparting up-to-date information and advanced data in this field. To ensure the same, a matchless editorial board was set up. Every individual on the board went through rigorous rounds of assessment to prove their worth. After which they invested a large part of their time researching and compiling the most relevant data for our readers.

The editorial board has been involved in producing this book since its inception. They have spent rigorous hours researching and exploring the diverse topics which have resulted in the successful publishing of this book. They have passed on their knowledge of decades through this book. To expedite this challenging task, the publisher supported the team at every step. A small team of assistant editors was also appointed to further simplify the editing procedure and attain best results for the readers.

Apart from the editorial board, the designing team has also invested a significant amount of their time in understanding the subject and creating the most relevant covers. They scrutinized every image to scout for the most suitable representation of the subject and create an appropriate cover for the book.

The publishing team has been an ardent support to the editorial, designing and production team. Their endless efforts to recruit the best for this project, has resulted in the accomplishment of this book. They are a veteran in the field of academics and their pool of knowledge is as vast as their experience in printing. Their expertise and guidance has proved useful at every step. Their uncompromising quality standards have made this book an exceptional effort. Their encouragement from time to time has been an inspiration for everyone.

The publisher and the editorial board hope that this book will prove to be a valuable piece of knowledge for researchers, students, practitioners and scholars across the globe.

List of Contributors

Saridi M, Toska A and Rekleiti M
Department of Nursing, General Hospital of Korinthos, Greece

Sarafis P
Faculty of Nursing, Technological Educational Institute, Lamia, Greece

Zoukas L
Department of Gynecology, General Hospital of Korinthos, Greece

Souliotis K
Faculty of Social Sciences, University of Peloponnese, Korinthos, Greece

Birbas K
Faculty of Nursing, National and Kapodistrian, University of Athens, Greece

Maria Scatigna, Maria De Felice, Anna R. Giuliani and Leila Fabiani
Department of Medicine, Health and Environmental Sciences, University of L'Aquila –Italy

Fabio Samani and Luigi Canciani
Health Search – Italy

Jin Xu, Yilu Zhou, Yinglin Wang and Hao Zhang
Department of Anesthesiology, Shanghai East Hospital, Tongji University School of Medicine, China

Samuel Abdu A, Habtamu Tesfaye M and Bekana FeKecha H
Department of Nursing, Jimma University, Ethiopia

Siti Nadzrah Y
Faculty of Medicine, University of Malaya, Malaysia

Zulkiflee AB and Prepageran N
Department of Otorhinolaryngology, Faculty of Medicine, University of Malaya, Malaysia

Vanessa Alvarado and Brigitte Liebig
University of Applied Sciences, Applied Psychology, Riggenbachstrasse 16, Olten, 4600, Switzerland

Caprice Knapp, Vanessa Madden and Hanny Lane
Department of Health Outcomes and Policy, Gainesville, FL, USA

Ruth Gubernick
Gubernick-RSG Consulting, Cherry Hill NJ, USA

Steven Kairys
School of Public Health, University of Medicine and Dentistry of New Jersey, Newark, NJ, USA

Cristina Pelaez-Velez
University of South Florida, Department of Pediatrics, Tampa, FL, USA

Lee Sanders
Center for Health Policy, Stanford University, Stanford, CA, USA

Lindsay Thompson
Department of Pediatrics and Health Outcomes and Policy, Gainesville, FL, USA

Vanishri Arun and Padma SK
Department of Information Science and Engineering, Sri Jayachamarajendra College of Engineering, Mysore– 570 006, India

Shyam V
Forus Health Private Ltd., Bengaluru – 560070, India

Joan Rosenbaum Asarnow, Jessica Harwood, Steven Shoptaw and Martin Anderson
UCLA School of Medicine, Los Angeles, California 90095, USA

Luis Roberto Zeledon and Anne LaBorde
Kaiser Permanente Los Angeles Medical Center, Los Angeles, USA

Elizabeth D'Amico
RAND, California, USA

Claudia Avina
Harbor-UCLA Medical Center, Torrance, CA 90502, USA

Talin Arslanian
UC Davis School of Medicine, Sacramento, CA 95817, USA

Minh-Chau Do
San Diego State/UCSD, San Diego, CA 92182, USA

Vassiliki Tzanetakou, Theodora Kanni and Evangelos Giamarellos-Bourboulis J
Department of Internal Medicine, University of Athens, Medical School, Greece

Kyriakoula Merakou and Anastasia Barbouni
Department of Public Health, National School of Public Health, Athens, Greece

Ervin K and Koschel A
Department of Rural Health, University of Melbourne, Graham St, Shepparton, 3630, Australia

Campi S
Violet Town Bush Nursing Centre, Cowslip St, Violet Town, 3669, Australia

K Nilvarangkul
Faculty of Nursing, Khon Kaen University, Thailand

T Phajan
Sirinthon College of Public Health, Khon Kaen, Thailand

U Inmuong, JF Smith and P Rithmark
Faculty of Public Health, Khon Kaen University, Thailand

Dalle Nogare N and Spiller R
Goulburn Valley Primary Care Partnership, Shepparton, Australia

Orr J
Goulburn Valley Health, Shepparton, Australia

Soutter E
Goulburn Valley Primary Care Partnership, Shepparton, Australia
Numurkah District Health Service, Numurkah, Australia

Qian Dai
Department of Centre for Psychological Health and Education, Sichuan University, China

Alexey Kalyagin and Maria Karnakova
Department of Propaedeutics of Internal Diseases, Irkutsk State Medical University, Russian Federation

Khalid A. Ansari and Hajed M. Al. Otaibi
University of Dammam, Department of Respiratory Care, Dammam, Saudi Arabia

Niall P. Keaney
Royal Hospital, Sunderland, Sunderland, Tyne & Wear, UK

Dien Gusta Anggraini N
Faculty of Medicine, Andalas University, Padang, Indonesia
Faculty of Public Health, Andalas University, Padang, Indonesia

Rizanda M and Eryati D
Faculty of Medicine, Andalas University, Padang, Indonesia

Nana M
Ministry of Health, Andalas University, Padang, Indonesia

Sarita Dhakal and Eun Woo Nam
Yonsei Global Health Center, Yonsei University, Wonju, Korea
Department of Health Administration, Graduate School, Yonsei University, Korea
Institute of Poverty Allivaiton and International Development, Yonsei University, Wonju, Korea

Young Suk Jun
West Africa Team, Korea International Cooperation Agency, Headquater, Korea

Ha Yun Kim and Jin Sung Song
Yonsei Global Health Center, Yonsei University, Wonju, Korea
Department of Health Administration, Graduate School, Yonsei University, Korea

Festus Adams
Ministry of Health, Ghana

Marie-Louise Mariager Pedersen
Queen Ingrid Primary Health Care Center, Nuuk, Greenland, Denmark

Michael Lynge Pedersen
Queen Ingrid Primary Health Care Center, Nuuk, Greenland, Denmark
Greenland Center for Health Research, Institute of Nursing and Health Science, University of Greenland, Denmark

Shantanu Sharma, Charu Kohli and Nandini Sharma
Department of Community Medicine, Maulana Azad Medical College, India

Devika Mehra
Department of Public Health, Sweden

Akanbi F
Department of Nursing, International Health Science University, Uganda

Afolabi KK
Department of Public Health, Cavendish University, Uganda

Aremu AB
Department of Community Medicine, Islamic University, Uganda

Ahmed Yasin Mohammed
Department of Public Health, College of Medicine and Health Science, Madawalabu University, Bale Goba, Ethiopia

Tomas Benti Tefera and Muktar Beshir Ahmed
Department of Nursing, College of Medicine and Health Science, Madawalabu University, Bale Goba, Ethiopi

Shibiru Tesema, Bayeta Disasa and Eliyas Kadi
Department of Pharmacy, college of health sciences, Jimma University, Jimma, Ethiopia

Selamu Kebamo
Department of pharmacy, college of medical and health sciences, Wollega University, Ethiopia

Tsegahun Worku Brhanie
Department of Public health, College of Medicine and Health Sciences, Bahir Dar University, Ethiopia

Habtamu Alemay Anteneh
Federal Ministry of Health, Ethiopia

Hassan MB, Hammam NA, Fuad AR, Bakr HA and Abdulrhman Ahmed G
Department of Medicine, Taibah University, Saudi Arabia

Inge M Verhoeven
The Hague University of Applied Sciences, Johanna Westerdijkplein 75, 2521 EN The Hague, The Netherlands Technical University, Jaffalaan 9, 2628 BX Delft, The Netherlands

Marjan J Klippel and Monique A M Berger
The Hague University of Applied Sciences, Johanna Westerdijkplein 75, 2521 EN The Hague, The Netherlands

Frederike van Markus
Sophia Rehabilitation, Vrederustlaan 180, 2543 SW The Hague, The Netherlands

Arend J de Kloet
The Hague University of Applied Sciences, Johanna Westerdijkplein 75, 2521 EN The Hague, The Netherlands Sophia Rehabilitation, Vrederustlaan 180, 2543 SW The Hague, The Netherlands

Micanti F, Pecoraro G, Mosca P, Riccio F and Galletta D
Department of Psychiatry, Universita degli Studi di Napoli Federico II Naples, Italy

Israel B
Department of Nursing, Faculty of Health Sciences, Jimma University, Ethiopia

Kifle W
Department of Epidemiology, Faculty of Health Sciences, Jimma University, Ethiopia

Tigist D
Department of Nursing, Faculty of Health Sciences, Jimma University, Ethiopia

Fantahun W
Specialized Teaching Hospital, Jimma University, Ethiopia

Mohammed-Durosinlorun Amina
Kaduna Polytechnic Clinic, Tudun Wada, Kaduna, Nigeria

Krishna Regmi
Department of Clinical Education and Leadership, University of Bedfordshire, UK

Abah AE
Department of Animal and Environmental Biology, University of Port Harcourt, Nigeria

Grey A and Onoja H
School of Science Laboratory Technology, University of Port Harcourt, Nigeria

Miek C Jong
Department Nutrition & Health, Louis Bolk Institute, Driebergen, Netherlands
Department of Nursing Science, Mid Sweden University, Sundsvall, Sweden
National Information and Knowledge Centre for Integrative Medicine (NIKIM), Netherlands

Martine Busch
National Information and Knowledge Centre for Integrative Medicine (NIKIM), Netherlands
Van Praag Institute, Utrecht, Netherlands

Lucy PL van de Vijver
Department Nutrition & Health, Louis Bolk Institute, Driebergen, Netherlands

Mats Jong
Department of Nursing Science, Mid Sweden University, Sundsvall, Sweden

Jolanda Fritsma
Zorgbelang Groningen, Groningen, Netherlands

Ruth Seldenrijk
Patiënten Platform Complementaire Gezondheidszorg, Netherlands

Angel Vila-Corcoles and Olga Ochoa-Gondar
Primary Health Care Service "Camp de Tarragona", Institut Catala de la Salut, Tarragona, Spain
Primary Care Research Institute (IDIAP Jordi Gol), Barcelona, Spain

Imma Hospital, Cinta de Diego and Eva Satue
Primary Health Care Service "Camp de Tarragona",
Institut Catala de la Salut, Tarragona, Spain

Maria Aragon
Information System for the Improvement of Research
in Primary Care (SIDIAP), Primary Care Research
Institute Jordi Gol, Universitat Autonoma de Barcelona,
Barcelona, Spain

Mohamed Salem Nasralla Saleh
Department of Family Medicine, Faculty of medicine
- Suez canal University – Egypt

**Zeliakha Alwahedi, Muna Taher, Ahmed Mostafa,
Mohamed Hashim and Hisham Almahdi**
Primary Health Care Corporation – Qatar

Khlid Al A and Nisha S
Department of Respiratory therapy, Inaya Medical
College, Riyadh, Saudi Arabia

Abbas Al M
Department of Nursing, Inaya Medical College, Riyadh,
Saudi Arabia

Hana Morrissey
Grad Cert Wound Care, Dip Hosp Pharm Admin,
Senior Lecturer in Pharmacy, MHFA Instructor, School
of Psychological and Clinical Sciences, Charles Darwin
University, Ellengowan Drive, Darwin NT 0909, Australia

Patrick Ball
Patrick Ball, Charles Darwin University, Ellengowan
Drive, Darwin NT 0909, Australia

Natasha Prosser
Department of Obstetrics and Gynaecology, Joondalup
Health Campus, Joondalup, WA 6027, Australia

Rodney Petersen
Women's and Babies Service, Women's and Children's
Hospital, North Adelaide, SA 5006, Australia

Julie Quinlivan
Department of Obstetrics and Gynaecology, Joondalup
Health Campus, Joondalup, WA 6027, Australia
Institute for Health Research, University of Notre
Dame Australia, Fremantle, 6160, WA, Australia

Kiflom Zegeye
Communicable disease control Team, Kellem Wollega
Zonal Health Department, Oromia Regional State,
Ethiopia

Abebaw Gebeyehu
Department of Reproductive Health, Institute of Public
Health, University of Gondar, Ethiopia

Tesfahun Melese
Department of Health Informatics, Institute of Public
Health, University of Gondar, Ethiopia

Mihiretu A and Elazar T
School of Public Health, College of Health Sciences
and Medicine, Wolaita Sodo University, Ethiopia

Negash T
Boloso Bombe Primary Hospital, Wolaita Zone,
Ethiopia

Ibanez G
Department of Education and Research in General
Medicine, Pierre-and-Marie-Curie, Sorbonne University,
France
Pierre Louis Institute of Epidemiology and Public Health,
Sorbonne University, France

**Khaled A, Renard JF, Rohani S, Robert S and
Chastang J**
Department of Education and Research in General
Medicine, Pierre-and-Marie-Curie, Sorbonne University,
France

Nizard J
Department of Obstetrics and Gynecology, Pitié
Salpêtrière Hospital, Sorbonne University, France

Baiz N
Department of Epidemiology, Allergic and Respiratory
Diseases, Pierre Louis Institute of Epidemiology and
Public Health, Sorbonne University, France

**Sena Belina Kitila, Ashagre Molla Asaye and Anuwar
Yusuf Issa**
Department of Nursing and Midwifery, College of
Health Science, Jimma University, Ethiopia

Index